Imaging of Epilepsy

John M. Stern • Noriko Salamon

Imaging of Epilepsy

A Clinical Atlas

Springer

John M. Stern
Department of Neurology
Geffen School of Medicine, University of California, Los Angeles
Los Angeles, CA, USA

Noriko Salamon
Department of Radiology
Geffen School of Medicine, University of California, Los Angeles
Los Angeles, CA, USA

ISBN 978-3-030-86671-6   ISBN 978-3-030-86672-3 (eBook)
https://doi.org/10.1007/978-3-030-86672-3

This Springer imprint is published by the registered company Springer Nature Switzerland AG
The registered company address is: Gewerbestrasse 11, 6330 Cham, Switzerland

"To the patients for all that they have taught us."
"To Jackie, my wife and partner in the adventure of life, with love and appreciation."
John Stern

"To Georges Salamon, who opened many doors for me."
Noriko Salamon

Preface

The clinical evaluation of epilepsy has evolved over the recent decades to increasingly integrate brain imaging as a complement to seizure semiology and electroencephalography (EEG). Although diagnosing epilepsy can rely entirely upon the history of unprovoked seizures, determining the specific epilepsy diagnosis, which may be an epilepsy syndrome for generalized epilepsies or a localization for focal epilepsies, depends upon the integration of imaging results and additional diagnostic information. The aim of identifying a specific epilepsy diagnosis is increasingly important because of the relevance to treatment selection, especially as treatment options have increased. In particular, imaging results can substantially impact treatment recommendations for those with medication-resistant epilepsy who are considering non-pharmacologic treatments. To provide best care, the epilepsy clinician's skills now include a sophisticated knowledge of epilepsy's imaging findings. The challenge in developing this skill arises from the broad range of findings from abnormalities that are small and subtle to obvious and extensive, and also includes findings that are either incidental or due to epilepsy treatment.

Achieving expertise in the interpretation of epilepsy imaging is helped by a knowledge of the collection of findings that are potentially related to epilepsy and the relationships of each to clinical situations. Although numerous types of imaging abnormality may cause epilepsy, the full scope is small within all radiologic abnormalities, and its review is achievable. With this perspective, we created a workshop for the American Epilepsy Society's annual meeting that reviewed the breadth of imaging findings related to epilepsy and presented the example images within their clinical contexts. Over several years, this workshop simulated a clinical case conference with clinical review alongside radiologic review. Essentially, we used a framework built upon a synthesis of clinical history and diagnostic modalities, which is the approach in conventional clinical practice, as an interactive educational program.

Transforming the workshop into a book was not initially considered, and we thank the publisher for proposing a reference book version of the workshop. The foundation of this book remains our experience that clinical context is invaluable when interpreting imaging, and this is especially important for epilepsy care with its inherent diagnostic challenges. This book provides a comprehensive review of epilepsy's imaging findings with the detailed clinical histories that make the findings relevant. By understanding patients' presentations and additional diagnostic testing, this radiologic review's purpose is to provide an education in imaging findings alongside insights into the integration of diagnostic information for epilepsy.

The book is divided into parts according to general categories for the imaging findings. Each imaging finding is presented as a collection of images across the relevant imaging modalities that relate to one patient, whose history accompanies the images. This detailed presentation of one finding can be supplemented by a review of the whole category to obtain a broader understanding of the finding in the context of related findings. Overall, the case-based organization with clinical history and multiple images is intended to provide a complete visual understanding of the imaging findings and the corresponding relationship of each finding to the clinical presentation, treatment, and outcome.

We are appreciative of our colleagues in the UCLA Seizure Disorder Center, who encompass the multiple disciplines needed for epilepsy care, including neurology, radiology, psychology, surgery, psychiatry, nursing, and clinical neurophysiology. We also feel honored by the patients, as they shared their experiences with us and entrusted us with helping them overcome epilepsy.

Los Angeles, CA, USA

John M. Stern, MD
Noriko Salamon, MD, PhD

Key Words List

Epilepsy
Seizure
Focal epilepsy
Neuroradiology
Brain imaging
Epilepsy imaging
MRI (Magnetic Resonance Imaging)
FDG - PET (Fluorodeoxyglucose Positron Emission Tomography)
CT (Computerized Tomography)
DTI (Diffusion Tensor Imaging)
DWI (Diffusion-weighted Imaging)

Contents

Part I
Hippocampal Sclerosis

The essential MRI findings for hippocampal sclerosis (HS) are a combination of reduced hippocampal volume, increased signal intensity with T2-weighted imaging, and disrupted internal architecture. Additional findings that are common but not essential are temporal lobe atrophy, asymmetric enlargement of the lateral ventricle's temporal horn, loss of the hippocampal head's digitations, atrophy of the white matter within the parahippocampal gyrus, atrophy of the fornix and mammillary body, and blurring of the junction between the gray matter and white matter within the ipsilateral temporal pole. These additional findings are less reliable as indicators for HS, and a unilateral, enlarged temporal horn occurs commonly in controls and should not be considered pathologic in isolation. HS does not have contrast enhancement.

The reduced hippocampal volume is more readily visualized with T1-weighted sequences, which provide greater anatomic detail, and the evident volume loss correlates to decreased neuronal cell counts. Classic HS has cell loss in fields CA1 and CA3, but severe HS may have more diffuse cell loss and include CA2. Cell loss that is limited to CA1 is a rare type of HS, and cell loss limited to CA4 can be caused by limbic encephalitis. Diagnosing the subtle intrahippocampal structural changes related to intrahippocampal regional differences requires high resolution MRI and the higher field strengths of 3 or 7 Tesla.

The increased signal intensity is evident with T2-weighted imaging but is more easily visualized with a fluid-attenuated inversion recovery (FLAIR) pulse sequence; however, the FLAIR sequence findings are more likely to produce a false-positive interpretation because of the increased signal due to field inhomogeneity artifacts. Moreover, hippocampal FLAIR hyperintensity without hippocampal atrophy occurs in about one third of normal controls, so it is not an abnormality when alone. Therefore, FLAIR findings must be confirmed with T2-weighted images, and the T2-weighted images provide a more detailed visualization of the internal architecture for visualization of its integrity. The increased T2 signal probably reflects gliosis and is possibly most influenced by gliosis in the dentate gyrus.

Bilateral HS that is symmetric and not severe can be difficult to visualize because the asymmetry in volume and signal are used for the visualization. When suspected, volumetric quantification can help with the identification. Hippocampal volume may be measured manually or with automated methods. Manual measurement of hippocampal volume requires segmenting the hippocampus on serial sections of a volumetric T1-weighted MR scan acquired perpendicular to the long axis of the hippocampus. Expert manual volumetry, which requires special training, is more sensitive than automated methods, but automated methods are a reasonable alternative.

Identifying HS with FDG-PET has greater dependence on visualizing asymmetry than MRI and quantitative approaches can have greater value. Because the mesial temporal lobe's normal metabolic signal is less than other cerebral regions, comparison to the contralateral temporal lobe is useful but less accurate when the abnormality is bilateral. The decreased metabolic signal of HS includes both the mesial temporal lobe and also the temporal pole and anterior-lateral temporal lobe because of functional integration with the hippocampus. That is, the spatial extent of hypometabolism does not necessarily indicate the spatial distribution of histopathologic abnormality.

Key References

Berkovic SF, Andermann F, Olivier A, et al. Hippocampal sclerosis in temporal lobe epilepsy demonstrated by magnetic resonance imaging. Ann Neurol. 1991;29:175–82.

Blumcke I, Coras R, Miyata H, Ozkara C. Defining clinico-neuropathological subtypes of mesial temporal lobe epilepsy with hippocampal sclerosis. Brain Pathol. 2012;22:402–11.

Briellmann RS, KalninsRM, Berkovic SF, JacksonGD. Hippocampal pathology in refractory temporal lobe epilepsy: T2-weighted signal change reflects dentate gliosis. Neurology. 2002;58:265–71.

Henry TR, Chupin M, Lehericy S, et al. Hippocampal sclerosis in temporal lobe epilepsy: Findings at 7 T. Radiology. 2011;261:199–209.

Malmgren TM. Hippocampal sclerosis: origins and imaging. Epilepsia. 2012;53(Suppl. 4):19–33.

1 Mild, Unilateral Hippocampal Sclerosis

Clinical History

The first recognized seizure was bilateral tonic-clonic at age 12 years. Soon after this seizure, episodes of staring and minor confusion were identified, and these are now believed to have been occurring for several years before the first recognized seizure.

The habitual seizures manifested as an aura of an abdominal sensation of butterflies or tingling followed by an intense and confusional fear that is described as similar to a disoriented awakening from a nightmare. During the aura, deep breathing was typical, and this progressed to impaired awareness and concentration. Oral automatisms and manual automatisms of the right, left, or both hands often occurred, but seizures also occurred without any motor activity. Sometimes, leftward gaze accompanied the impairment. The seizure duration was typically 30 seconds, and resolution was accompanied by fatigue and an immediate return to verbal ability. Seizures progressing to bilateral tonic-clonic were rare. Treatment included multiple anti-seizure medications with a seizure frequency of 2–3 seizures monthly.

The epilepsy risk factor was a family history of one aunt with epilepsy.

Neurological examination was normal. Neuropsychological testing identified mild difficulty with visual reasoning, normal verbal reasoning and language, and normal verbal and visual episodic memory.

Interictal EEG depicted epileptiform discharges independently over the right and left temporal lobes. Video-EEG monitoring recorded seizures manifested as restlessness, confused facial expression, right-hand motor automatisms, and sometimes oral automatisms. The ictal EEG's seizure onset was across the right anterior temporal region.

MRI identified mild right hippocampal sclerosis. PET identified right temporal hypometabolism. Functional MRI of language identified left hemispheric dominance for language with bilateral basal temporal language areas and Wernicke's areas. For the epilepsy surgery evaluation, an intracarotid amobarbital test was performed, and it identified left hemispheric dominance for language with the presence of significant right hemispheric language function as evident in continued counting aloud during the left intracarotid injection. Episodic memory was fully intact with both the right- and left-sided injections.

The history and evaluation indicate right mesial temporal lobe epilepsy. The aura has characteristic limbic features of an epigastric sensation and an emotional experience, and limbic epilepsy also is supported by the occurrence of focal seizures with impaired awareness that rarely progress to bilateral tonic-clonic. Lateralization is evident in the EEG's right temporal seizure onsets, MRI evidence of hippocampal sclerosis, PET evidence of right temporal hypometabolism, and right hemispheric cognitive dysfunction. The leftward head turning can be consistent with a right-sided ictal onset, but head turning is not always a reliable lateralizing feature during focal seizures that do not progress to bilateral tonic-clonic. The non-lateralized manual automatisms; the bilateral, independent interictal epileptiform discharges; and the bilaterally intact hippocampal memory systems do not contribute to the lateralization. The intact visual memory function may be related to the hippocampal sclerosis being mild, as evident with MRI.

Because of the medication resistance and diagnostic test results, a right anterior-mesial temporal lobe resection was provided as treatment. Histopathological examination identified mild hippocampal sclerosis and focal cortical dysplasia, type IIIa, of the adjacent temporal pole. The mild extent of the sclerosis corresponds to the MRI and the integrity of the memory function. Seizures have not occurred for the 2 years since the surgery.

J. M. Stern, N. Salamon, *Imaging of Epilepsy*, https://doi.org/10.1007/978-3-030-86672-3_1

Imaging

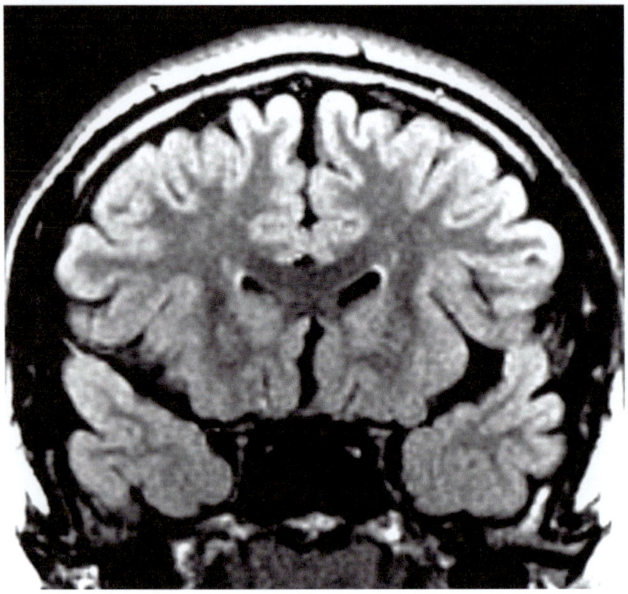

Fig. 1.1 MRI coronal FLAIR sequence at a temporal pole level. The right temporal pole is slightly smaller than the left. Within both temporal poles, gray-white differentiation is normal, and there is no signal abnormality within the gray matter or white matter

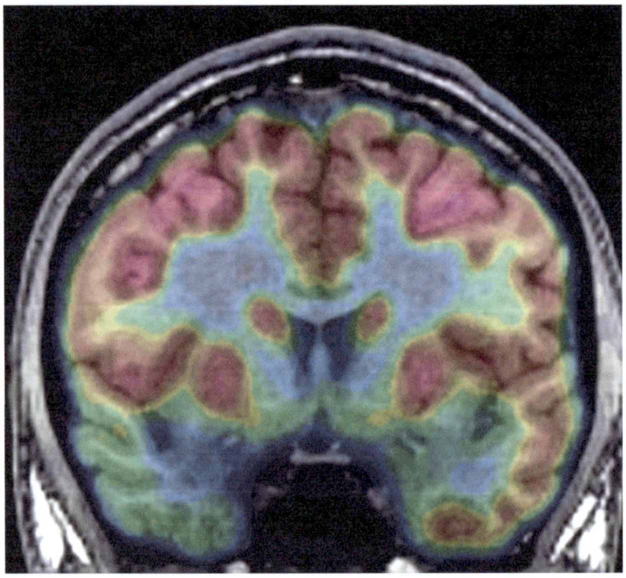

Fig. 1.2 PET-MRI co-registration with color-scale FDG tracer in a coronal plane at the same temporal pole level as Fig. 1.1. The right temporal pole is markedly hypometabolic mesially. Less pronounced hypometabolism is present in the right temporal pole's lateral and inferior cortices. The left temporal pole is normal

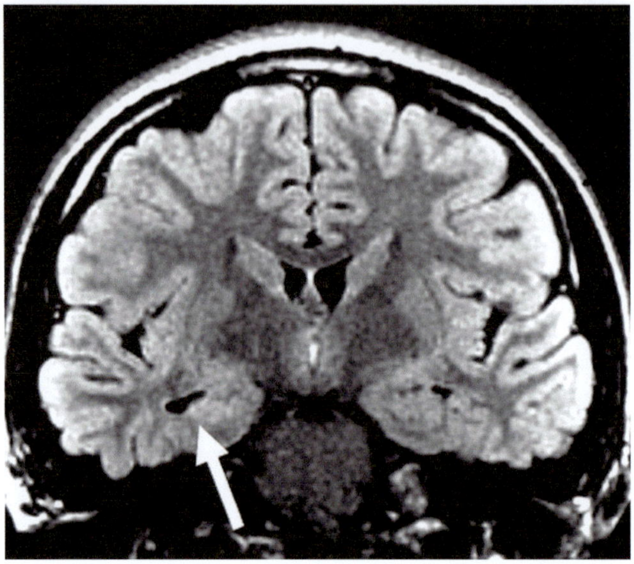

Fig. 1.3 MRI coronal FLAIR sequence at a hippocampal head level. The right hippocampal head is abnormally hyperintense (arrow), and the right temporal lobe is atrophic, as is evident in the larger right temporal horn. The gray-white differentiation along the inferior and lateral temporal lobe is normal bilaterally

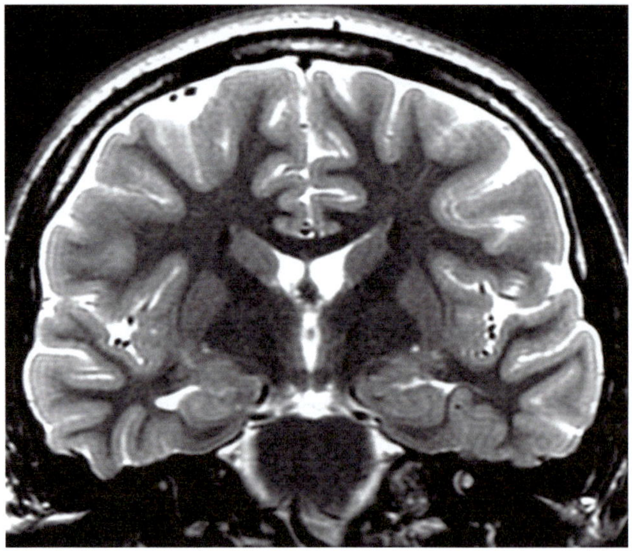

Fig. 1.4 MRI coronal T2 sequence at the same hippocampal head level as Fig. 1.3. The hippocampal heads are asymmetric with the right hippocampus demonstrating subtly increased signal, blurring of the internal architecture, and smoothing of the superior indentations when compared to the left. The gray-white differentiation is normal and symmetric

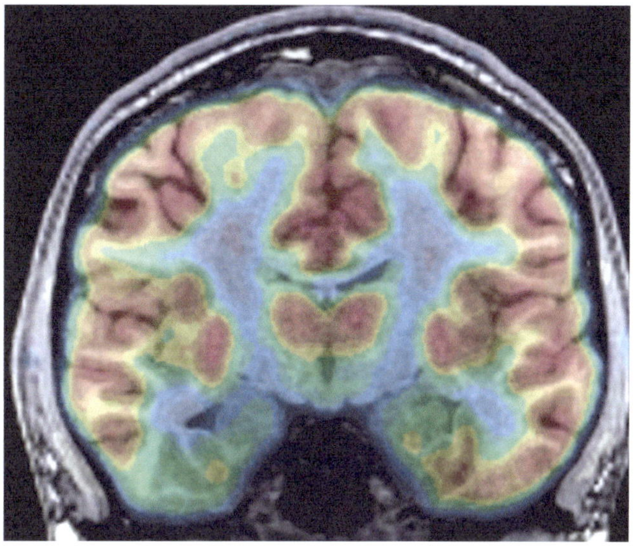

Fig. 1.5 PET-MRI co-registration with color-scale FDG tracer in a coronal plane at the same hippocampal head level as Figs. 1.3 and 1.4. Hypometabolism is evident in the right hippocampal head, parahippocampal gyrus, fusiform gyrus, and inferior temporal gyrus. The left hippocampal head metabolism is normal

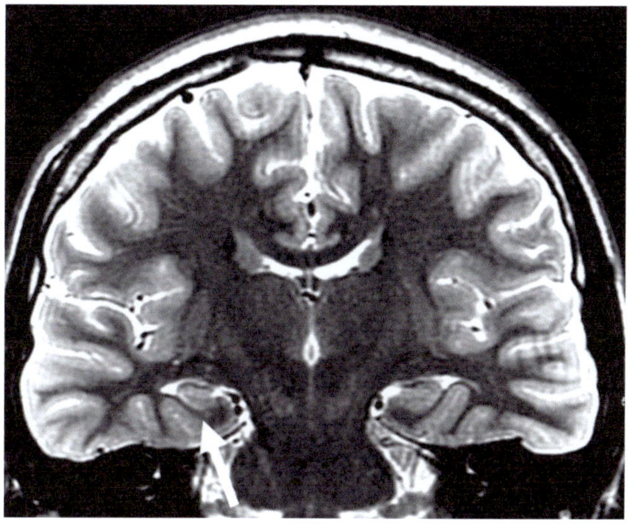

Fig. 1.7 MRI coronal T2 sequence at the same body of the hippocampus level as Fig. 1.6. Mildly increased signal is evident in CA1 of the right hippocampus, and the right hippocampus also is slightly smaller than left. Gray-white differentiation is clear (arrow) in the right mesial temporal lobe

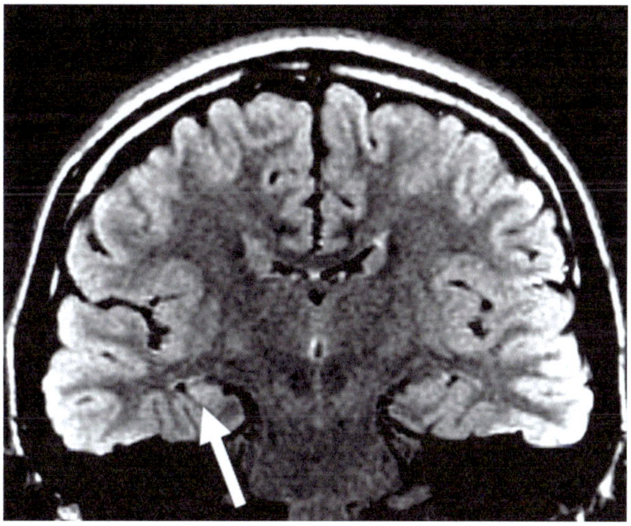

Fig. 1.6 MRI coronal FLAIR sequence at a body of the hippocampus level. Increased signal is evident within the right hippocampus (arrow). The gray-white differentiation is normal bilaterally, and the temporal lobes are symmetric in size

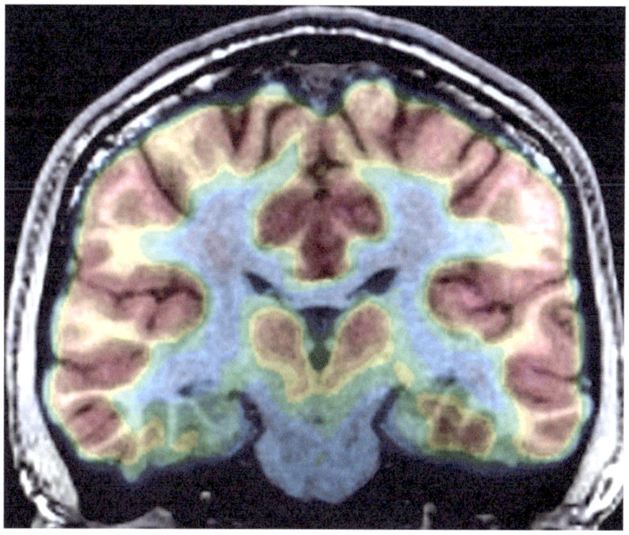

Fig. 1.8 PET-MRI co-registration with color-scale FDG tracer in a coronal plane at a posterior hippocampus level. Hypometabolism is evident in the right mesial temporal lobe, including the hippocampus and inferior temporal cortex. The lateral temporal lobe is normal bilaterally. The right thalamus has mildly decreased metabolism

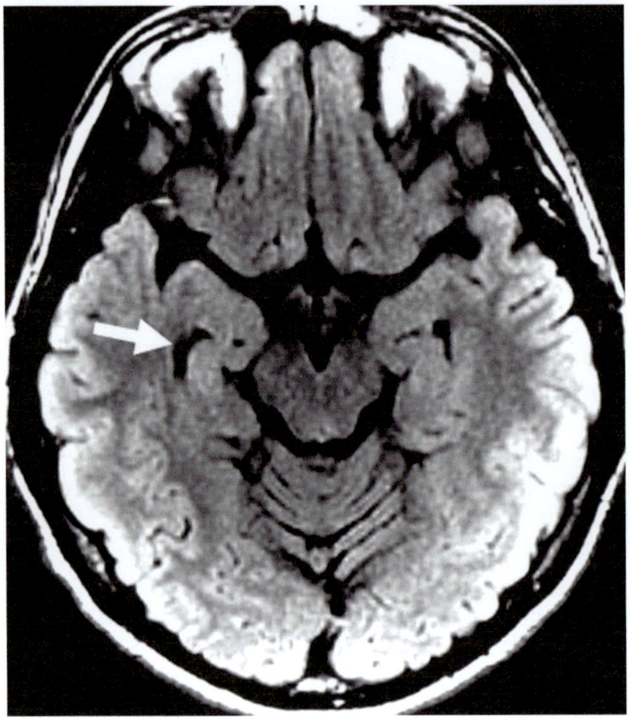

Fig. 1.9 MRI axial FLAIR sequence at a hippocampal level. The right hippocampus is atrophic and has abnormally increased signal. Because of the atrophy, the right temporal horn is larger (arrow)

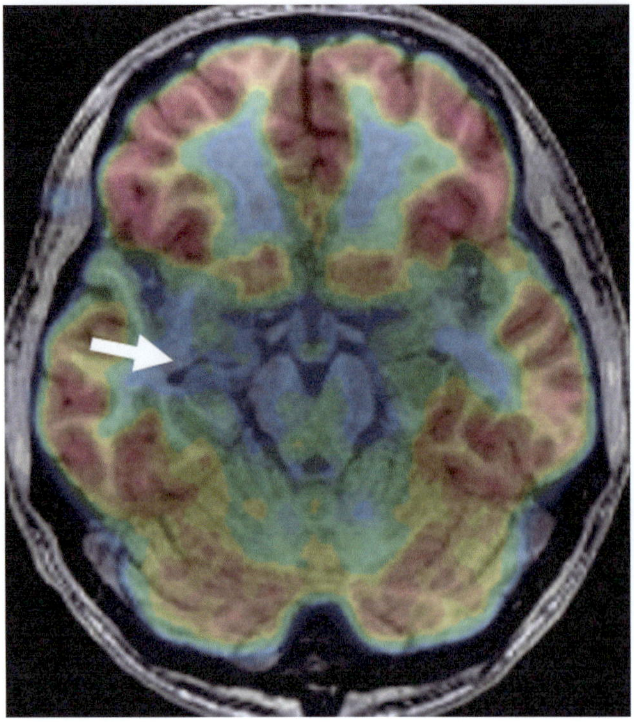

Fig. 1.10 PET-MRI co-registration with color-scale FDG tracer in an axial plane at a hippocampal head level similar to Fig. 1.9. The right hippocampal head is hypometabolic, and marked hypometabolism extends within the right hippocampus (arrow) compared to the left. The lateral temporal metabolism is normal bilaterally

Moderate, Unilateral Hippocampal Sclerosis

2

Clinical History

The first recognized seizure occurred at age 7 years as an episode of seeing stars and that progressed to shaking.

The habitual seizures followed an aura of a rising sensation in the abdomen that became shortness of breath and then sometimes progressed to a lapse in awareness and a memory gap with oral automatisms and purposeless wandering. The seizure duration was about 1–2 minutes and postictal fear and headache follows. About half of the seizures were an aura in isolation. In contrast, bilateral tonic-clonic seizures were rare, occurring only when not taking anti-seizure medications. Treatment included multiple anti-seizure medications with a seizure frequency of one seizure weekly.

No epilepsy risk factors were present. Neurological examination was normal.

Interictal EEG depicted bilateral, independent anterior temporal epileptiform discharges that were more frequent on the left. Video-EEG monitoring recorded 15 seizures that followed the habitual aura and were manifested as bilateral manual automatisms, non-versive turning to the left, and sometimes dystonic posturing of the left hand. Ictal EEG's seizure onset was across the left anterior temporal region for nine seizures and right anterior temporal region for six. The left-hand dystonic posturing occurred during some of the seizures with the right-sided onset and none of the seizures with the left-sided onset.

MRI identified left hippocampal atrophy and signal abnormality. PET identified mild left temporal hypometabolism.

The history and evaluation are consistent with mesial temporal lobe epilepsy. The aura includes limbic features that support mesial temporal lobe epilepsy, but the features do not indicate lateralization or whether the epilepsy is unilateral or bilateral. The imaging supports left mesial temporal lobe epilepsy, but the video-EEG monitoring recorded both left- and right-sided seizure onsets. The presence of bilateral independent anterior temporal interictal epileptiform abnormality does not necessarily indicate bilateral mesial temporal lobe, and the greater number of the left-sided discharges is consistent with the imaging in supporting left mesial temporal lobe epilepsy. Additional testing is warranted to determine whether epilepsy surgery would be beneficial for control of the habitual seizures, as the MRI and PET findings alone cannot establish this.

J. M. Stern, N. Salamon, *Imaging of Epilepsy*, https://doi.org/10.1007/978-3-030-86672-3_2

Imaging

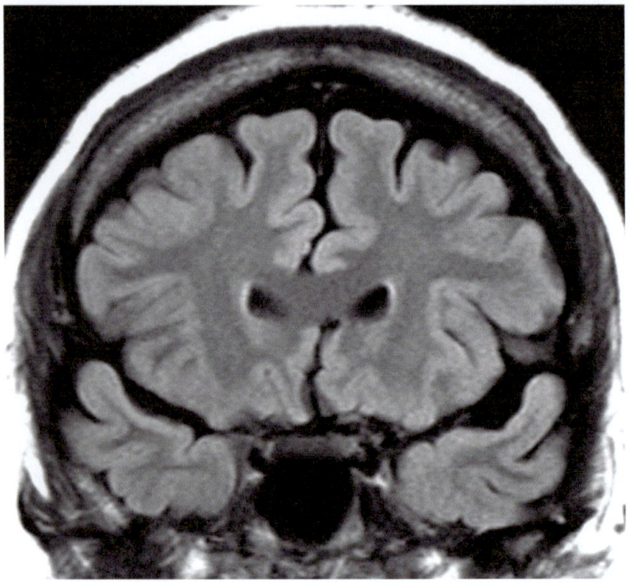

Fig. 2.1 MRI coronal FLAIR sequence at a temporal pole level. The gray-white junction is blurred along the mesial surface of the left temporal pole. The lateral and inferior arborization of the white matter and the gray-white junction is normal bilaterally

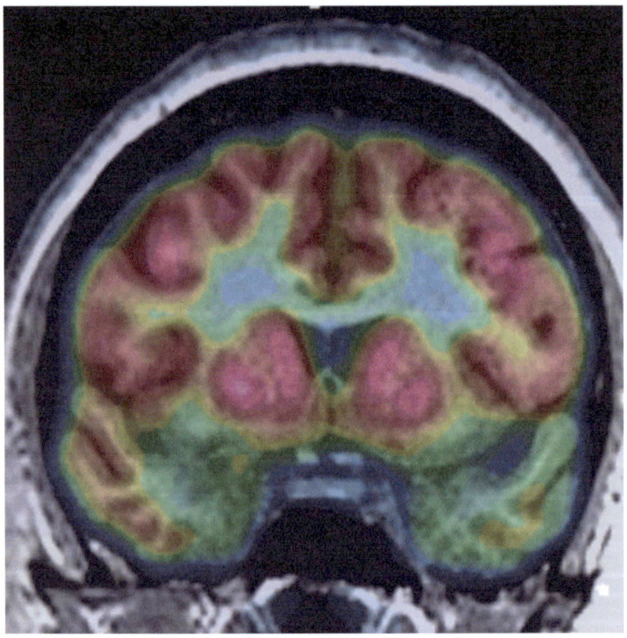

Fig. 2.2 PET-MRI co-registration with color-scale FDG tracer in a coronal plane at the same temporal pole level as Fig. 2.1. Hypometabolism is evident in the left superior, middle, inferior temporal gyri. The mesial temporal poles have symmetric metabolic signal

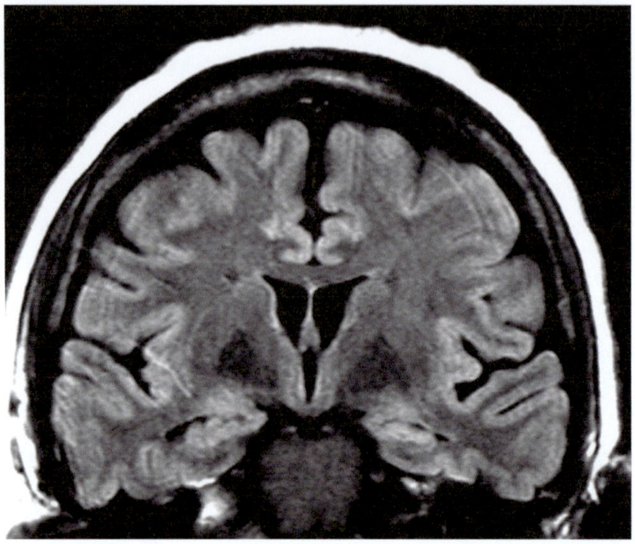

Fig. 2.3 MRI coronal FLAIR sequence at a hippocampal head level. The left hippocampus is smaller and has abnormally increased signal intensity with a flattening of the superior surface. In comparison, the right hippocampus' superior surface has clear indentations. The gray-white differentiation is preserved bilaterally

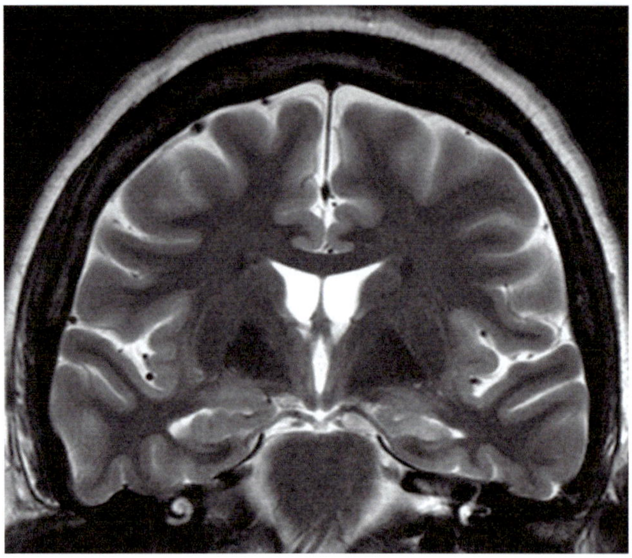

Fig. 2.4 MRI coronal T2 sequence at the same hippocampal head level as Fig. 2.3. The left hippocampus is smaller and has increased signal intensity and a flattening of the superior surface. The gray-white differentiation is preserved bilaterally. The findings are the same as Fig. 2.3 with differences in appearance because of the different MRI sequence

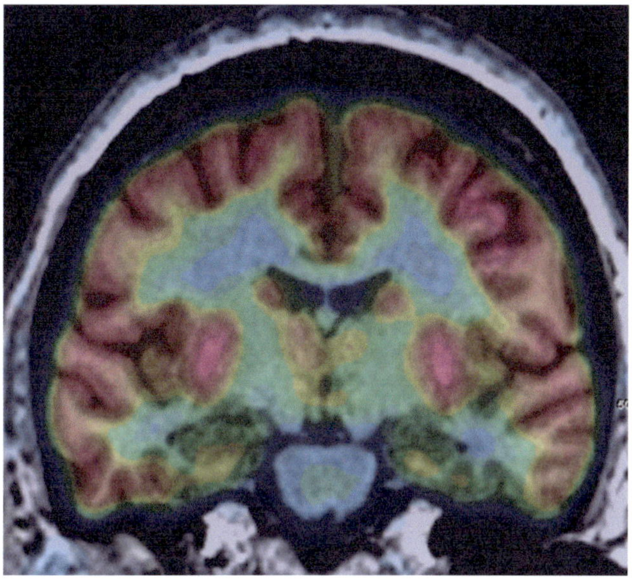

Fig. 2.5 PET-MRI co-registration with color-scale FDG tracer in a coronal plane at a hippocampal head level similar to Figs. 2.3 and 2.4. Asymmetrically greater hypometabolism is evident in the left entorhinal cortex and along the left temporal lobe's inferior surface. The left thalamus also is hypometabolic

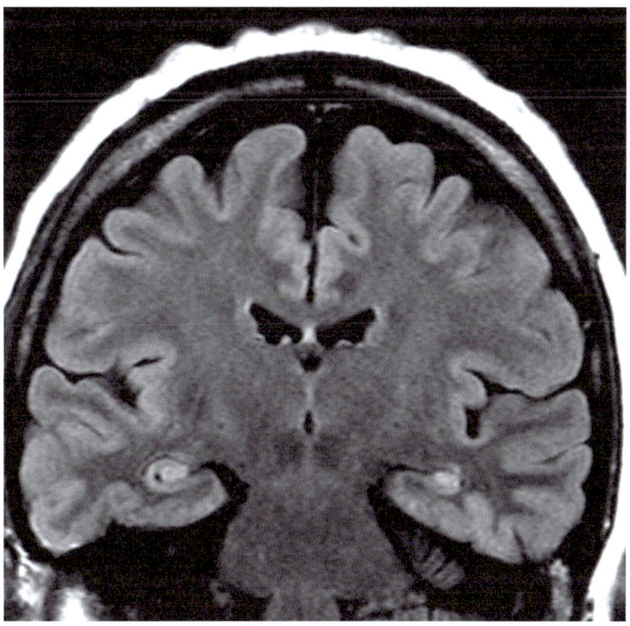

Fig. 2.6 MRI coronal FLAIR sequence at a body of the hippocampus level. The left hippocampus is hyperintense and markedly smaller than the right. The gray-white differentiation is normal bilaterally

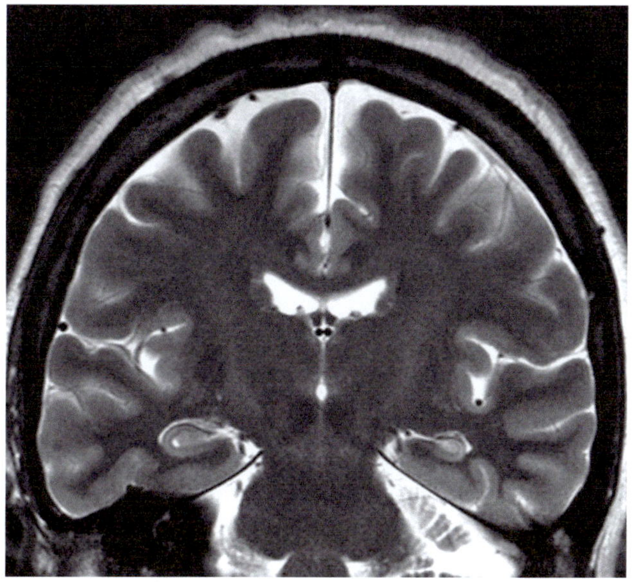

Fig. 2.7 MRI coronal T2 sequence at the same body of the hippocampus level as Fig. 2.6. The left hippocampus is small and has increased signal. Its internal architecture is diminished compared to the right hippocampus. Nevertheless, the left hippocampus' CA1, dentate gyrus, and subiculum are visible, with the left CA1 and dentate gyrus in particular demonstrating higher signal than on the right

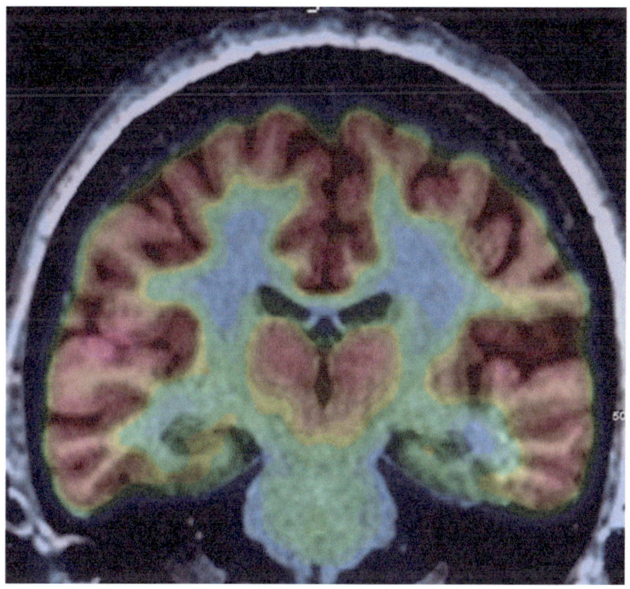

Fig. 2.8 PET-MRI co-registration with color-scale FDG tracer in a coronal plane at the same hippocampus level as Figs. 2.6 and 2.7. The left hippocampus and inferior temporal cortex are hypometabolic. The lateral temporal cortex and the thalamus have symmetric metabolic signal

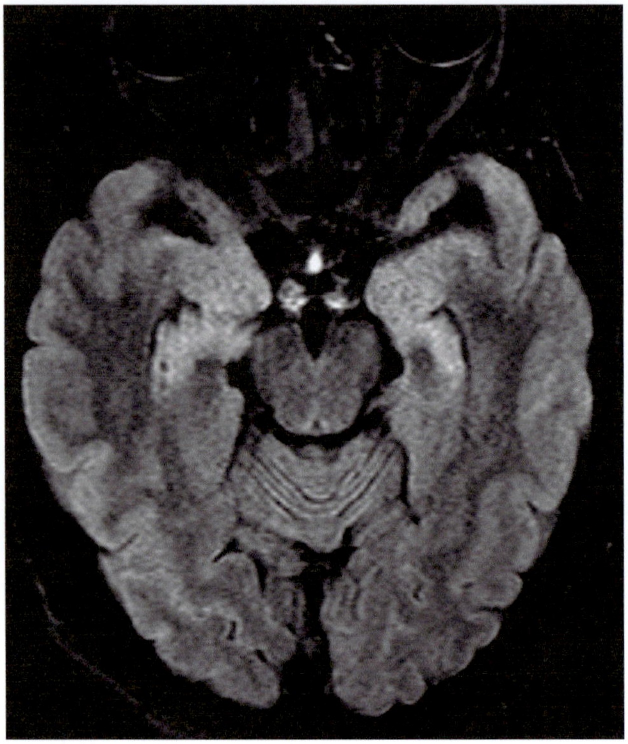

Fig. 2.9 MRI axial FLAIR sequence at a hippocampal head level. The normal hippocampal indentations are visible across the right hippocampal head. In comparison, abnormal smoothing is evident along the left hippocampal head. The hippocampal signals and volumes are bilaterally symmetric

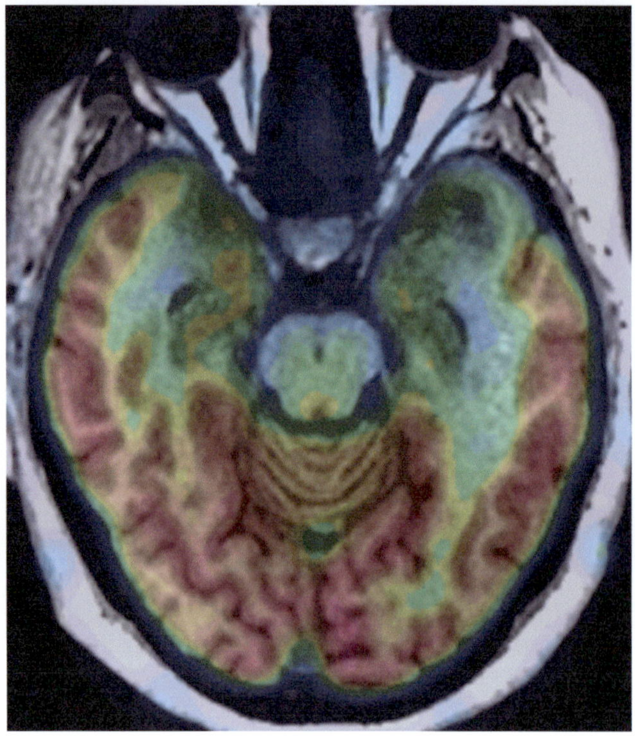

Fig. 2.10 PET-MRI co-registration with color-scale FDG tracer in an axial plane at a hippocampal head level similar to Fig. 2.9. The left temporal pole, amygdala, and hippocampus are hypometabolic. The lateral temporal lobes have normal, symmetric metabolism

3 Severe, Unilateral Hippocampal Sclerosis

Clinical History

The first recognized seizure occurred in early childhood as an episode of staring and mumbling with repetitive opening and closing of the hands. The episode recurred many times in later childhood, but the episodes were not recognized as seizures, so an evaluation and treatment were not undertaken until adulthood.

The habitual seizures did not included an aura. The ictal behavior was similar to the behavior present in childhood except for progression to evident confusion that lasts several minutes. If alone, the patient was unaware of these seizures. Rarely, a seizure progressed to bilateral tonic-clonic. The tonic-clonic seizures also occurred without an aura and they have not been witnessed to include lateralizing features. A total of 4 or 5 were believed to have occurred. Treatment included multiple anti-seizure medications with an estimated seizure frequency of 1 or 2 monthly, but the actual frequency was believed to be higher.

No epilepsy risk factor was present.

Neurological examination was abnormal because of impaired cognitive performance. Neuropsychological testing identified low borderline global function with asymmetrically greater left hemispheric dysfunction. The language dominant temporal lobe had both mesial and lateral dysfunction with relatively greater lateral temporal abnormality. Medical history included cryptogenic onset hepatic disease with cirrhosis that required a liver transplant in early childhood.

Interictal electroencephalography (EEG) depicted rare left anterior temporal epileptiform discharges. Video-EEG monitoring recorded focal seizures with ictal EEG's seizure onset across the left temporal region.

MRI identified marked left hippocampal sclerosis and PET identified concordant left temporal hypometabolism along with left thalamic hypometabolism. An intracarotid amobarbital test was performed in consideration of epilepsy surgery, and it identified left hemispheric language dominance, intact memory function with both the right and left injections, and better memory performance with the right-sided injection.

The history and diagnostic evaluation support a diagnosis of left temporal lobe epilepsy, as evident in the ictal EEG's seizure onset; however, the other diagnostic tests include features of both mesial and lateral temporal lobe epilepsy. The occurrence of focal seizures with impaired awareness as the habitual seizure and rare bilateral tonic-clonic seizures supports mesial temporal lobe epilepsy and this is further supported by the MRI evidence of left hippocampal sclerosis and the concordant PET hypometabolism. In addition, the lack of an aura and the significant left lateral temporal dysfunction extend the localization to the temporal neocortex. In contrast, the neuropsychological testing evidence for bilateral temporal dysfunction and the intracarotid amobarbital test identification of intact episodic memory function in both right and left hippocampal systems suggest mild, bilateral mesial temporal dysfunction. Because of the uncertainty for the epileptogenic zone and the risk of an anterior temporal lobe resection producing a memory deficit, resective surgery was not offered.

J. M. Stern, N. Salamon, *Imaging of Epilepsy*, https://doi.org/10.1007/978-3-030-86672-3_3

Imaging

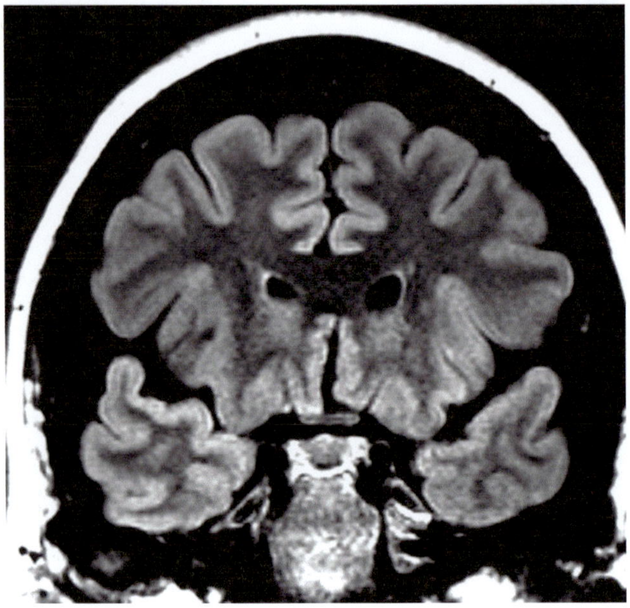

Fig. 3.1 MRI coronal FLAIR sequence at a temporal pole level. The left temporal pole is smaller with blurring of the gray-white differentiation across the medial-inferior portion. The gray-white differentiation is normal in the right temporal pole

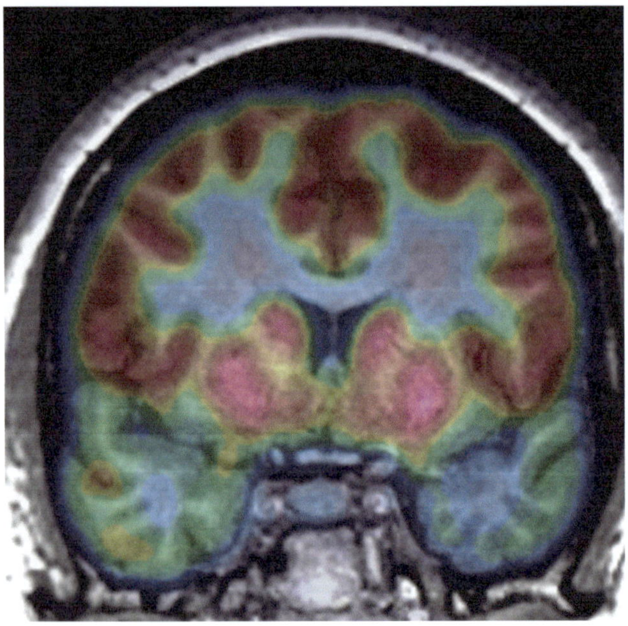

Fig. 3.2 PET-MRI co-registration with color scale fluoro-deoxyglucose (FDG) tracer in a coronal plane at the temporal pole level in Fig. 3.1. The left temporal pole is smaller with marked hypometabolism of its medial and inferior cortex. The left lateral temporal cortex has less prominent hypometabolism as compared to the right

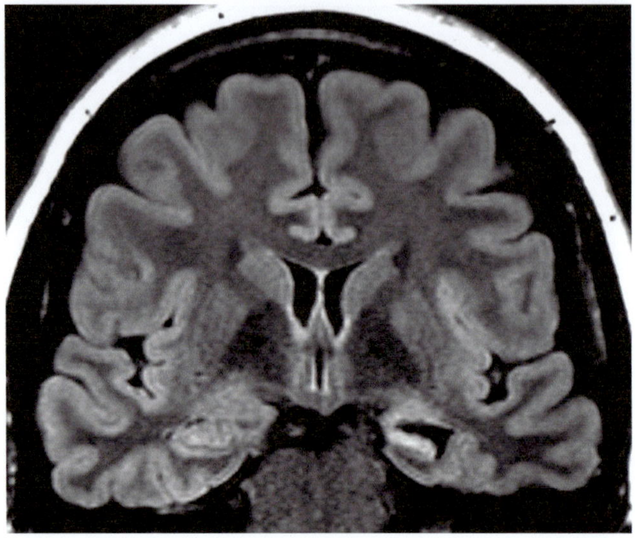

Fig. 3.3 MRI coronal FLAIR sequence at a hippocampal head level. The left hippocampal head has marked atrophy and increased signal with loss of the superior surface indentations. Due to the hippocampal volume loss, the left temporal horn is prominent. The right hippocampal head and the bilateral gray-white differentiation are normal

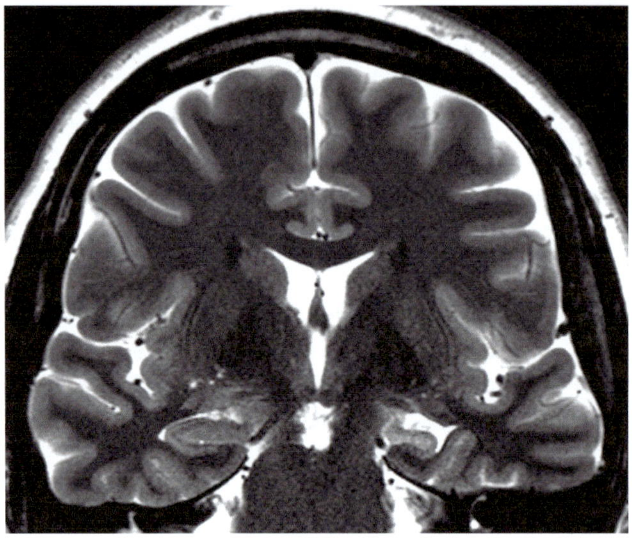

Fig. 3.4 MRI coronal T2 sequence at a hippocampal head level similar to Fig. 3.3. The left hippocampal head has marked atrophy and loss of the internal architecture's demarcation. With the atrophy, the left temporal horn is prominent. The right hippocampal head demonstrates the normal stripe of the hippocampal internal architecture. The gray-white differentiation is normal bilaterally

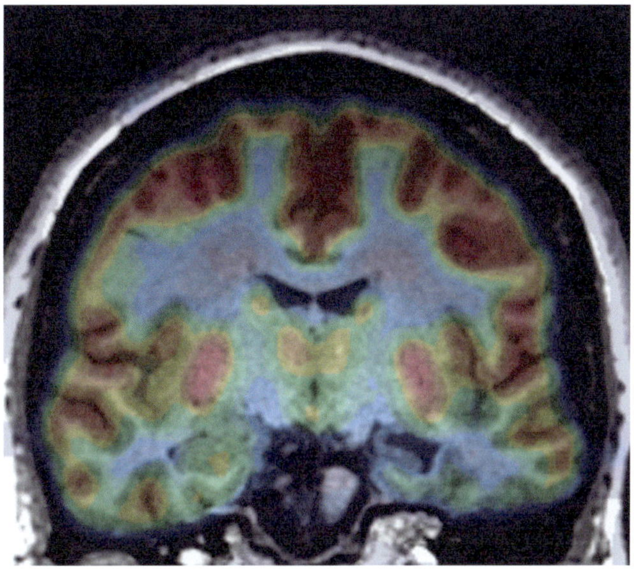

Fig. 3.5 PET-MRI co-registration with color scale FDG tracer in a coronal plane at a hippocampal head level similar to Figs. 3.3 and 3.4. Marked hypometabolism of the left hippocampal head is evident with less substantial hypometabolism of the inferior left temporal surface. The left thalamus is slightly hypometabolic when compared to the right

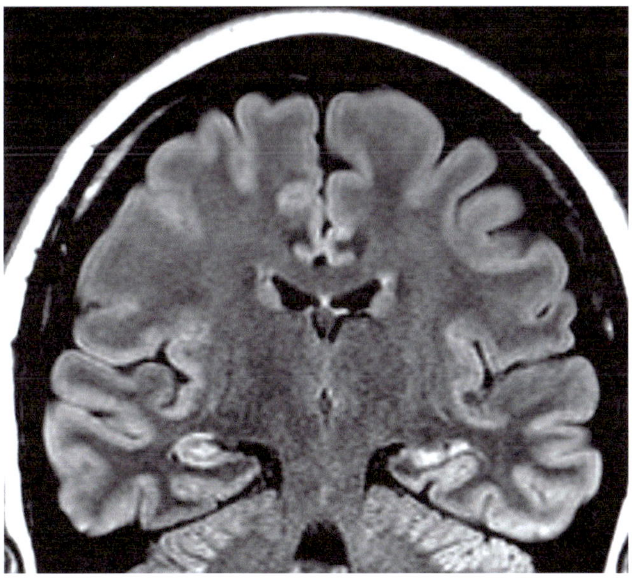

Fig. 3.6 MRI coronal FLAIR sequence at a body of the hippocampus level. The left hippocampus is atrophic and has abnormally increased signal. Its internal architecture is obscured compared to the right hippocampal body. The gray-white differentiation is normal bilaterally

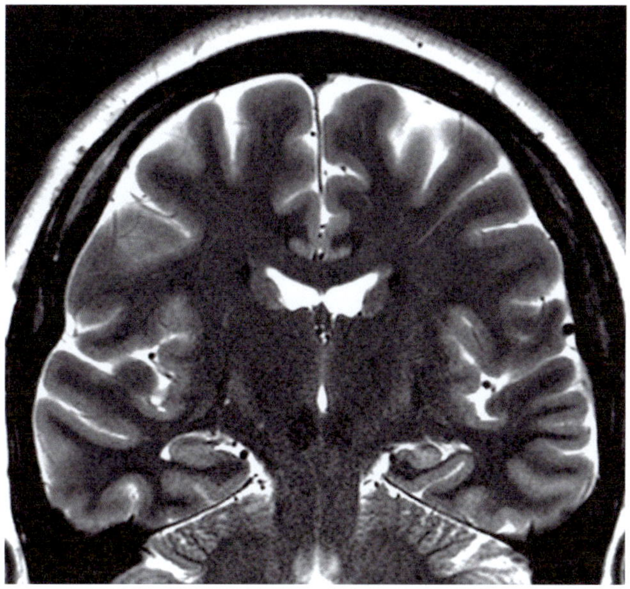

Fig. 3.7 MRI coronal T2 sequence at a body of the hippocampus level similar to Fig. 3.6. The left hippocampus is atrophic and abnormally hyperintense with loss of detailed internal architecture. The subtlety of the right hippocampus's internal architecture is apparent and normal. The gray-white differentiation is normal bilaterally

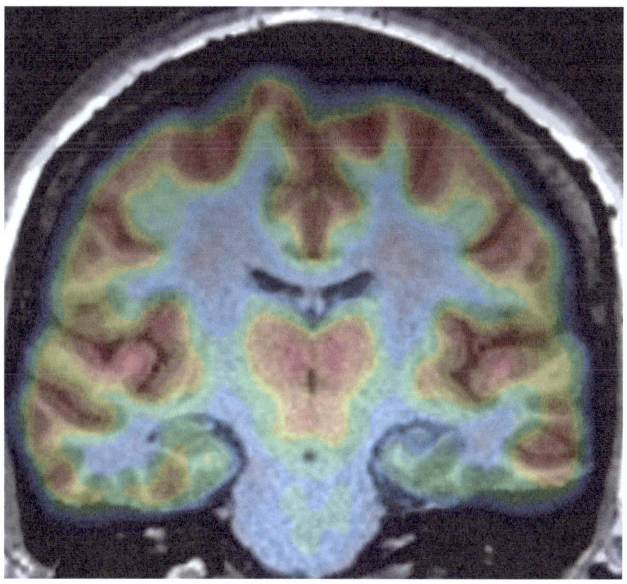

Fig. 3.8 PET-MRI co-registration with color scale FDG tracer in a coronal plane at a body of the hippocampus level similar to Figs. 3.6 and 3.7. Marked hypometabolism is evident within the left hippocampal body and the medial and inferior left temporal lobe. The thalamus is symmetric at this level. Metabolism across the right temporal cortex is normal

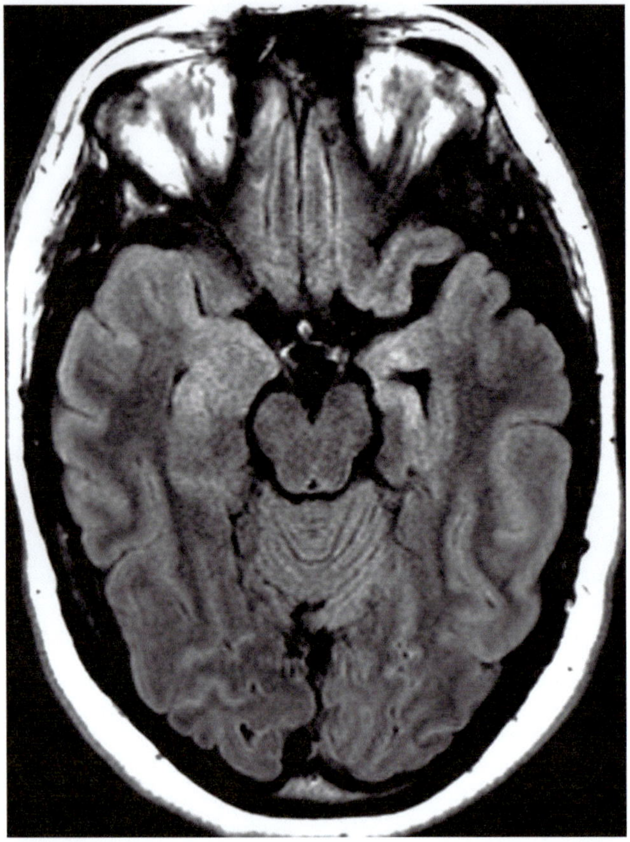

Fig. 3.9 MRI axial FLAIR sequence at a hippocampal head level. The left hippocampal head is atrophic and hyperintense with a prominent temporal horn of the lateral ventricle. Atrophy of the left amygdala and minor atrophy of the left temporal pole also are evident

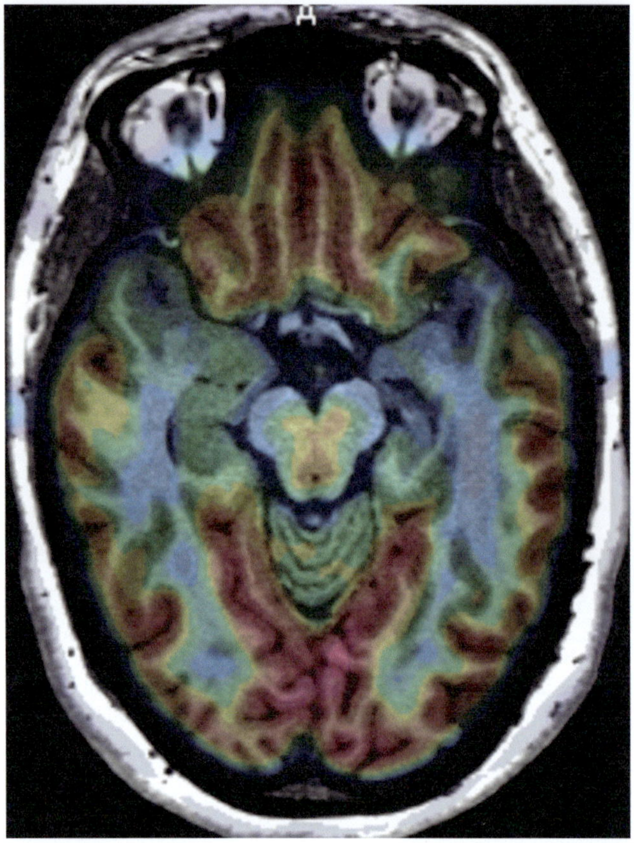

Fig. 3.10 PET-MRI co-registration with color scale FDG tracer in an axial plane at a hippocampal head level similar to Fig. 3.9. The left hippocampal head and amygdala are markedly hypometabolic. Hypometabolism also is present across the left temporal pole. The lateral temporal lobes have normal, symmetric metabolism

Mild, Bilateral Hippocampal Sclerosis

4

Clinical History

The first recognized seizure was at age 18 years as a bilateral tonic-clonic seizure that occurred months after a major traumatic brain injury.

The habitual seizures manifested with four ictal behaviors. The first manifestation to have occurred was a bilateral tonic-clonic seizure that did not follow an aura. The duration was 1–3 minutes with postictal sleep for 1 hour. These were infrequent with seizure-free periods of several years. The second manifestation was staring with impaired awareness and turning to the right followed by right-sided shaking and occasionally urinary incontinence. These did not follow an aura and had durations of 30 to 60 seconds with postictal confusion for an hour. The frequency of this seizure was 1–3 weekly except for catamenial clustering of 5–10 daily. The third seizure manifestation was an experience of déjà vu, epigastric rising, and intensified clarity of perception that produced a brief respiratory arrest. There was limitation in responsiveness with the retained one-word answers, and, occasionally, oral automatisms. Postictally, weariness was present for a few minutes. These seizures occurred one to dozens of times daily. The fourth seizure manifestation first developed recently. It occurred during sleep and appeared as nonsensical talking with right-hand clenching that lasted 30 seconds. The frequency was 1–2 times weekly. Treatment included multiple anti-seizure medications and the vagus nerve stimulator.

The epilepsy risk factor was a traumatic brain injury from a motor vehicle accident. The injury produced left temporal lobe edema and a left posterior Sylvian fissure hemorrhage. Retrograde amnesia was present for the year prior to the accident.

Neurological examination identified impairment of recent memory that was further characterized with neuropsychological testing that identified deficits in executive functioning and verbal and nonverbal learning with intact visuospatial abilities.

Interictal EEG depicted bilateral, independent temporal slowing and bilateral, independent temporal epileptiform discharges that were more often on the left. Video-EEG monitoring recorded all four of the ictal behaviors, and ictal EEG identified seizure onsets independently across both the right and left temporal regions with the majority occurring across the right.

MRI identified mild bilateral hippocampal sclerosis, and PET identified bilateral but asymmetric temporal lobe hypometabolism with greater hypometabolism on the right. In consideration of epilepsy surgery, an intracarotid amobarbital test was performed. It identified left hemispheric dominance for language and dependence on the left mesial temporal structures for episodic memory.

The history and evaluation indicate an epilepsy that possibly has more than one epileptogenic zone, which is plausible in the context of the major head trauma. The frequent bilateral tonic-clonic seizures and the asymmetric motor seizures are consistent with neocortical onsets. The asymmetric motor seizures may be propagating into medial frontal cortex as a cause of the urinary incontinence. In contrast, the occurrence of auras with limbic features and focal seizures with impairment that do not progress to bilateral tonic-clonic suggests limbic onsets without extensive propagation. The ictal EEG and neuropsychological testing further support the possibility of more than one epileptogenic zone and bilateral epilepsy.

Because of the disability and morbidity associated with the seizures, a palliative epilepsy surgery was considered. The ictal EEG, PET, and intracarotid amobarbital test findings supported the possibility of benefit and safety from a right anterior-mesial temporal lobe resection, which was performed without the expectation of full seizure control. Histopathological examination of the resected tissue identified mild focal cortical dysplasia and no evidence of traumatic injury.

Following surgery, memory impairment and anxiety increased. Because of a concern for subtle seizures, video-EEG monitoring was performed, and it identified ictal EEG's seizure onsets across the left temporal region that did not have an obvious behavioral change. With education, the family was subsequently able to identify these behavioral seizures,

J. M. Stern, N. Salamon, *Imaging of Epilepsy*, https://doi.org/10.1007/978-3-030-86672-3_4

and the frequency was found to be five monthly, which was a marked reduction to the frequency prior to epilepsy surgery. Years later, a responsive neurostimulator was implanted with electrodes in the left entorhinal cortex and hippocampal head. Intracranial recordings identified left anterior temporal seizures, and stimulation has subsequently reduced the seizure frequency to two monthly.

Imaging

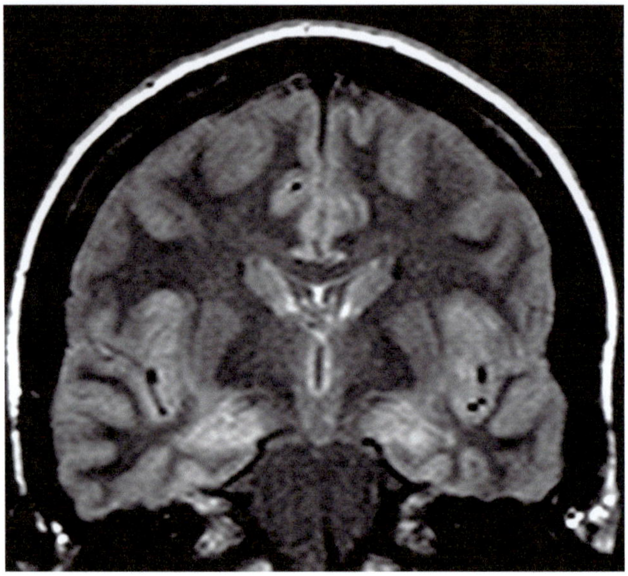

Fig. 4.1 MRI coronal FLAIR sequence at a hippocampal head level. Bilateral hippocampal heads demonstrate abnormal hyperintensity without atrophy. However, FLAIR does not depict hippocampal head volumes as clearly as with T2 of T1 sequences. The temporal lobes are normal volume with clear gray-white differentiation

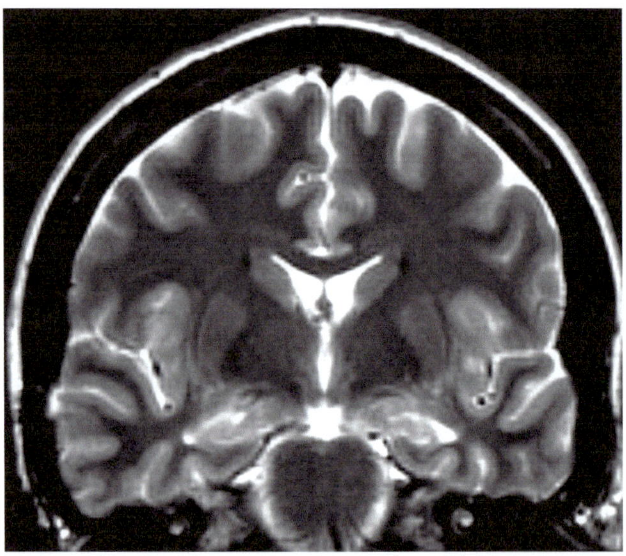

Fig. 4.2 MRI coronal T2 sequence at the hippocampal head level in Fig. 4.1. Bilateral hippocampal heads demonstrate both hyperintensity and atrophy with prominent temporal horns of the lateral ventricles. The internal architecture of both hippocampi is blurred. The temporal lobes are otherwise normal with clear gray-white differentiation

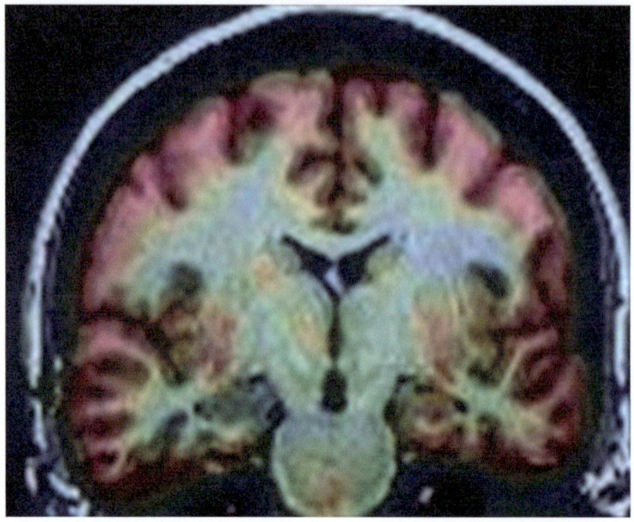

Fig. 4.3 PET-MRI co-registration with color-scale FDG tracer in a coronal plane at the hippocampal head level in Figs. 4.1 and 4.2. Bilateral hippocampal head hypometabolism is present with more pronounced hypometabolism on the right. The right temporal lobe also has asymmetrically greater hypometabolism within the parahippocampal gyrus. Thalamic hypometabolism also is evident, but it is asymmetrically greater on the left

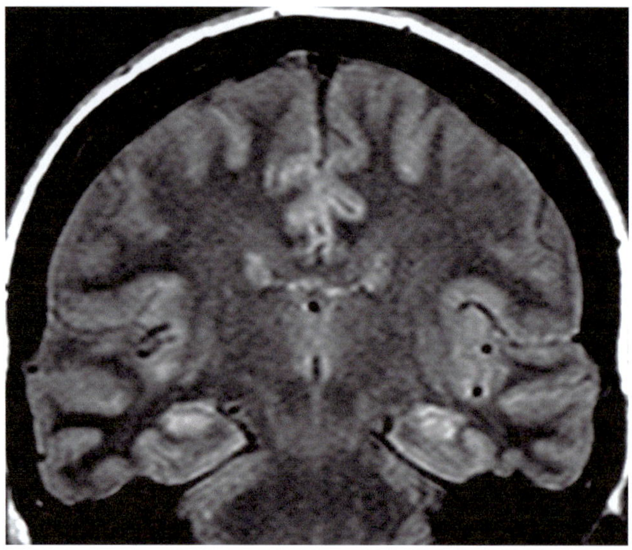

Fig. 4.4 MRI coronal FLAIR sequence at a hippocampal body level. Bilateral hippocampal bodies are abnormally hyperintense and have blurring of their internal architecture

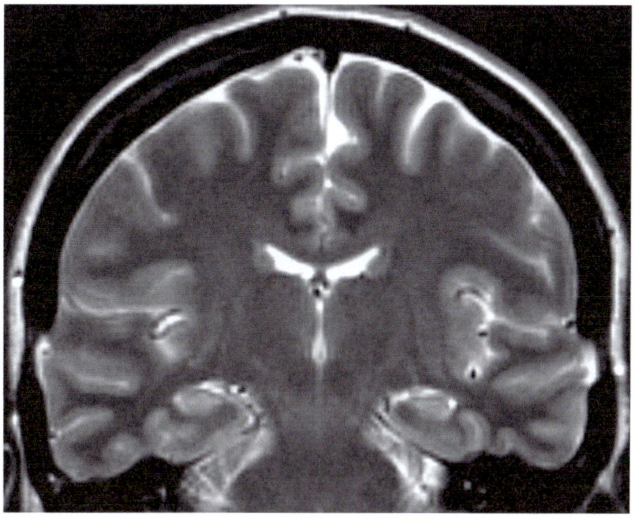

Fig. 4.5 MRI coronal T2 sequence at a hippocampal body level similar to Fig. 4.4. Bilateral hippocampal atrophy is present with blurring of the internal architecture and a mildly increased signal

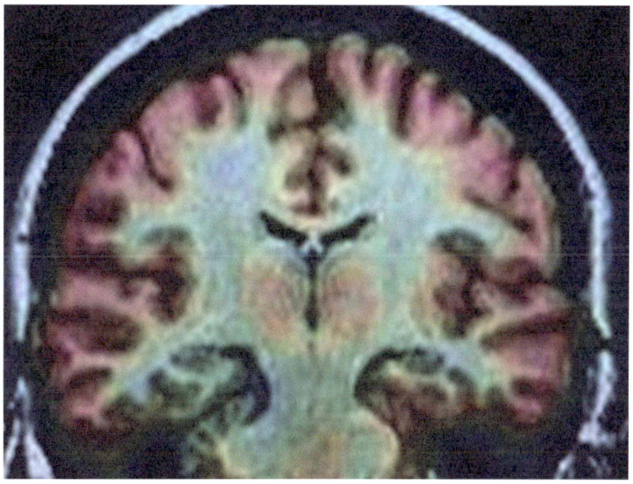

Fig. 4.6 PET-MRI co-registration with color-scale FDG tracer in a coronal plane at a hippocampal body level similar to Figs. 4.4 and 4.5. Bilateral hippocampal body hypometabolism is evident with more extensive hypometabolism across the right inferior temporal lobe. The thalamus is symmetric

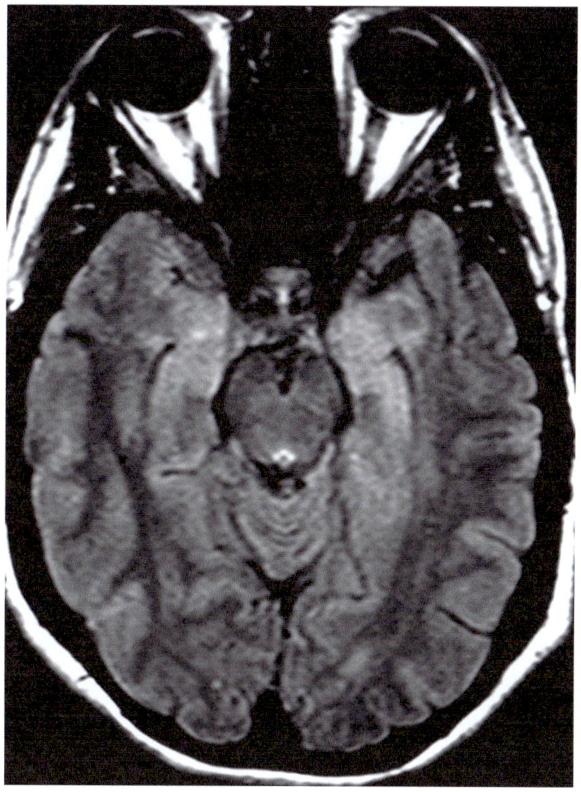

Fig. 4.7 MRI axial FLAIR sequence at a hippocampal head level. The hippocampal heads and amygdalae are bilaterally hyperintense but are normal in volume. The temporal poles are bilaterally normal in volume and gray-white differentiation

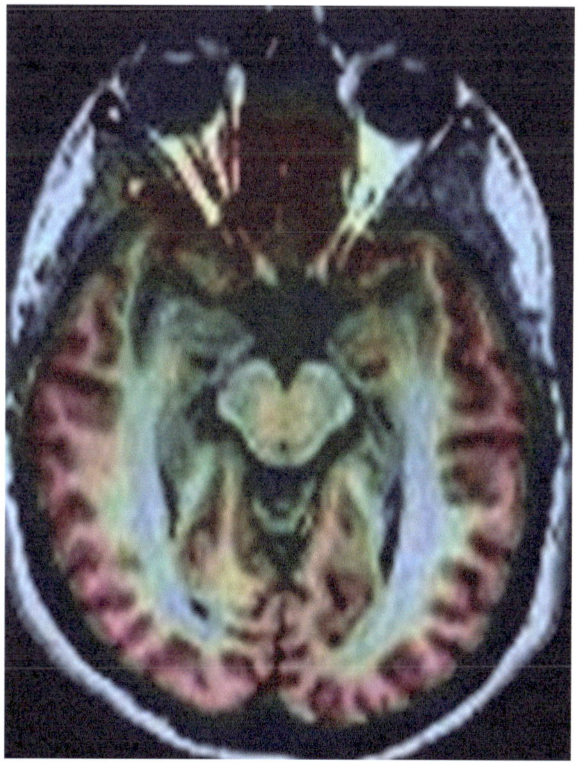

Fig. 4.8 PET-MRI co-registration with color-scale FDG tracer in an axial plane at a hippocampal head level similar to Fig. 4.7. Bilateral hippocampal hypometabolism and right amygdala hypometabolism are evident. The lateral temporal cortex is normal

5 Severe, Bilateral Hippocampal Sclerosis

Clinical History

The first recognized seizure occurred at age 20 years as an episode of impaired awareness with shaking consistent with tonic-clonic movements.

The habitual seizures manifested as an aura of tingling and chills in bilateral arms with a choking or throat closing sensation. This was followed by staring with oral automatisms and unresponsiveness for about 30 seconds. Progression to forced gaze deviation upward and bilateral tonic-clonic movements did not occur for many years, but it was typical during the first year after the onset of epilepsy. Treatment included multiple anti-seizure medications with a seizure frequency of one to two monthly.

The epilepsy risk factor was one close relative with epilepsy.

Neurological examination was normal. Neuropsychological testing identified impaired verbal and nonverbal memory with poor learning and rapid forgetting. Visuo-perceptual function also was impaired, suggestive of lateral temporal dysfunction. Medical history includes treatment for depression.

Interictal EEG depicted mildly abnormal generalized slowing with bilateral, independent anterior temporal epileptiform sharp waves. Video-EEG monitoring recorded focal seizures sometimes manifested as minimal behavioral change and sometimes with oral automatisms. Ictal EEG's seizure onsets were bilaterally independent over the anterior temporal regions.

MRI identified bilateral hippocampal sclerosis and PET identified symmetric hypometabolism of bilateral anterior temporal regions.

The history and evaluation indicate bilateral mesial temporal lobe epilepsy. The aura has limbic features, including the possibility of insular involvement with the choking sensation and the diffuse somatosensory experience. The bilaterally independent ictal onsets are concordant with the evidence of bilateral hippocampal abnormality on MRI, PET, and neuropsychological testing. Based on the evaluation, resective epilepsy surgery candidacy was not evident. Neurostimulation was offered with either responsive neurostimulation to bilateral anterior temporal lobes or vagus nerve stimulation. The patient chose vagus nerve stimulation, and this has provided 4 years of a substantial decrease in seizure severity along with improved mood.

J. M. Stern, N. Salamon, *Imaging of Epilepsy*, https://doi.org/10.1007/978-3-030-86672-3_5

Imaging

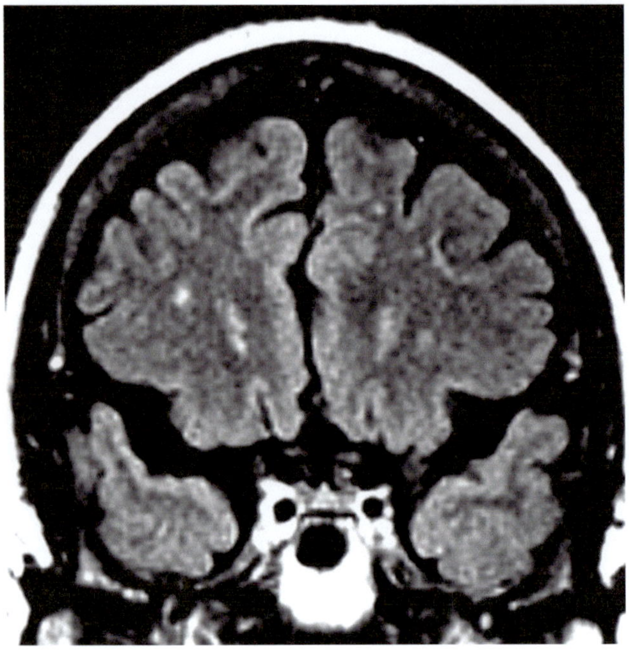

Fig. 5.1 MRI coronal FLAIR sequence at a temporal pole level. The gray-white differentiation is obscured in the medial portion of bilateral temporal poles

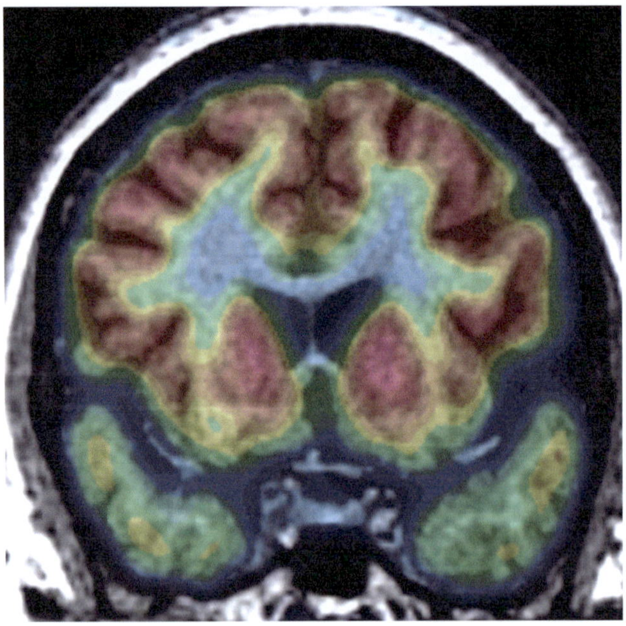

Fig. 5.2 PET-MRI co-registration with color-scale FDG tracer in a coronal plane at the temporal pole level in Fig. 5.1. Bilateral temporal poles demonstrate hypometabolism that includes the temporal lobes' medial and lateral surfaces

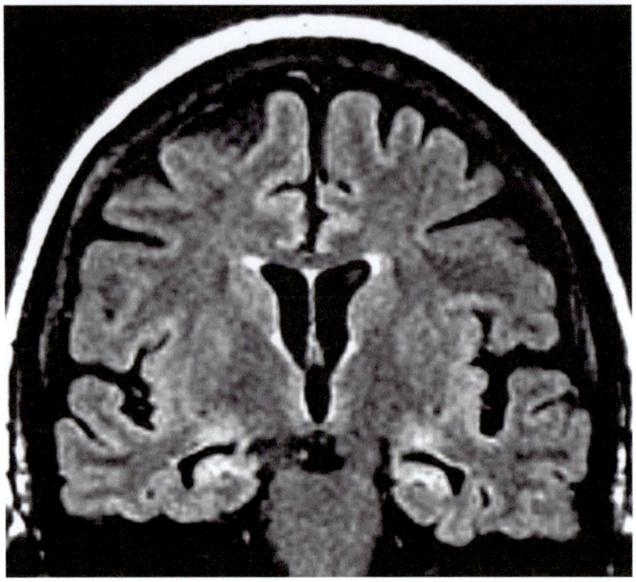

Fig. 5.3 MRI coronal FLAIR sequence at a hippocampal head level. Bilateral hippocampal heads demonstrate marked atrophy and hyperintensity. The superior surfaces of bilateral hippocampal heads are abnormally straight due to loss of the hippocampal indentations. Mild, bilateral cerebral atrophy also is present

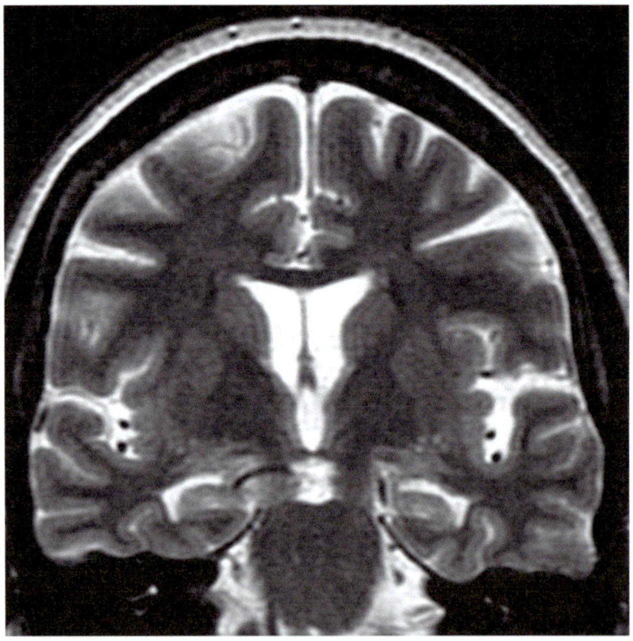

Fig. 5.4 MRI coronal T2 sequence at the hippocampal head level in Fig. 5.3. Bilateral hippocampal head atrophy is present with obscuration of the hippocampi internal architecture. The temporal horns are bilaterally prominent. The extra-hippocampal temporal lobes are normal bilaterally with clear gray-white differentiation. Mild, bilateral cerebral atrophy also is present

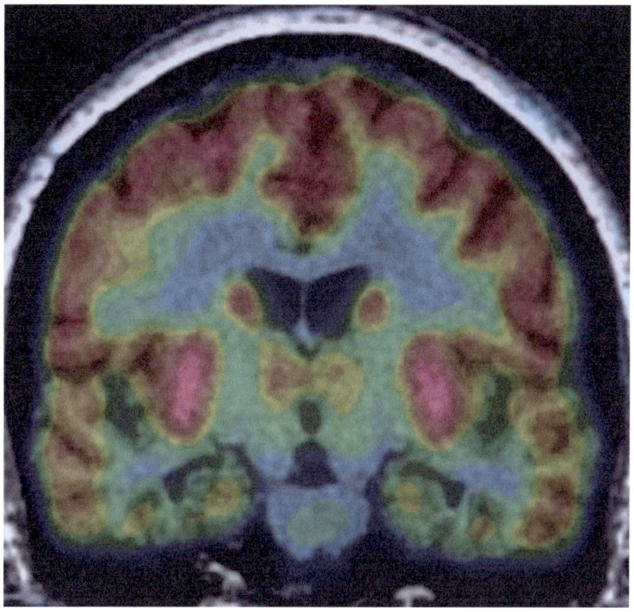

Fig. 5.5 PET-MRI co-registration with color-scale FDG tracer in a coronal plane at the hippocampal head level in Figs. 5.3 and 5.4. Bilaterally symmetric hypometabolism is present in the hippocampi and inferior temporal lobes. The left thalamus has mildly decreased metabolism compared to the right

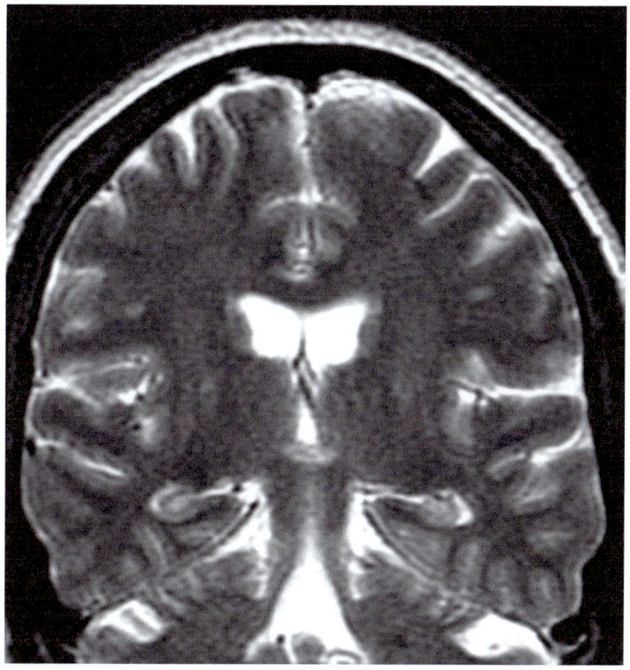

Fig. 5.7 MRI coronal T2 sequence at the hippocampal body level in Fig. 5.6. The hippocampi are bilaterally atrophic and hyperintense with prominence of bilateral temporal horns. The gray-white junction is normal in bilateral temporal lobes

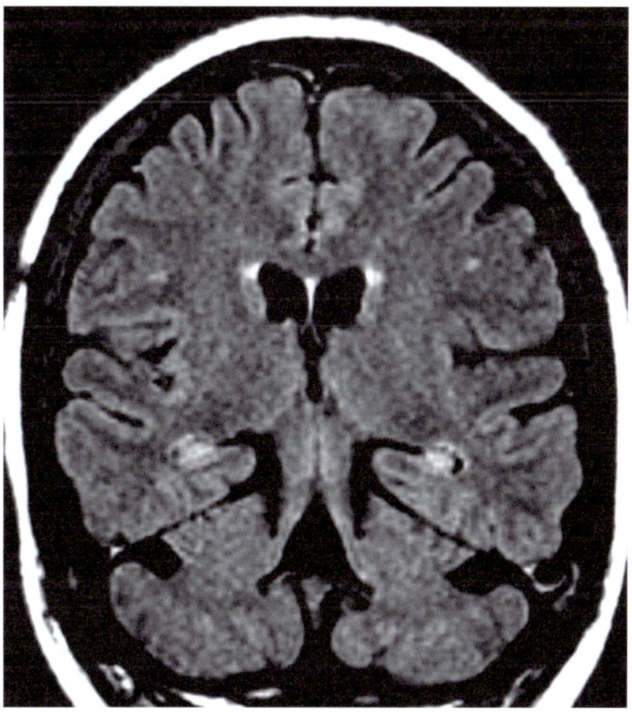

Fig. 5.6 MRI coronal FLAIR sequence at a hippocampal body level. The hippocampi are markedly atrophic bilaterally and are symmetric in volume and signal

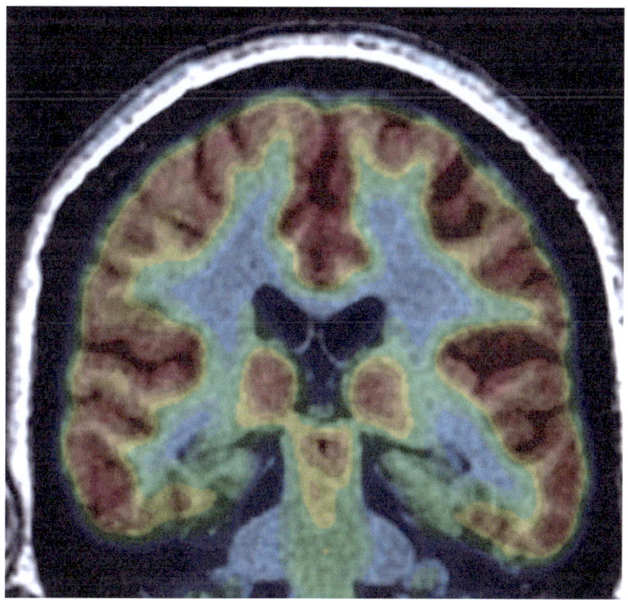

Fig. 5.8 PET-MRI co-registration with color-scale FDG tracer in a coronal plane at a hippocampal body level similar to Figs. 5.6 and 5.7. The hippocampal bodies and mesial temporal lobes have bilaterally symmetric hypometabolism. Less prominent hypometabolism is evident in bilateral inferior temporal lobes. The thalami are symmetric and normal in metabolism

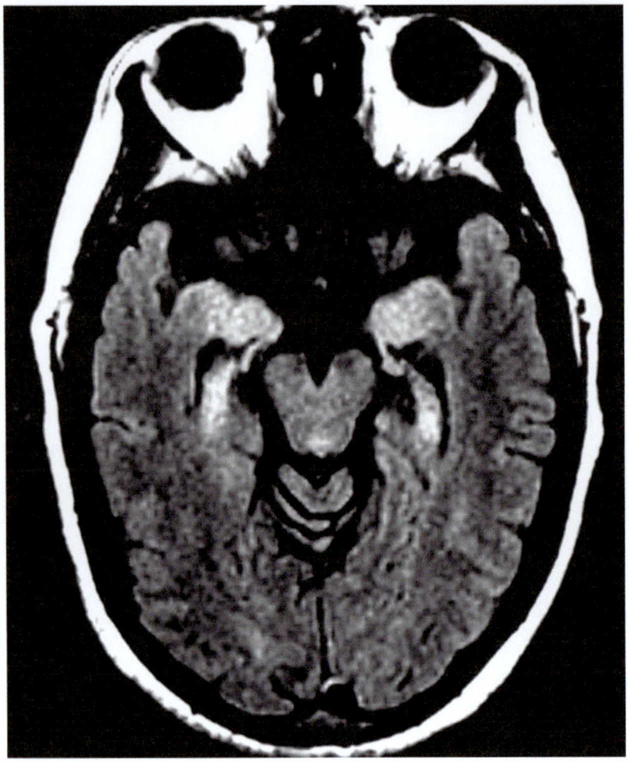

Fig. 5.9 MRI axial FLAIR sequence at a hippocampal head level. Bilateral hippocampal heads are markedly atrophic and hyperintense. The amygdalae are bilaterally hyperintense but not atrophic

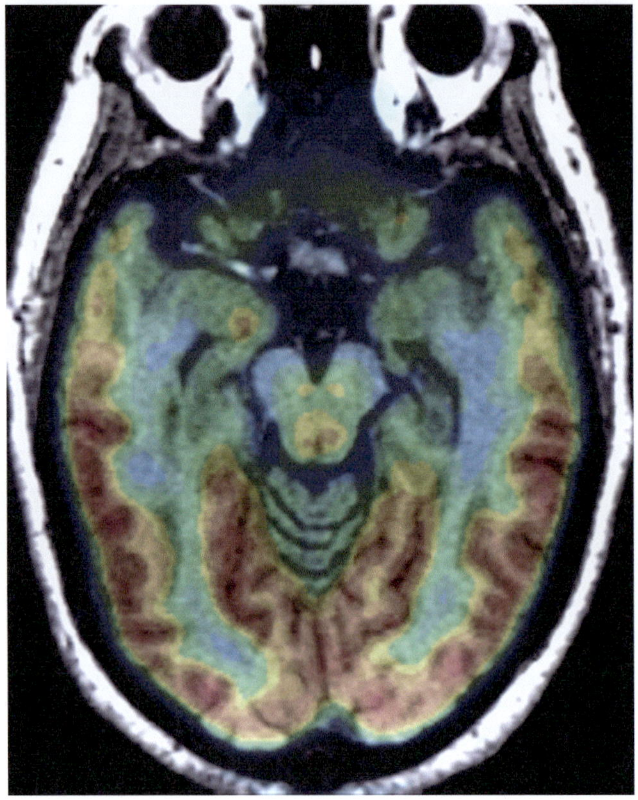

Fig. 5.10 PET-MRI co-registration with color-scale FDG tracer in an axial plane at a hippocampal head level similar to Fig. 5.9. Bilateral hippocampi and amygdalae are hypometabolic with slightly greater hypometabolism of the left hippocampus and amygdala

Hippocampal Sclerosis with Normal MRI and Abnormal PET

6

Clinical History

The first recognized seizure occurred at age 7 years as a bilateral tonic-clonic seizure that was accompanied by a fever. Epilepsy was diagnosed with seizure recurrence and the development of the habitual seizures at age 30 years.

The habitual seizures initially manifested as exclusively nocturnal bilateral tonic-clonic seizures that occurred approximately weekly until treatment was begun. With anti-seizure medication, seizures were exclusively during wakefulness. These seizures followed an aura of an emotion and sense in the pit of the stomach that are experienced as something horrible has happened or is about to happen. The aura was followed by an impairment of awareness and interaction that was accompanied by a blank stare and drooling. The seizure duration was 1 minute. Treatment included multiple anti-seizure medications with a seizure frequency of about three seizures weekly.

The only epilepsy risk factor was a childhood illness with a fever of 107 °F that produced a bilateral tonic-clonic seizure.

Neurological examination was normal. Neuropsychological testing identified mild weakness in visuospatial memory with above-average verbal memory.

Interictal EEG depicted frequent left anterior temporal epileptiform discharges and occasional right anterior temporal epileptiform discharges. Video-EEG monitoring recorded focal seizures manifested as oral automatisms with right-hand dystonic posturing that progressed to right facial contraction and versive turning to the right. Ictal EEG's seizure onset was across the left anterior temporal region.

MRI was normal and PET identified hypometabolism of the left anterior temporal lobe. MEG identified epileptiform dipoles over the left mesial temporal region. An intracarotid amobarbital test identified left hemispheric language dominance, intact memory with a left-sided injection, and no recall with a right-sided injection.

The history and evaluation indicate left mesial temporal lobe epilepsy. A limbic localization is suggested by the aura's characteristic emotional features and by the occurrence of focal seizures without progression to bilateral tonic-clonic. The dystonic posturing, versive turning, and lateralized ictal EEG's seizure onset are concordant and suggest a left-sided lateralization. Although the neuropsychological testing identified mild, nonverbal memory impairment, the intracarotid amobarbital test identified impairment of the left hippocampal memory system, suggesting an atypical lateralization for episodic memory. The PET provided further confirmation of left temporal lobe epilepsy localization despite no evidence of hippocampal sclerosis on the MRI. In addition to the normal MRI, the predominance of nocturnal tonic-clonic seizures before beginning treatment is another atypical feature for mesial temporal lobe epilepsy.

Consideration of epilepsy surgery included concern for a decline in verbal memory after an anterior temporal lobe resection because of the normal MRI and the intact verbal memory. As such, a stereotactic laser ablation of the left hippocampus was performed based on the intracarotid amobarbital test results and the ablation's potentially lower risk to verbal memory as compared to a standard anterior-mesial temporal lobe resection. The lower risk was considered as justification for the possibility of the ablation's reduced likelihood of seizure freedom. Seizure control has improved from three focal seizures with impairment weekly to several nocturnal tonic-clonic seizures in total during the 2 years since surgery. Surgery produced a meaningful success with freedom from seizures during wakefulness despite the lack of complete seizure freedom. The return of nocturnal tonic-clonic seizures furthers the original impression of atypical mesial temporal lobe epilepsy.

J. M. Stern, N. Salamon, *Imaging of Epilepsy*, https://doi.org/10.1007/978-3-030-86672-3_6

Imaging

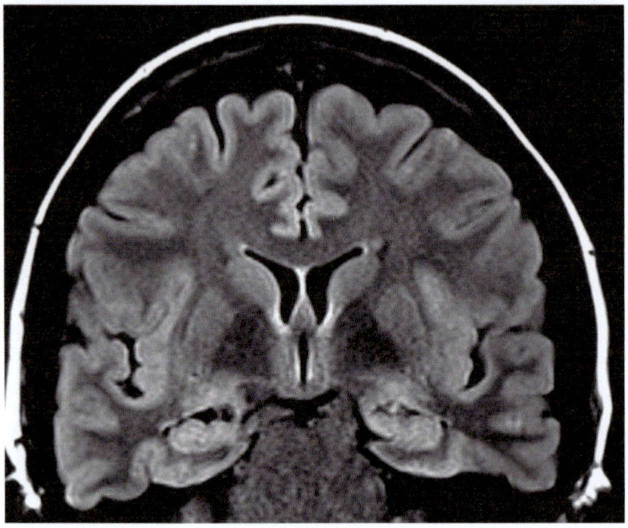

Fig. 6.1 MRI coronal FLAIR sequence at a hippocampal head level. The hippocampi are bilaterally normal in signal and volume. The internal architecture is subtly evident on the right and not abnormal on the left. The hippocampi's superior indentations are present bilaterally

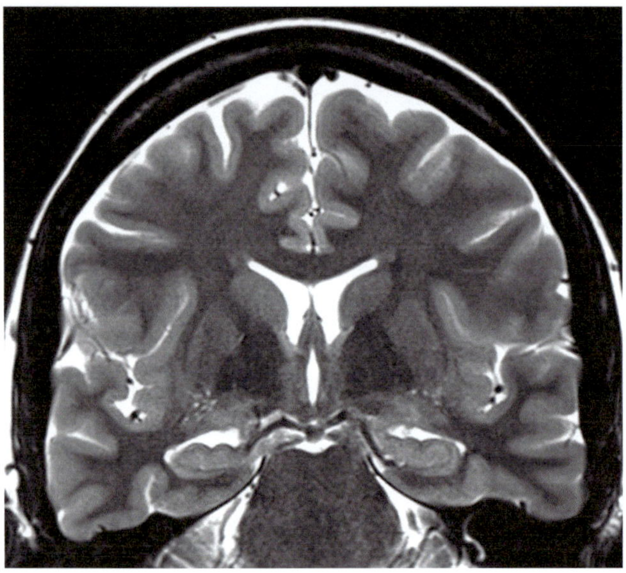

Fig. 6.2 MRI coronal T2 sequence at the hippocampal head level in Fig. 6.1. The hippocampi are bilaterally normal in signal and volume with normal internal architecture bilaterally. The temporal horns are bilaterally prominent but not abnormal. Normal gray-white differentiation is present in bilateral temporal lobes

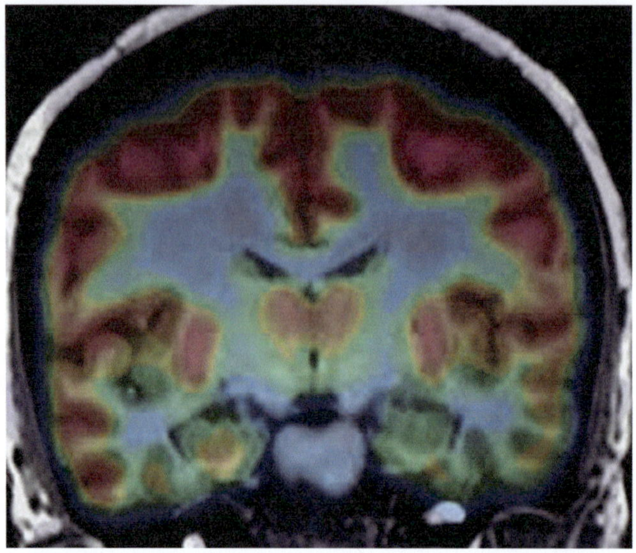

Fig. 6.3 PET-MRI co-registration with color-scale FDG tracer in a coronal plane at a hippocampal head level similar to Figs. 6.1 and 6.2. The left hippocampal head and inferior temporal lobe demonstrate asymmetrically greater hypometabolism, and the left lateral temporal lobe demonstrates less prominent asymmetric hypometabolism. The thalami are symmetric

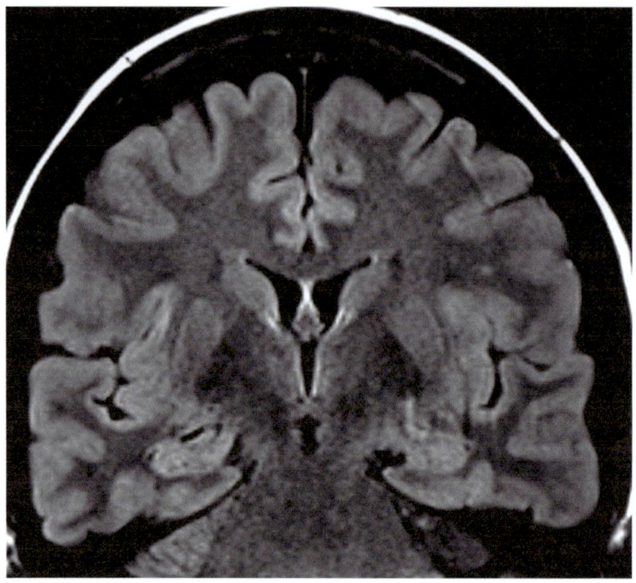

Fig. 6.4 MRI coronal FLAIR sequence at a hippocampal body level. The hippocampi are symmetric in signal and volume, and the temporal lobes are also symmetric with normal gray-white differentiation

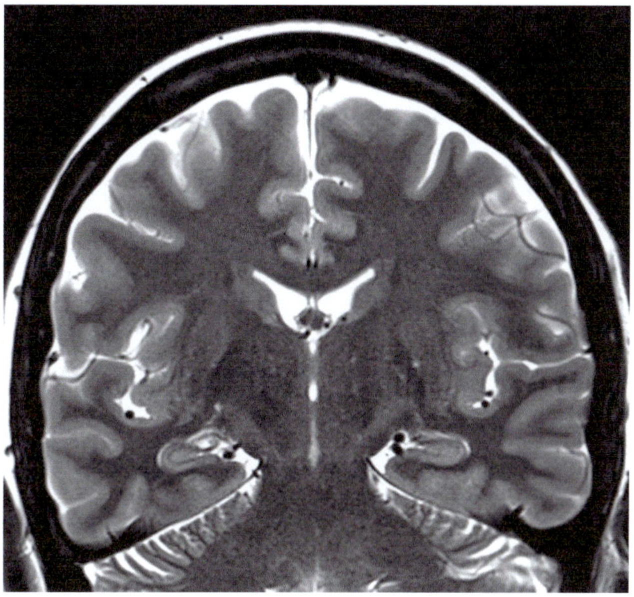

Fig. 6.5 MRI coronal T2 sequence at a hippocampal body level similar to Fig. 6.4. The hippocampi are symmetric in signal and volume, and the temporal lobes are also symmetric with normal gray-white differentiation

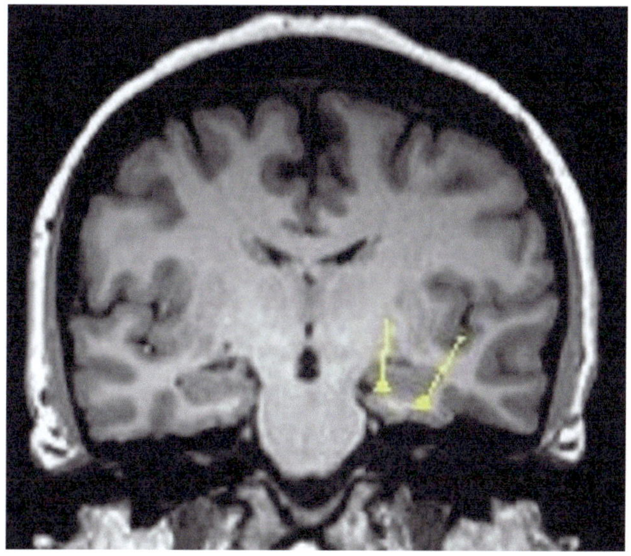

Fig. 6.7 MEG co-registered to MRI coronal T1 sequence at a hippocampal body level. MEG epileptiform dipole source analysis indicates mapping of two dipoles to the left parahippocampal gyrus

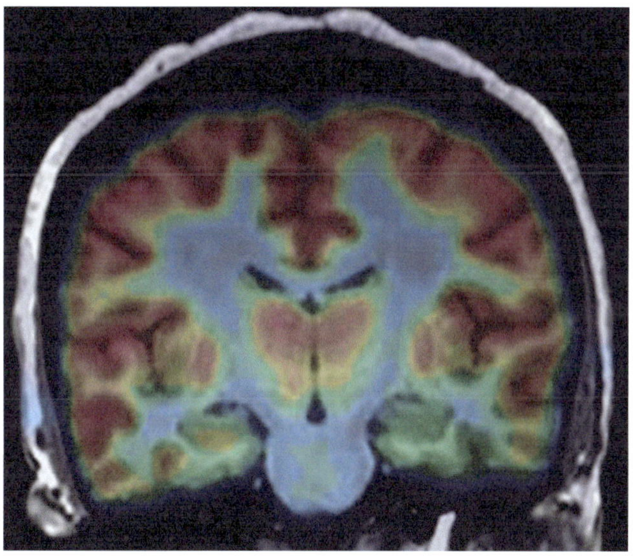

Fig. 6.6 PET-MRI co-registration with color-scale FDG tracer in a coronal plane at a hippocampal body level similar to Figs. 6.4 and 6.5. The left hippocampal body and inferior temporal lobe demonstrate asymmetrically greater hypometabolism. The thalami are symmetric

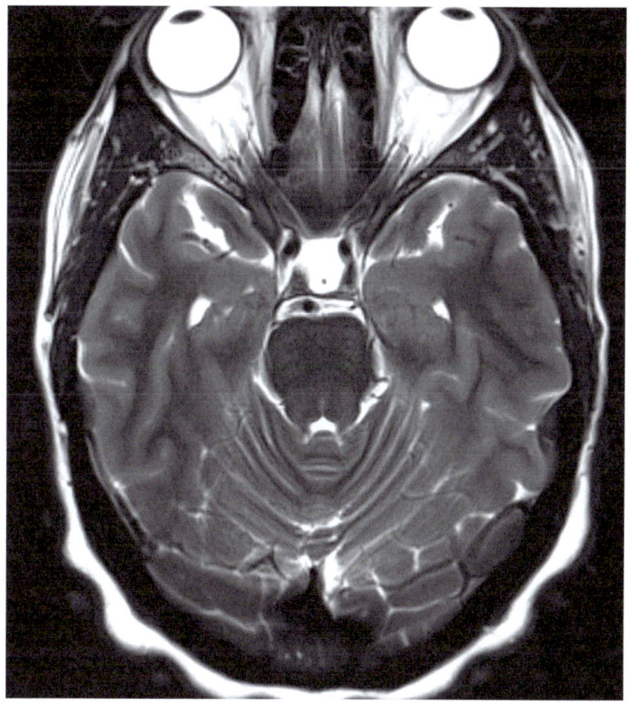

Fig. 6.8 MRI axial T2 sequence at a hippocampal head level. The hippocampi, amygdalae, and temporal poles are bilaterally normal

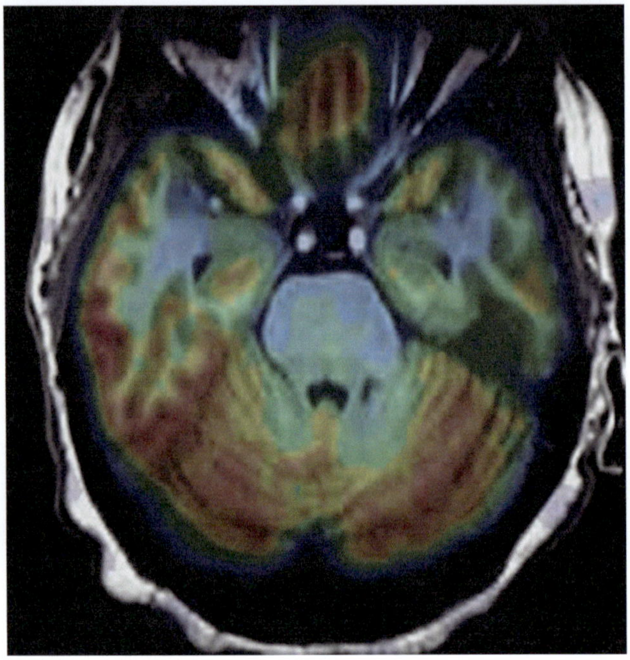

Fig. 6.9 PET-MRI co-registration with color-scale FDG tracer in an axial plane at a hippocampal head level immediately inferior to Fig. 6.8. Asymmetrically greater hypometabolism is evident in the left hippocampal head, temporal pole, and lateral temporal lobe

Part II

Cerebral Malformations

According to the International League Against Epilepsy's classification, focal cortical dysplasias (FCD) are divided into three types. Type I is defined histologically as cerebral cortex neuronal layering abnormality that is radial (Type 1a), tangential (Type Ib), or both radial and tangential (Type Ic). For Type I FCDs, the epilepsy onset is often in adulthood and the dysplasia is often in the temporal pole. Type II FCD is defined as cortical dyslamination combined with dysmorphic neurons and is divided into IIa and IIb, with IIb indicating the presence of balloon cells. Type II is often extra-temporal and has a predilection for the frontal lobe. Epilepsy due to a Type II FCD often presents in childhood. Type III FCD is a combination of a Type I FCD and a structural abnormality associated with epilepsy, which can be hippocampal sclerosis (Type IIIa), glial or glioneuronal tumors (Type IIIb), vascular malformations (Type IIIc), or another malformation from early life, such as from ischemia, encephalitis, or trauma (Type IIId).

Brain MRI often does not identify Type I FCD, but the co-registration to FDG-PET can increase the imaging sensitivity for this abnormality. In comparison, most Type II FCDs are usually evident with MRI. However, Types I and II have similar imaging features when Type I is visible. These features include: neocortical thickening, blurring of the margin between white matter and gray matter, abnormal signal within the subcortical layer, abnormal signal within white matter occurring with abnormal signal in adjacent cortex (transmantle sign), increased T2 signal within gray matter, abnormal sulcal or gyral pattern, and segmental atrophy. The increased signal from gray matter on T2-weighted images is more easily observed in Type II than Type I. Type III is often within the ipsilateral temporal pole when it is associated with hippocampal sclerosis. When it is associated with tumors, such as DNET or ganglioglioma, it is adjacent to the tumor.

Heterotopia

Gray matter heterotopia arise from premature arrest of neuronal migration from the germinal matrix along the walls of the lateral ventricles to the developing cerebral cortex. The three major categories are band heterotopia, periventricular gray matter heterotopia, and nodular subcortical heterotopia. Each is identified by the presence of gray matter signal indicating abnormality along the peri-ventricular margin or the cerebral white matter. When occurring in the subcortical white matter, the heterotopia can appear as a duplicate (double) cortex parallel to the surface cortex.

Polymicrogyria

Polymicrogyria is a developmental disorder or injury that occurs between gestational weeks 17 and 26 and sometimes relates to a genetic abnormality. When patients are younger than 12 months, polymicrogyria appears as a small undulating cortex. When older than 12 months, the cortex has a bumpy contour and appears abnormally thick. The difference between the two appearances relates to the myelination of underlying white matter.

Schizencephaly

Schizencephaly is a developmental malformation characterized by an abnormal slit or cleft in the cerebral hemispheres with an orientation toward the ventricular system. Polymicrogyria usually spans the cleft with sulcation abnormalities that vary from the scale of a fissure to minor cortical surface indentations.

Lissencephaly

Lissencephaly is a set of rare brain disorders characterized by abnormal smoothness to the entirety or aspects of the cerebral surface. The abnormality arises from defective neuronal migration during gestational weeks 12 to 24 with a resulting in a lack of development of gyri and sulci.

Hemimegalencephaly

Hemimegalencephaly is hamartomatous overgrowth of one hemisphere as a proliferative anomaly during cortical development with dysmorphic neurons. When the ipsilateral brainstem and cerebellum are also enlarged, the term total hemimegalencephaly is used. Before age 6 months, hypermyelination of the affected hemisphere's white matter is a characteristic feature.

After age 6 months, the myelination within the unaffected hemisphere exceeds the affected hemisphere, so the affected hemisphere appears hypomyelinated. The affected hemisphere also may have band heterotopia, polymicrogyria, and lissencephalic features. Occasionally, the unaffected hemisphere may have relatively minor abnormalities, including heterotopic gray matter or mild focal cortical dysplasia. Syndromic anomaly can be associated with hemimegalencephaly, including Klippel–Trenaunay-Weber, hypomelanosis of Ito, linear sebaceous nevus, neurofibromatosis, tuberous sclerosis complex, epidermal nevus, and Proteus syndromes.

Encephalocele

Encephaloceles are gaps in the bone that are typically congenital and allow protrusion of the cerebrum beyond the normal cerebral contour. The protrusion can vary from subtle to extension beyond the skull's outer table. The cerebral tissue may demonstrate signal abnormality at the site of the encephalocele, but this is not essential and normal signal does not exclude the possibility of focal histologic abnormality. CT more clearly identifies encephaloceles because of its superior depiction of bone.

Key References

Barkovich AJ. Current concept of polymicrogyria. Neuroradiology. 2010;52:479–87.

Barkovich AJ, Koch TK, Carrol CL. The spectrum of Iissencephaly: report of ten patients analyzed by magnetic resonance imaging. Ann Neurol. 1991;30:139–46.

Blumcke I, Thom M, Aronica E, et al. The clinicopathologic spectrum of focal cortical dysplasias: a consensus classification proposed by an ad hoc Task Force of the ILAE Diagnostic Methods Commission. Epilepsia 2011;52:158–74.

Flores-Sarnat L. Hemimegalencephaly: part 1. Genetic, clinical, and imaging aspects. J Child Neurol. 2002;17:373–84.

Salamon N, Kung J, Shaw SJ, et al. FDG-PET/MRI coregistration improves detection of cortical dysplasia in patients with epilepsy. Neurology. 2008;71:1594–601.

Focal Cortical Dysplasia, Type I

7

Clinical History

The first recognized seizures occurred at age 3 years as stereotyped episodes of staring that followed a frightened or anxious appearance. The first episodes were not noted as abnormal, and presentation for evaluation was after multiple stereotyped recurrences. In retrospect, another seizure manifestation may have been present at age 7 months and manifested as 15-second episodes of gaze deviation to the right with eyelid fluttering. The episodes during infancy spontaneously resolved after several weeks and were not brought for medical attention.

The habitual seizures manifested as oral automatisms with grunting and sometimes manual automatisms. No aura or warning was evident. The seizure duration was 1–2 minutes followed by 2 hours of fatigue or sleeping. No bilateral tonic-clonic seizures occurred. Treatment included multiple anti-seizure medications without seizure freedom.

The epilepsy risk factor was encephalitis at age 2 years. An infectious organism was not identified, and the encephalitis was presumed to be viral. However, the episodes during infancy suggested a possibility of epilepsy prior to the encephalitis.

Neurological examination was normal; however, neuropsychological testing identified an auditory processing disorder with mild learning disability.

Interictal EEG depicted bifrontal, polyspike discharges and right frontal and temporal focal discharges. An interictal EEG at age 5 years depicted slowing and attenuation over the right frontal region. Video-EEG monitoring recorded seizures manifested as abrupt staring with unresponsiveness and left facial twitching and dystonic posturing of the left hand. The ictal EEG's seizure onset had a broad distribution across the right frontal-temporal region.

MRI was reported normal at age 5 years. MRI at age 7 years identified signal abnormality in the subcortical white matter of the right temporal lobe from the pole to approximately 5.5 cm posteriorly and including the supramarginal gyrus. PET at ages 5 years and 8 years identified hypometabolism of the right superior temporal lobe and right anterior parietal lobe. MEG at age 8 years identified interictal dipoles across bilateral perisylvian regions with a substantial predominance of the right side.

The history and evaluation indicate right temporal lobe epilepsy. The fearful or anxious facial expression, non-forced lateral gaze deviation, and lack of bilateral tonic-clonic or other convulsive seizures suggest a limbic onset. However, the early age of onset and interictal EEG with bifrontal, polyspike epileptiform discharges suggest a neocortical epilepsy. The MRI, PET, and MEG confirm an abnormality beyond the hippocampus and temporal pole, although much of the abnormality is within the right temporal lobe.

Based on the diagnostic testing, a right temporal resection was performed with posterior boundaries that extended beyond the standard resection for mesial temporal lobe epilepsy. The resection extended to 8 cm from the temporal pole and spared the supramarginal gyrus abnormality because of functional concerns. Histopathological examination identified mild, focal crowding of neurons in the deeper layers with cortical dyslamination. Heterotopic neurons were present in subcortical white matter. No dysmorphic neurons were present.

Following the resection, seizures decreased in frequency, increased in duration, and more often occurred without an impaired awareness. At age 10 years, video-EEG monitoring identified a seizure onset that was maximum over the posterior right temporal lobe, indicating the possibility of an epileptogenic zone adjacent to the resection margin. Because of concerns for a functional deficit, additional surgery was not performed, and treatment has involved alterations in medications.

J. M. Stern, N. Salamon, *Imaging of Epilepsy*, https://doi.org/10.1007/978-3-030-86672-3_7

Imaging

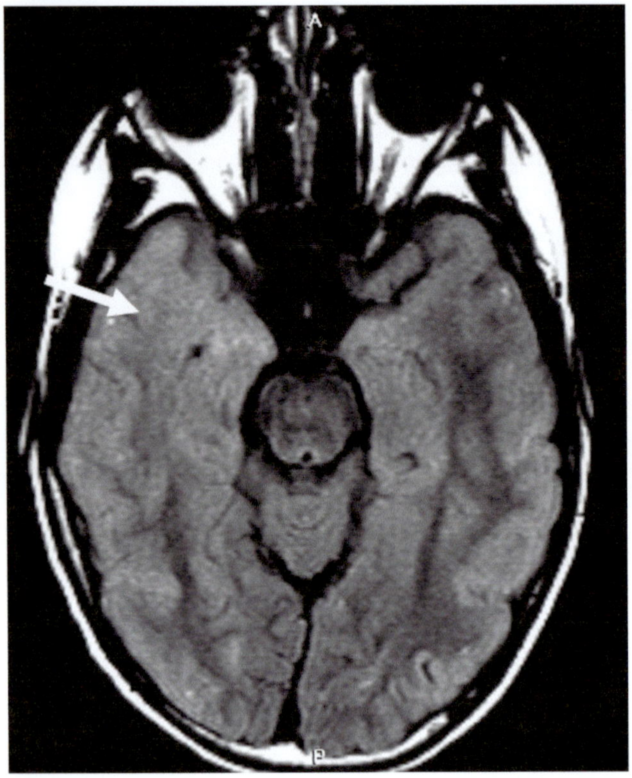

Fig. 7.1 MRI axial FLAIR sequence at the temporal lobe level. The gray-white differentiation of right anterior temporal lobe (arrow) is blurred without abnormal signal in cortical gray matter. Hippocampi are normal and symmetrical in volume and signal

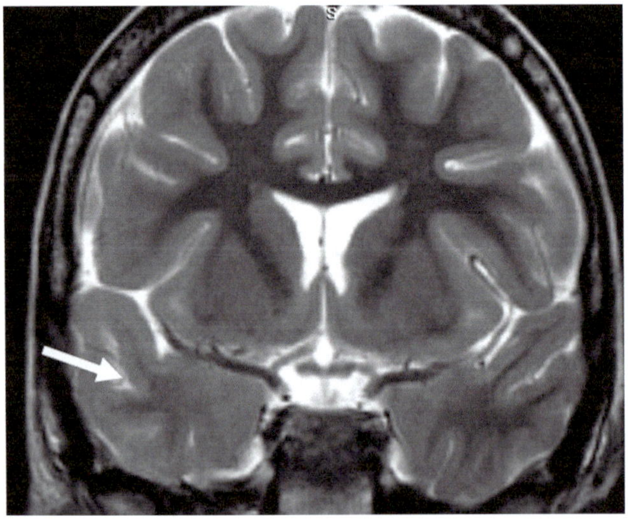

Fig. 7.2 MRI coronal T2 sequence at the anterior temporal lobe level. The gray-white junction is blurred at the temporal pole lateral to the right amygdala. Anterior amygdalae are visible and normal. Increased signal appears as gray in the white matter within the superior (arrow) and middle temporal gyrus

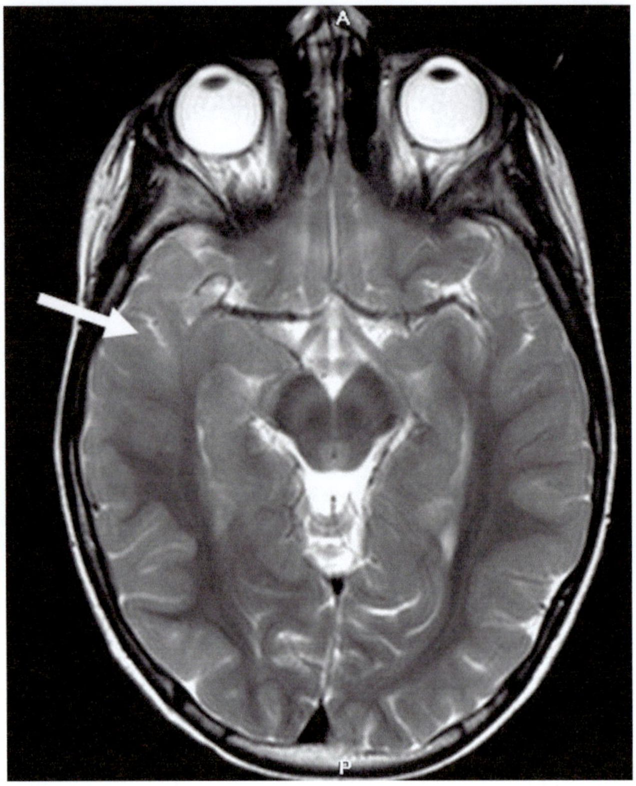

Fig. 7.3 MRI axial T2 sequence at the midbrain level, slightly superior to Fig. 7.1. The gray-white junction is blurred in the right middle temporal gyrus (arrow). The temporal lobes are symmetric in volume. Both hippocampi and amygdalae are normal

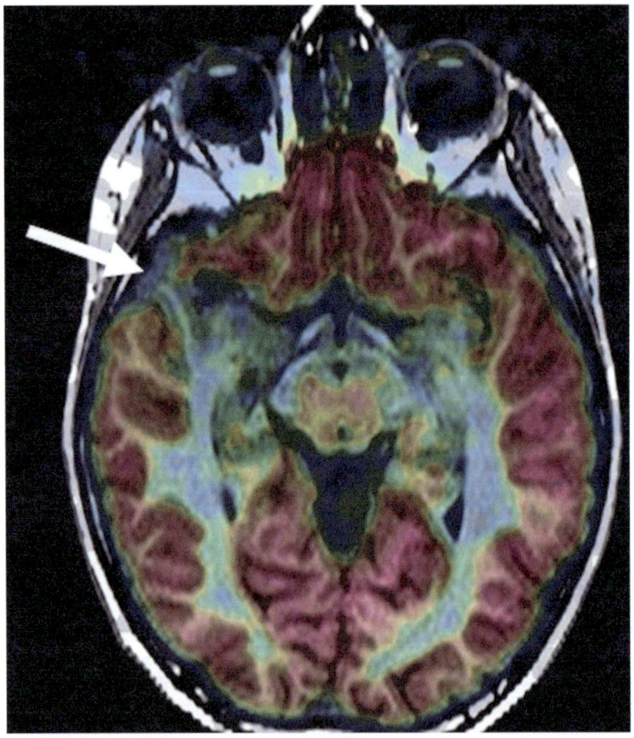

Fig. 7.4 PET-MRI co-registration with color-scale FDG tracer in the axial plane at the temporal lobe level. Hypometabolism is evident in the right middle temporal gyrus' anterior portion (arrow) with clear metabolic demarcation. The region immediately posterior is asymmetrically hypometabolic when compared to the left, but less abnormal

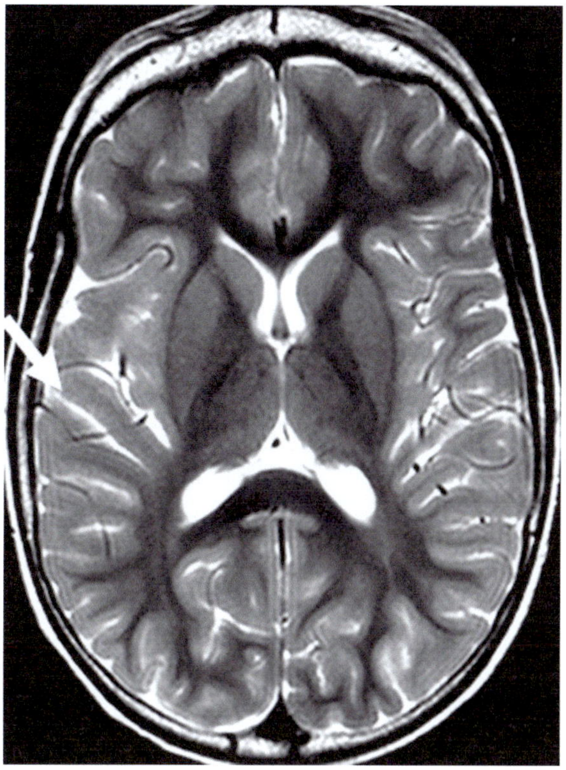

Fig. 7.5 MRI axial T2 sequence at the insular level. The gray-white differentiation is blurred in the right superior temporal gyrus (arrow). The adjacent posterior opercular region also is blurred and lacks white matter arborization into the gyri, especially when compared to the left opercular region. Gray-white differentiation and white mater arborization are more evident posterior to the superior temporal gyrus

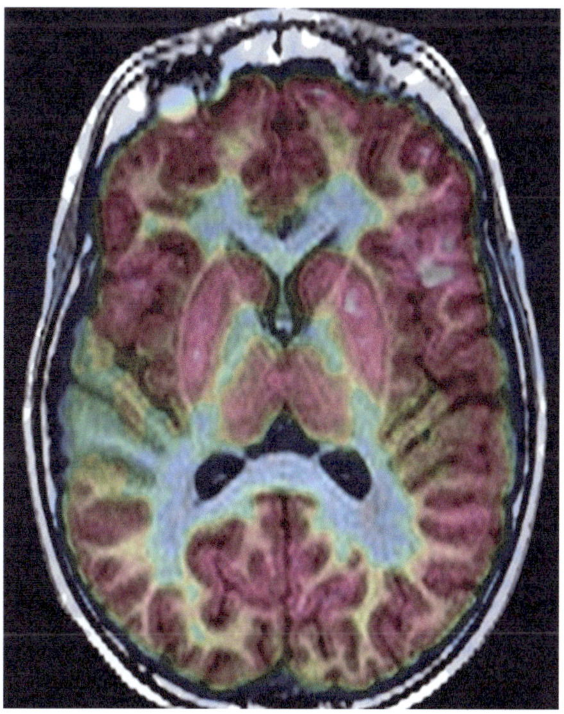

Fig. 7.6 PET-MRI co-registration with color-scale FDG tracer in the axial plane at the insular level, similar to Fig. 7.5. Hypometabolism of the right superior temporal gyrus and supramarginal gyrus is evident. The right insula and operculum are normal and symmetric with the left homotopic region

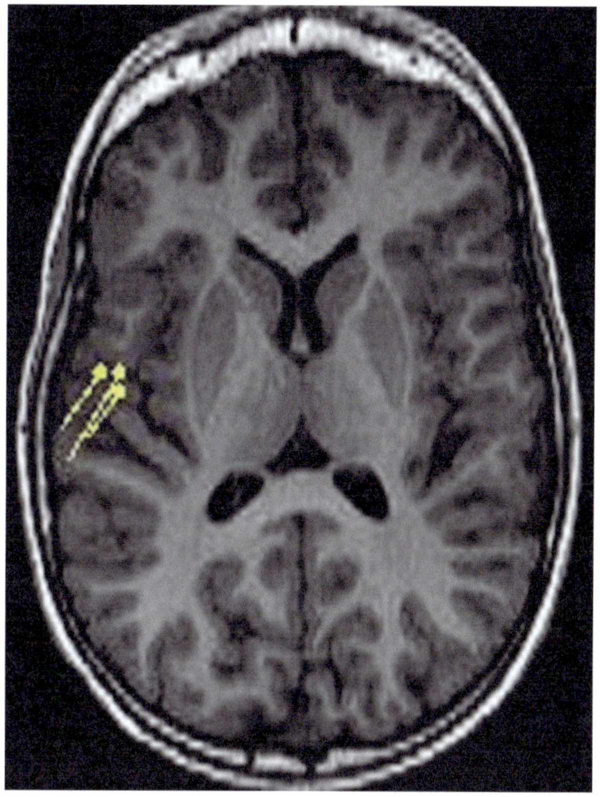

Fig. 7.7 MEG co-registered to MRI axial T1 sequence at the insular level. MEG epileptiform dipole source analysis indicates localization of the three interictal dipoles within the right superior temporal gyrus

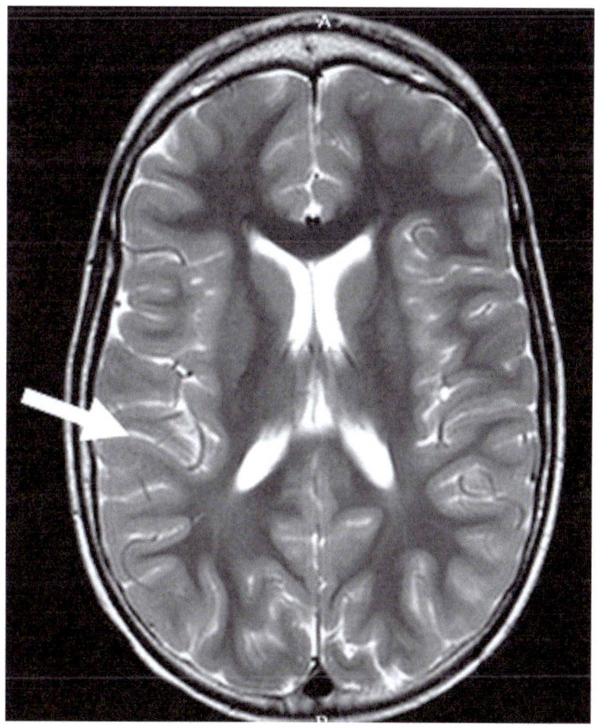

Fig. 7.8 MRI axial T2 sequence slightly superior to level in Fig. 7.5. The gray-white junction between the superior temporal gyrus and supramarginal gyrus is blurred (arrow). The right operculum is normal with normal gray-white differentiation and symmetry to left operculum

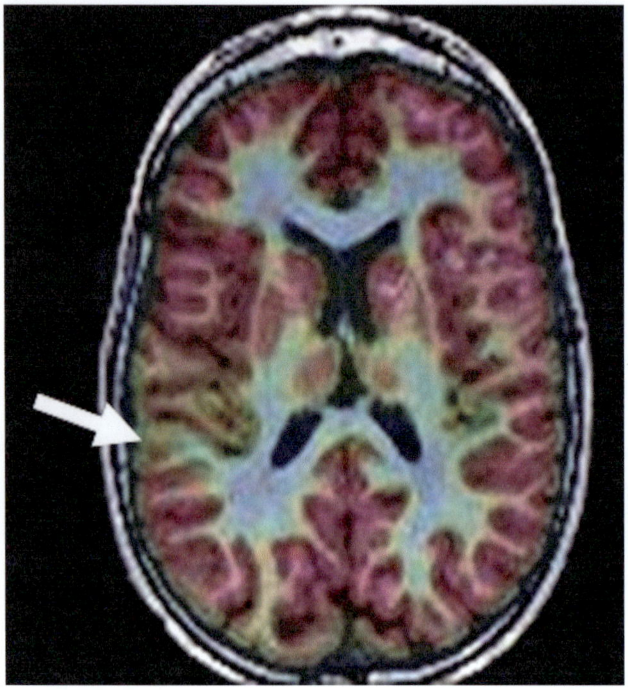

Fig. 7.9 PET-MEG co-registration with color-scale FDG tracer in the axial plane at the level of Fig. 7.8. Hypometabolism is evident in the right superior temporal gyrus and supramarginal gyrus (arrow)

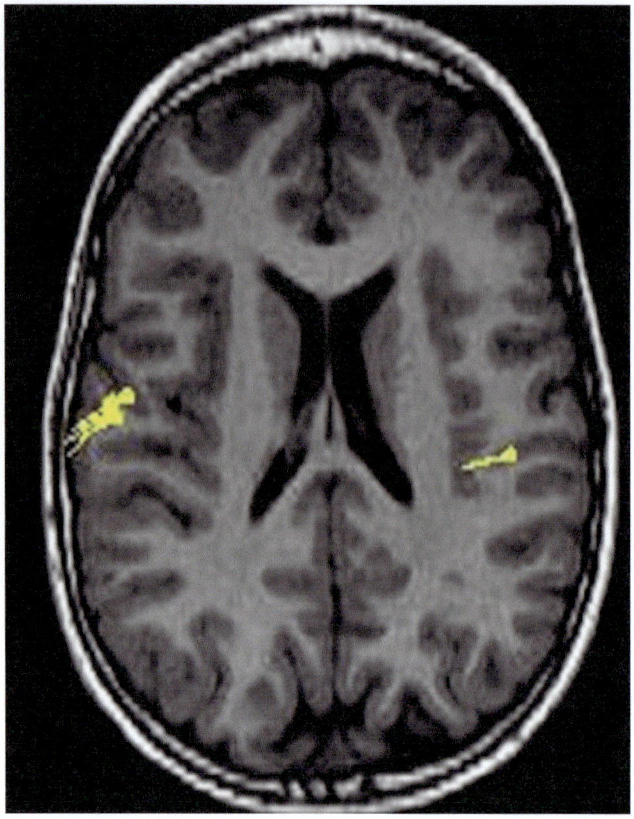

Fig. 7.10 MEG co-registered to MRI axial T1 sequence at the level in Figs. 7.8 and 7.9. Source analysis indicates localization of a cluster of overlapping epileptiform dipoles in the right parietal operculum and one dipole in the left supramarginal gyrus

8 Focal Cortical Dysplasia, Type IIa

Clinical History

The first recognized seizure occurred at age 11 years as an episode of right leg sensory abnormality and tonic posturing.

The habitual seizures were similar and occurred as right leg tonic posturing with a sensory experience that was a combination of decreased sensation and either tickling or pain. If tickling occurred, laughter resulted. During these sensory-motor seizures, awareness and interactions were normal. Some seizures progressed with extension of the sensory experience to the right arm and, more rarely, to become bilateral tonic-clonic with loss of awareness. Treatment included multiple anti-seizure medications with a seizure frequency of four or five seizures daily.

No epilepsy risk factor was identified. Neurological examination was normal.

Medical history was otherwise normal.

Interictal EEG was normal, and video-EEG monitoring recorded focal seizures visible as right leg posturing. Ictal EEG's seizure onset did not identify a correlating epileptiform abnormality.

MRI identified subtle cortical dysplasia involving the left anterior paracentral lobule and posterior left superior frontal gyrus. A prominent draining vein in the left central sulcus also was evident. Angiography confirmed a deep left paramedian developmental venous anomaly. PET identified hypometabolism in the region of the cortical dysplasia.

The history and evaluation indicate neocortical epilepsy with a left central localization. The focal sensory and motor seizures with normal mentation suggest this localization, and the MRI supports it with the identification of a structural abnormality. The normal EEG does not alter the likely diagnosis because of EEG's insensitivity to midline neocortical seizures and seizures without impaired of awareness.

In consideration of epilepsy surgery, intracranial EEG was performed with subdural grid electrodes over the region of hypometabolism and coverage of the structural abnormality and the surrounding functional abnormality. Focal seizures were recorded with an onset in the frontal region, and a resection was performed with margins defined by electrocorticographic interictal and ictal epileptiform abnormality.

Histopathological examination identified blurring of the gray-white junction with disorganized cortical architecture, neuronal crowding, and focal cytomegalic neurons. No balloon cells were present. As such, the resected tissue was consistent with cortical dysplasia, type IIa. Seizures have not occurred for 7 years since surgery, and anti-seizure medications were discontinued 3 years ago.

J. M. Stern, N. Salamon, *Imaging of Epilepsy*, https://doi.org/10.1007/978-3-030-86672-3_8

Imaging

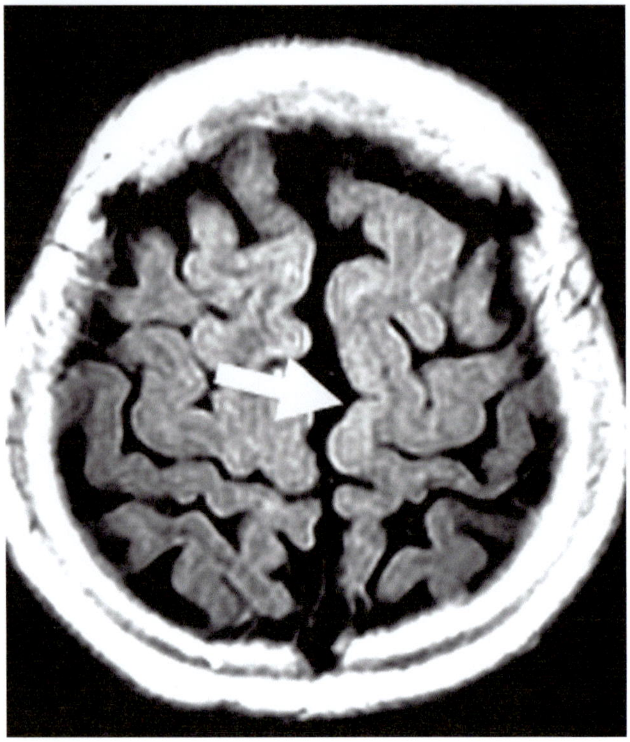

Fig. 8.1 MRI axial FLAIR sequence at a high convexity level. Abnormally increased signal within gray matter of posterior portion superior frontal gyrus and left paracentral lobule (arrow). Minor atrophy of these structures is evident

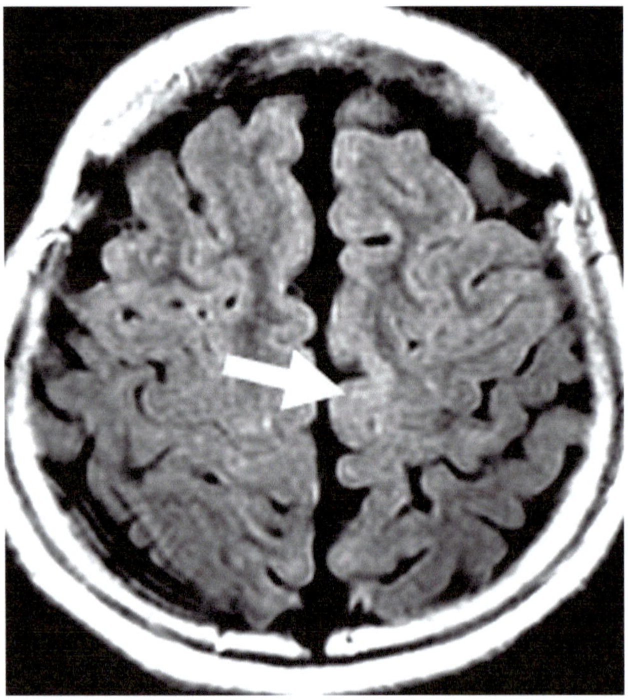

Fig. 8.2 MRI axial FLAIR sequence at a high convexity level slightly inferior to Fig. 8.1. Abnormally increased signal of the anterior portion of the left paracentral lobule is evident (arrow). Changing the window level settings during image review improves visualization of this finding. Gray-white differentiation is normal in the surrounding frontal lobe tissue

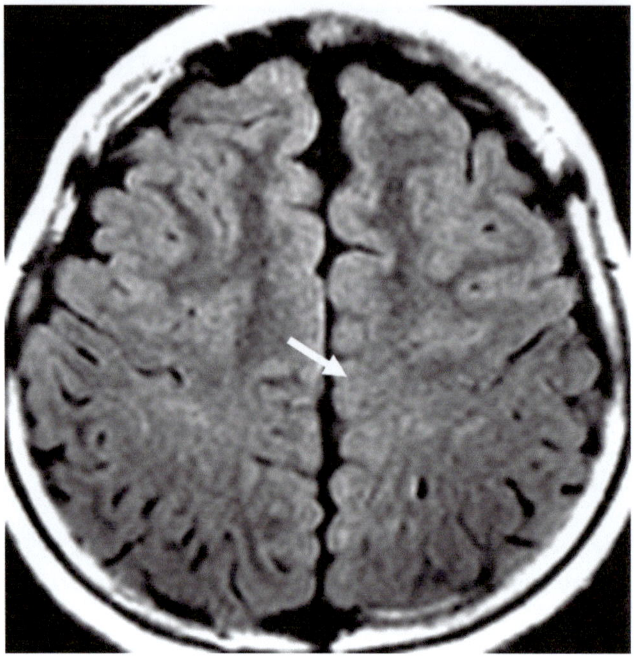

Fig. 8.3 MRI axial FLAIR sequence at a centrum semi-ovale level, slightly inferior to Fig. 8.2. The inferior boundary of the abnormality is identified with normal gray-white differentiation and signal intensity (arrow)

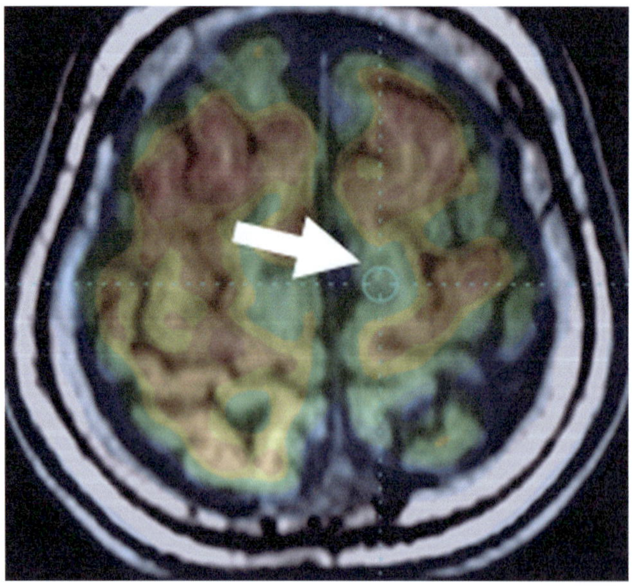

Fig. 8.4 PET-MRI co-registration with color-scale FDG tracer in the axial plane at a high convexity level similar to Fig. 8.1. Hypometabolism is evident in the posterior superior frontal gyrus and left paracentral lobule (arrow) with extension posteriorly into the superior parietal lobule. The contralateral superior frontal gyrus and paracentral lobule also are hypometabolic, but the hypometabolism does not extend posteriorly

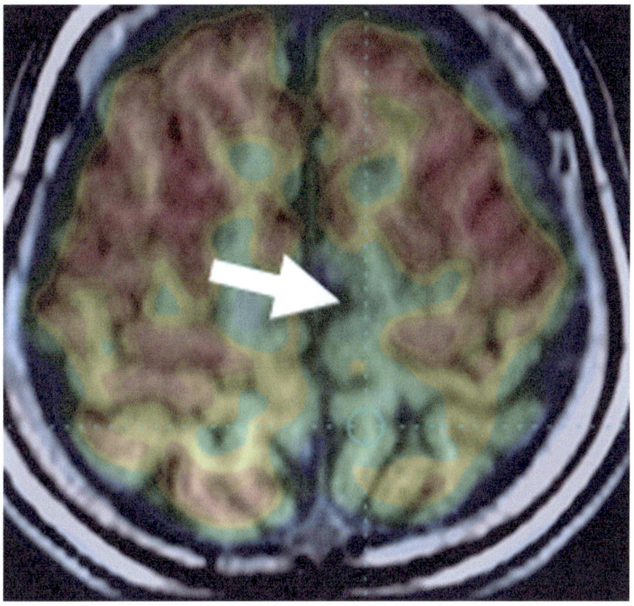

Fig. 8.5 PET-MRI co-registration with color-scale FDG tracer in the axial plane at a high convexity level similar to Fig. 8.2. Hypometabolism of left paracentral lobule and superior parietal lobule is evident. The right paracentral lobule demonstrates more minor hypometabolism that does not extend into the superior parietal lobule

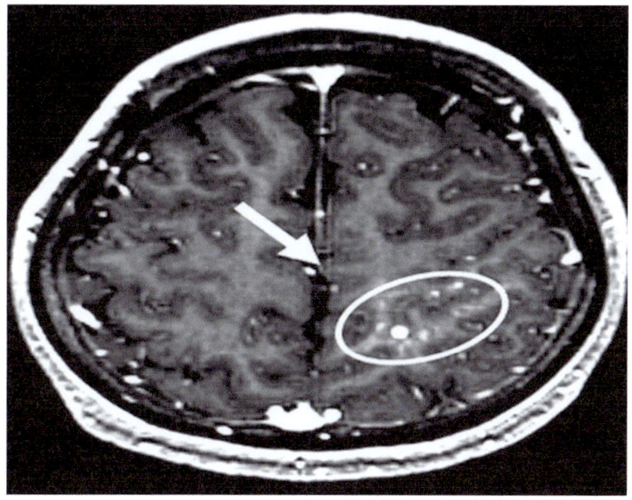

Fig. 8.7 MRI axial T1 sequence at a high convexity level after administration of intravenous contrast. The region that was found to be abnormal with T2 sequence and PET is indicated by the arrow and appears normal in the T1 sequence. Multiple, punctuate foci of enhancement (oval) are within the left parietal region, which is consistent with a developmental venous anomaly

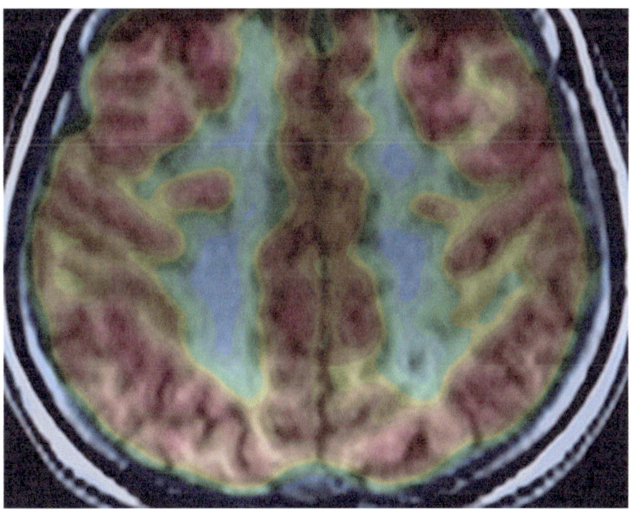

Fig. 8.6 PET-MRI co-registration with color-scale FDG tracer in the axial plane at a centrum semi-ovale level similar to Fig. 8.3. Normal metabolism is present bilaterally, including within the paramedian cortex and parietal lobe

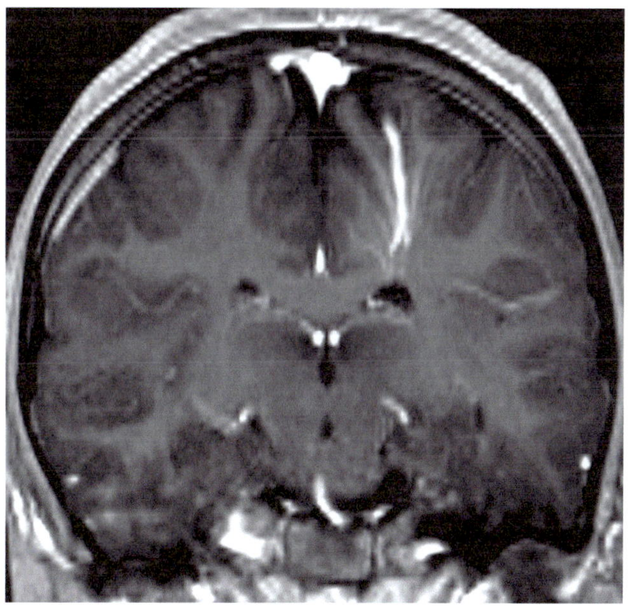

Fig. 8.8 MRI coronal T1 sequence at a parietal level after administration of intravenous contrast. A line of hyperintensity due to the contrast is evident in the left parietal lobe and is due to a draining vein from the developmental venous anomaly

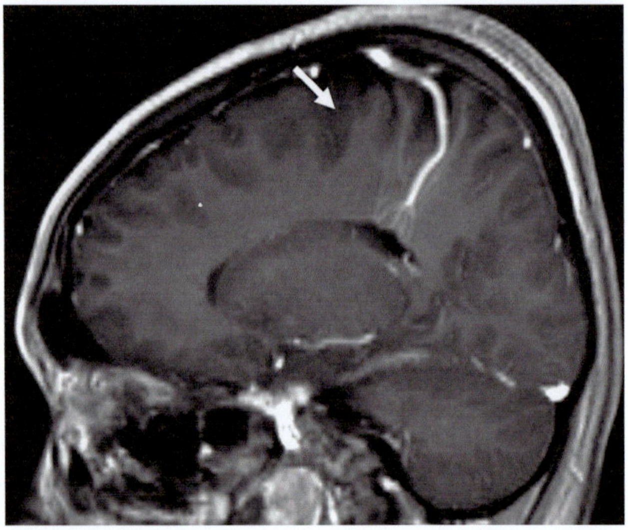

Fig. 8.9 MRI T1 sequence in a left parasagittal level after administration of intravenous contrast. A curving line of contrast enhancement is evident in the parietal lobe. The inferior portion branches into multiple intramedullary venules that connect to the ependymal surface. A parasagittal sulcus within the paracentral lobule corresponds to the focal cortical dysplasia (arrow)

9 Focal Cortical Dysplasia, Type IIb

Clinical History

The first recognized seizures occurred at age 5 years as episodes of right arm stiffening that sometimes included impaired awareness.

The habitual seizures were similar and recognized to having two distinct manifestations. One manifestation was right arm stiffening with a mild right facial droop and no impaired awareness. Its duration was 30–45 seconds. The other manifestation included the same right arm stiffening and an impaired awareness accompanied by repetitive verbalizations or clearing of the throat. Its duration was several minutes. Neither seizure had postictal confusion. The first manifestation occurred daily and the second occurred once monthly. Seizures with bilateral tonic-clonic activity have not occurred. Treatment included multiple anti-seizure medications without seizure freedom.

No epilepsy risk factor was identified, and the routine neurological examination was normal. Neuropsychological testing identified impairments in attention and perceptual reasoning.

Interictal EEG depicted left-sided slowing and generalized epileptiform spikes with a consistently left-sided asymmetry at the discharge onset. Focal epileptiform discharges with multiple locations across the central and left lateral regions occurred less often. Video-EEG monitoring recorded the habitual seizures with right facial droop. Ictal EEG's seizure onset for these seizures was generalized. MRI identified blurring of the gray-white junction in the posterior left middle and inferior temporal gyri. PET identified a corresponding region of hypometabolism.

The history and evaluation indicate a left-sided epilepsy that has both neocortical and limbic features. The focal motor seizures without impaired awareness and postictal confusion suggests a left neocortical localization. The interictal EEG evidence of left-sided slowing, broadly distributed left-sided focal discharges, and the left-sided lead-in to the generalized discharges support the left-sided neocortical localization and suggest that the generalized ictal EEG finding is not indicating a generalized epilepsy. The habitual progression to oral-pharyngeal automatisms suggests a propagation into the limbic system instead of a neocortical spread with rapid development of a bilateral tonic-clonic seizure. The temporal neocortex imaging abnormalities provide a plausible explanation for these neocortical features with limbic propagation.

Based on the EEG and imaging, a left temporal lobe resection was considered. An intracarotid amobarbital test identified right-hemispheric dominance for language, which is consistent with the left-handedness and apparent epilepsy localization. A left posterior temporal lobe resection was performed at age 9 years. Histopathological examination identified severely disorganized cortical architecture with multifocal loss of the laminar pattern. Cortical and subcortical neurons had varying degrees of cytomegaly and dysmorphism. Balloon cells were present in the subcortical white matter. No seizures have occurred for the 6 years since surgery, and verbal function has not been impacted.

J. M. Stern, N. Salamon, *Imaging of Epilepsy*, https://doi.org/10.1007/978-3-030-86672-3_9

Imaging

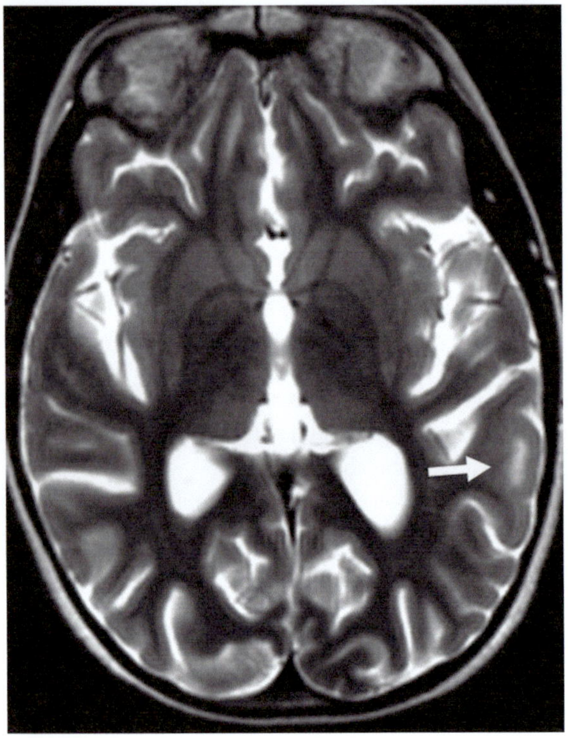

Fig. 9.1 MRI axial T2 sequence at a superior temporal gyrus level. Abnormal, increased signal (arrow) is present in the subcortical white matter of the most posterior portion of left superior temporal gyrus. This abnormality overlaps with Wernicke's area. The gray-white differentiation is normal in the tissue surrounding the abnormality

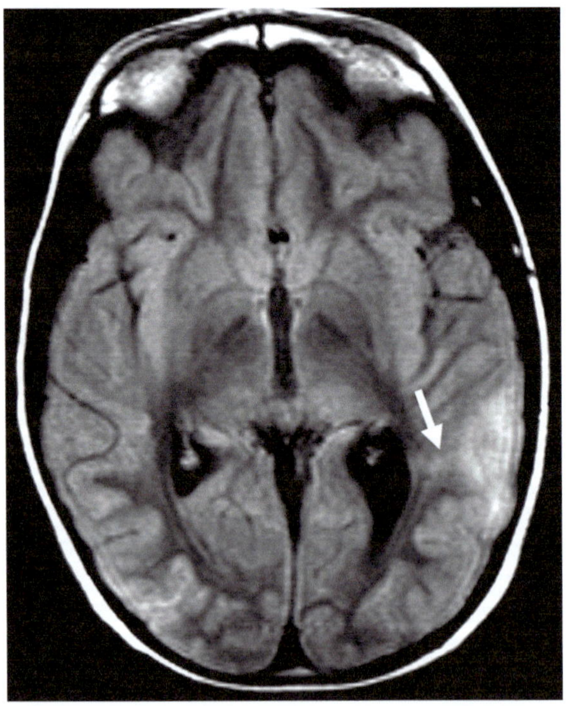

Fig. 9.2 MRI axial FLAIR sequence at the superior temporal gyrus level in Fig. 9.1. Abnormally increased signal is present in the cortex and subcortical white matter of the posterior left superior temporal gyrus. The abnormality, which is a transmantle sign, extends (arrow) as a tail to the ventricular margin. The gray-white differentiation is blurred, which is an additional abnormality and differs from the T2 sequence in Fig. 9.1

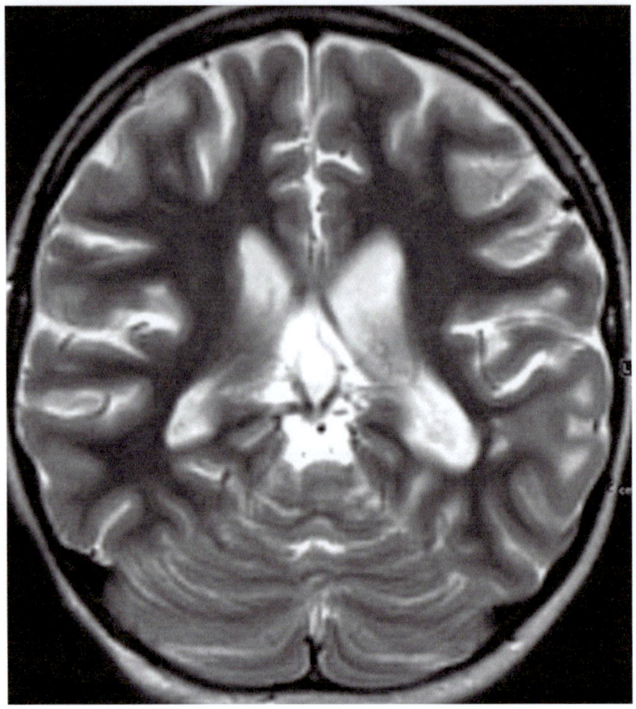

Fig. 9.3 MRI coronal T2 sequence at a ventricular atrium level. Abnormally increased signal is evident in two gyri of the left temporal lobe. The superior temporal sulcus between these two gyri is abnormally shallow and the transmantle sign is evident between the sulcus and the ventricle

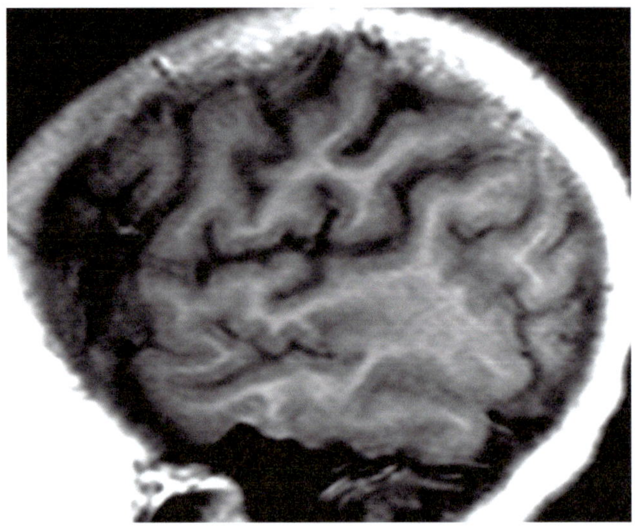

Fig. 9.4 MRI sagittal T1 sequence at a left temporal lobe level. The division into the superior and middle temporal gyri is abnormal with confluence of the two gyri over the posterior temporal lobe. This depiction of abnormal sulcation with hypointense signal corresponds to the transmantle sign, as is more clearly evident in Fig. 9.3

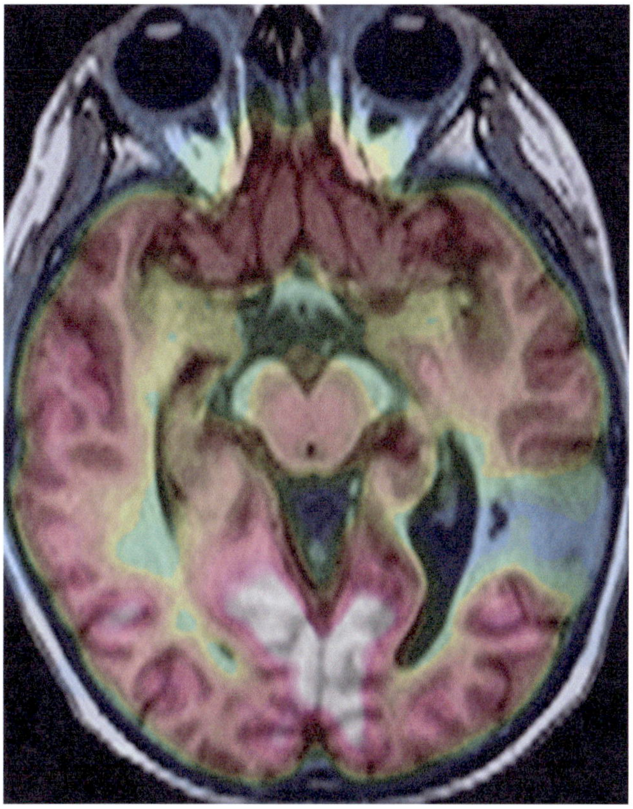

Fig. 9.5 PET-MRI co-registration with color-scale FDG tracer in an axial plane at hippocampus level. A region of clearly demarcated hypometabolism is present in the left posterior temporal lobe. The metabolic abnormality is uniform through the region and corresponds to the MRI abnormality. Neighboring cortex is normal

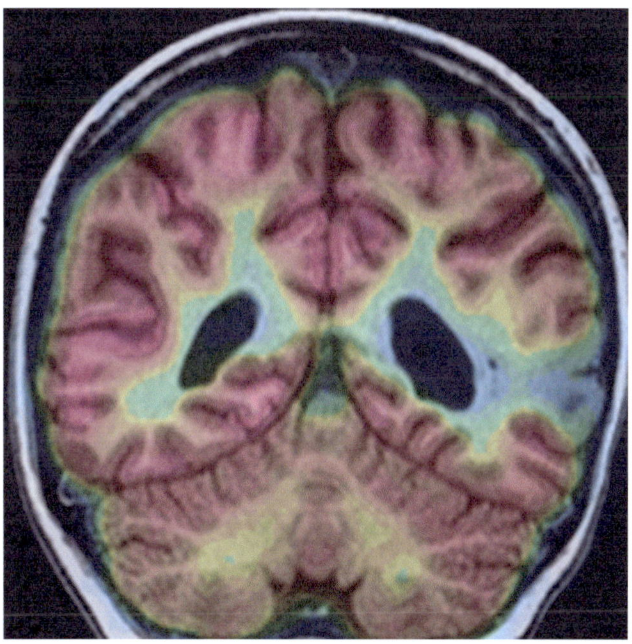

Fig. 9.6 PET-MRI co-registration with color-scale FDG tracer in a coronal plane at a ventricular atrium level. The region of clearly demarcated hypometabolism includes the left superior and middle temporal gyri evident in Fig. 9.3

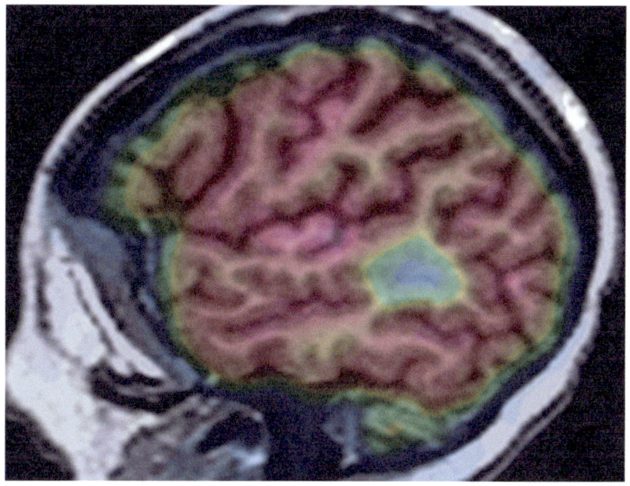

Fig. 9.7 PET-MRI co-registration with color-scale FDG tracer in a sagittal plane at a left temporal lobe level. An oval region of markedly hypometabolism is evident across the posterior temporal lobe and corresponds to region identified in Fig. 9.4. Adjacent cortex is normal

Focal Cortical Dysplasia, Type IIIb

10

Clinical History

The first recognized seizure occurred at age 34 years as an episode of self-identified disorientation with amnesia for the preceding minutes.

The habitual seizures manifested as a blank facial expression, no verbal production, and occasionally oral automatisms. An aura of anxiety preceded about half of the seizures. The seizure duration was 2–3 minutes followed by 10 minutes of postictal confusion. Generalized seizures have not occurred. Treatment has included multiple anti-seizure medications with seizure frequencies that averaged two monthly and varied from three weekly to one annually.

The known epilepsy risk factor was a fall at age 15 years that produced head injury and a 30-minute loss of consciousness. Routine neurological examination was normal. Neuropsychological testing identified left lateral temporal and left frontal lobe dysfunction. Memory deficits were not present.

Interictal EEG depicted mild abnormal slowing across the left temporal region with epileptiform sharp waves over the left anterior temporal region. Video-EEG monitoring recorded focal seizures manifested as staring with unresponsiveness lasting 2 minutes. Ictal EEG's seizure onset was initially broadly across the left temporal region and evolved to become focal over the left anterior temporal region.

MRI identified an irregular cystic lesion in the left posterior inferior temporal lobe with surrounding disorganized and gliotic gray matter. The hippocampi were normal. PET identified focal hypometabolism co-localizing to the MRI abnormality.

The history and EEG evaluation indicate left temporal lobe epilepsy. The aura and seizure behavior suggest a limbic localization with the occurrence of anxiety followed by unresponsiveness without progression to bilateral tonic-clonic movements. However, the imaging and neuropsychological testing suggest left lateral temporal lobe epilepsy with sparing of the hippocampus. As such, the limbic seizure features were considered due to propagation from a neocortical temporal lobe epileptogenic lesion.

A left inferior temporal gyrus resection was performed at age 44 years with a resection that was tailored to the imaging abnormalities and intraoperative language mapping. Histopathological examination identified neuronal disorganization with dysplastic features indicating cortical dysplasia and focal atypical, non-proliferative cells indicating ganglioglioma. Seizures after epilepsy surgery has been limited to when anti-seizure medication was not taken with an overall frequency of once every 9 months.

J. M. Stern, N. Salamon, *Imaging of Epilepsy*, https://doi.org/10.1007/978-3-030-86672-3_10

Imaging

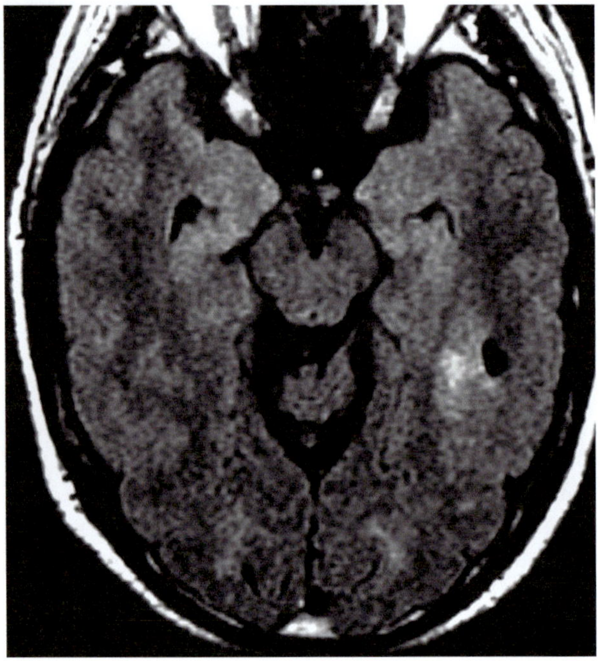

Fig. 10.1 MRI axial FLAIR sequence at a hippocampal head level. The left middle temporal gyrus includes a cystic abnormality with medially adjacent hyperintense signal that extends into the fusiform gyrus. The surrounding haziness with blurring of gray-white differentiation suggests focal cortical dysplasia. The left temporal pole is abnormal due to hyperintensity that is evident when compared to the right temporal pole. The hippocampi are normal bilaterally

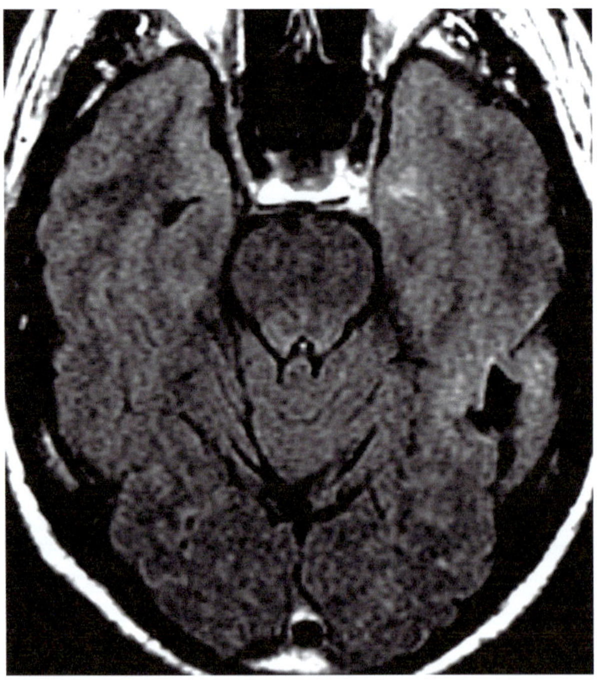

Fig. 10.2 MRI axial FLAIR sequence inferior to the level in Fig. 10.1 at a parahippocampal gyrus level. At this level, the cystic abnormality in the left inferior temporal gyrus has an irregular shape and has abnormal, hyperintense signal surrounding it both medially and laterally. Extension into the fusiform gyrus is evident, similar to Fig. 10.1. Abnormal hyperintensity of the left temporal pole is clearer than in Fig. 10.1

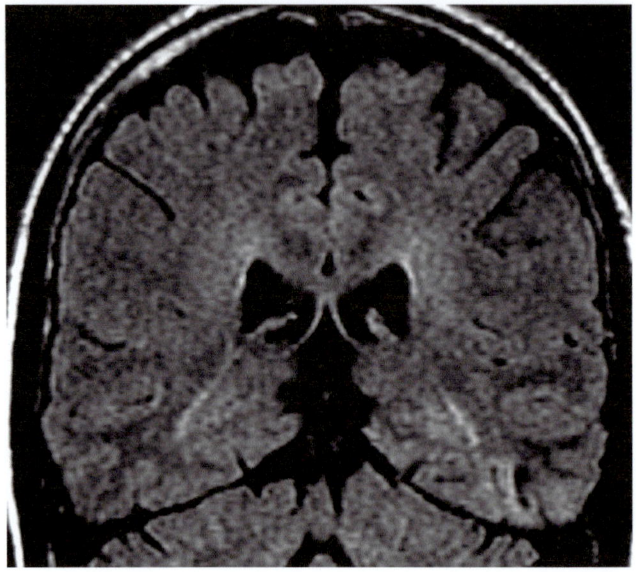

Fig. 10.3 MRI coronal FLAIR sequence at a pulvinar level. The left, inferior temporal gyrus and adjacent fusiform gyrus have abnormal hyperintensity and an indistinct gray-white differentiation. The cystic abnormality in the inferior temporal gyrus is linear and smaller in this level

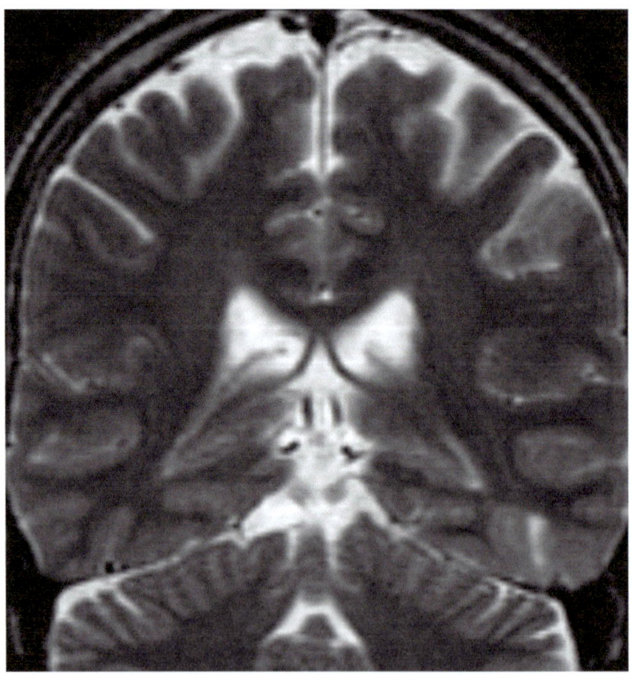

Fig. 10.4 MRI coronal T2 at the pulvinar level in Fig. 10.3. The left inferior temporal gyrus cystic abnormality appears as a linear hyperintensity with surrounding abnormally hyperintense gray matter that extends to the lateral aspect of fusiform gyrus. The left middle temporal gyrus is normal

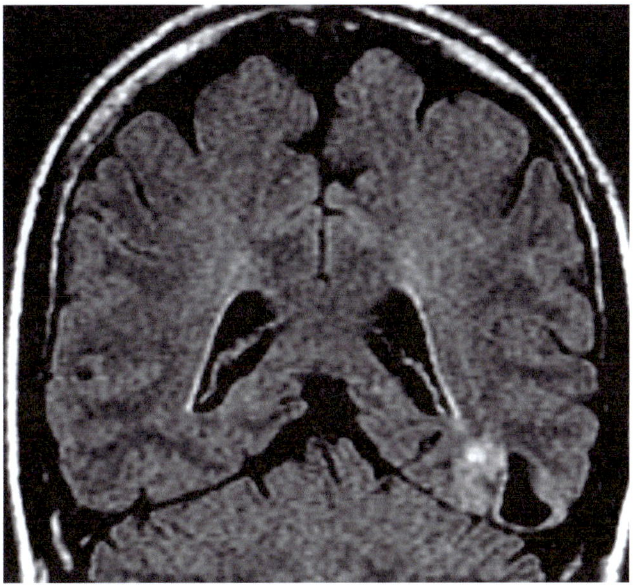

Fig. 10.5 MRI coronal FLAIR sequence at a splenium of the corpus callosum level. The cystic abnormality in this level reaches the surface of the left inferior temporal gyrus, and it has more focal hyperintense abnormality superior-medial to it. The gray-white differentiation within the left inferior temporal gyrus is blurred. The lateral temporal lobe is normal

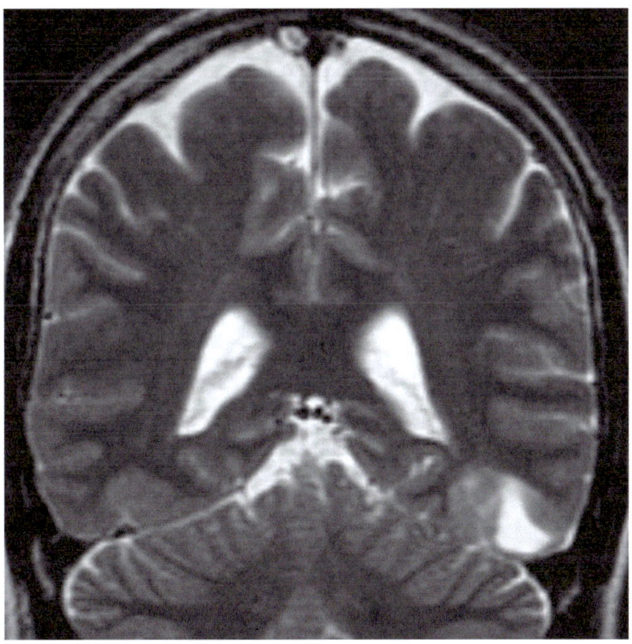

Fig. 10.6 MRI coronal T2 sequence at the splenium of the corpus callosum level in Fig. 10.5. The cystic abnormality is hyperintense with surrounding hyperintensity that is most prominent medially but also present laterally. The adjacent middle temporal gyrus is normal

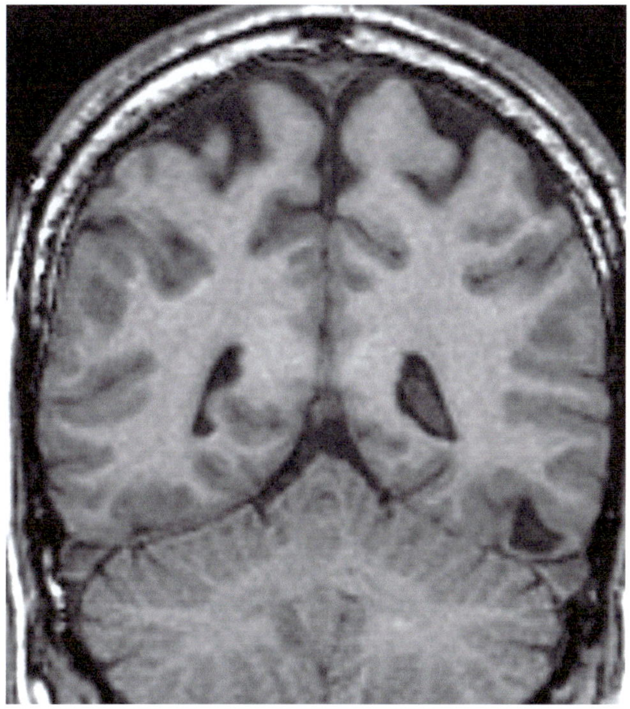

Fig. 10.7 MRI coronal T1 sequence at a ventricular atrium level. The left inferior temporal gyrus cystic abnormality is triangular in this level and is surrounded by gray matter with indistinct gray-white differentiation. This gives the appearance of thickened cortex

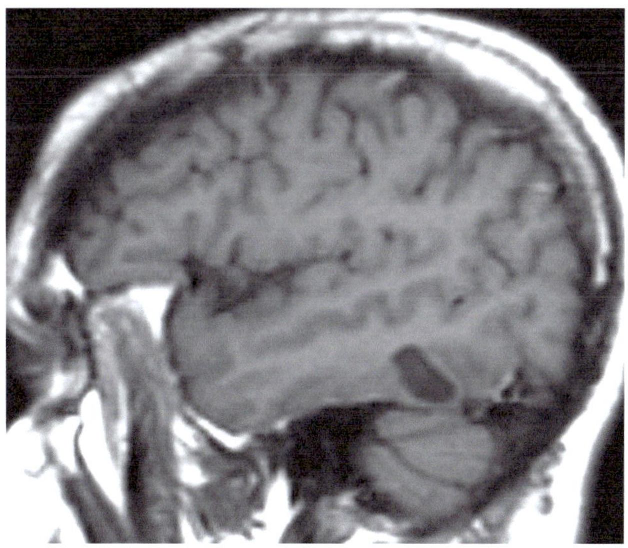

Fig. 10.8 MRI sagittal T1 sequence at a Sylvian fissure level. The left inferior temporal gyrus cystic abnormality has an oblong shape with surrounding blurring of the gray-white differentiation. The superior temporal sulcus is normal

Focal Cortical Dysplasia with the Transmantle Sign

11

Clinical History

The first recognized seizure occurred at age 27 years as a nocturnal episode of staring with unresponsiveness accompanied by bilateral stiffening and shaking. An evaluation with MRI and EEG at that time was normal, and epilepsy treatment was not begun. A second seizure occurred at age 29 years with the subsequent development of the habitual seizures in wakefulness. The habitual seizures manifested as a tingling across the back of the head followed by behavioral arrest, impaired awareness, and turning of the head or gaze to the left. The seizure duration has been about 10 seconds. Treatment included multiple anti-seizure medications with a seizure frequency of several seizures within a day on 1 day each week.

An epilepsy risk factor was not present. Neurological examination was normal.

Interictal EEG identified rare epileptiform sharp waves over the left mid-temporal region. Video-EEG monitoring recorded focal seizures manifested as confusion with oral and manual automatisms and non-versive turning to the left. Ictal EEG's seizure onset was evolving, rhythmic slowing over the left temporal region.

MRI identified a focal cortical dysplasia of the right superior frontal gyrus. PET was normal. MEG identified epileptiform dipoles within the right frontal and bilateral parietal lobes.

The ictal behavior supports a diagnosis of focal seizures, but it does not suggest a likely localization. The midline tingling is nonspecific and can occur with both limbic and neocortical seizures. Furthermore, the non-versive leftward deviation does not reliably lateralize the seizure onset. As such, the video-EEG recordings provided the seizure onset localization and thereby a left temporal lobe epilepsy diagnosis. However, the MRI and MEG abnormalities suggested the alternative epilepsy diagnosis of right frontal lobe epilepsy, as right frontal lobe epilepsy also may produce the patient's ictal behavior.

Because the diagnostic tests were not concordant, video-EEG monitoring with intracranial depth electrodes was performed. Electrodes were placed in bilateral frontal and temporal lobes, including the mesial temporal structures, lateral temporal lobe, and the cortical dysplasia identified by MRI. Seizures during the intracranial EEG monitoring were behaviorally similar to those during the scalp EEG monitoring and had seizure onsets localized to the right frontal neocortical electrodes that were closest to the cortical dysplasia. As such, the scalp EEG seizure onsets were found to be misleading.

A resection of the right frontal cortical dysplasia was performed. Electrocorticography during the epilepsy surgery identified epileptiform discharges and abnormal slowing of the exposed right frontal lobe. Histopathological examination identified dysmorphic neurons and balloon cells, indicating a type IIb focal cortical dysplasia. The postoperative seizure control is not known at this time.

J. M. Stern, N. Salamon, *Imaging of Epilepsy*, https://doi.org/10.1007/978-3-030-86672-3_11

Imaging

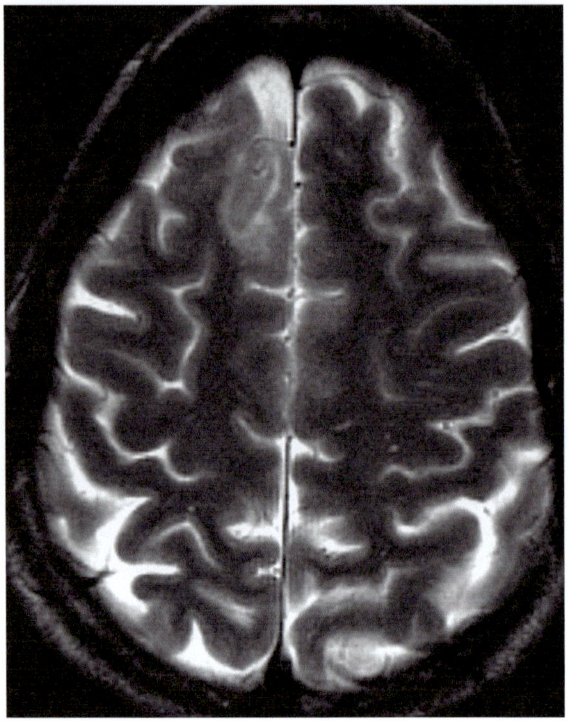

Fig. 11.1 MRI axial T2 sequence at a high convexity level. Abnormal hyperintensity is present in the subcortical white matter of the right superior frontal gyrus. The anterior right superior frontal gyrus has a region of focal atrophy

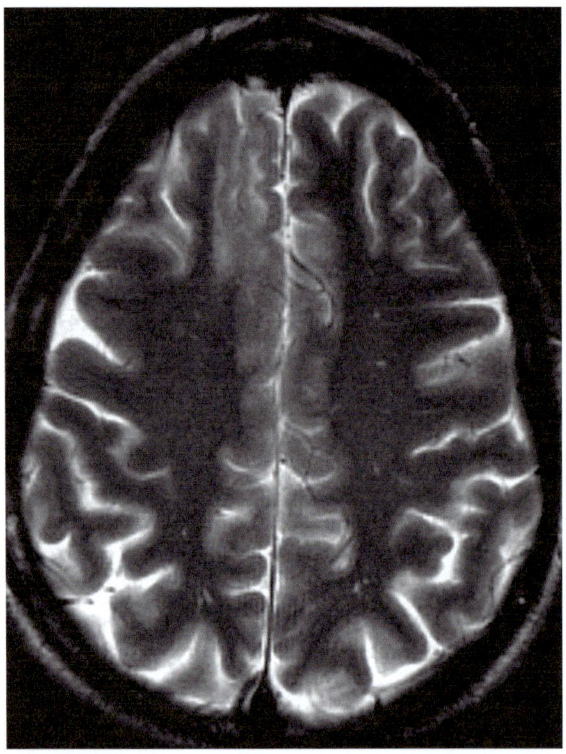

Fig. 11.2 MRI axial T2 sequence at a centrum semi-ovale level. The abnormal hyperintensity in the right superior frontal gyrus is more apparent than in Fig. 11.1. The adjacent anterior cingulate gyrus and middle frontal gyrus are normal with clear gray-white differentiation

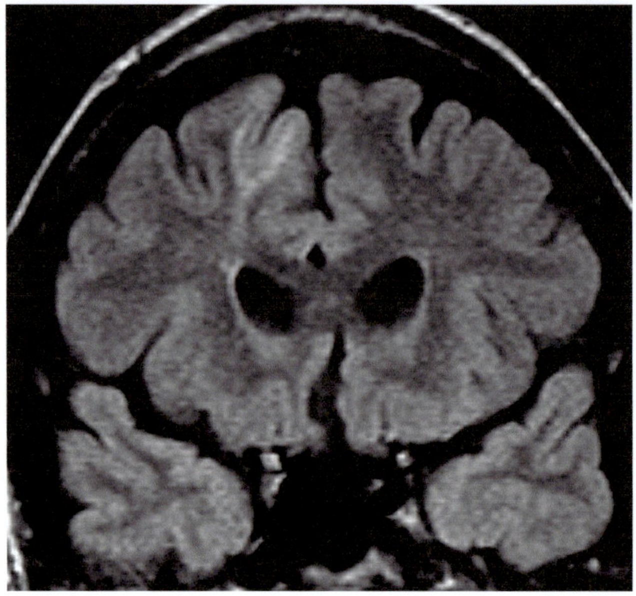

Fig. 11.3 MRI coronal FLAIR sequence at a temporal pole level. Abnormal hyperintensity is present in the medial right superior frontal gyrus with merging of the subcortical hyperintensity into one line directed toward the lateral ventricle, which is the transmantle sign. The linear signal along the ventricular margin is normal and bilaterally symmetric. The lateral superior frontal gyrus gray-white differentiation is normal

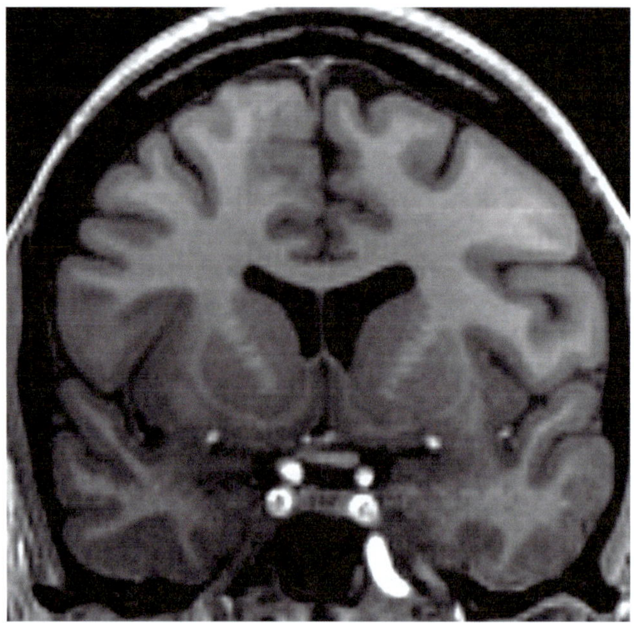

Fig. 11.4 MRI coronal T1 sequence at a temporal pole level slightly posterior to Fig. 11.3. The gray-white differentiation within the medial right superior frontal gyrus is indistinct; however, no abnormality is present in the deep white matter. Unlike the FLAIR sequence in Fig. 11.3, the transmantle sign is not visible

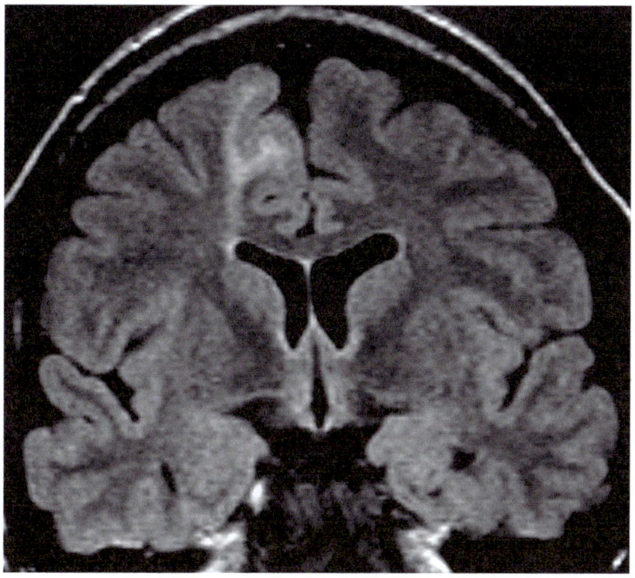

Fig. 11.5 MRI coronal FLAIR sequence at an amygdala level. Abnormal hyperintensity extends from the medial right superior frontal gyrus to the lateral ventricle as a transmantle sign. The gray-white differentiation in the lateral right superior frontal gyrus is not as clear as in Fig. 11.3 because of volume averaging

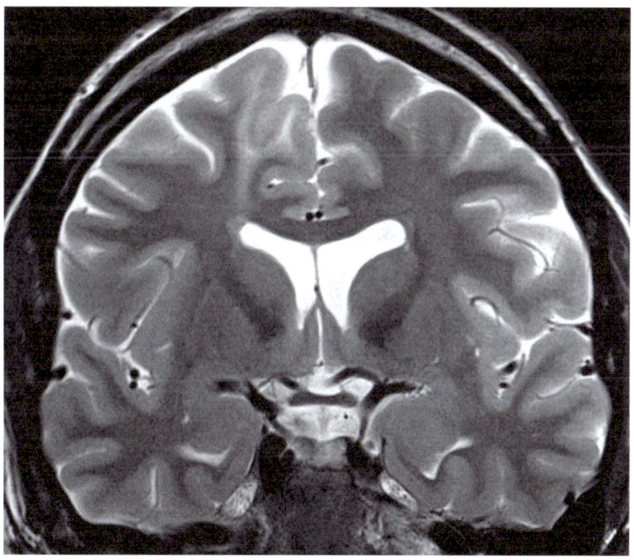

Fig. 11.6 MRI coronal T2 sequence at the amygdala level in Fig. 11.5. Hyperintensity of medial half of the right superior frontal gyrus tapers as it extends through the white matter to the surface of the lateral ventricle. The signal along the edge of the ventricular horn is normal and without evidence of periventricular gray matter heterotopia. The right cingulate gyrus is normal

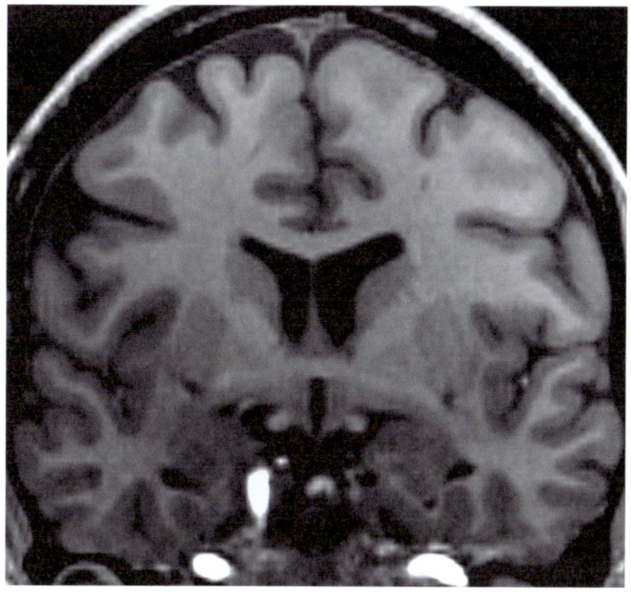

Fig. 11.7 MRI coronal T1 sequence at an amygdala level similar to Figs. 11.5 and 11.6. The transmantle sign is not visible, and the gray-white differentiation is clear across the right superior frontal gyrus. The subcortical white matter in the right superior frontal gyrus also has normal signal

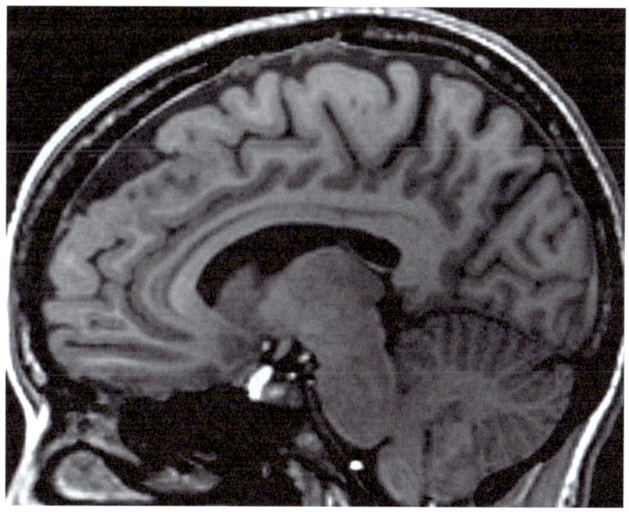

Fig. 11.8 MRI sagittal T1 sequence at corpus callosum level slightly right of the midline. The anterior superior frontal gyrus has marked atrophy with mixed signal in the gray matter

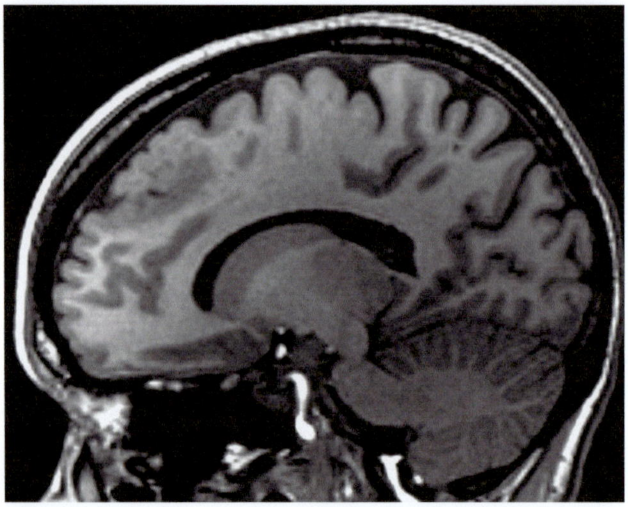

Fig. 11.9 MRI sagittal T1 sequence at a corpus callosum level that is slightly lateral to Fig. 11.8. The gray-white differentiation is indistinct within the superior frontal gyrus. The subcortical white matter of the superior frontal gyrus is obscured, but a transmantle sign is not visible

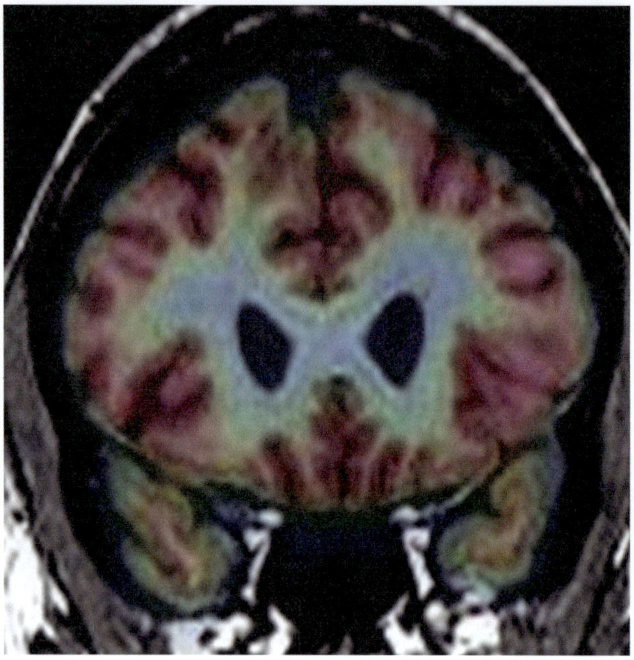

Fig. 11.10 PET-MRI co-registration with color-scale FDG tracer in a coronal plane at a temporal pole level. The medial half of right superior frontal gyrus has a minor, abnormal decrease in cortical ribbon metabolism. The metabolic signal in the right superior frontal gyrus' subcortical region is normal and has the appearance of volume averaging

12 Focal Cortical Dysplasia with Bottom of the Sulcus Abnormality

Clinical History

The first recognized seizure was an episode of loss of awareness at age 10 years. Similar episodes recurred within a short time, and epilepsy was diagnosed soon after the first seizure.

The habitual seizures were manifested as an appearance of inattention with bilateral raising of the arms. If standing, a fall sometimes occurred late in the seizure. An aura of a sense of being "spaced out" accompanied by a tingling across the left leg commonly preceded the loss of awareness. The seizure duration was 10–30 seconds with postictal confusion that lasted a few seconds. Treatment included multiple anti-seizure medications with a seizure frequency of about two to three seizures daily.

An epilepsy risk factor was not identified.

Neurological examination was normal.

Interictal EEG depicted epileptiform discharges over the right central-parietal region. Video-EEG monitoring recorded focal seizures manifested as staring with arm raising. Ictal EEG's seizure onset was slowing over the right central region with evolution to focal slowing over the right mid-temporal region.

MRI was normal with initial imaging, but T2 sequences on a later MRI identified a subtle thickening of the right supramarginal gyrus. MRI with a bilateral parietal surface coil confirmed an abnormal signal and irregular thickening of the right supramarginal gyrus with an uneven contour at the gray-white junction. PET identified subtle hypometabolism within the right supramarginal gyrus and no other abnormality. MEG identified a cluster of epileptiform dipoles across the right supramarginal gyrus.

The history and evaluation indicate right central-parietal neocortical epilepsy. The aura of unilateral, limb tingling suggests a primary somatosensory symptomatogenic zone, and a right central localization is further supported by the ictal EEG onset. Imaging supported the localization with identification of a right supramarginal gyrus structural and functional abnormality. Epilepsy surgery was performed with a right temporal-parietal junction resection at age 19 years. Histopathological examination identified non-laminar, hypercellularity with numerous, dysmorphic cells. No seizures have occurred over the 1 year since surgery.

J. M. Stern, N. Salamon, *Imaging of Epilepsy*, https://doi.org/10.1007/978-3-030-86672-3_12

Imaging

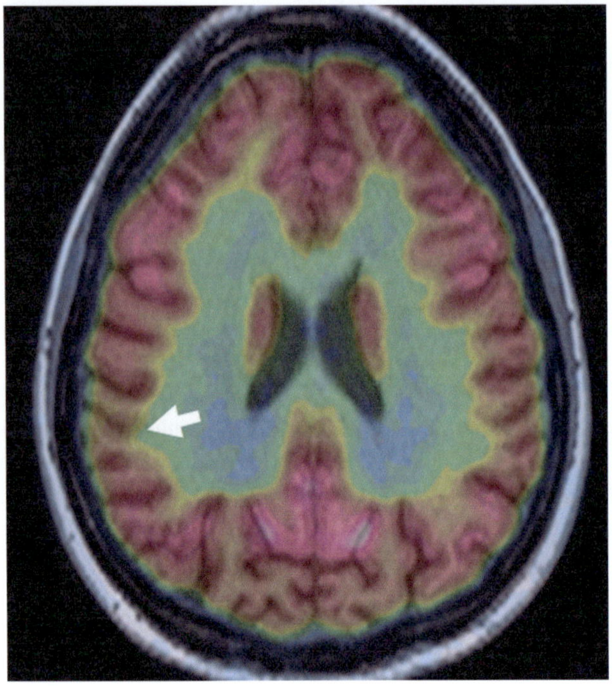

Fig. 12.1 PET-MRI co-registration with color-scale FDG tracer in an axial plane at a lateral ventricle level. Focal hypometabolism (arrow) of the supramarginal gyrus is evident. The cortical metabolism is otherwise normal and has normal contour and thickness. Metabolism from the caudate bodies is present lateral to the ventricles

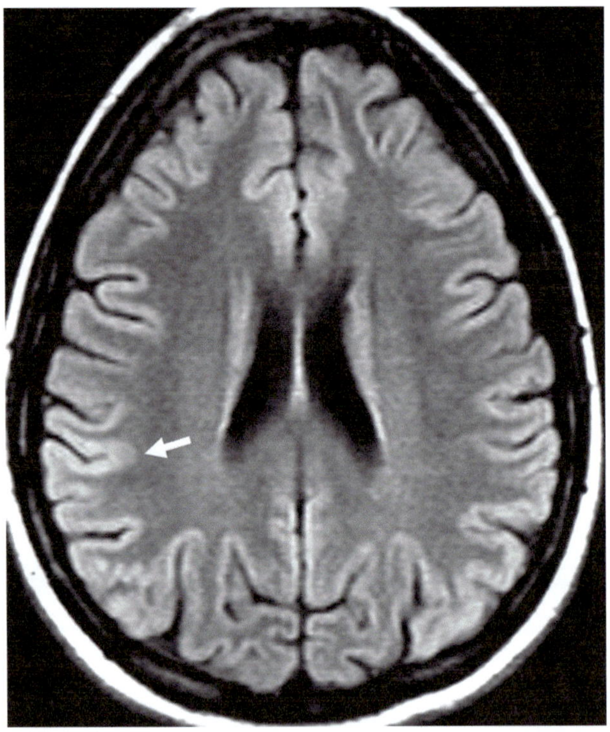

Fig. 12.2 MRI axial FLAIR sequence at a lateral ventricle level similar to Fig. 12.1. The sulcal depth (arrow) within the supramarginal gyrus is slightly thickened. The cortical ribbon has otherwise normal gray-white differentiation. No signal abnormality is present in the subcortical white matter

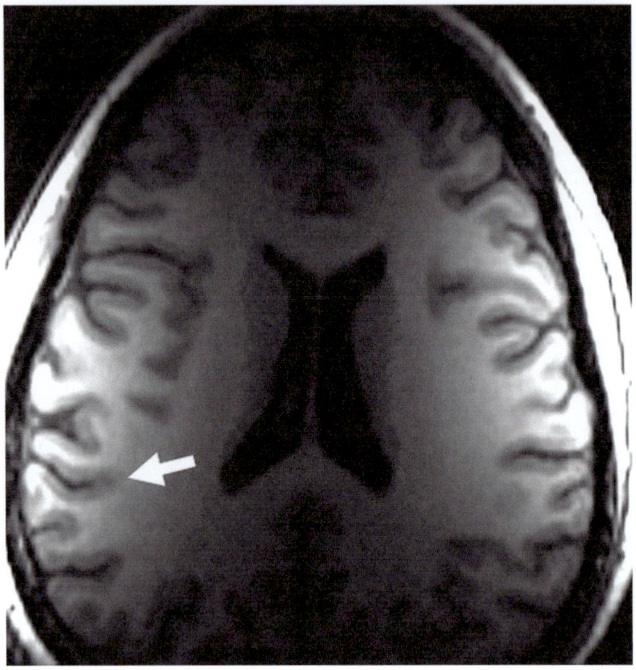

Fig. 12.3 MRI axial T1 sequence at a lateral ventricle level similar to Fig. 12.1. The sulcus of the supramarginal gyrus (arrow) is not abnormal in thickness or signal. The increased brightness of the bilateral posterior regions of the head is due to the use of a surface coil to increase the resolution in these regions

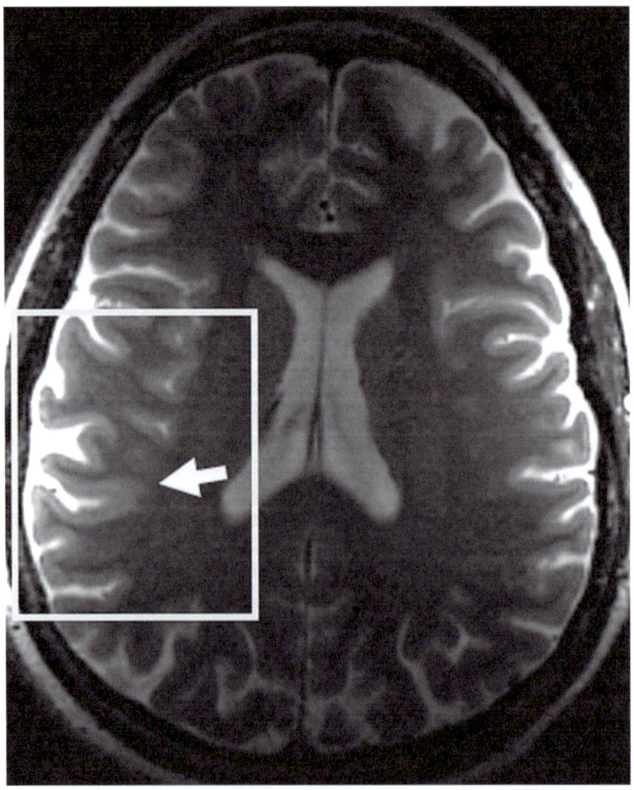

Fig. 12.4 MRI axial T2 sequence at a lateral ventricle level similar to Figs. 12.1 and 12.3. The sulcus of the supramarginal gyrus (arrow) is thickened but has normal gray-white differentiation. The increased brightness adjacent to the abnormality is due to a surface coil

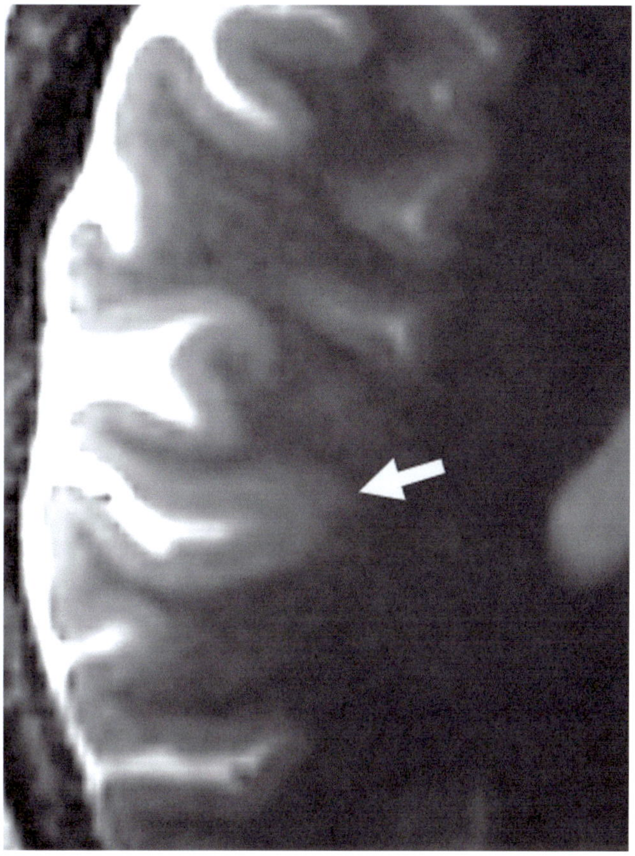

Fig. 12.5 MRI axial T2 sequence at the lateral ventricle level in Fig. 12.4 with an enlargement of the boxed region in Fig. 12.4. The contour of the depth of the sulcus appears irregular and thickened (arrow) when enlarged and examined more closely

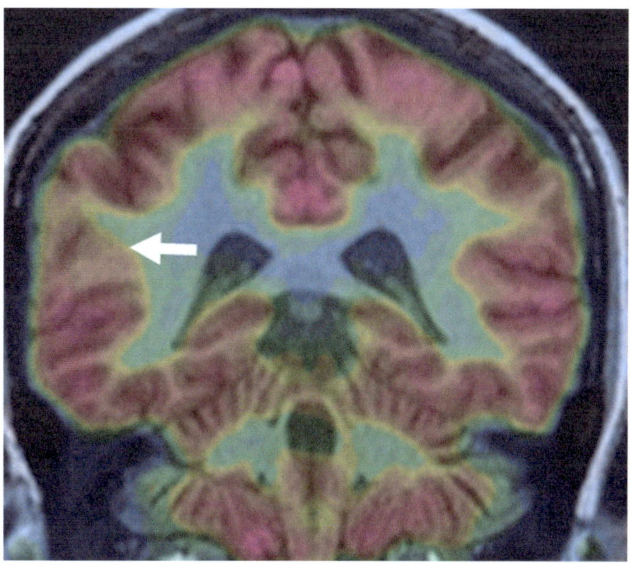

Fig. 12.6 PET-MRI co-registration with color-scale FDG tracer in a coronal plane at a splenium of the corpus callosum level. A focal region of hypometabolism (arrow) is present in the right supramarginal gyrus. The contour of the cortical ribbon is normal

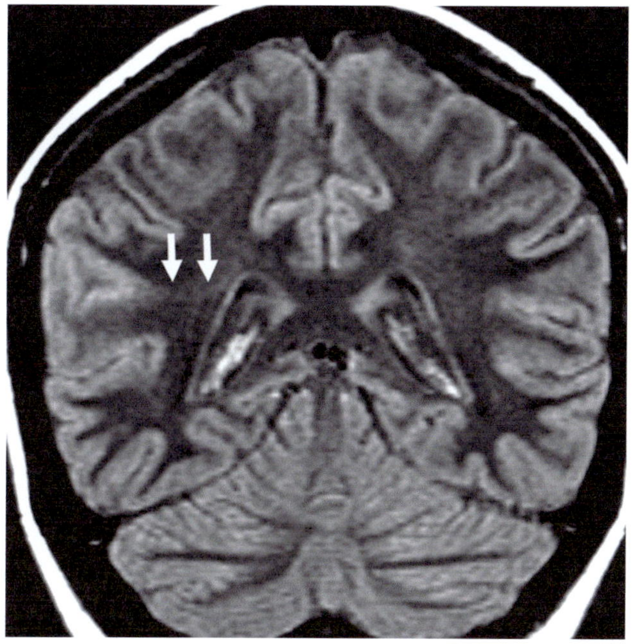

Fig. 12.7 MRI coronal FLAIR sequence at a splenium of the corpus callosum level with a cerebral region similar to Fig. 12.6. A subtle blurring of the gray-white junction is present at the depth of the right parietal sulcus with mildly increased signal (arrows) from the cortical ribbon to the ventricular margin

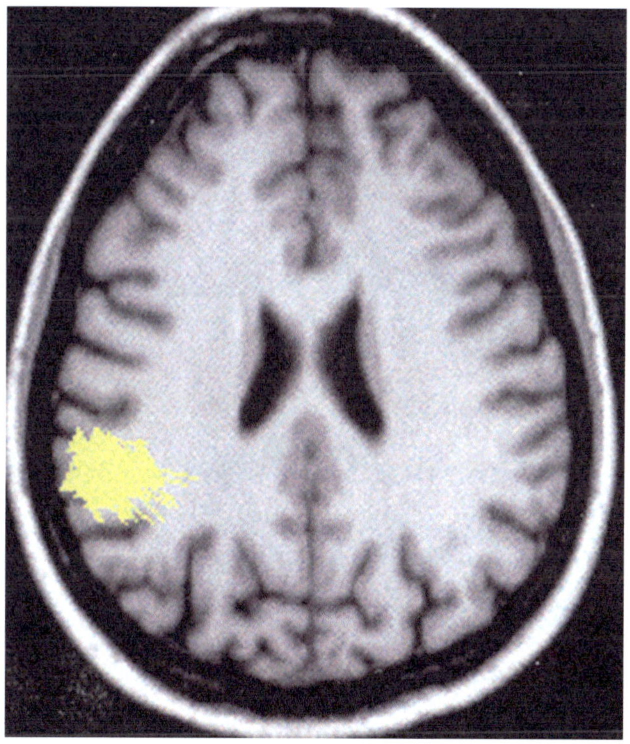

Fig. 12.8 MEG co-registered to MRI axial T1 sequence at a lateral ventricle level most similar to Fig. 12.1. Many epileptiform dipoles overlap with varying dipole orientations in the region of the supramarginal gyrus

Focal Cortical Dysplasia with Gray-White Junction Blurring

13

Clinical History

The first recognized seizure occurred at age 3 years with an episode of staring and rightward turning. Recurrent, stereotyped seizures developed soon after the first.

The habitual seizures manifested as a blank stare, turning of the head to the right, flexing or jerking of the right arm, and sometimes an accompanying extension of the left arm. There was no loss of postural tone. Awareness and interaction were intact throughout each seizure, but confusion was typically evident. The total seizure duration was 1–2 minutes, and fatigue was present postictally. Treatment included multiple anti-seizure medications with a seizure frequency of six to eight daily.

The epilepsy risk factor was developmental delay. Neurological examination was abnormal with impaired verbal expression. At age 6 years, language function was similar to a 3-year-old.

Interictal EEG depicted abnormal right-sided slowing and multifocal, independent epileptiform spikes over bilateral frontal and temporal regions. Video-EEG monitoring recorded focal seizures that were consistent with the habitual episodes. Ictal EEG's seizure onset was broadly across the right anterior quadrant with some spread to include the left anterior region also.

MRI identified blurring of the cortical-subcortical junction within the right superior frontal gyrus with an anterior-posterior dimension of 3.5 cm. PET was normal. MEG identified epileptiform dipoles within the right superior and middle frontal gyri.

The seizure behavior supports the likelihood of focal seizures with the stereotyped, asymmetric motor features. The maintenance of interaction during the prominent motor seizures suggests a neocortical epilepsy and most likely a frontal or parietal localization. The ictal EEG is compatible with the ictal behavior and suggests right frontal lobe epilepsy, which both the MEG and MRI also support.

Based on the evaluation, a right frontal lobe resection was performed at age 6 years. Electrocorticography during the operation identified diffuse slowing and frequent epileptiform spikes and paroxysmal fast activity across the frontal and posterior temporal regions. Histopathological examination identified mild disorganization of the cerebral cortex with scattered heterotopic neurons and a diagnosis of focal cortical dysplasia, type I. Postoperative seizure control cannot be determined because of an insufficient observation period.

J. M. Stern, N. Salamon, *Imaging of Epilepsy*, https://doi.org/10.1007/978-3-030-86672-3_13

Imaging

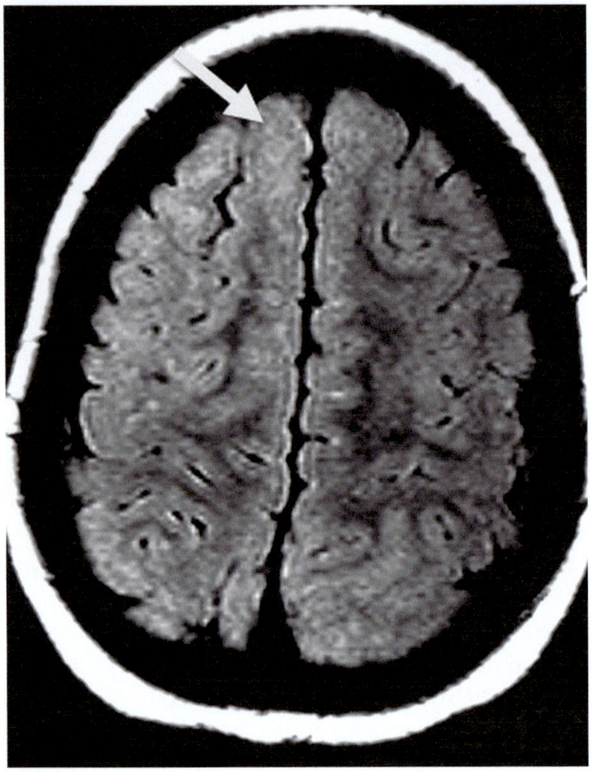

Fig. 13.1 MRI axial FLAIR sequence at a high convexity level. Abnormal gray-white differentiation is evident in the anterior, right superior frontal gyrus (arrow). The posterior half of the right superior frontal gyrus is less abnormally hyperintense, but it also has blurring, as is evident when compared to the left posterior superior frontal gyrus. The right middle frontal gyrus also has abnormal gray-white differentiation at this level when compared to the left middle frontal gyrus

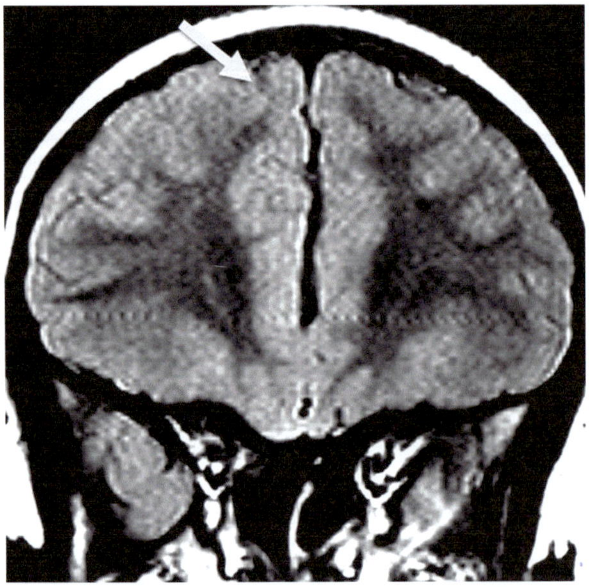

Fig. 13.2 MRI coronal FLAIR sequence at an orbitofrontal level. Abnormal gray-white differentiation is evident along the superior surface of the right superior and middle frontal gyri (arrow). Gray-white differentiation of the left superior and middle frontal gyri is normal. Gray-white differentiation also is normal within the cingulate gyri bilaterally

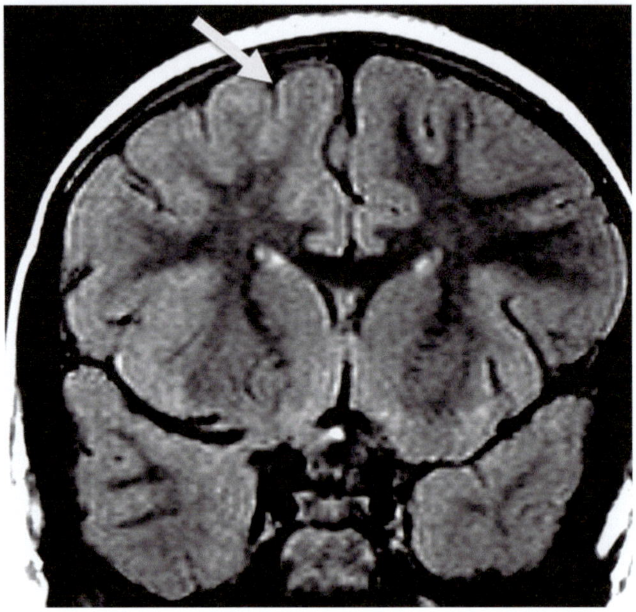

Fig. 13.3 MRI coronal FLAIR sequence at a temporal pole level, slightly posterior to Fig. 13.2. The gray-white differentiation is blurred in the right superior and middle frontal gyri (arrow). The cortical ribbon thickness is normal bilaterally but appears thickened on the right because of the FLAIR sequence

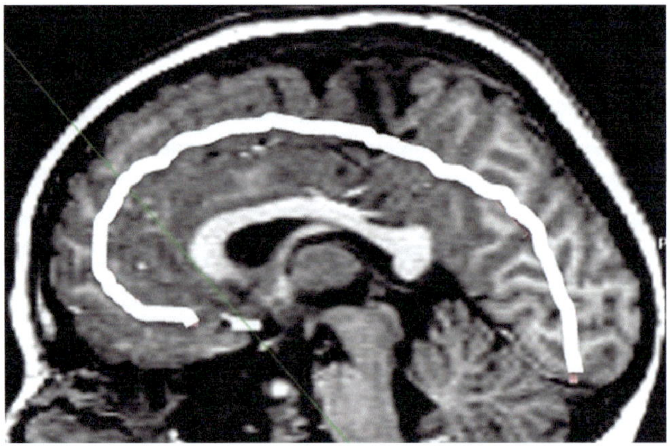

Fig. 13.4 MRI sagittal T1 sequence at the midline. The white line indicates the curved surface that is reformatted as a flat surface in Fig. 13.5

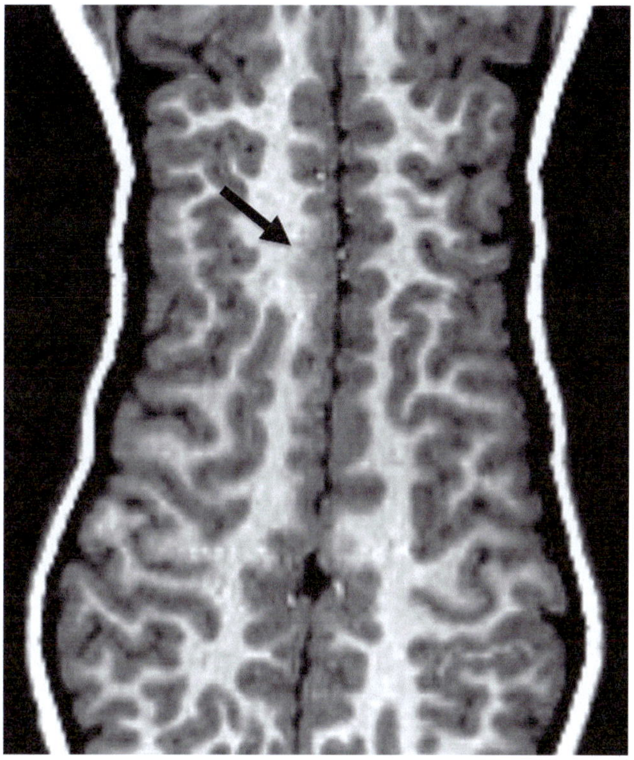

Fig. 13.5 MRI T1 sequence with reformatted frontal and parietal lobes as a flat image. Blurring of the gray-white differentiation (arrow) is evident, especially in comparison to the contralateral, homotopic gray-white junction. The cortex is not thickened at the region of blurring

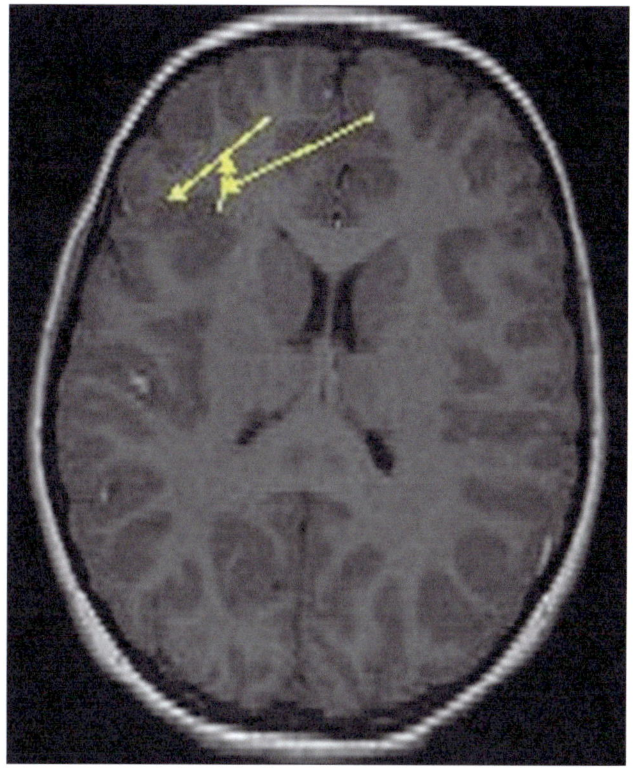

Fig. 13.7 MEG co-registered to MRI axial T1 sequence at a basal ganglia level. Multiple epileptiform dipoles localize to the right inferior frontal gyrus

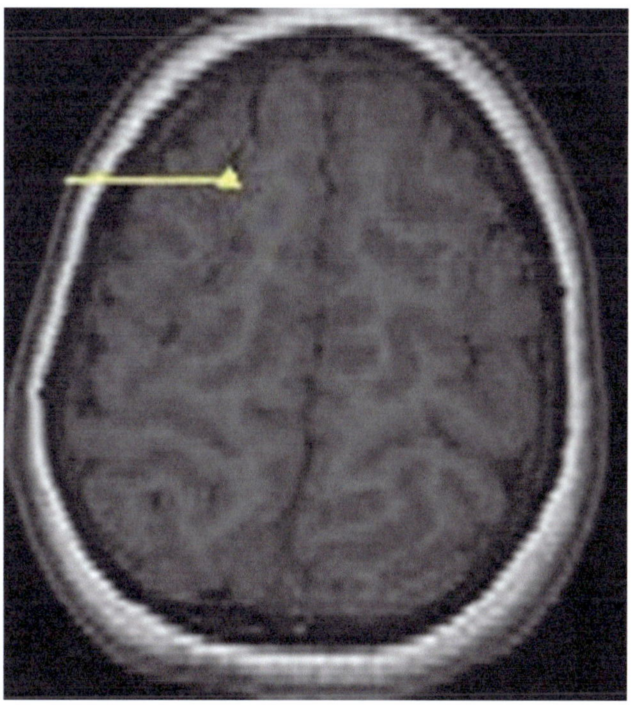

Fig. 13.6 MEG co-registered to MRI axial T1 sequence at a high convexity level. An epileptiform dipole localizes to the junction of the right superior and middle frontal gyri

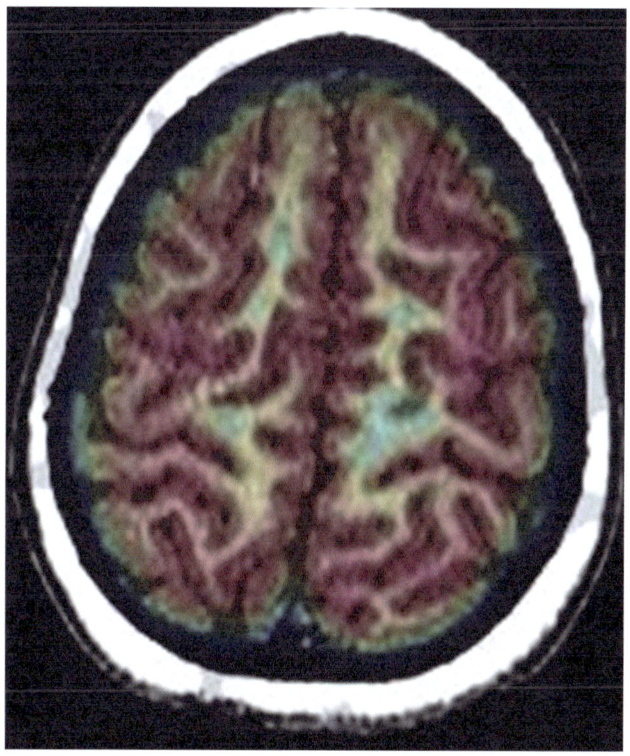

Fig. 13.8 PET-MRI co-registration with color-scale FDG tracer in an axial plane at the same high convexity level as Fig. 13.1. The right superior and middle frontal gyri are hypometabolic with the most evident hypometabolic abnormality evident in the anterior right superior frontal gyrus

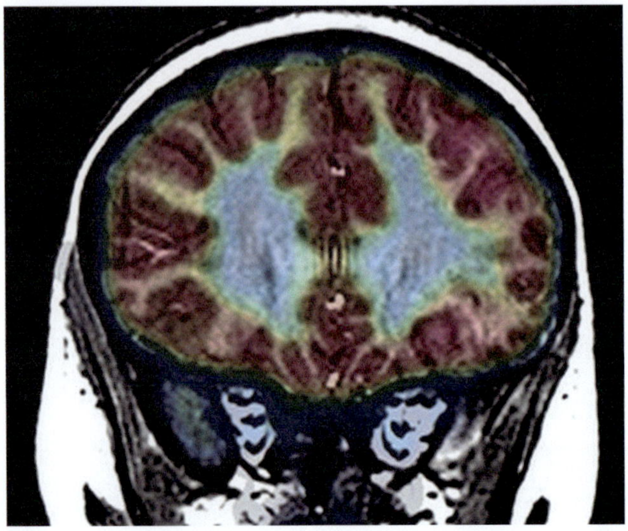

Fig. 13.9 PET-MRI co-registration with color-scale FDG tracer in a coronal plane at the same orbitofrontal level as Fig. 13.2. Hypometabolism is evident in the right superior frontal gyrus. The right middle frontal gyrus is normal although slightly asymmetric when compared to the left middle frontal gyrus

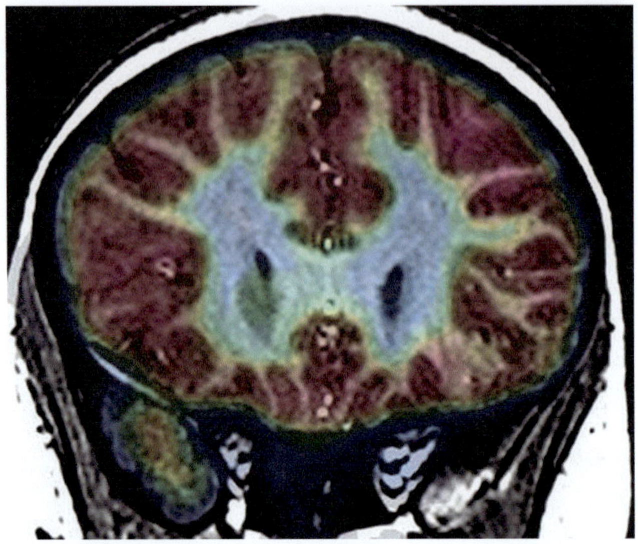

Fig. 13.10 PET-MRI co-registration with color-scale FDG tracer in a coronal plane at a genu of corpus callosum level between Figs. 13.2 and 13.3. Hypometabolism is present in the right superior frontal gyrus and is most evident at the crown of the gyrus. The right middle frontal gyrus is normal

Focal Cortical Dysplasia with Normal MRI and Abnormal PET

14

Clinical History

The first recognized seizure occurred at age 17 years as a lapse in awareness that was later recognized as the habitual ictal behavior.

The seizures manifested as staring and confusion with amnesia that followed an aura of midline facial tingling, vertigo, and nausea. Some seizures progressed to include spitting or vomiting. The aura also occurred in isolation with about half of the auras progressing to an impaired awareness. The seizure duration was typically several minutes. Seizures with bilateral tonic-clonic activity occurred

several times and only when anti-seizure medication was not taken. Treatment included multiple anti-seizure medications with a seizure frequency of 12 monthly.

The epilepsy risk factor was head trauma with loss of consciousness that occurred at age 8 years. Neurological examination was normal.

Interictal EEG depicted epileptiform sharp and slow-wave complexes over the right temporal-parietal junction. Video-EEG monitoring recorded focal seizures manifested as impaired awareness with an ictal EEG's seizure onset over the right mid- and posterior temporal lobe.

MRI was normal. PET identified right inferior parietal hypometabolism with clear boundaries. Functional MRI of language identified left-sided dominance with some activation in the right Broca's area.

The aura of vertiginous spinning suggests a neocortical sympatomatogenic zone in the region of the posterior temporal lobe or the temporal-parietal-occipital junction, and seizures with this localization often manifest as impaired awareness without convulsive activity. This localization was supported by the ictal EEG and the PET scan. Language function was dependent on contralateral regions, which was especially important to establish because of the ambidexterity.

Based on concordant diagnostic results, a right inferior parietal lobe resection was performed. Electrocorticography during the operation identified epileptiform discharges over the inferior parietal lobe and the resection eliminated the discharges. Histopathological examination identified neuronal crowding and gliosis but without sufficient abnormality to diagnose dysplasia. No seizures occurred for several months after surgery and then habitual seizures returned. However, the frequency was half of the prior frequency with six monthly.

One year after epilepsy surgery, additional diagnostic testing was performed.

Video-EEG monitoring at that time recorded focal seizures with impaired awareness that were behaviorally similar to the seizures recorded during the first evaluation, and the ictal EEG's seizure onset for these seizures was similarly over the right posterior quadrant. However, a breach effect was present, which can produce a misleading localization. MRI depicted the prior resection, and PET identified.

hypometabolism in the region of the resection. Because the PET abnormality was altered by the resection, determination of retained dysplasia through a margin of hypometabolism was not possible. Overall, the postoperative evaluation did not identify a cause for the return of the seizures, but it also did not identify an alternative localization for the epileptogenic zone.

Based on the second evaluation, an extension of the right inferior parietal lobe resection was performed. Histopathological examination of the tissue from the additional resection identified crowding without dyslamination or dysmorphic neurons and was considered to be diagnostic of focal cortical dysplasia. Seizure freedom has been present for the 1 year since the second epilepsy surgery.

J. M. Stern, N. Salamon, *Imaging of Epilepsy*, https://doi.org/10.1007/978-3-030-86672-3_14

Imaging

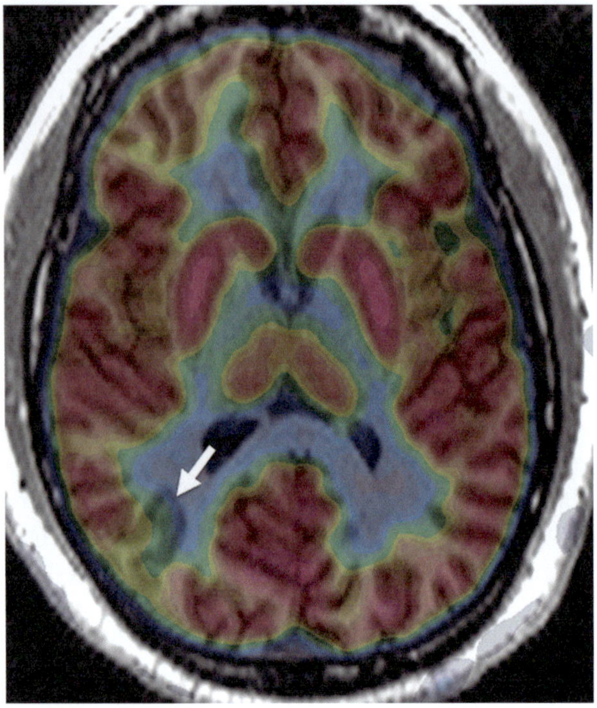

Fig. 14.1 PET-MRI co-registration with color-scale FDG tracer in an axial plane at a basal ganglia level. Focal hypometabolism is present within the cortex of the right, inferior parietal lobe. The hypometabolism extends into the sulcus (arrow) that is deep to the cortical abnormality

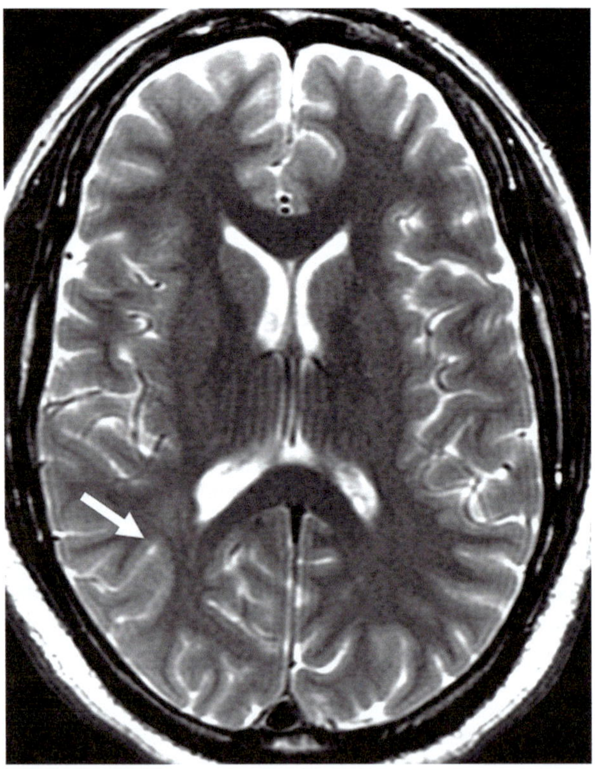

Fig. 14.2 MRI axial T2 sequence at the same basal ganglia as Fig. 14.1. The area of hypometabolism (arrow) appears as normal gray-white differentiation and subcortical white matter. The gyral and sulcal anatomy also are normal. The posterior horn of the right lateral ventricle, which is deep to the hypometabolism, is enlarged

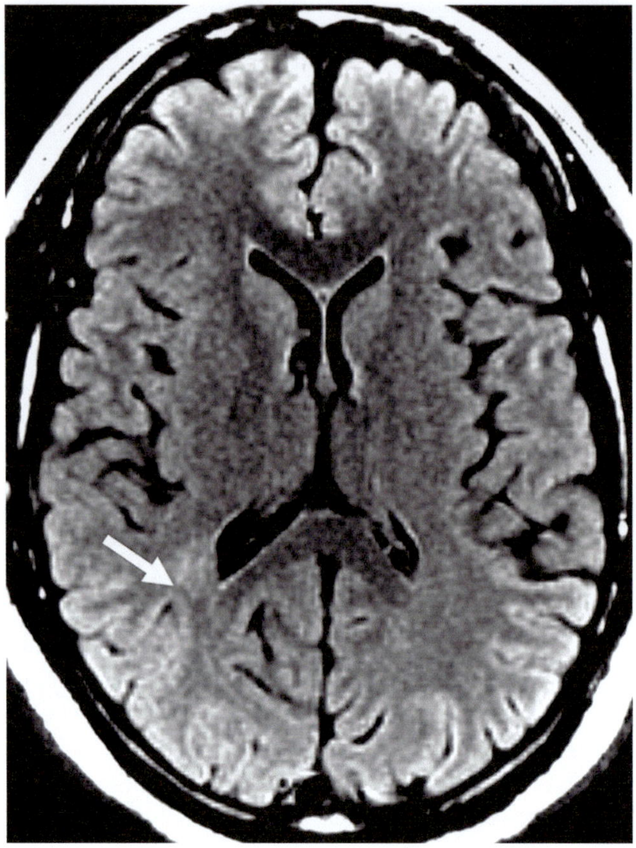

Fig. 14.3 MRI axial FLAIR sequence at the same basal ganglia level as Figs. 14.1 and 14.2. The area of hypometabolism (arrow) does not correspond to abnormal signal, but gyral and sulcal anatomy are less clear with this imaging sequence. The posterior horn of the lateral ventricle is enlarged, and the white matter adjacent to the ventricle has slightly increased signal, which is a nonspecific finding

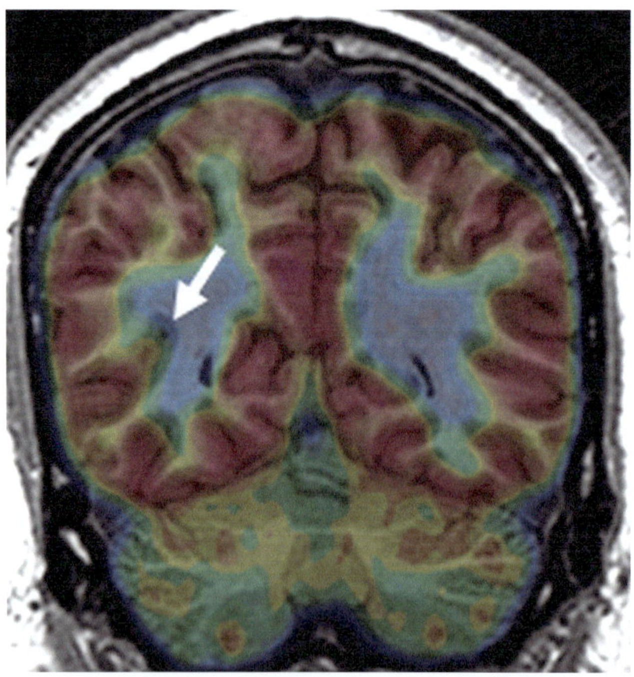

Fig. 14.4 PET-MRI co-registration with color-scale FDG tracer in a coronal plane at an occipital horn level. Focal hypometabolism (arrow) is evident at the sulcal depth within the right inferior parietal lobe

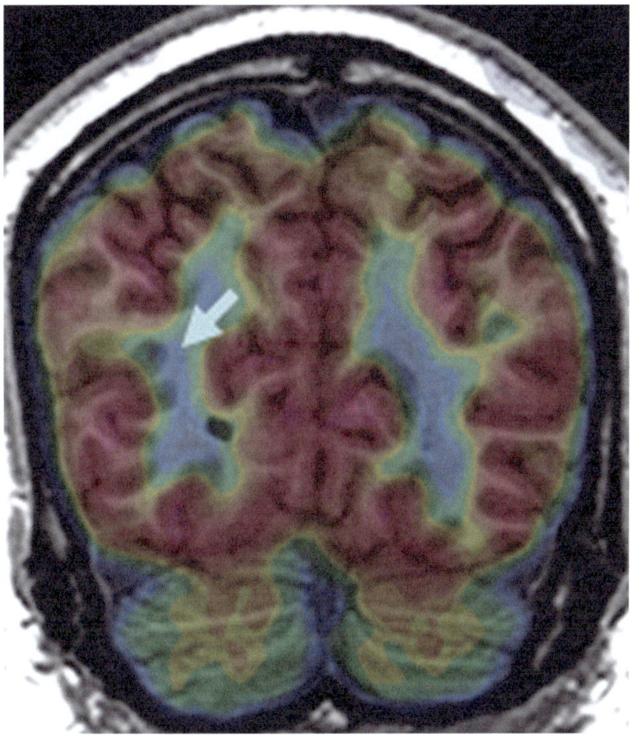

Fig. 14.5 PET-MRI co-registration with color-scale FDG tracer in a coronal plane at a posterior cerebellum level. Two regions of hypometabolism (arrow at superior region) correspond to sulci within the right inferior parietal lobe at the parietal-occipital junction. The inferior hypometabolism is within the superior occipital lobe

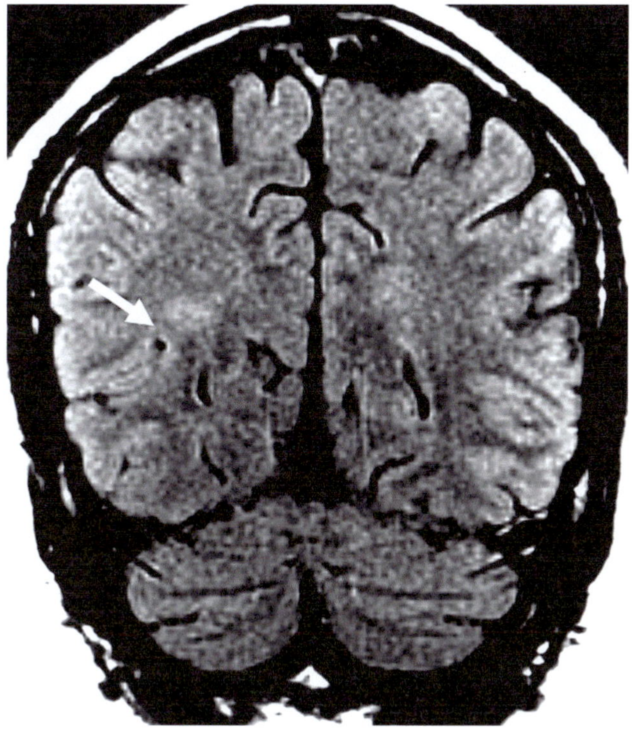

Fig. 14.7 MRI coronal FLAIR sequence at a posterior cerebellum level similar to Fig. 14.5. No abnormal signal or cortical contour is present. A region of hyperintensity (immediately medial to arrow) corresponds to the nonspecific white matter hyperintensity in Fig. 14.3

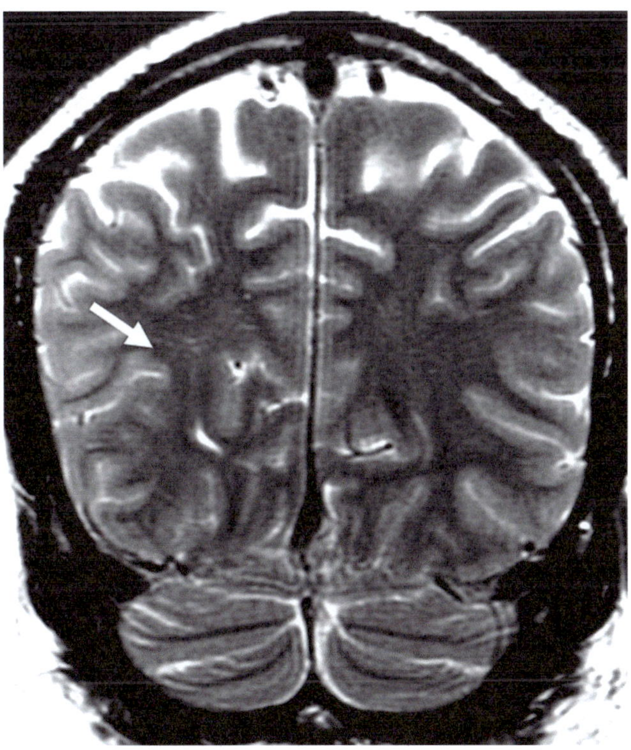

Fig. 14.6 MRI coronal T2 sequence at a posterior cerebellum level similar to Fig. 14.5. The sulcus at the parietal-occipital junction has normal gray-white differentiation (arrow), and the subcortical white matter has normal signal

Focal Cortical Dysplasia of the Temporal Pole

15

Clinical History

The first recognized seizure occurred at age 8 years with a lapse in awareness accompanied by bilateral purposeless movements.

The habitual seizures manifested as an aura of an auditory hallucination of a single word repeated with an echo quality that behaviorally progressed to gasping and oral automatisms and then to hypermotor activity of bilateral arms and legs. Sometimes, sudden jumping to a standing position was a component of the ictal behavior. Seizure duration was approximately 1 minute followed by postictal sleepiness for approximately 1 hour. Treatment included multiple anti-seizure medications with a seizure frequency of three monthly.

No epilepsy risk factor was identified. Neurological examination was normal.

Neuropsychological testing identified impairments in language, verbal learning, and verbal memory.

Interictal EEG depicted rare left anterior temporal lobe epileptiform discharges. Video-EEG monitoring recorded focal seizures during wakefulness manifested as a sense of brief cognitive change. During sleep, seizures manifested as sudden full body movements with kicking. Ictal EEG's seizure onset was over the left temporal region.

MRI identified a focal cortical dysplasia of the left temporal pole. The hippocampi were normal. Functional MRI mapping of language identified left hemispheric dominance. PET identified hypometabolism of the anterior left temporal lobe.

The history and evaluation indicate left anterior temporal lobe epilepsy. The focal seizures with impaired awareness and automatisms are typical for limbic epilepsy, and the ictal EEG and verbal memory impairment support this possibility, but hypermotor activity is atypical for mesial temporal lobe epilepsy, and the imaging suggests a more anterior localization. In consideration of the risks of including resection of the mesial temporal structures in an epilepsy surgery, an intracarotid amobarbital test was performed, and it identified intact episodic memory after both left and right injections.

Based on the imaging and cognitive testing findings, a left temporal pole resection with sparing of the hippocampus was performed at age 15 years. Histopathological examination identified dyslamination with neuronal crowding and enlarged, dysmorphic neurons indicating a diagnosis of cortical dysplasia, type IIa. No seizures with impaired awareness have occurred for 1.5 years since surgery, but auras occasionally occur.

J. M. Stern, N. Salamon, *Imaging of Epilepsy*, https://doi.org/10.1007/978-3-030-86672-3_15

Imaging

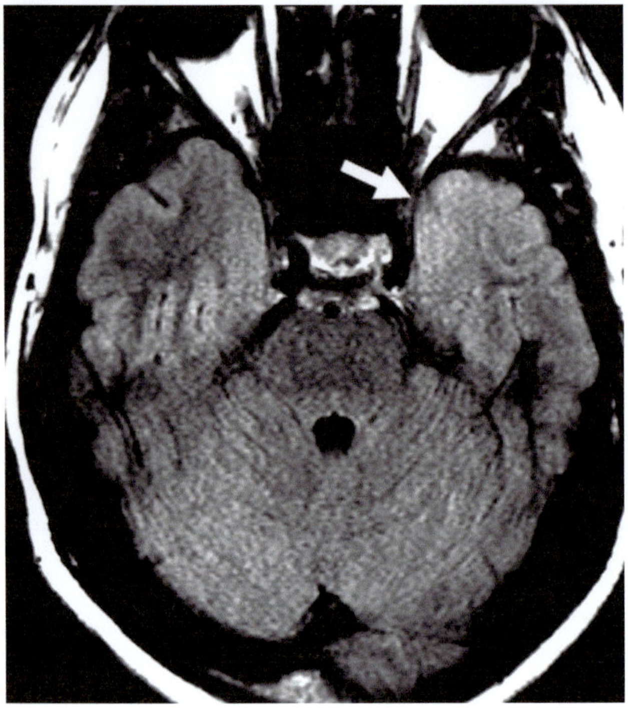

Fig. 15.1 MRI axial FLAIR sequence at a temporal pole level. Anterior and mesial left temporal pole hyperintensity (arrow) is present. Abnormal blurring of the left lateral temporal pole's gray-white junction also is evident. As a whole, the left temporal pole is smaller than the right

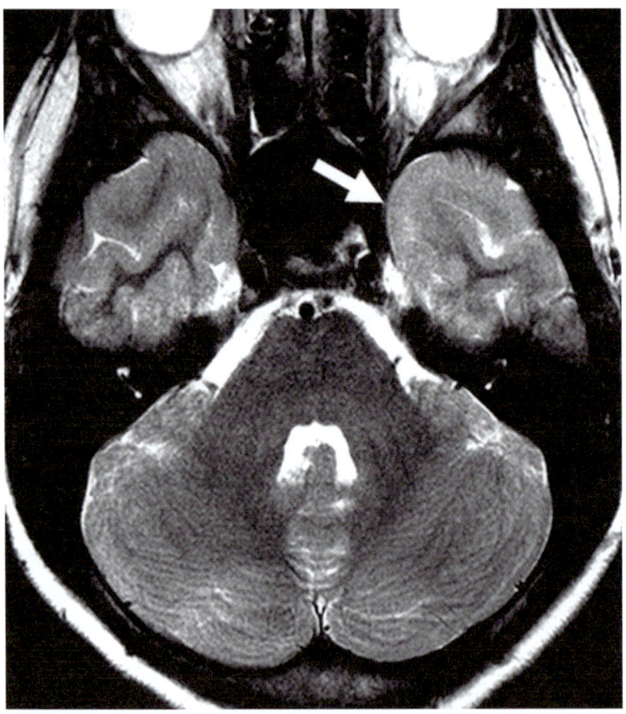

Fig. 15.2 MRI axial T2 sequence at a temporal pole level that is inferior to Fig. 15.1. With the T2 sequence, blurring of the gray-white junction is more clearly depicted (arrow) along the anterior and mesial left temporal lobe

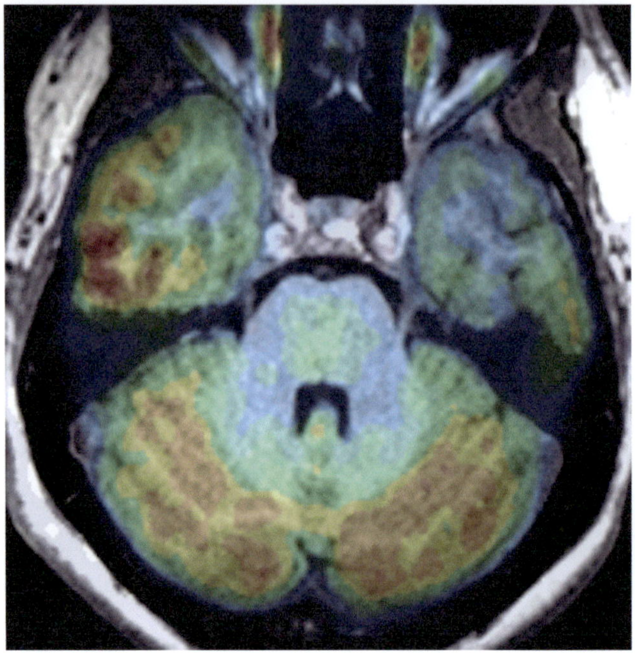

Fig. 15.3 PET-MRI co-registration with color-scale FDG tracer in an axial plane at a temporal pole level that is similar to Figs. 15.1 and 15.2. The left temporal pole is hypometabolic, including both the mesial and lateral aspects

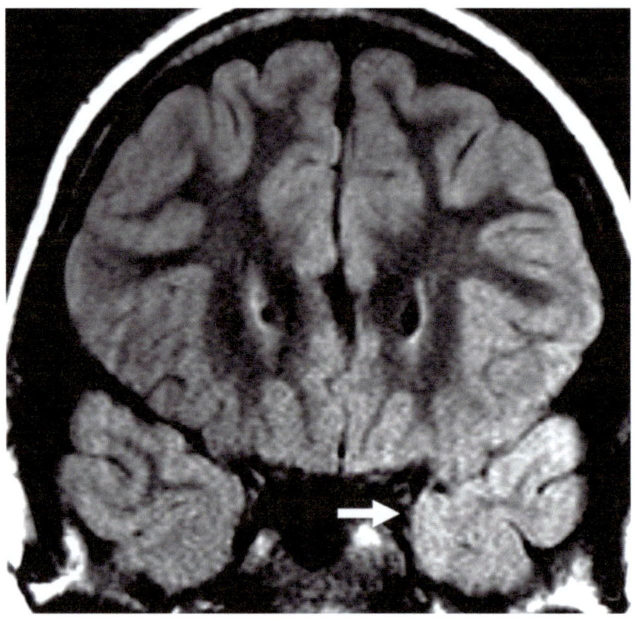

Fig. 15.4 MRI coronal FLAIR sequence at a temporal pole level. Abnormal hyperintensity of the mesial left temporal lobe (arrow) is prominent. Abnormal blurring of the left lateral temporal lobe's gray-white junction also is evident. At this level, the left temporal lobe is slightly smaller than the right

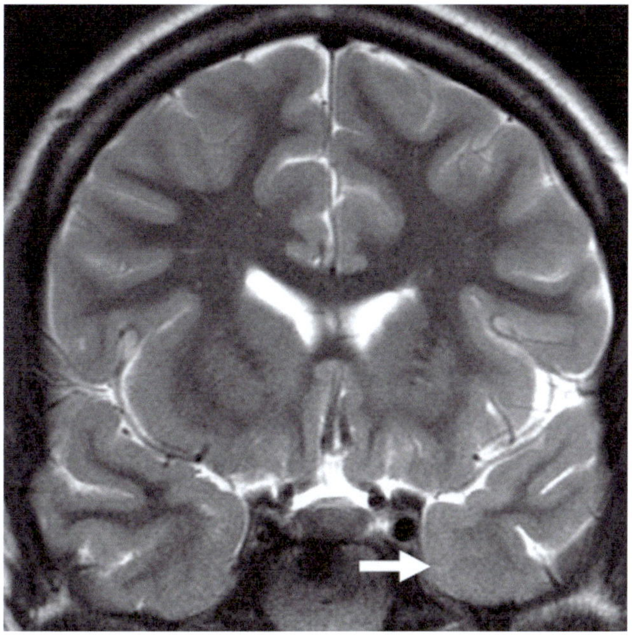

Fig. 15.5 MRI coronal T2 sequence at a temporal pole level that is posterior to Fig. 15.2. Gray-white differentiation is not present along the mesial (arrow) and inferior aspects of the left temporal pole. Differentiation at the gray-white junction at the crown of the middle and superior temporal gyri is slightly diminished, compared to the right

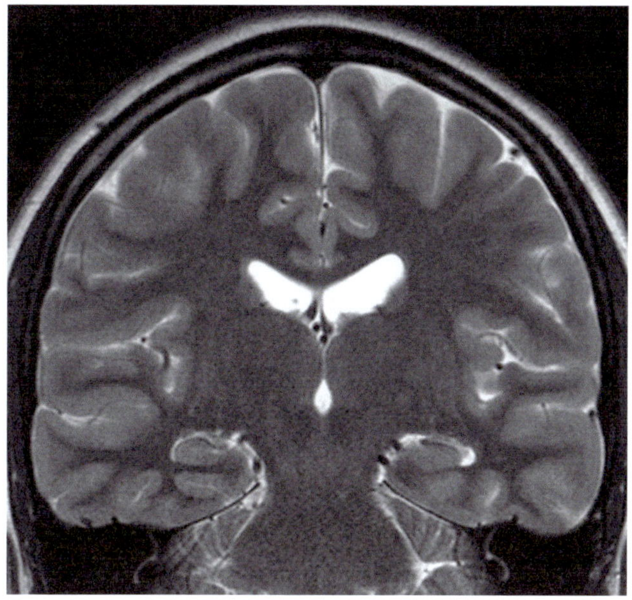

Fig. 15.7 MRI coronal T2 sequence at a hippocampal body level. The gray-white junctions within the left parahippocampal and fusiform gyri are blurred. The hippocampi are bilaterally normal in volume and signal

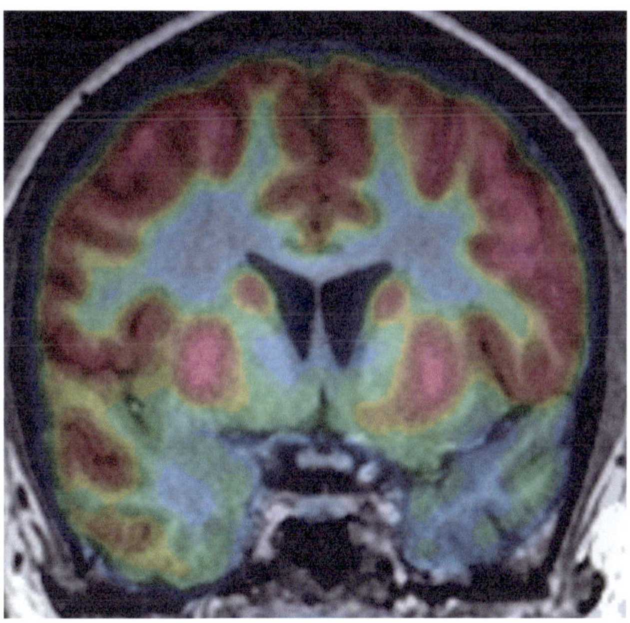

Fig. 15.6 PET-MRI co-registration with color-scale FDG tracer in a coronal plane at a temporal pole level that is similar to Figs. 15.4 and 15.5. The entire visible temporal lobe is hypometabolic. The mesial regions of blurred gray-white junction demonstrate greater hypometabolism than the less blurred regions in the superior and middle temporal gyri

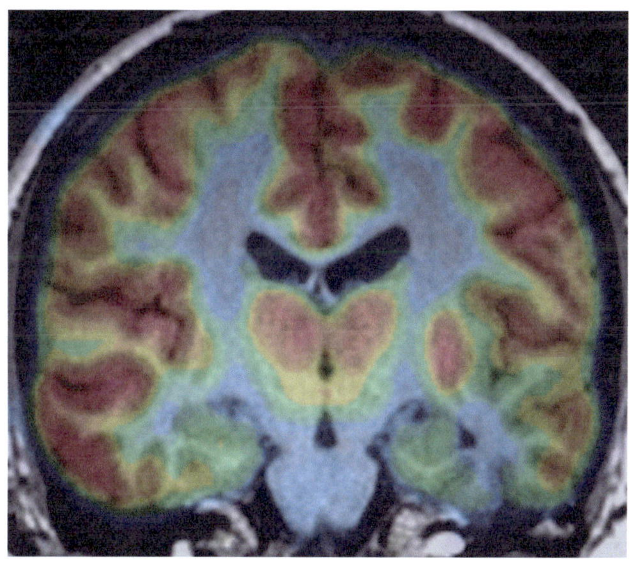

Fig. 15.8 PET-MRI co-registration with color-scale FDG tracer in a coronal plane at a hippocampal body level that is similar to Fig. 15.7. The left parahippocampal and fusiform gyri demonstrate prominent hypometabolism. The superior, middle, and inferior temporal gyri also are hypometabolic when compared to the right temporal lobe, but the hypometabolism is not as prominent as within the mesial and inferior structures. The hippocampi are symmetric in metabolism

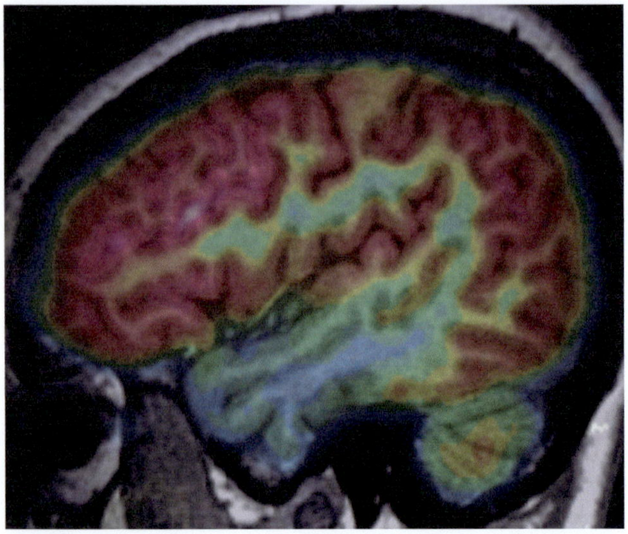

Fig. 15.9 PET-MRI co-registration with color-scale FDG tracer in a parasagittal plane at a left temporal pole level. The temporal pole demonstrates prominent hypometabolism. Hypometabolism of the superior temporal gyrus spares Heschl's gyrus

16 Focal Cortical Dysplasia of the Amygdala

Clinical History

The first recognized seizure occurred in early childhood as an episode of unresponsiveness followed by confusion.

The habitual seizures did not change after late childhood and manifested as a sense of moving backward in time through a tunnel with auditory hallucinations of familiar voices. The aura occasionally also included déjà vu. Unresponsiveness and impaired awareness followed the aura, and this sometimes included eyelid flutter. The total seizure duration was 1–3 minutes followed by postictal confusion. Treatment included multiple anti-seizure medications with a seizure frequency of two to three seizures weekly.

Epilepsy risk factors were birth at 3 months premature and possibly a febrile convulsion. Neurological examination was normal. Neuropsychological testing identified impaired verbal memory with intact visual memory and language function. Medical history was significant for depression.

Interictal EEG depicted epileptiform sharp waves over the left temporal region. Video-EEG monitoring recorded focal seizures manifested as staring. Ictal EEG was rhythmic slowing across the left temporal region during several of the seizures.

MRI identified abnormal signal within the left amygdala and normal bilateral hippocampi. PET identified left amygdala hypometabolism.

The history and evaluation indicate left mesial temporal lobe epilepsy. The aura of a distortion of time and memory is typical for limbic epilepsy. Curiously, the aura did not include emotional features characteristic of amygdalar involvement. With evidence of verbal memory impairment, a left anterior-mesial temporal lobe resection was considered, and an intracarotid amobarbital test was performed. This identified left hemispheric dominance for language and episodic memory function during both left and right injections.

Because the imaging abnormality did not include the hippocampi and episodic memory was intact during a right intracarotid amobarbital injection, intracranial EEG monitoring with depth electrodes was performed for consideration of a left anterior temporal lobe resection that spares the hippocampus. Intracranial electrode coverage was bilateral temporal and frontal lobes, and EEG's seizure onset was within the left mesial temporal lobe, including the amygdala, for most seizures but sometimes within the anterior temporal neocortex.

Based on the intracranial EEG results, a left anterior-mesial temporal lobe resection was considered necessary for seizure freedom, and a risk for memory impairment was discussed with the patient. A left anterior-mesial temporal lobe resection was performed at age 53 years. Histopathological examination identified increased vascularity and gliosis within the amygdala. No seizures with impaired awareness have occurred for the 7 years since epilepsy surgery. Auras lasting about 1 second occasionally occur. The resection did not produce a significant change to memory function.

J. M. Stern, N. Salamon, *Imaging of Epilepsy*, https://doi.org/10.1007/978-3-030-86672-3_16

Imaging

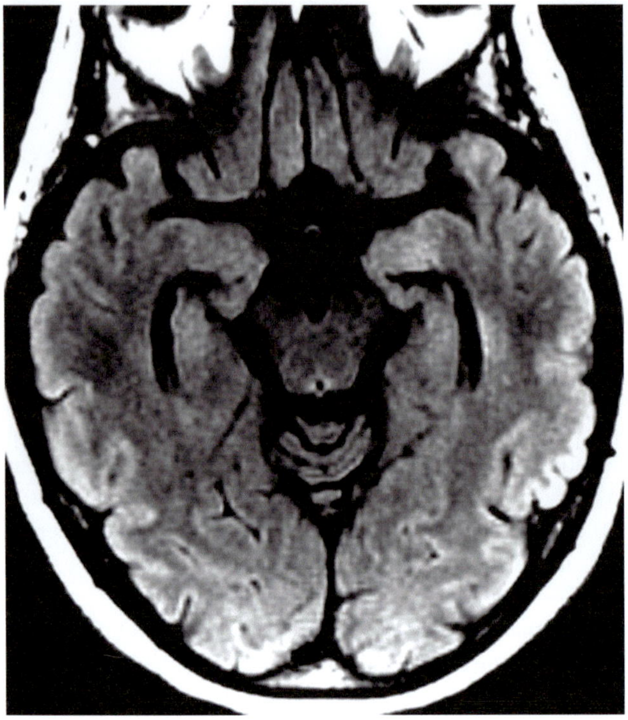

Fig. 16.1 MRI axial FLAIR sequence at an amygdala and hippocampal head level. The left amygdala demonstrates hyperintense signal abnormality, and the hippocampi are bilaterally normal in size and signal

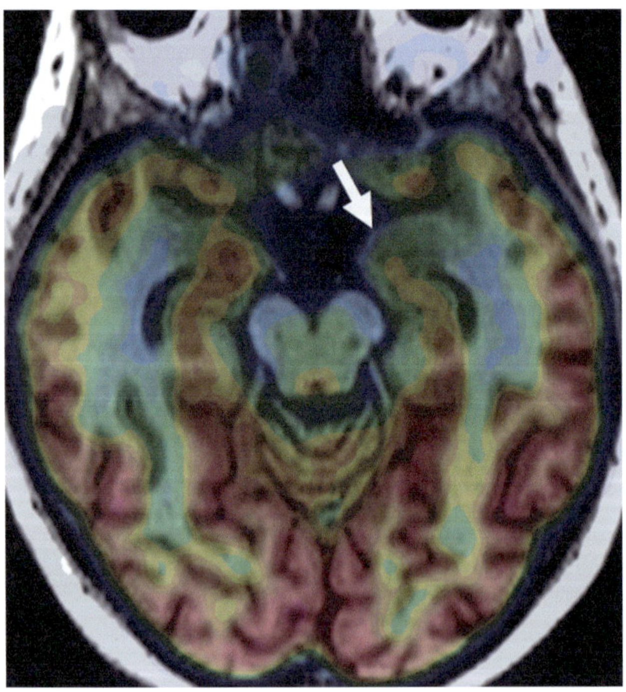

Fig. 16.2 PET-MRI co-registration with color-scale FDG tracer in an axial plane at the same level as Fig. 16.1. The left amygdala is markedly hypometabolic (arrow), especially when compared to the right amygdala. The hippocampi are symmetric and normal in metabolic signal

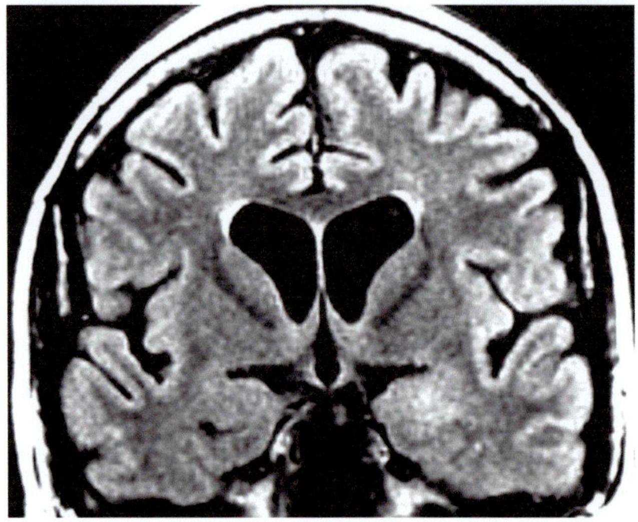

Fig. 16.3 MRI coronal FLAIR sequence at an amygdala level. The left amygdala demonstrates abnormal hyperintensity and has normal volume with bilateral amygdalae symmetric in volume. The asymmetrically greater signal along the left lateral frontal and temporal cortical ribbon is due to magnetic field inhomogeneity and does not indicate abnormality

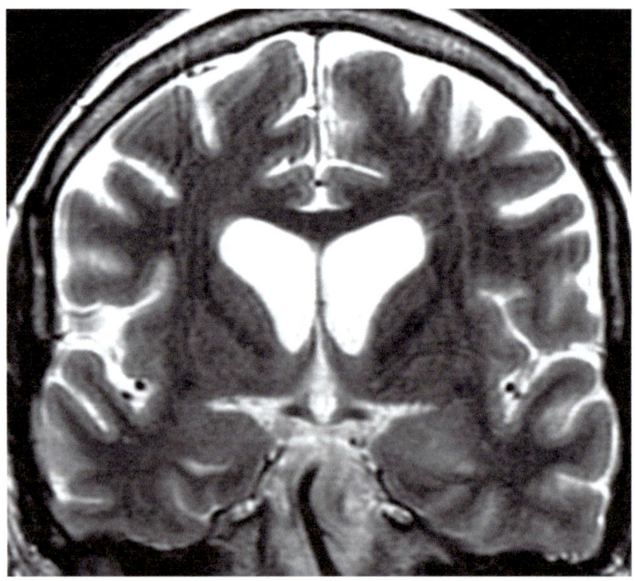

Fig. 16.4 MRI coronal T2 sequence at the same amygdala level as in Fig. 16.3. Abnormal hyperintensity is evident within the left amygdala, and the amygdalae are not significantly different in volume. The temporal lobes are otherwise normal

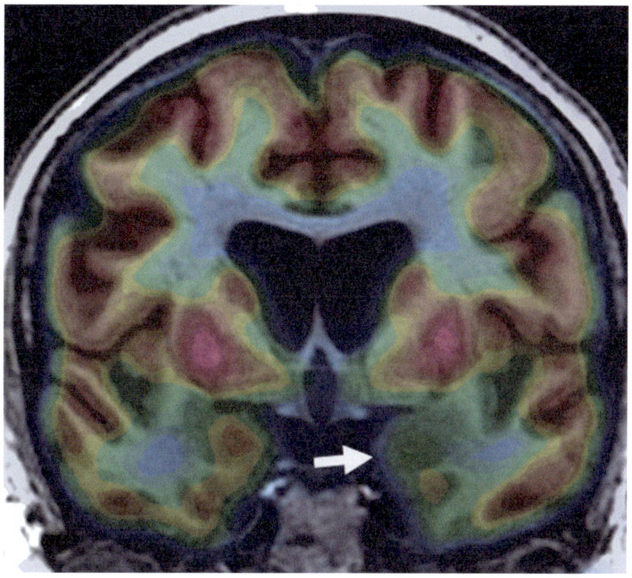

Fig. 16.5 PET-MRI co-registration with color-scale FDG tracer in a coronal plane at a similar amygdala level as Figs. 16.3 and 16.4. Marked hypometabolism of the left amygdala (arrow) is evident with a region of additional hypometabolism within the left parahippocampal gyrus. The lateral temporal lobes are symmetric and normal

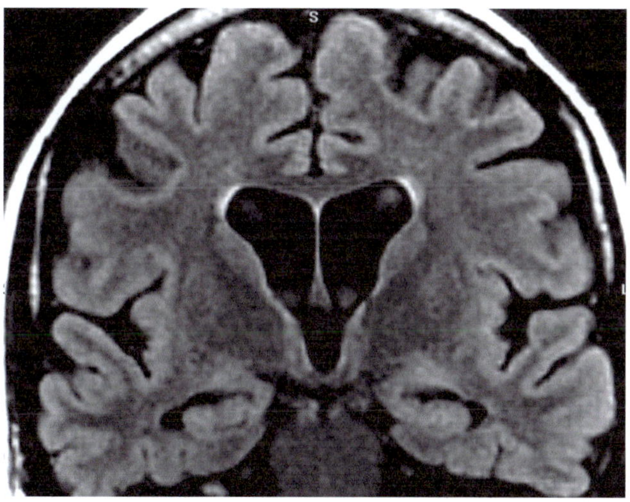

Fig. 16.6 MRI coronal FLAIR sequence at a hippocampal head level. The hippocampi are normal with symmetric size and signal. The lateral and third ventricles are prominent with unclear clinical significance

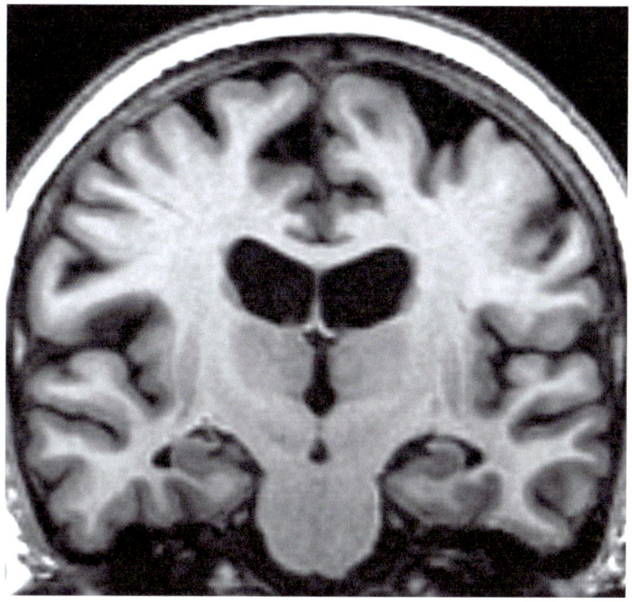

Fig. 16.7 MRI coronal T1 sequence at a hippocampal body level. The hippocampi are normal with symmetric size. The cortical ribbon and gray-white junction are normal across bilateral temporal lobes

17 Diffuse Periventricular Heterotopia

Clinical History

The first recognized seizure was generalized tonic-clonic at age 20 years, but this seizure followed a stereotyped experience that was retrospectively recognized to have been occurring since about age 15 years.

The stereotyped experience was a habitual seizures manifested as déjà vu with a specific forced memory followed by impaired awareness with left hand automatisms and sometimes also verbal automatisms. The aura occasionally also included nausea or epigastric discomfort. The seizure duration was 2 minutes, followed by postictal headache and fatigue for 20 minutes. Tonic-clonic seizures occurred very rarely. None occurred in more than 10 years, and about four have occurred in total. The habitual seizure was retrospectively estimated to have occurred once every few weeks to every few months for the 5 years from the first occurrence to the epilepsy diagnosis and treatment. The seizure frequency increased over the years since diagnosis to several seizures weekly. Treatment included multiple anti-seizure medications and vagus nerve stimulation.

An epilepsy risk factor was not present, but a contributing genetic factor was evident. Both the patient and her daughter have periventricular nodular heterotopia. Neurological examination was normal.

Interictal EEG depicted right temporal epileptiform discharges. Video-EEG monitoring recorded seizures with impaired awareness that were consistent with the habitual seizures. Ictal EEG's seizure onset was not localized.

MRI identified extensive, symmetrical subependymal gray matter heterotopia along the lateral aspects to the occipital horns of the lateral ventricles.

The ictal behavior suggests limbic epilepsy with mesial temporal memory and insular features. The motor features are not lateralizing, and the EEG also did not indicate an epileptogenic zone. This clinical presentation of focal features without clear localization is compatible with bilateral, periventricular heterotopia. Because resective epilepsy surgery is not feasible with this epileptogenic abnormality, additional diagnostic testing was not pursued at the time of the evaluation. However, intracranial EEG would be considered in the current era because of the benefits of better localization toward seizure control when treated with stereotactic ablation or responsive neurostimulation, which are now routinely offered treatment options.

J. M. Stern, N. Salamon, *Imaging of Epilepsy*, https://doi.org/10.1007/978-3-030-86672-3_17

Imaging

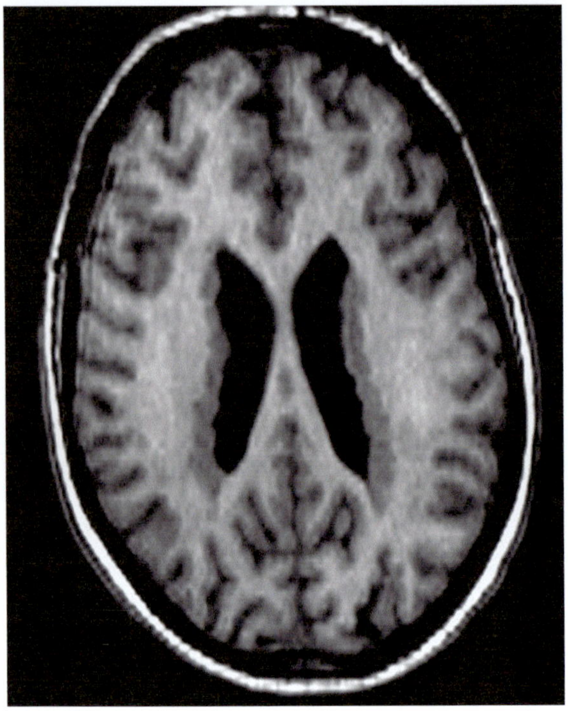

Fig. 17.1 MRI axial T1 sequence at a lateral ventricle level. Nodular heterotopic gray matter are evident along the lateral walls of both lateral ventricles. The surrounding white matter and its overlying cortical ribbon are normal

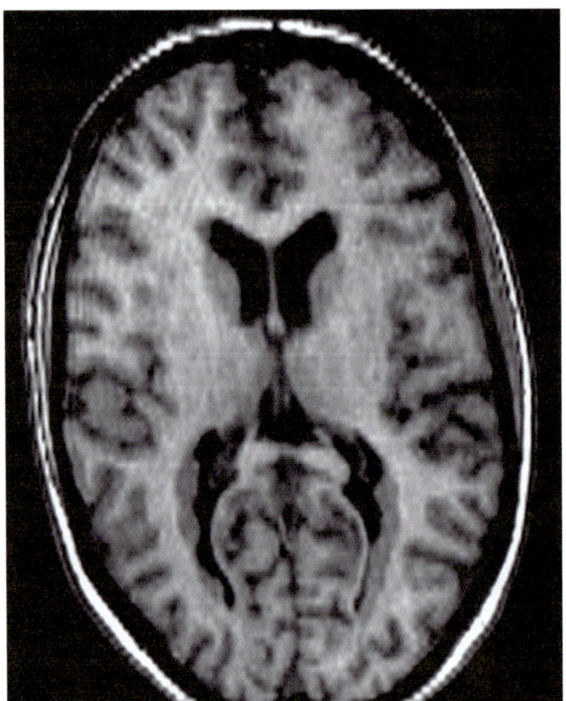

Fig. 17.2 MRI axial T1 sequence at a ventricular atrium level. Nodular heterotopic gray matter are evident along the lateral portions of the atrium to the occipital horns bilaterally. The frontal horns, the cerebral white matter, and the cortical ribbon are normal

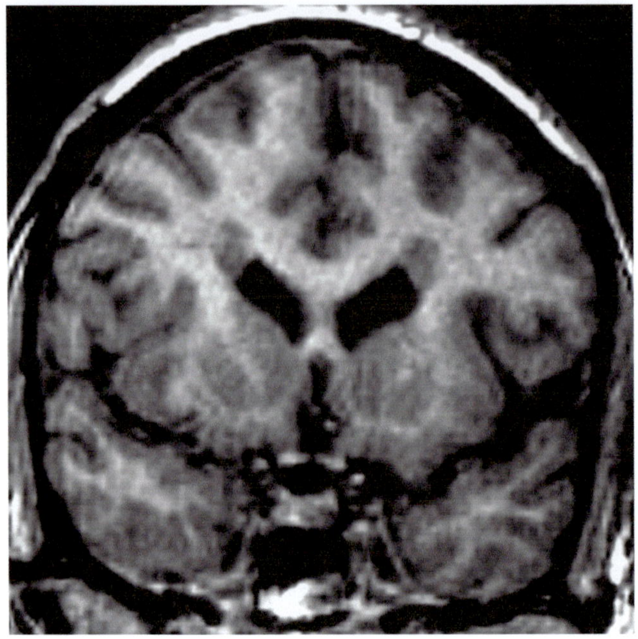

Fig. 17.3 MRI coronal T1 sequence at a temporal pole level. Gray matter heterotopia are evident along the lateral aspects of the frontal horns of both lateral ventricles

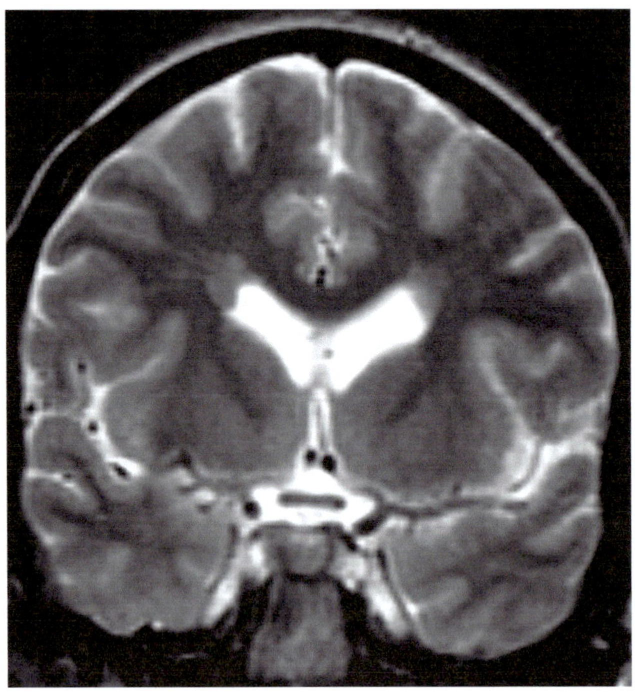

Fig. 17.4 MRI coronal T2 sequence at the same temporal pole level as Fig. 17.3. Gray matter heterotopia are present along the lateral aspects of the frontal horns bilaterally. Linear perivascular spaces are evident in the white matter and directed perpendicularly from the frontal horn heterotopia. In this image, the perivascular spaces are more prominent in the right cerebrum. Unlike a transmantle sign, they do not taper toward the ventricle, and they do not appear as gray matter on T1 sequence image

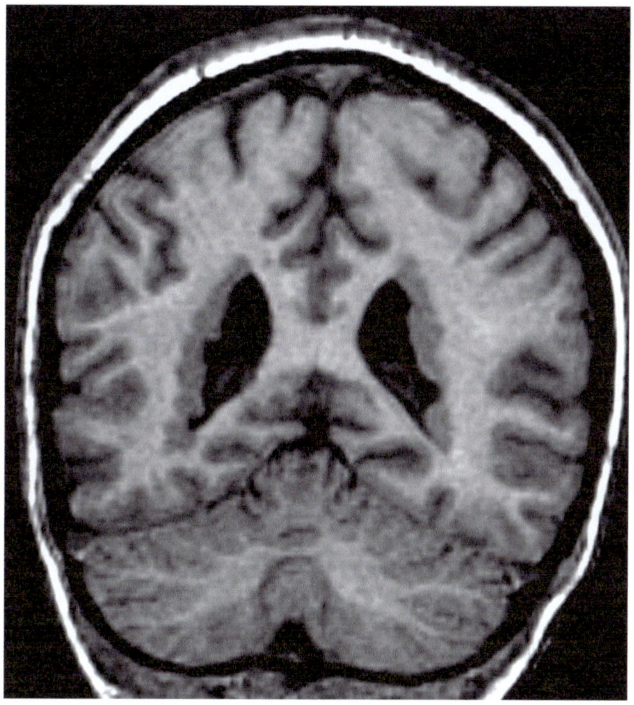

Fig. 17.5 MRI coronal T1 sequence at a splenium of the corpus callosum level. Nodular gray matter heterotopia are confluent along the lateral aspects of the posterior lateral ventricles bilaterally. The medial aspects, including both the superior and inferior portions, of the lateral ventricles are normal

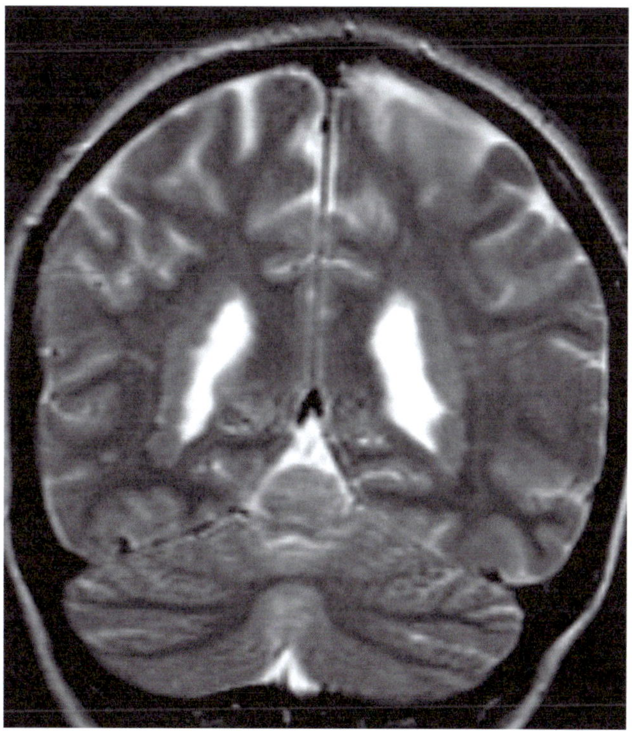

Fig. 17.6 MRI coronal T2 sequence at a posterior to the splenium of the corpus callosum level. Nodular gray matter heterotopia are confluent along the lateral aspects of the posterior lateral ventricles bilaterally. Perivascular spaces are visible bilaterally as linear signals that are parallel to each other and are perpendicular from the heterotopia's lateral surfaces

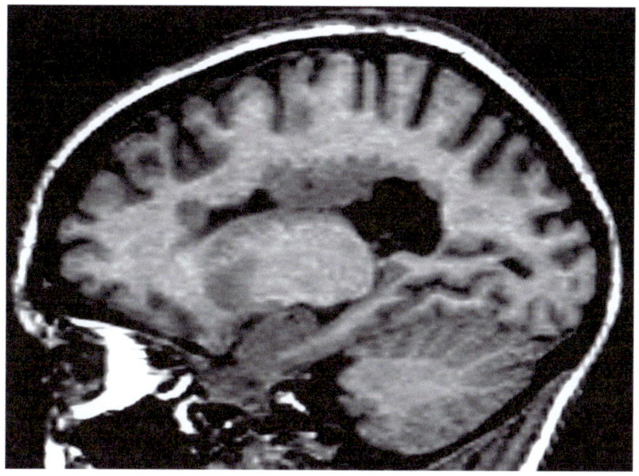

Fig. 17.7 MRI sagittal T1 sequence at a left thalamus level. Gray matter heterotopia are evident along the superior margin of the lateral ventricle with a more nodular surface near the frontal horn, as seen in Figs. 17.3 and 17.4. The cortical ribbon and white matter are normal

Multifocal Periventricular Heterotopia

18

Clinical History

The first recognized seizure occurred at age 7 years as a sudden blackening of vision that recurred over months with each occurrence lasting several minutes and some including forced gaze to the right.

The subsequent habitual seizures manifested as either (1) a flash of light in the right visual field followed by a loss of vision for several seconds; (2) a dimming of central vision that expands outward and is associated with anxiety, amnesia, and repetitive questioning for 30 to 60 seconds; or (3) a bilateral tonic-clonic convulsion. Treatment included multiple anti-seizure medications with focal visual seizures occurring about seven times daily and seizures with impaired awareness and memory occurring about five times monthly. Bilateral tonic-clonic seizures have not occurred in more than 5 years.

An epilepsy risk factor was not present. Neurological examination was normal, including visual fields as assessed with automated testing.

Interictal EEG depicted intermittent and independent slowing over the temporal regions and the left posterior quadrant, multifocal epileptiform sharp waves across bilateral central and temporal regions and the left occipital region, and epileptiform discharges over the left occipital region during photic stimulation. Video-EEG monitoring recorded focal seizures manifested as right-sided vision changes due to blurring or hallucinations of flashes. Some seizures progressed to unresponsiveness with manual automatisms. Ictal EEG's seizure onset was evolving, rhythmic slowing that was maximal over the left occipital region.

MRI identified small foci of heterotopic gray matter along the ependymal surface of the occipital horns with a greater presence on the left. PET identified small, corresponding regions of hypometabolism along the ependymal surface of the occipital horns.

The seizure experience of right-sided primary visual hallucinations with forced gaze and the ictal EEG's onset suggest a left occipital epileptogenic region. This is supported by the structural and metabolic abnormality along the left occipital horn, but additional abnormality is present along the right occipital horn and the interictal EEG identifies more diffuse epileptiform abnormality. Based on this evidence, additional diagnostic testing was performed to further assess the localization and the corresponding deficit risk of a resection.

Interictal EEG source analysis localized 90% of the epileptiform discharges to either the left occipital lobe, left posterior parietal lobe, or left inferior-lateral temporal lobe. MEG identified epileptiform dipoles across the left temporal lobe and left temporal-parietal-occipital junction.

Functional MRI of vision was normal, and functional MRI of language identified left hemispheric dominance with the basal temporal naming area close to the heterotopia. Neuropsychological testing identified impairments in verbal and visual episodic memory and in visuospatial perception and reasoning.

The functional assessment provided further support for a left occipital epileptogenic region with likely involvement of the left occipital horn heterotopia. To avoid significant visual field deficits, surgical treatment was performed with stereotactic laser thermo-ablation (see 81 in the Treatment Related Findings section). Following this treatment, the focal visual seizures and the seizures with impaired awareness have been reduced to about half of their preoperative frequency. At 1 year after surgery, automated visual field testing demonstrated no change and neuropsychological testing identified improved visuospatial perception and reasoning.

J. M. Stern, N. Salamon, *Imaging of Epilepsy*, https://doi.org/10.1007/978-3-030-86672-3_18

Imaging

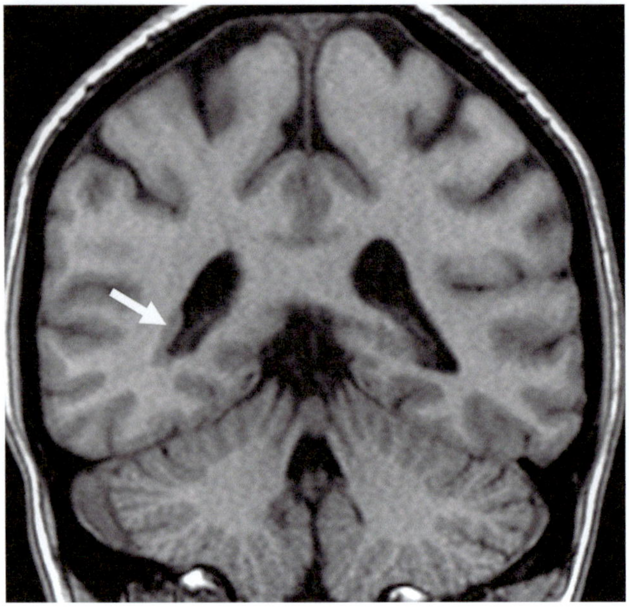

Fig. 18.1 MRI coronal T1 sequence at a splenium of the corpus callosum level. Heterotopic gray matter (arrow) is evident along the lateral inferior wall of the right lateral ventricle. The overlying neocortical ribbon and its gray-white differentiation are normal bilaterally

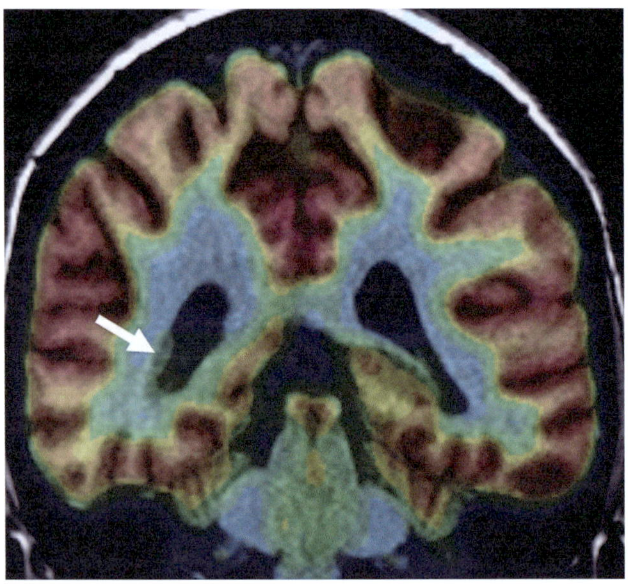

Fig. 18.2 PET-MRI co-registration with color-scale FDG tracer in a coronal plane at the same splenium of the corpus callosum level as Fig. 18.1. The heterotopic gray matter (arrow) is hypometabolic compared to normal gray matter metabolism, which is evident in the neocortical ribbon. However, the heterotopia's metabolism is slightly greater than the surrounding white matter

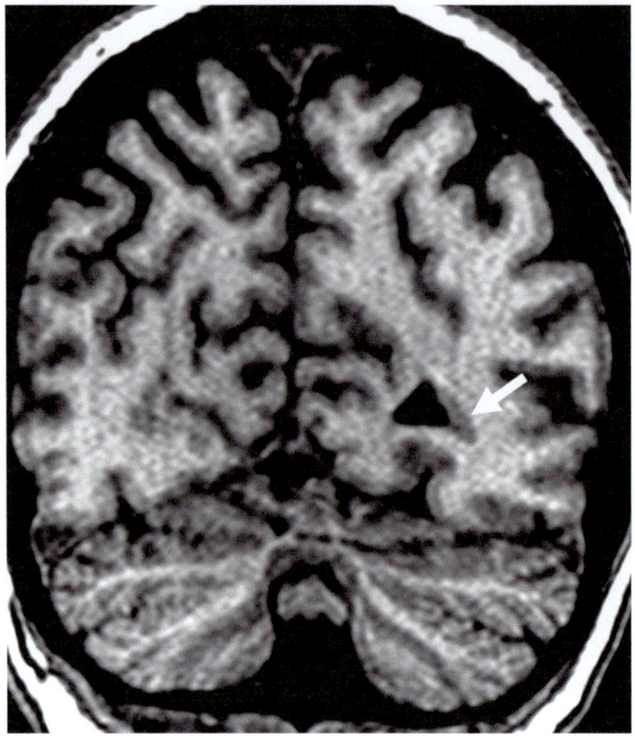

Fig. 18.3 MRI coronal T1 sequence at an occipital horn level. Heterotopic gray matter (arrow) is evident along the lateral wall of the left lateral ventricle near the left occipital horn. The overlying neocortical ribbon is normal. The right occipital horn is not visible, and the gray matter signal that is evident contralaterally symmetric to the heterotopia is normal gyral anatomy

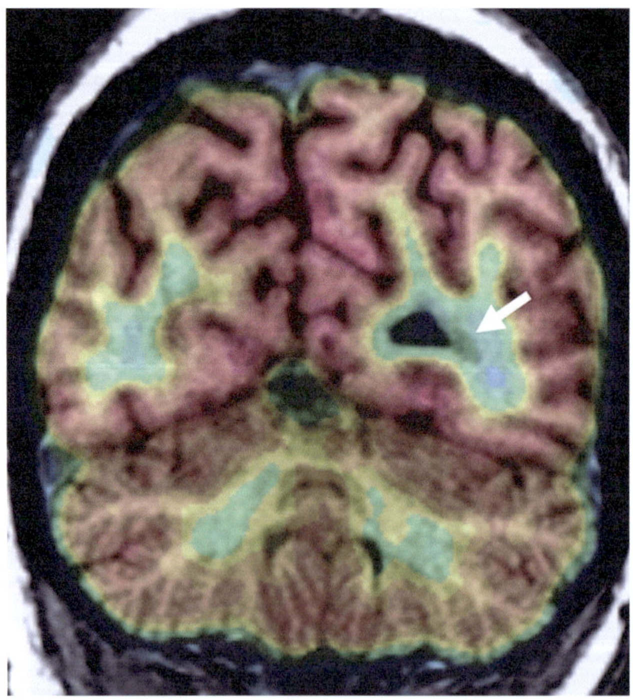

Fig. 18.4 PET-MRI co-registration with color-scale FDG tracer in a coronal plane at a similar occipital horn level as Fig. 18.3. Heterotopic gray matter (arrow) is evident along the lateral aspect of the left lateral ventricle. This nodule is hypometabolic compared to neocortex and mildly increased compared to white matter

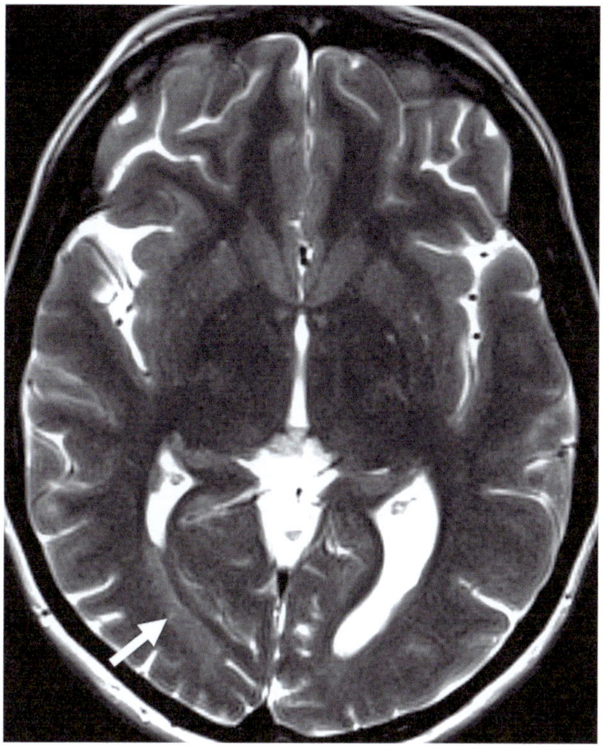

Fig. 18.5 MRI axial T2 sequence at a thalamus level. An elongated gray matter signal (arrow) is evident along the margin of the occipital horn of the right lateral ventricle. The signal of the heterotopic gray matter is slightly higher than the surrounding white matter. A subtle irregularity of the contour to the left lateral ventricle's lateral wall is due to a smaller heterotopic abnormality

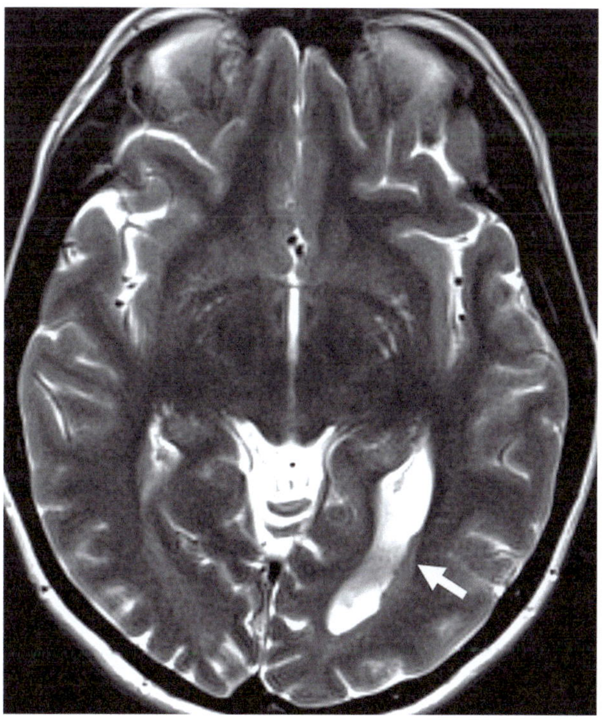

Fig. 18.6 MRI axial T2 sequence at a superior colliculus level that is slightly inferior to Fig. 18.5. Heterotopic gray matter is present along the lateral wall of the left lateral ventricle. It is contiguous with the subtle left ventricular wall abnormality in Fig. 18.5. The overlying neocortex is normal

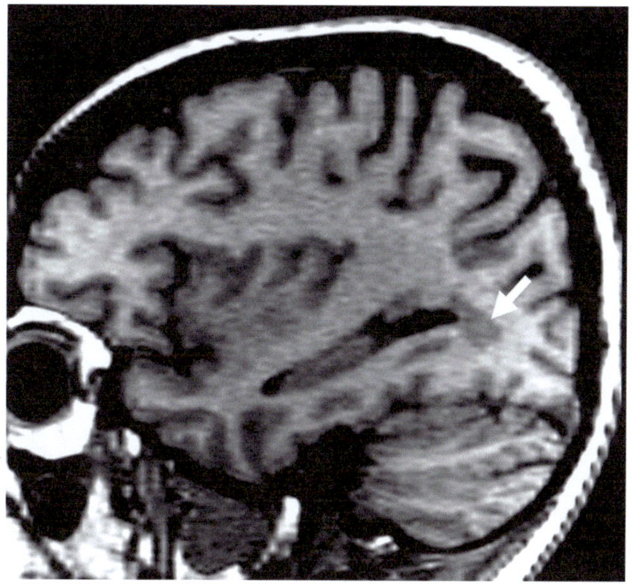

Fig. 18.7 MRI sagittal T1 sequence at a right insula level. Heterotopic gray matter (arrow) is present at the posterior margin of the occipital horn of the right lateral ventricle. Additional heterotopic gray matter is present immediately anterior to the most superior extent of the ventricle. The two gray matter signal islands inferior to the ventricle are normal deep portions of the collateral sulcus

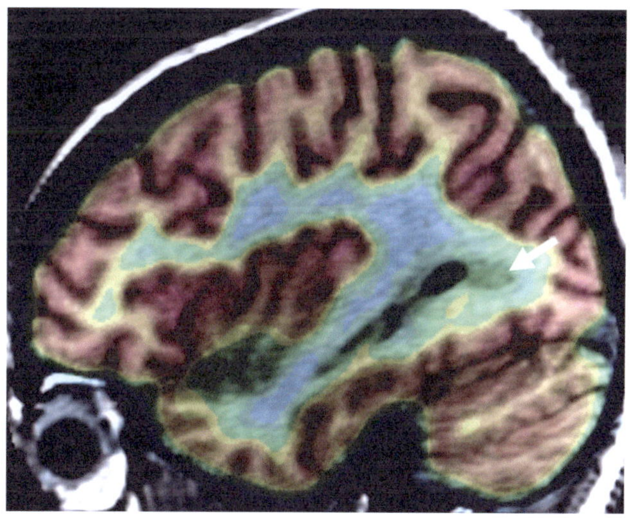

Fig. 18.8 PET-MRI co-registration with color-scale FDG tracer in a sagittal plane at a similar right insular level as Fig. 18.7. Gray matter signal (arrow) is present at the posterior of margin of the occipital horn of the right lateral ventricle. Additional heterotopic gray matter is evident along the ventricle's superior margin. The heterotopia's metabolic signal is slightly more than the white matter and less than the gray matter along the cortical ribbon and the yellow signal inferior to the ventricle that corresponds to the depth of the collateral sulcus

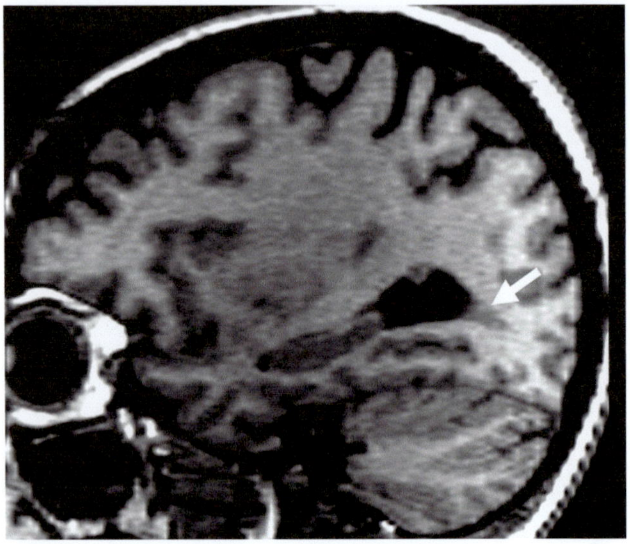

Fig. 18.9 MRI sagittal T1 sequence at a left hippocampus level that is slightly lateral to the level in Fig. 18.7. Heterotopic gray matter (arrow) is present at the posterior margin of the occipital horn of the right lateral ventricle. An additional nodule is present at the superior extent of the ventricle

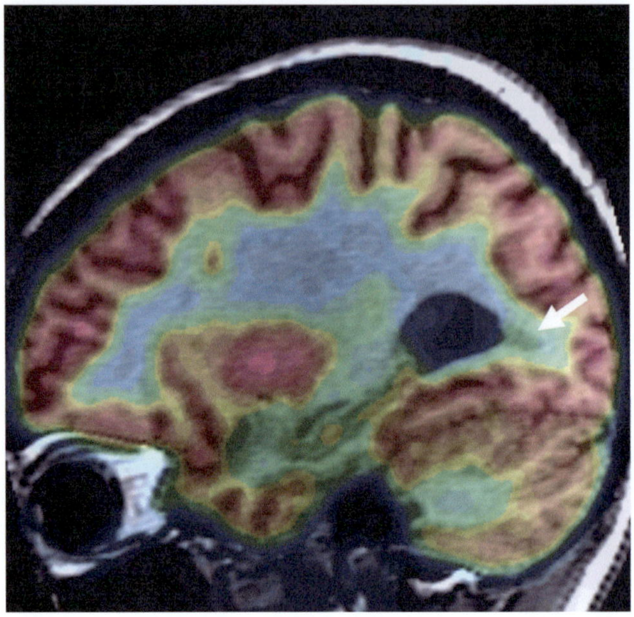

Fig. 18.10 PET-MRI co-registration with color-scale FDG tracer in a sagittal plane at a similar right hippocampus level as Fig. 18.9. Heterotopic gray matter (arrow) is present at the posterior margin of the occipital horn. The superior nodule is not evident because the level is slightly lateral to the level in Fig. 18.9

Band Heterotopia

19

Clinical History

The first recognized seizure occurred at age 12 years as an episode of non-vertiginous dizziness, anxiety, and fear followed by impairment of awareness with oral and manual automatisms.

The habitual seizures were similar to first seizure, but a minority progressed to a bilateral tonic-clonic seizure. Treatment included multiple anti-seizure medications with a seizure frequency that is typically 12 to 15 monthly. Up to four seizures occurred within a day.

The epilepsy risk factor was a family history of epilepsy, but relevant details were not known.

Neurological examination was significant for mild intellectual disability, and medical history included depression.

Interictal EEG depicted mild, generalized slowing with asymmetrically greater slowing across the left temporal region. Epileptiform sharp waves were present broadly over the left temporal region and independently over the anterior right temporal region. Video-EEG monitoring recorded focal seizures manifested as lapses in awareness that became tonic-clonic seizures with inconsistently lateralized versive movements. The ictal EEG's seizure onsets also were inconsistently lateralized with some having an onset over the right temporal region and others having an onset over the left posterior quadrant with subsequent propagation to the left temporal region.

MRI identified bilateral symmetric, confluent, bands of gray matter in the parietal-occipital and posterior temporal regions. PET identified abnormal metabolic signal consistent with the band heterotopia.

Although the history suggests one seizure localization because of a reported stereotyped ictal experience and manifestation, the evaluation indicated bilaterally independent focal seizures, as evident in both left and right versive movements and right and left ictal EEG's seizure onset lateralization. The bilateral band heterotopia provides an etiologic explanation for the bilateral, independent focal seizures, and the band heterotopia asymmetry suggests an explanation for the ictal EEG's seizure onset patterns also differing between the right and left seizures. However, these differences did not produce differing auras or automatisms before progressing to bilateral tonic-clonic. Surgical treatment was not pursued.

J. M. Stern, N. Salamon, *Imaging of Epilepsy*, https://doi.org/10.1007/978-3-030-86672-3_19

Imaging

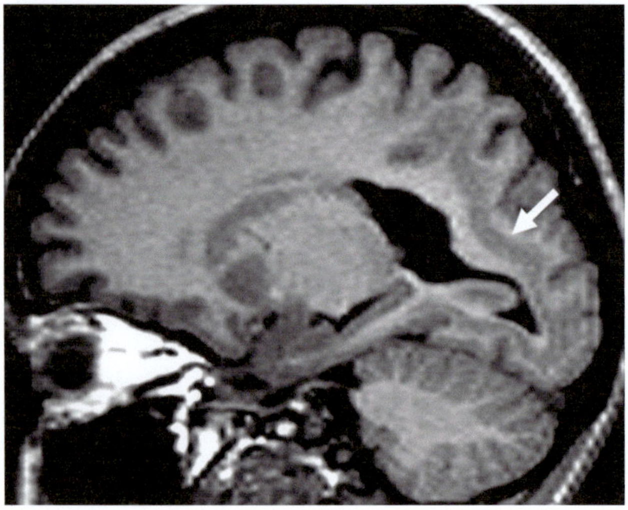

Fig. 19.1 MRI sagittal T1 sequence at a left thalamus level. A band of gray matter signal (arrow) extends across the parietal-occipital region below the cortex with white matter separating it from the cortex. The cortical ribbon is normal

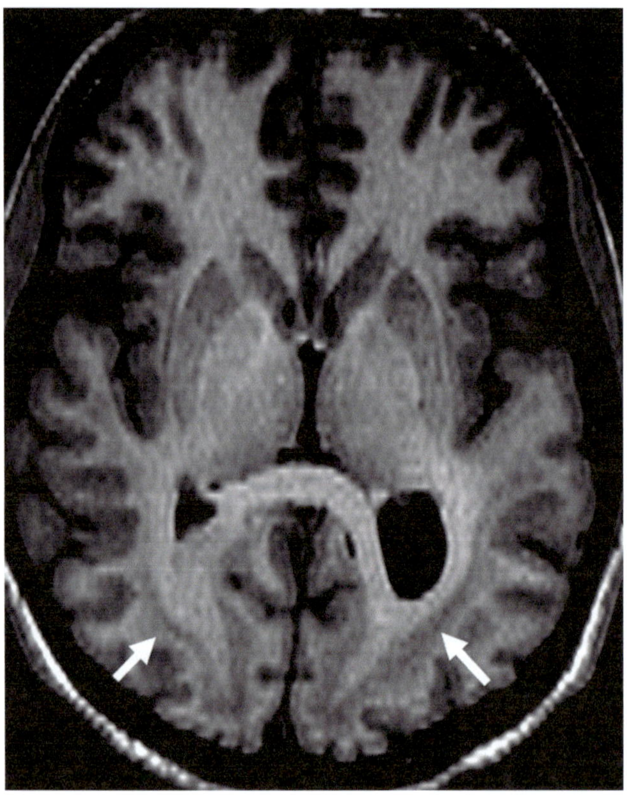

Fig. 19.2 MRI axial T1 sequence at a thalamus level. Bands of gray matter signal (arrows) are present bilaterally in the temporal-occipital region and turn at the occipital pole with continuation anteriorly in the medial occipital lobe. The bands are asymmetric and wider in the left occipital lobe

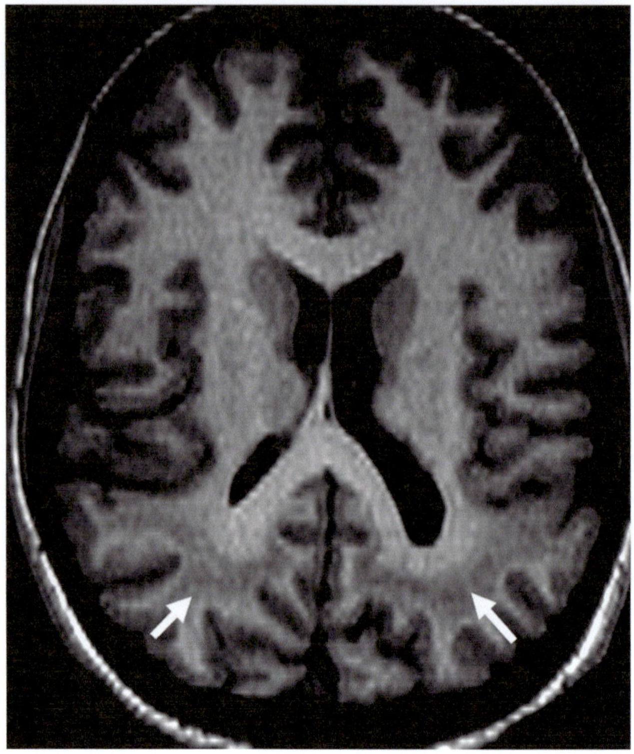

Fig. 19.3 MRI axial T1 sequence at a superior caudate level. Bilateral bands of heterotopic gray matter (arrows) curve from the inferior parietal regions toward the superior parietal regions and extending into the posterior cingulate gyrus. The bands are asymmetric in their differentiation from the surrounding white matter with greater blurring of the junction in the left occipital lobe

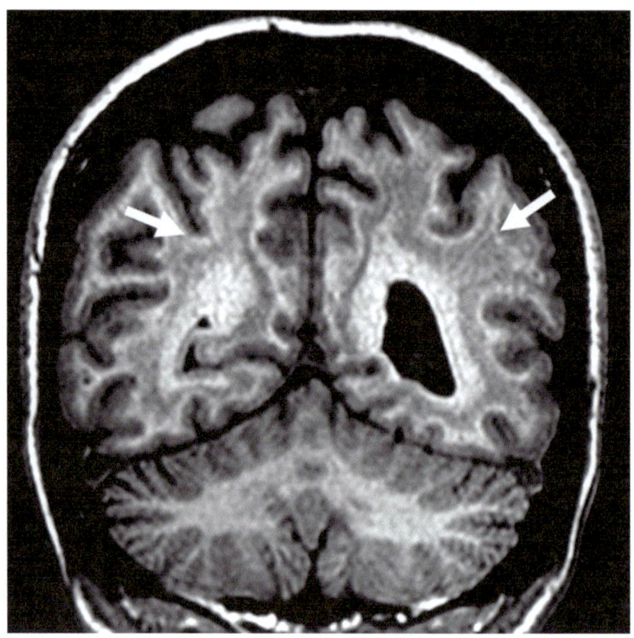

Fig. 19.4 MRI coronal T1 sequence at an atrium of the lateral ventricles level. At this level, the band heterotopia (arrows) is much wider and extend across much of the white matter space between the ventricles and the cortical ribbon

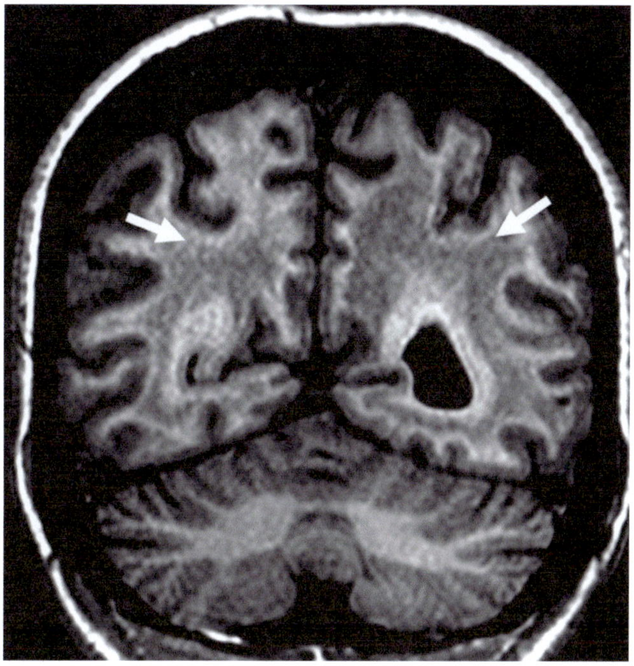

Fig. 19.5 MRI coronal T1 sequence at an atrium of the lateral ventricles level immediately posterior to Fig. 19.4. Band heterotopia surrounds the left lateral ventricle at this level with a wider dimension laterally (left parietal arrow) and a narrower dimension adjacent to the posterior cingulate gyrus. On the right, the heterotopia also is present medially and laterally, but the abnormality is not as wide (right parietal arrow) as on the left

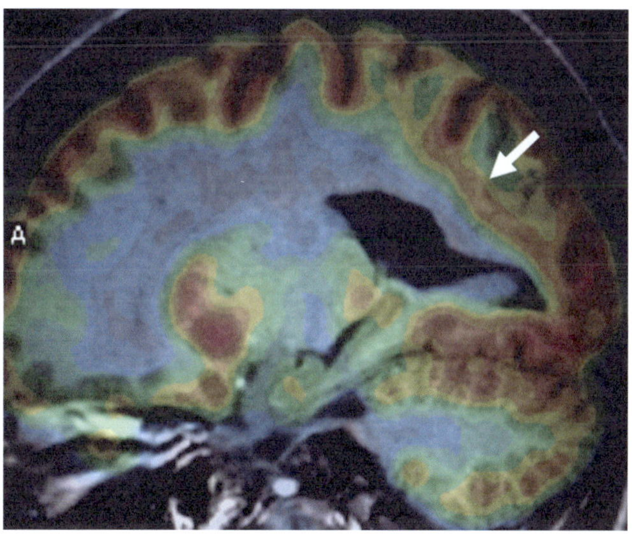

Fig. 19.6 PET-MRI co-registration with color-scale FDG tracer in a sagittal plane at a left thalamic level similar to Fig. 19.1. Gray matter metabolism is evident as a subcortical band (arrow) with a metabolic signal that is slightly less than the cortex. Because of the PET spatial resolution, the band has the false appearance of being contiguous with the cortex

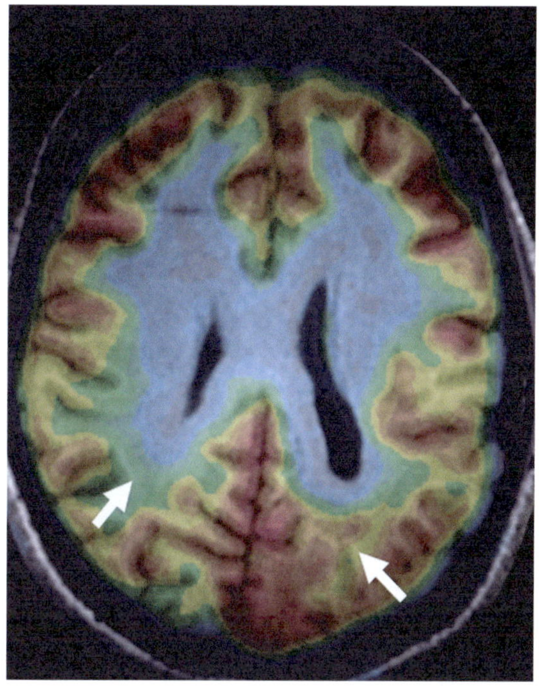

Fig. 19.7 PET-MRI co-registration with color-scale FDG tracer in an axial plane at a corpus callosum level superior to Fig. 19.2. The left parietal heterotopia (arrow) has a metabolic signal that is close to the signal of the cortex and, because of the PET's spatial resolution, appears to be part of the cortex. The image does not accurately differentiate the two. The right parietal heterotopia (arrow) has a lower signal than the cortex and appears as an extension of the cortex with lower metabolic signal. The lateral cortex at the parietal-occipital junction is abnormally hypometabolic, as compared to the left frontal cortex and right parietal-occipital cortex, indicating abnormality beyond the band heterotopia

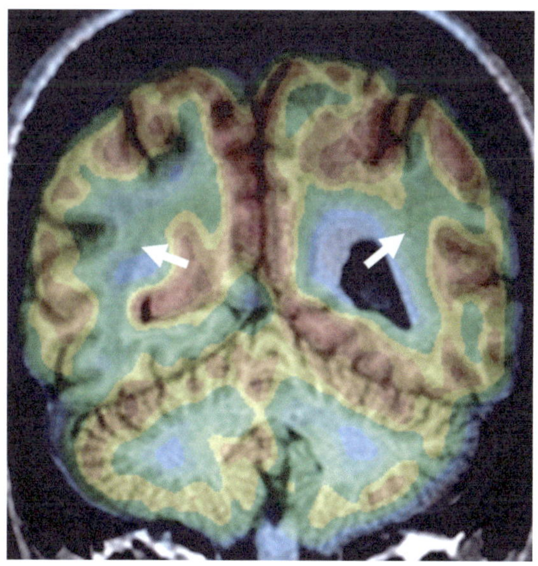

Fig. 19.8 PET-MRI co-registration with color-scale FDG tracer in a coronal plane at an atrium of the lateral ventricles level similar to Fig. 19.4. The band heterotopia's metabolic signal is similar bilaterally (arrows), but the signal within the left heterotopia is more heterogeneous. In the left heterotopia's superior aspect, the metabolic signal includes portions that are similar to normal neocortex. The right occipital lobe's inferior cortex is abnormally hypometabolic and indicates additional abnormality beyond the band heterotopia

20 Heterotopia Within Cerebral White Matter

Clinical History

The first recognized seizure occurred at age 16 years as a collapse with loss of consciousness, but other episodes of loss of consciousness occurred since age 9 years and the aura preceding these episodes occurred since age 6 years.

The habitual seizures were similar to the ones that occurred in childhood and adolescence. An aura experienced as a stereotyped achy somatosensory experience across the right face and scalp preceded some seizures and also occurred in isolation. In particular, the aura preceded the seizures that manifested as a lapse in awareness and responsiveness with oral automatisms and sometimes also left arm tonic posturing. These seizures lasted 10 to 60 seconds. Seizures that manifested as bilateral tonic-clonic convulsions did not followed the aura, and they were more likely to be nocturnal. Historically, the focal seizures with impaired awareness occurred between several weekly and several monthly. The bilateral tonic-clonic seizures were much less frequent.

An epilepsy risk factor was not present.

Neurological examination was normal. Neuropsychological testing identified normal performance overall with verbal memory that was superior to nonverbal memory.

Interictal EEG depicted multiple, bilaterally independent, temporal epileptiform sharp waves. Video-EEG monitoring recorded auras in isolation, and they did not have an epileptiform EEG correlate. Focal seizures with progression to bilateral tonic-clonic convulsions had broad EEG onsets with some occurring across the right temporal region and others across the left temporal region. MEG depicted a few, scattered epileptiform discharges over left anterior and mid-temporal region and, independently, a tight cluster of epileptiform discharges over right anterior, middle, and posterior temporal and adjacent parietal regions.

MRI identified extensive polymicrogyria of the right parietal and temporal lobes with periventricular heterotopia across right lateral ventricle and extension to the right parahippocampal gyrus. PET identified diffuse, patchy hypometabolism of right cerebral cortex. An intracarotid amobarbital test identified left hemispheric dominance for language and bilaterally intact episodic memory function.

The seizure manifestation and imaging abnormalities suggest epilepsy with a localization in the region of the right temporal and parietal lobes. The somatosensory aura's headache aspect may be consistent with both a limbic and a parietal localization, and the left-sided posturing, diminished nonverbal memory, and MEG dipole clustering suggest the right-sided lateralization. The occurrence of impaired awareness and automatisms and left-sided posturing suggests progression into the limbic system, but the imaging indicates a larger epileptogenic region. However, the scalp ictal EEG recordings raised concern for bilateral epilepsy.

To narrow the localization in consideration of epilepsy surgery, video-EEG monitoring was repeated after implantation of bilateral depth electrodes within bilateral temporal and parietal lobes. Habitual seizures were recorded with slightly differing ictal onsets. Some seizures had onsets at the right mesial entorhinal and amygdala contacts, and some had onsets at the right mesial entorhinal contacts without the amygdala contacts and with greater involvement of the right posterior temporal contacts.

Overall, the diagnostic evaluation indicated right temporal lobe epilepsy with an unusually larger distribution. Based on this, a right temporal lobe resection was performed with extension posteriorly beyond the typical margins for mesial temporal lobe epilepsy. The patient understood that including the mesial temporal structures would likely improve the seizure control, but it also would compromise nonverbal memory function. Histopathological examination identified focal cortical dysplasia, type IIa.

Seizure control improved postoperatively to one monthly for 12 months, and then seizure freedom was present for 1 year until anti-seizure medications were missed. Since then, treatment has been consistent, and seizure freedom has been present for 2.5 years. Neuropsychological testing at 2.5 years after surgery identified a new nonverbal memory deficit and no other clinically relevant change.

J. M. Stern, N. Salamon, *Imaging of Epilepsy*, https://doi.org/10.1007/978-3-030-86672-3_20

Imaging

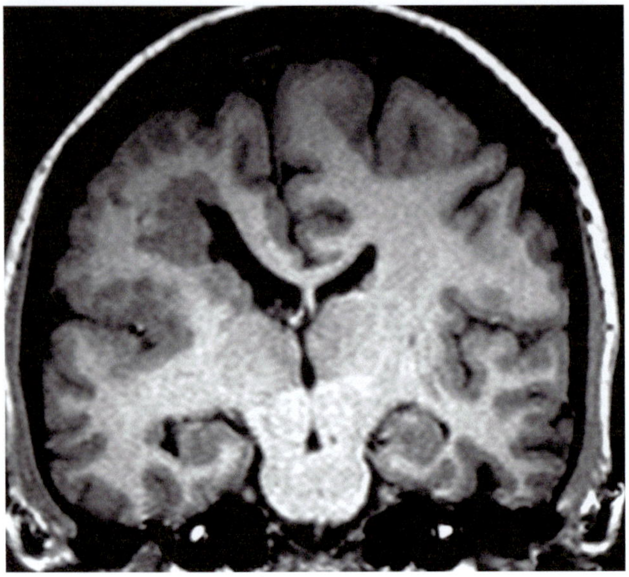

Fig. 20.1 MRI coronal T1 sequence at a hippocampal body level. Conglomerated heterotopic gray matter are present in the right periventricular region with enlargement and deformation of the right lateral ventricle. The right Sylvian cortex is abnormal due to polymicrogyria. Smaller periventricular heterotopic gray matter is present along the right temporal horn. The hippocampi are normal

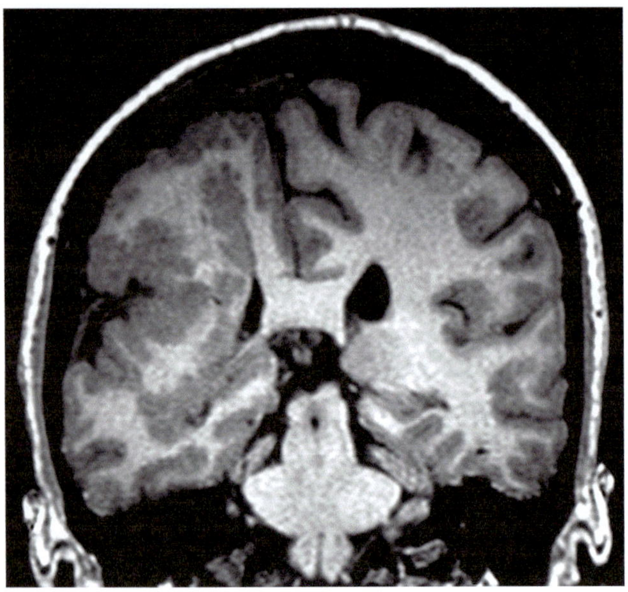

Fig. 20.2 MRI coronal T1 sequence at a splenium of the corpus callosum level. Extensive periventricular heterotopic gray matter projects superiorly and extends along wall of right lateral ventricle. Perisylvian polymicrogyria are present with an open Sylvian fissure. Sulcation of the posterior temporal lobe also is abnormal. Thickened cortex of left Sylvian fissure is normal gyral anatomy, and its appearance is related to the imaging plane and volume averaging

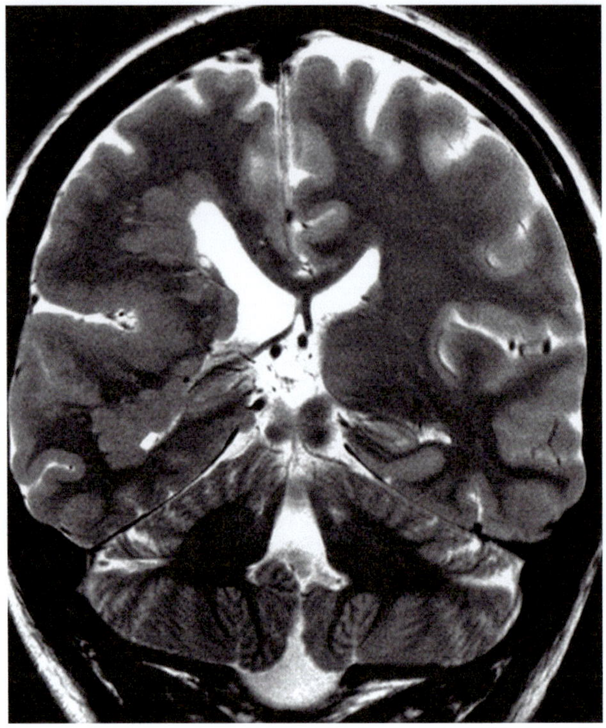

Fig. 20.3 MRI coronal T2 sequence at a collicular level between Figs. 20.1 and 20.2. Right periventricular heterotopic gray matter is present along the margin of right lateral ventricle and includes the inferior region near the trigone. The heterotopia is associated with ventricular deformity. Polymicrogyria is present along the posterior Sylvian fissure. The left hemisphere is normal

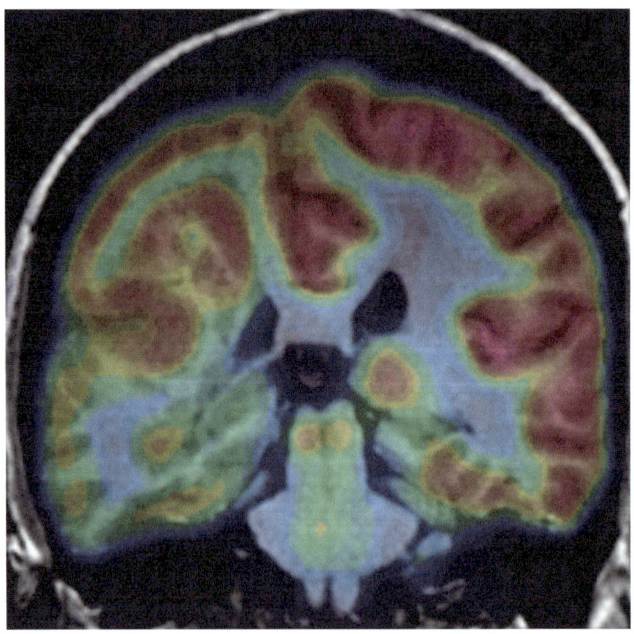

Fig. 20.4 PET-MRI co-registration with color-scale FDG tracer in a coronal plane at the same level as Fig. 20.2. The right hemisphere is diffusely hypometabolic with relatively greater metabolism in the superior portion of the gray matter heterotopia. The temporal lobe portion of the heterotopia is more hypometabolic than the superior portion. Similarly, the right temporal neocortex is more hypometabolic than the right frontal lobe. Metabolism of the left hemisphere, including the left thalamus, is normal. The right thalamus is not visible because of the level position and anterior displacement of the right thalamus

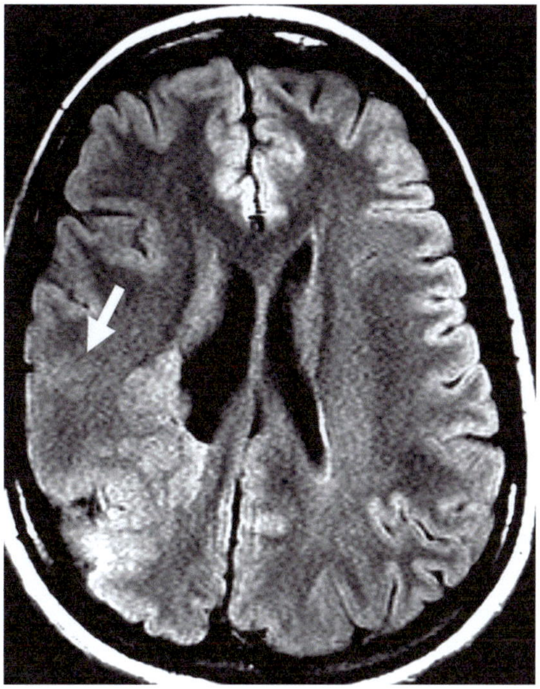

Fig. 20.5 MRI axial FLAIR sequence at a lateral ventricles level. The right ventricle is enlarged with multi-lobulated, extensive heterotopic gray matter along the posterior-lateral aspect of right ventricle. Polymicrogyria is evident along the lateral surface of the right frontal lobe, lateral to the heterotopic gray matter. Regions of more subtle heterotopia (arrow) are evident between the ventricular surface and cerebral surface

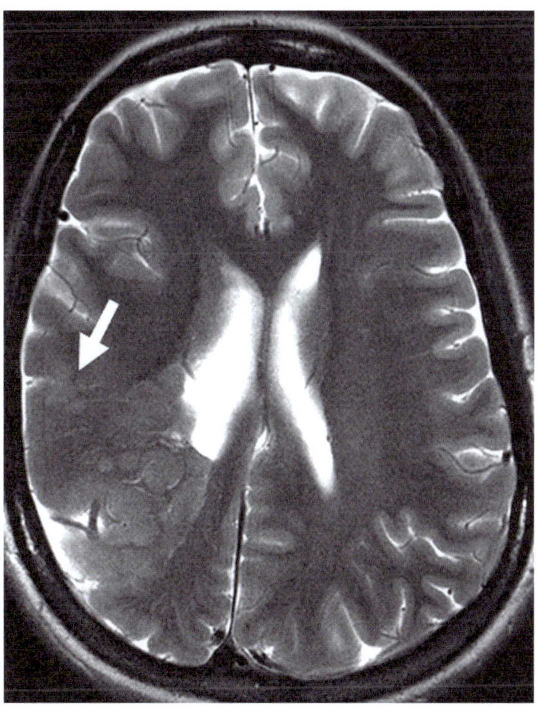

Fig. 20.6 MRI axial T2 sequence at the same level as Fig. 20.5. The findings are similar to Fig. 20.5, but the difference in imaging sequence produces differences in signal. The T2 sequence produces greater anatomic detail, but the heterotopia does not differ as much in signal intensity from the surrounding white matter. For both T2 and FLAIR sequences, the heterotopia signal is similar to cerebral cortex gray matter

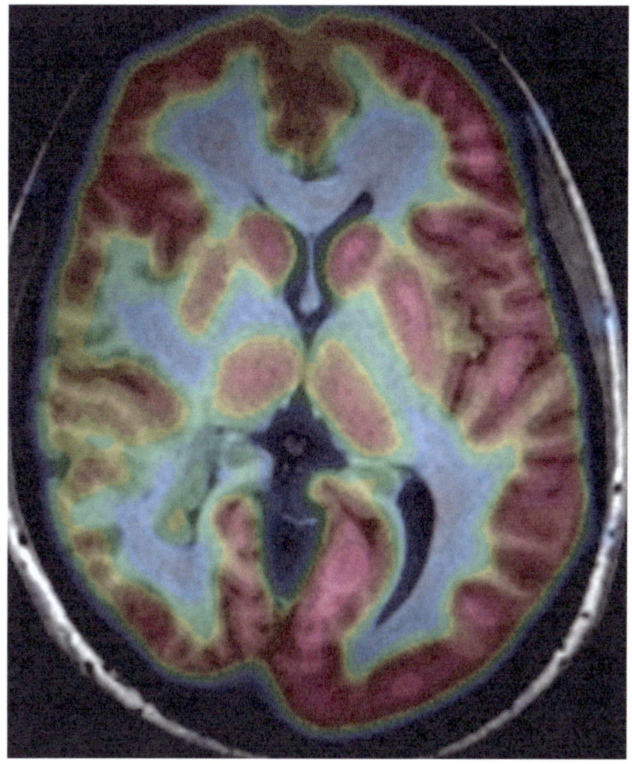

Fig. 20.7 PET-MRI co-registration with color-scale FDG tracer in an axial plane at an insula level. Periventricular heterotopic gray matter is evident as metabolic signal along the ventricular atrium. The cerebral cortex along the posterior frontal and parietal lobes is clearly hypometabolic when compared to the contralateral, homotopic cortex. The right thalamus is anteriorly displaced, as was seen in Fig. 20.4, but it is otherwise normal. Right cerebral hemispheric atrophy is evident at this level

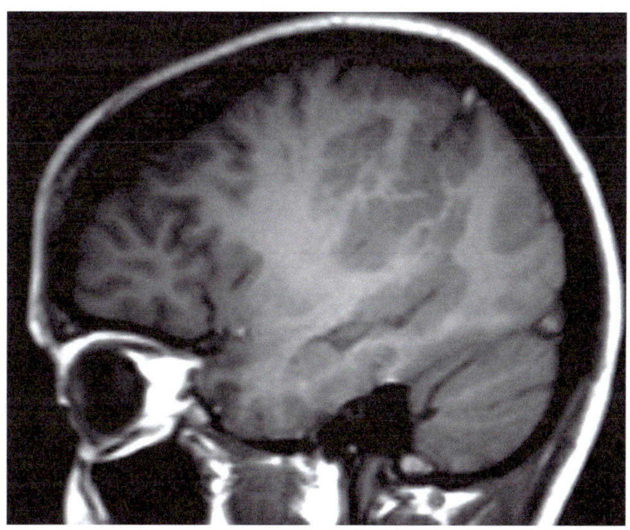

Fig. 20.8 MRI parasagittal T1 sequence at a right hippocampus level. The parietal lobe demonstrates abnormal sulcation with polymicrogyria and multi-lobulated gray matter heterotopia in the white matter. Periventricular heterotopic gray matter is evident along temporal horn of the right lateral ventricle. A parietal cleft is present at the cerebral surface level of the heterotopia

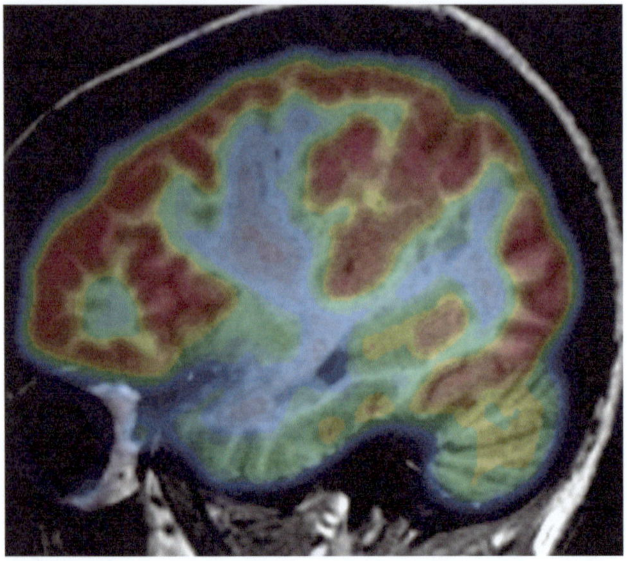

Fig. 20.9 PET-MRI co-registration with color-scale FDG tracer in a parasagittal plane at a right hippocampus level similar to Fig. 20.8. Metabolic signal is normal for gray matter within the large parietal heterotopia. Hypometabolism is evident in the periventricular heterotopia along the temporal horn. The temporal lobe also is hypometabolic

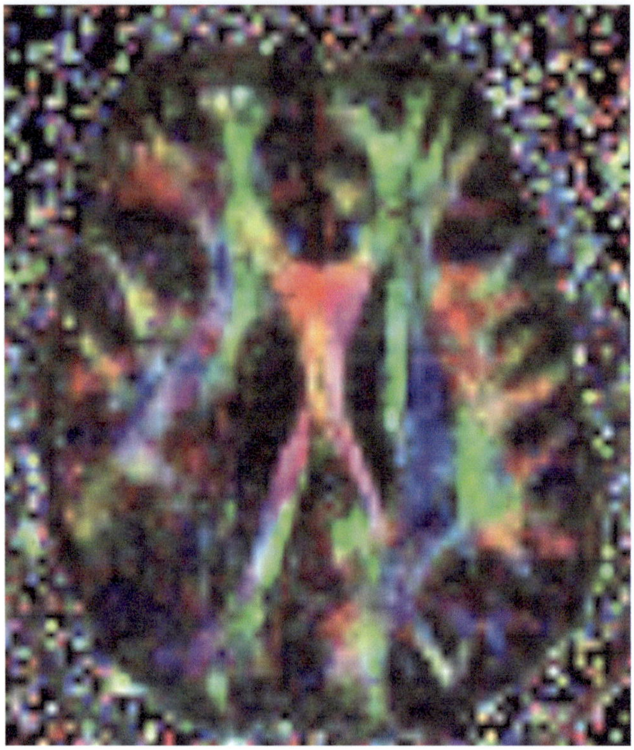

Fig. 20.10 MRI with axial diffusion tensor imaging at a corpus callosum level. The right parietal region has loss of normal white matter organization that co-localizes with the right periventricular gray matter heterotopia

21 Polymicrogyria Without Schizencephaly

Clinical History

The first recognized seizure occurred at age 12 years as a gustatory hallucination of a metallic taste followed by a loss of consciousness.

The habitual seizures occurred since age 12 years and reliably followed the gustatory hallucination aura. They were manifested as lapses in awareness and responsiveness with impairment of speech and left-hand motor ability for several seconds. The aura never occurred in isolation. Some seizures progressed to left arm jerking, but seizures that progress to tonic-clonic convulsions were rare with eight in total. Treatment included multiple anti-seizure medications with a seizure frequency of four weekly.

The epilepsy risk factor was a family history of seizures. Neurological examination was significant for a left pronator drift with mildly decreased left-hand fine finger movements. Neuropsychological testing identified reduced visuospatial organization and impaired set shifting with impaired ability to block distracters.

Interictal EEG depicted abnormal slowing in the right posterior temporal region and epileptiform discharges across the right posterior temporal and parietal region or simultaneously across bilateral posterior temporal and parietal regions. Video-EEG monitoring recorded focal seizures manifested as non-versive head turning to the right followed by versive movement to the left with left face contraction and left arm jerking prior to bilateral tonic-clonic movements. Postictal confusion was not present when seizures ended prior to the bilateral tonic-clonic activity. Ictal EEG's seizure onset was across the right central-temporal region.

MRI identified polymicrogyria within the right frontal operculum with architectural distortion of the underlying white matter. PET was normal. MEG identified a cluster of epileptiform dipoles across the right temporal, central-frontal, and parietal regions.

The history and evaluation indicate right neocortical epilepsy with propagation into the limbic and motor systems. In particular, the immediate return to normal mentation postictally supports the neocortical onset despite the gustatory hallucination aura.

Because of the extensive region of structural abnormality and possibility of co-localized function, subdural grid electrodes were placed for mapping of function and seizure onset. Coverage included a grid across the right posterior frontal, anterior parietal, and superior temporal regions and strips across the regions superior, posterior, and inferior to the grid. Based on the subdural recordings, a right parietal-temporal resection was performed. Histopathological examination identified polymicrogyria and mild disorganization of the cortical lamination. Long-term postoperative seizure control is not known at this time.

J. M. Stern, N. Salamon, *Imaging of Epilepsy*, https://doi.org/10.1007/978-3-030-86672-3_21

Imaging

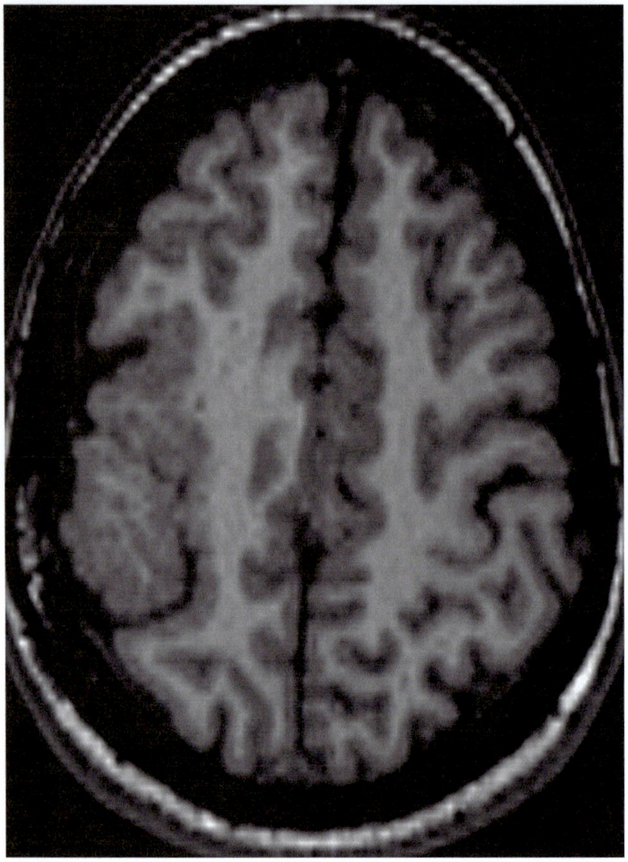

Fig. 21.1 MRI axial T1 sequence at a centrum semi-ovale level. Polymicrogyria along the surface of the right frontal and parietal lobes is evident in the distorted cortical ribbon and abnormal sulcation. The right central sulcus is abnormally oriented with a turn into the anterior to posterior direction

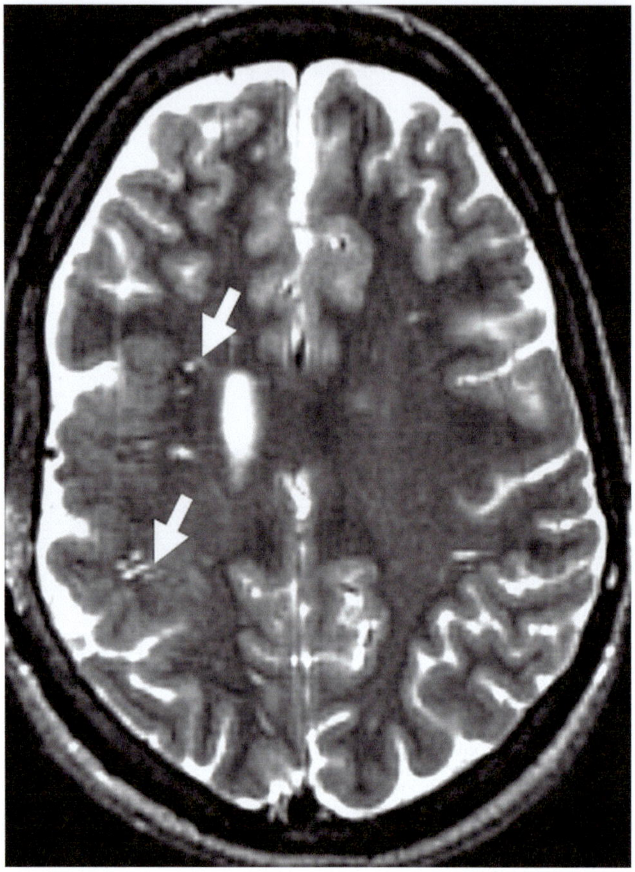

Fig. 21.2 MRI axial T2 sequence at a central semi-ovale level that is slightly inferior to Fig. 21.1 and tilted to include the superior portion of the right lateral ventricle. Polymicrogyria is present in the right frontal and parietal operculum. Small gyri are less visible with this sequence, so the cortex appears thicker than with a T1 sequence. Prominent perivascular spaces (arrows) are more apparent because of their high T2 signal

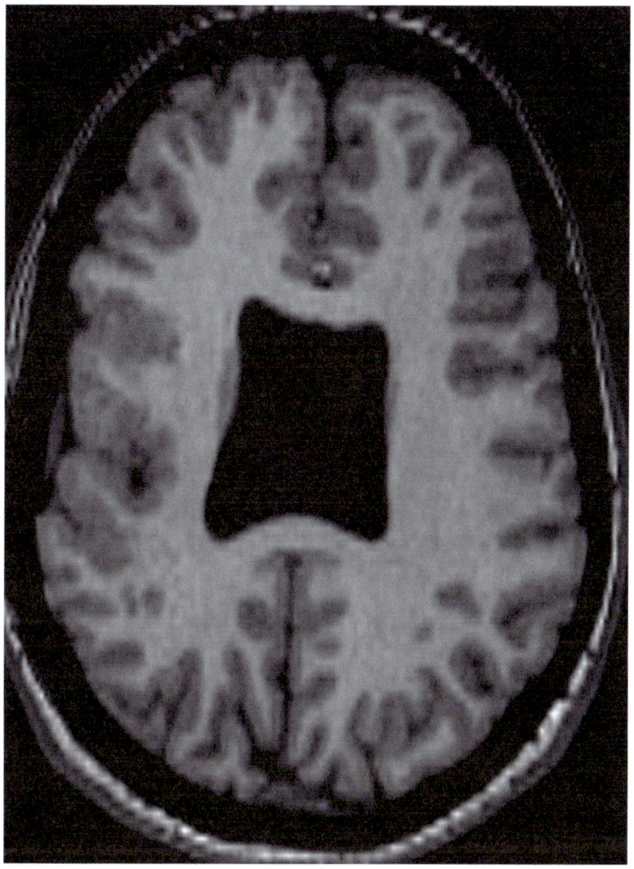

Fig. 21.3 MRI axial T1 sequence at a lateral ventricle level. The septum pellucidum is absent, and the lateral ventricles have a rectangular distortion. Widespread polymicrogyria is present across the right opercular region. The cortex within the polymicrogyria is thickened with multiple small gyri, but the gray-white junction is normal

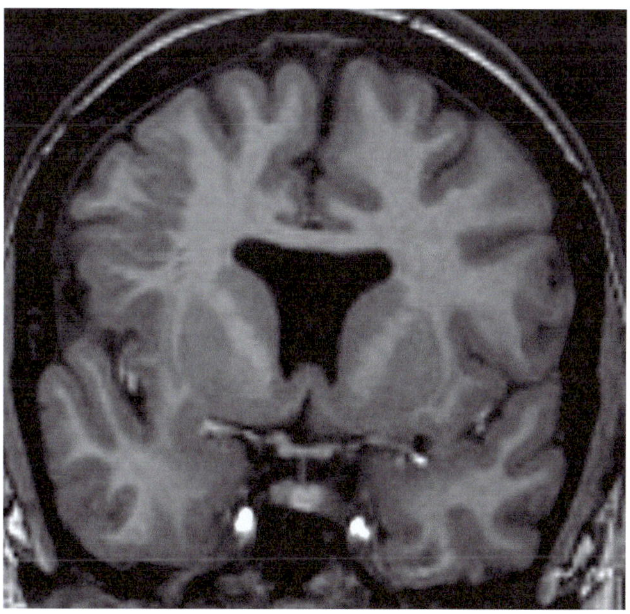

Fig. 21.4 MRI coronal T1 sequence at an optic chiasm level. The septum pellucidum is absent, and polymicrogyria is evident across the right frontal opercular region. The right superior frontal gyrus is normal. The polymicrogyria begins in within the right middle frontal gyrus and extends to include the right inferior frontal gyrus. The temporal lobes are normal bilaterally at this level

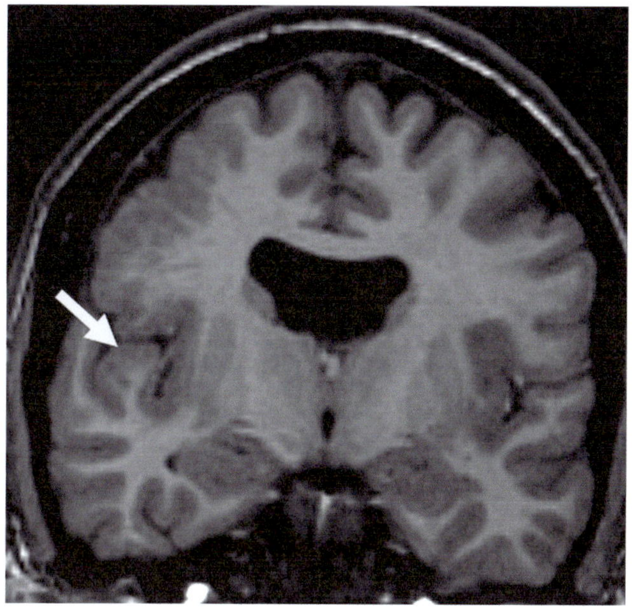

Fig. 21.5 MRI coronal T1 sequence at a hippocampal head level. Similar to the more anterior level in Fig. 21.3, the polymicrogyria is present throughout the right middle frontal gyrus and continues to include the inferior frontal gyrus. However, Heschl's gyrus (arrow) also demonstrates polymicrogyria. The remainder of the temporal lobe is normal

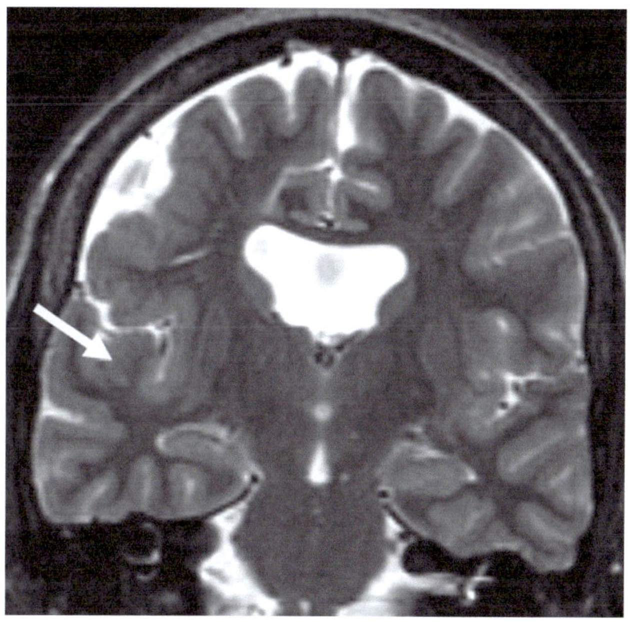

Fig. 21.6 MRI coronal T2 sequence at an anterior hippocampus level that is slightly posterior to Fig. 21.5. Polymicrogyria begins in the right middle frontal gyrus and extends inferiorly to the frontal operculum and involves Heschl's gyrus (arrow). The right insular is distorted with a straightening of the normal curvature. The normal insula curvature is evident on the left

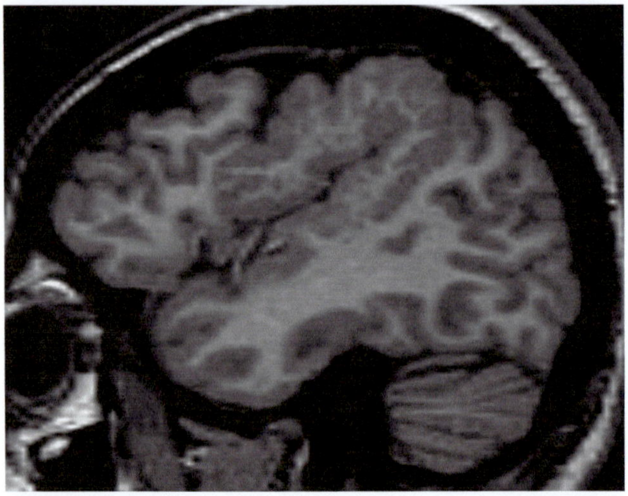

Fig. 21.7 MRI right parasagittal T1 sequence at a perisylvian level. Polymicrogyria is evident along the margins of the Sylvian fissure with involvement of the frontal and parietal opercula and the posterior portion of the superior temporal gyrus. Thickened cortex with multiple smaller gyri is visible within each gyrus

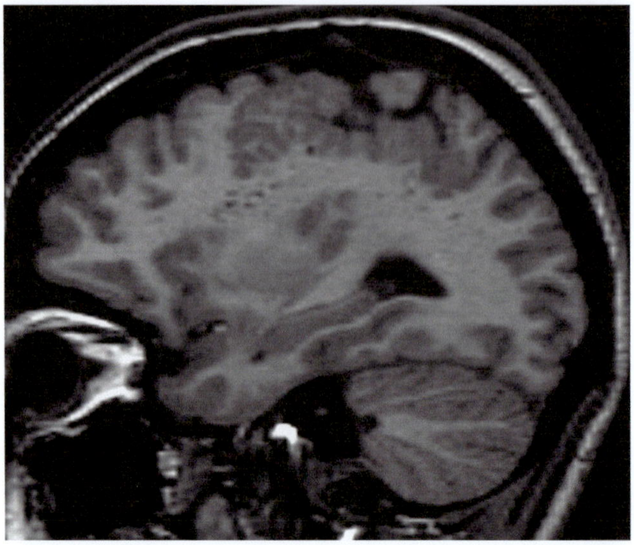

Fig. 21.8 MRI right parasagittal T1 sequence at an insula level that is medial to the level in Fig. 21.7. The right frontal and parietal cortex are distorted in the region of the central sulcus with prominent perivascular spaces in the subcortical white matter. At this level, the temporal lobe is normal

22 Polymicrogyria with Closed-Lip Schizencephaly

Clinical History

The first recognized seizure occurred at age 12 years as loss of awareness with bilateral movements that lasted 2 minutes and resolved without postictal confusion.

The habitual seizures were identical to the first seizure for several years until a new seizure manifestation presented at age 27 years. The new seizure produced sensory loss across the right arm and leg followed by jerking of the right leg and then a sudden fall with bilateral tonic posturing. Awareness and subsequent recall were not altered during the seizure, and postictal confusion was not present. The total seizure duration was unchanged at 2 minutes. Treatment included multiple anti-seizure medications with a seizure frequency of three to four seizures over several days every few weeks to months.

The epilepsy risk factor was a family history. The patient's mother has seizures with a sensory aura that progressesed to bilateral tonic activity without loss of awareness. Her diagnostic evaluation results are not known.

Neurological examination was normal.

Interictal EEG depicted generalized slowing and focal epileptiform discharges over the right mid-frontal and left mid-temporal regions. The interictal EEG also included bursts of evolving, central sharp waves in runs that lasted several seconds. Video-EEG monitoring recorded right arm myoclonic jerks and bilateral tonic-clonic seizures. Both the myoclonus and the tonic-clonic seizures had seizure onsets of repetitive focal discharges over the left frontal-central region.

MRI identified a closed-lip schizencephaly extending from the left lateral ventricular body to the overlying posterior frontal lobe. Extensive abnormal thickening of the gray matter was present along the margins of the cleft and the adjacent frontal and parietal lobes. Polymicrogyria across the frontal and parietal lobes also was present.

The history and evaluation indicate neocortical epilepsy localized to the left central region. This localization is supported by the manifestation as sudden unilateral or bilateral motor activity, clonus that produces falls, sudden resolution, and no ictal or postictal alteration of mentation. The localization also is evident in the focal EEG seizure onset and broad region of central epileptiform abnormality. The schizencephaly and polymicrogyria structural abnormality is a corresponding, relatively large region with epileptogenic potential. Despite the structural malformation, this patient's neurological exam is normal, as may occur with schizencephaly.

Because of the extensive, irregular cerebral surface and expected atypical functional organization, intracranial mapping for both function and epileptiform abnormality was recommended before an epilepsy surgery to maximize both the benefit and the safety. Based on patient preference, surgical evaluation and treatment were not undertaken.

J. M. Stern, N. Salamon, *Imaging of Epilepsy*, https://doi.org/10.1007/978-3-030-86672-3_22

Imaging

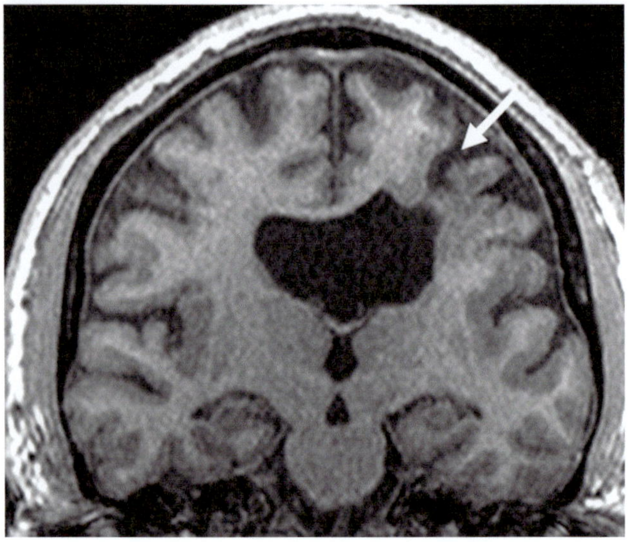

Fig. 22.1 MRI coronal T1 sequence at a hippocampal body level. A schizencephalic cleft is present lateral to the left superior frontal gyrus (arrow). Gray matter lines both banks of the cleft, which are in immediate opposition and extend to the ependymal surface with lateral ventricle communication. Abnormally increased gyral contouring is present along the left middle frontal gyrus, indicating polymicrogyria. The left lateral ventricle is deformed and a septum pellucidum is absent

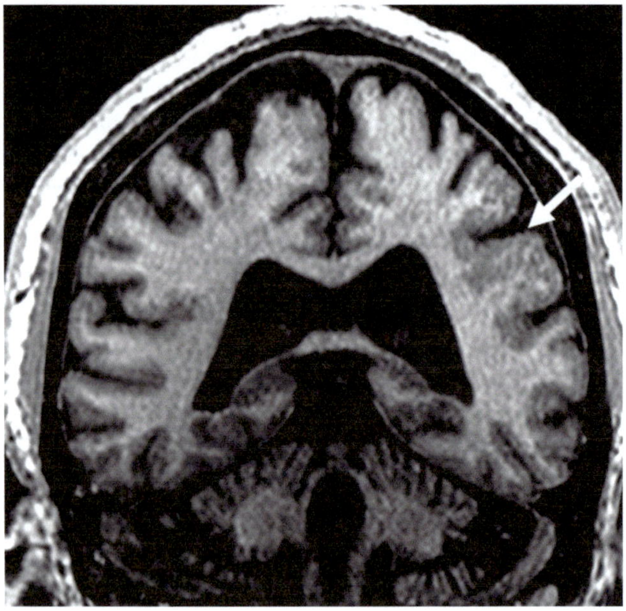

Fig. 22.2 MRI coronal T1 sequence at a trigone level. Increased gyral contouring is present across the supramarginal gyrus (arrow) with thickening of the cortical ribbon. A minor asymmetry of the lateral ventricles is present with a subtle enlargement of the left lateral ventricle

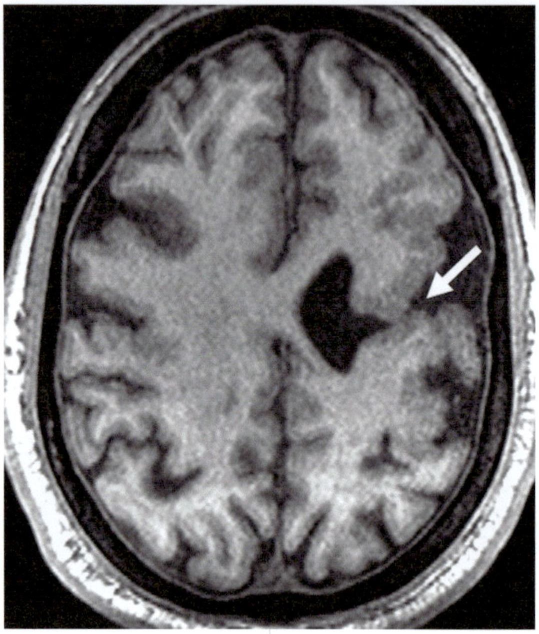

Fig. 22.3 MRI axial T1 sequence at a centrum semi-ovale level. The left lateral ventricle enlargement results in the ventricle's presence at this superior level. The ventricle's lateral margin is a continuation of the schizencephalic cleft (arrow), although communication to the cleft is not visible in this image. The lateral frontal lobe surface anterior and posterior to the cleft has polymicrogyria

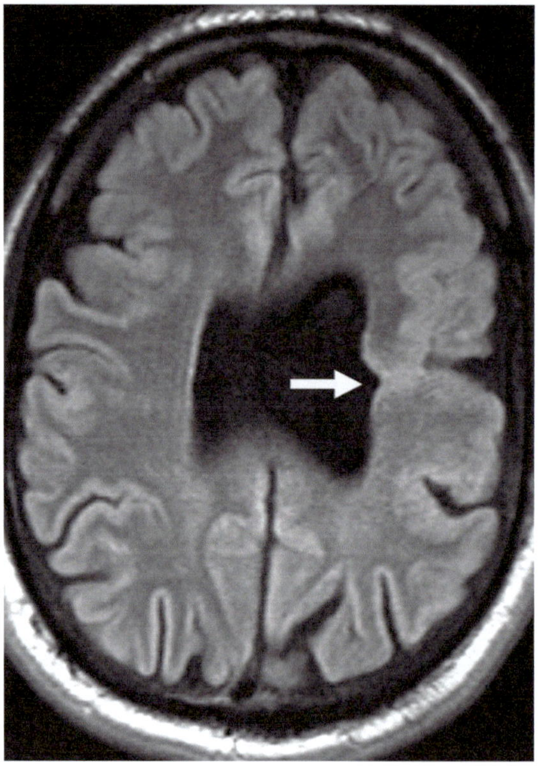

Fig. 22.4 MRI axial FLAIR sequence at a ventricular level slightly inferior to Fig. 22.3. Compared to Fig. 22.2, the two banks of the schizencephalic cleft are opposed over a greater dimension, and the cleft is not as deep. An indentation from the lateral ventricle toward the cleft is visible (arrow). Because FLAIR sequences do not provide as the anatomic detail of T1, the polymicrogyria posterior to the cleft is not as clearly evident

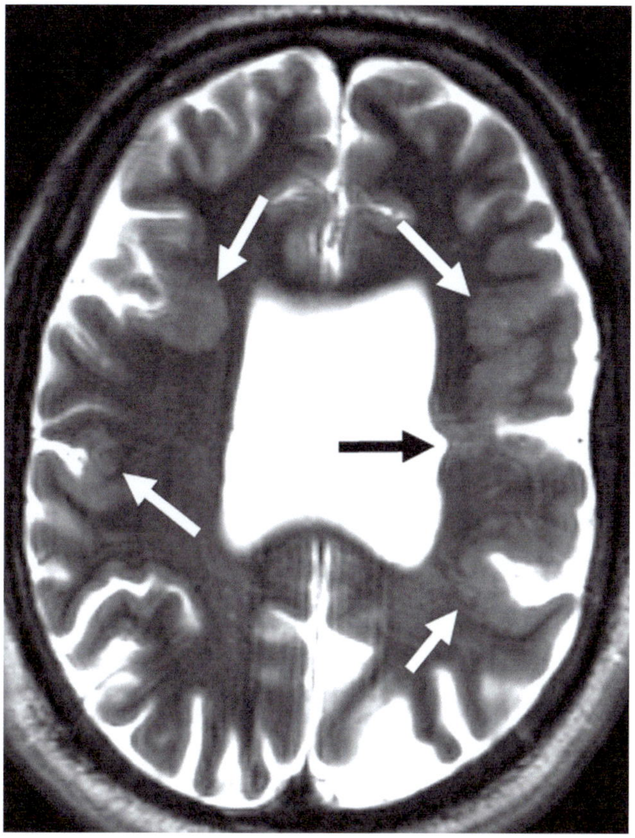

Fig. 22.5 MRI axial T2 sequence at a lower ventricular level slightly inferior to Fig. 22.4. The ventricular indentation that is the continuation of the cleft is evident (black arrow) without signal to indicate communication between the cleft and the lateral ventricle. An abnormally thickened cortical ribbon is present bilaterally in the frontal and parietal lobes (white arrows), indicating another malformation of cortical development manifestation

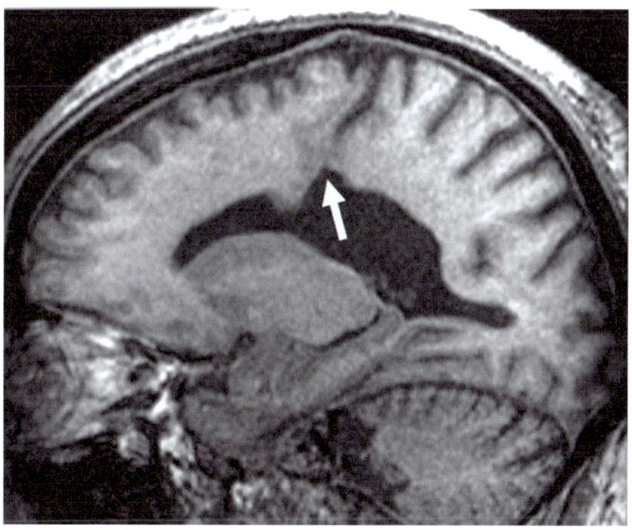

Fig. 22.6 MRI sagittal T1 sequence at a left lateral ventricular level. The deep schizencephalic cleft is evident a ventricular indentation (arrow) and gray matter along both the anterior and posterior banks

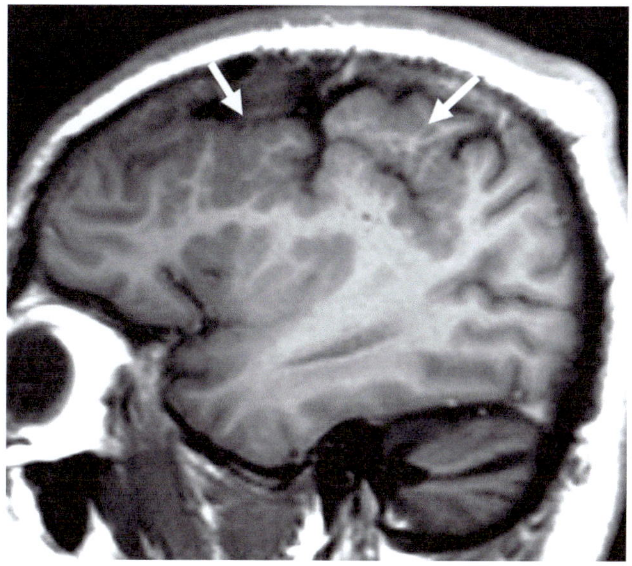

Fig. 22.7 MRI sagittal T1 sequence at a left insular level. Extensive polymicrogyria is evident across the frontal and parietal lobes around the schizencephalic cleft. In particular, the cortical ribbon is thickened with numerous microgyri along the surface (arrows)

23 Polymicrogyria with Open Lip Schizencephaly

Clinical History

The first recognized seizure occurred at age 11 years as an abnormal sensory experience across the left face and arm that progressed to forced gaze to the left and left-sided jerking. None of the seizures since age 12 years have included any motor features.

The habitual seizures manifested as tingling or numbness of the left face and arm with a typical duration of 5–10 seconds and maximum duration of 1 minute. The seizure frequency was twice weekly. Treatment included multiple anti-seizure medications without seizure freedom, but the seizures were not disabling.

The only identified epilepsy risk factor was cerebral palsy. Neurological examination identified bilateral dystonic posturing that was greater on the left and bilaterally increased deep tendon reflexes that also were greater on the left. Gait was mildly asymmetric due to left hemiparesis. Intellectual development was normal.

Interictal EEG at age 21 years identified epileptiform sharp discharges over the right temporal region and paroxysmal fast activity over a broad, right-sided distribution. Diffuse slowing also was present and was asymmetrically greater on the right. Video-EEG monitoring recorded focal seizures that were confirmed to be sensory experiences without impairment of awareness. Ictal EEG did not identify an epileptiform abnormality.

MRIs at age 11 years and at 22 years identified extensive polymicrogyria with an open lip schizencephaly on the right and a closed lip schizencephaly on the left. Cortical dysplasia was present within both frontal lobes cortex and extended on the right to the insula. Dysgenesis of the splenium of the corpus callosum also was present.

The history and evaluation indicate a focal epilepsy that is likely localized to the right central or insular region. An epileptogenic abnormality in either of these regions may produce a focal sensory experience, but propagation into either of these regions also is possible. However, the occurrence of the habitual seizures, without progression to motor features or impaired awareness, suggests a confined epileptogenic zone that is functionally isolated and smaller than the broad interictal abnormality evident with scalp EEG. The lack of an ictal pattern with scalp EEG is consistent with a confined, focal seizure that does not impair awareness, and it does not alter the epilepsy diagnosis. The cerebral malformation indicates a potential localization for the epileptogenic zone, but the localization is complicated by its extensive distribution and the likelihood of altered functional organization within it. Because the seizures are not disabling, intracranial evaluation was not undertaken, so a more detailed localization was not obtained.

J. M. Stern, N. Salamon, *Imaging of Epilepsy*, https://doi.org/10.1007/978-3-030-86672-3_23

Imaging

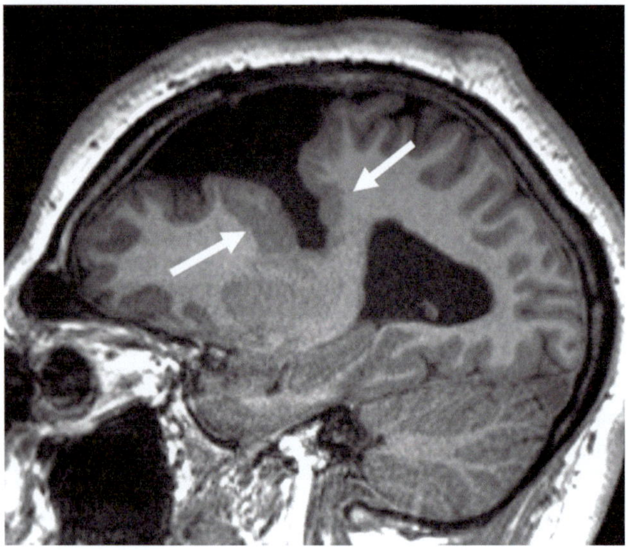

Fig. 23.1 MRI sagittal T1 sequence at a right hippocampus level. An open lip schizencephaly is evident as polymicrogyria (arrows) along the banks of a frontal lobe cleft with the absence of normal sulcation. As additional abnormalities, gray matter signal is present at the deepest portion of the cleft as a faint signal, and the trigone is abnormally enlarged. Sulcation is normal outside of the cleft, including the indentation across the anterior, superior frontal lobe

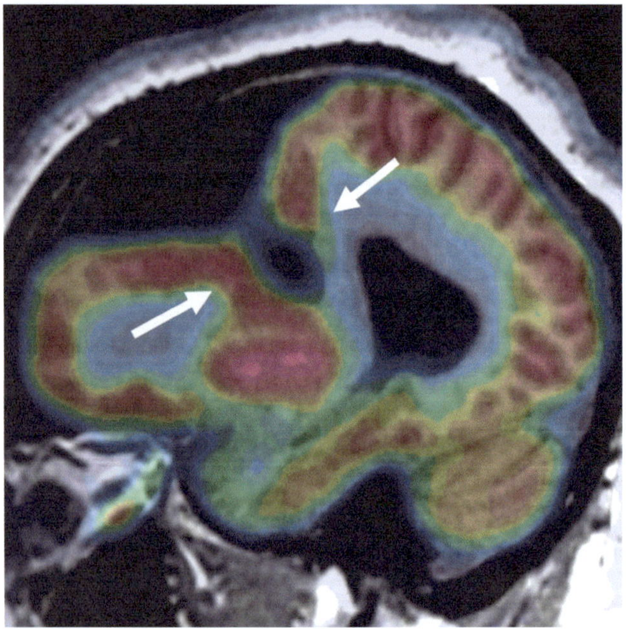

Fig. 23.2 PET-MRI co-registration with color-scale FDG tracer in a sagittal plane at the same level as Fig. 23.1. The posterior inferior portion of the frontal lobe cleft is abnormally hypometabolic. In contrast, the anterior, inferior, and posterior superior portions have normal metabolism, and this includes the gray matter that is faintly seen on the MRI at the deepest portion of the cleft. The temporal pole is also hypometabolic, and the remaining cortical metabolism is normal. The region of increased metabolism inferior to the cleft is normal basal ganglia

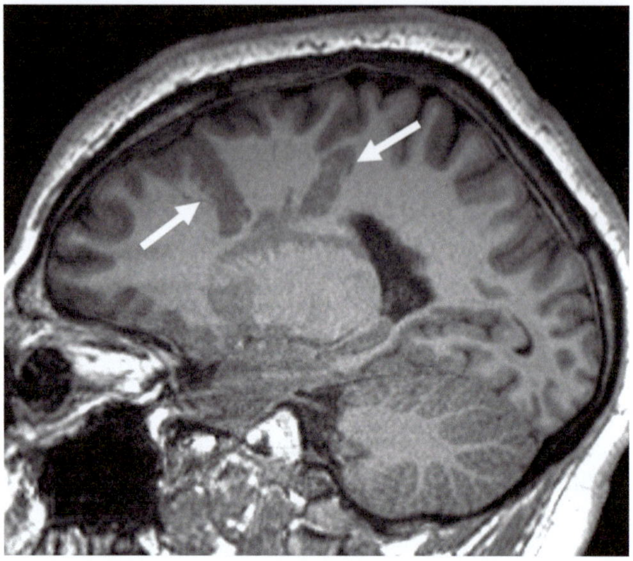

Fig. 23.3 MRI sagittal T1 sequence at a left hippocampus level. A closed lip schizencephaly is present in the frontal lobe (anterior arrow) with polymicrogyria along both the anterior and posterior aspects. A separate closed lip schizencephaly is present in the parietal lobe (posterior arrow). It also has polymicrogyria, but it does not reach the neocortical surface in this imaging level

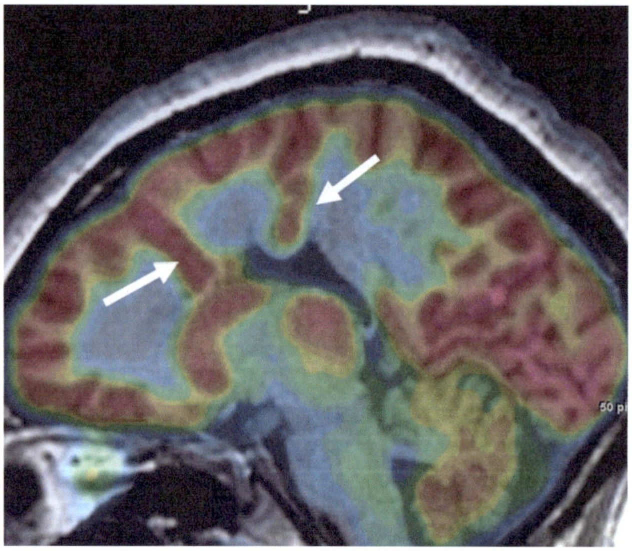

Fig. 23.4 PET-MRI co-registration with color-scale FDG tracer in a sagittal plane at the same level as Fig. 23.3. The polymicrogyria within both the frontal and parietal cleft has normal metabolism (arrows). Each of the two clefts appears as one region of metabolism because of the adjacency of each cleft's two opposing surfaces

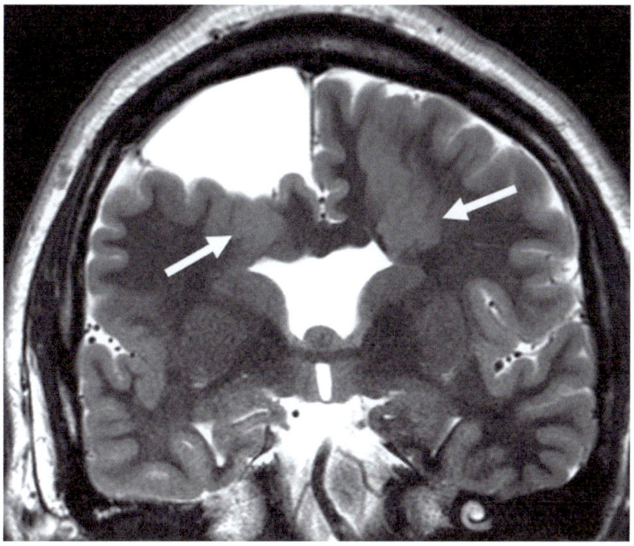

Fig. 23.5 MRI coronal T2 sequence at an anterior commissure level. Polymicrogyria with extension to the ependymal surfaces is present in both frontal lobes (arrows). The left frontal lobe cleft with its opposing polymicrogyria surfaces is not visible in this image, but faint contours are evident that suggest the gray matter is polymicrogyria. In addition, the frontal horns of the lateral ventricles have an atypical boxed shape and septum pellucidum is absent. The round structure at the base of the lateral ventricles is the fusion of the two fornices

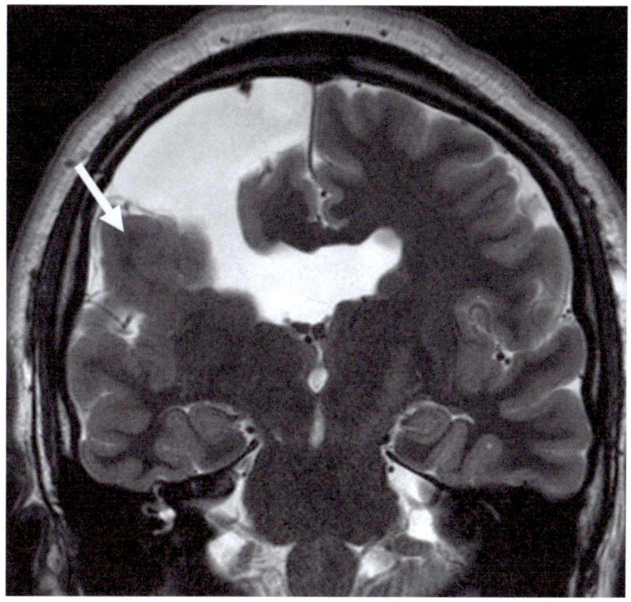

Fig. 23.7 MRI coronal T2 sequence at a body of the hippocampus level. Polymicrogyria is present along both aspects of the right frontal cleft with extension across the cleft's inferior border (arrow). Both temporal lobes and the left frontal lobe are normal

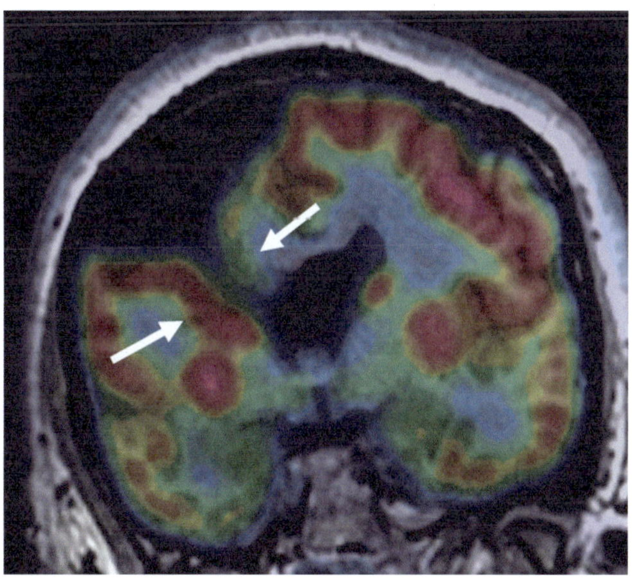

Fig. 23.6 PET-MRI co-registration with color-scale FDG tracer in a coronal plane at an anterior commissure level. Compared to Fig. 23.5, the plane is obliquely angled with the inferior portion more anterior and superior portion more posterior. The right frontal lobe schizencephaly has normal metabolism along the inferior cleft and hypometabolism along the superior cleft (arrows). The cleft in this level is contiguous with the right lateral ventricle. The left-sided polymicrogyria is not in this imaging level

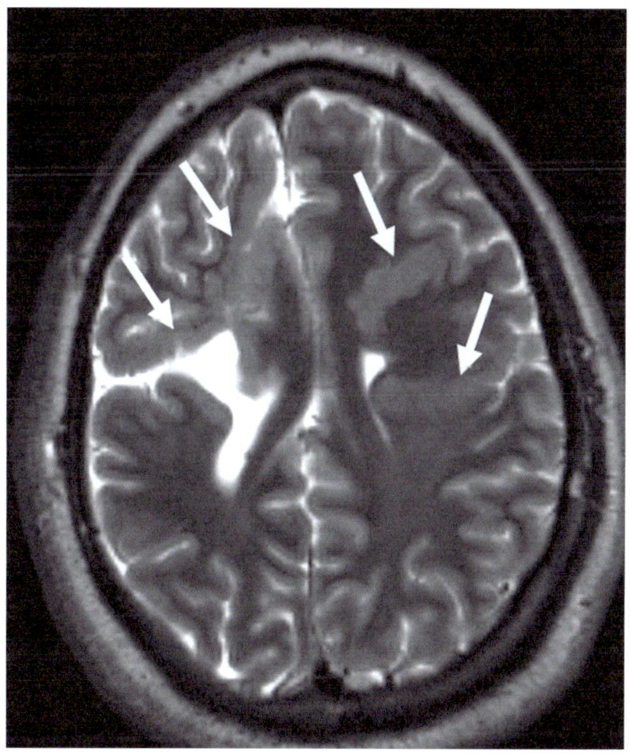

Fig. 23.8 MRI axial T2 sequence at a lateral ventricle level. Polymicrogyria is present in the right frontal lobe along the anterior aspect of the cleft and across the superior frontal gyrus (right-sided arrows). The cleft is contiguous with the right lateral ventricle. Polymicrogyria also is present in the left frontal lobe and is evident as two regions of gray matter signal that indicate two closed lip schizencephalies (left-sided arrows). The posterior left-sided cleft indents into the left lateral ventricle but is not contiguous with it. The posterior cerebral sulcation is normal

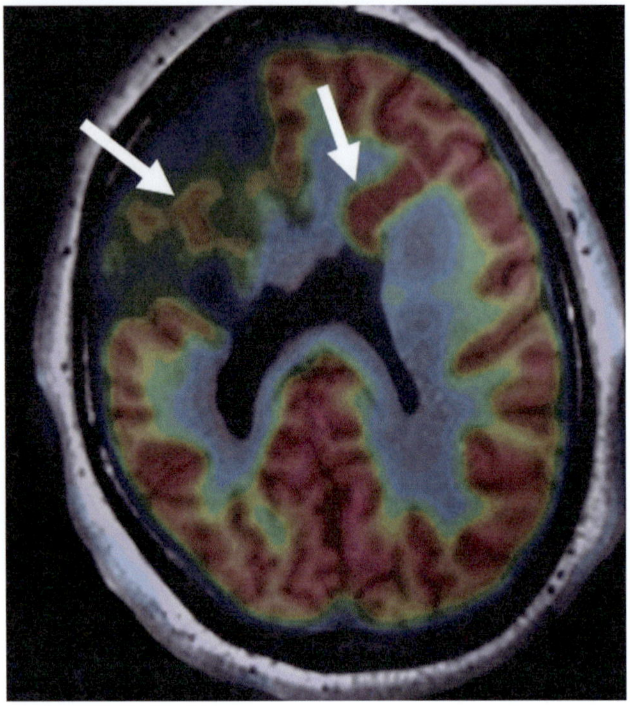

Fig. 23.9 PET-MRI co-registration with FDG tracer in an axial plane at level that is slightly inferior to the level in Fig. 23.8. Right frontal lobe polymicrogyria has heterogeneous metabolism (right-sided arrow) in the anterior cleft. The ametabolic region anterior to the cleft and lateral to the right superior frontal gyrus is the enlarged subarachnoid space that is evident in Fig. 23.1. Metabolism in the right frontal lobe's posterior cleft is normal. The left frontal lobe's anterior polymicrogyria (left-sided arrow) has normal metabolism. The posterior polymicrogyria is not visible in the level. The remaining left cerebral sulcation is normal

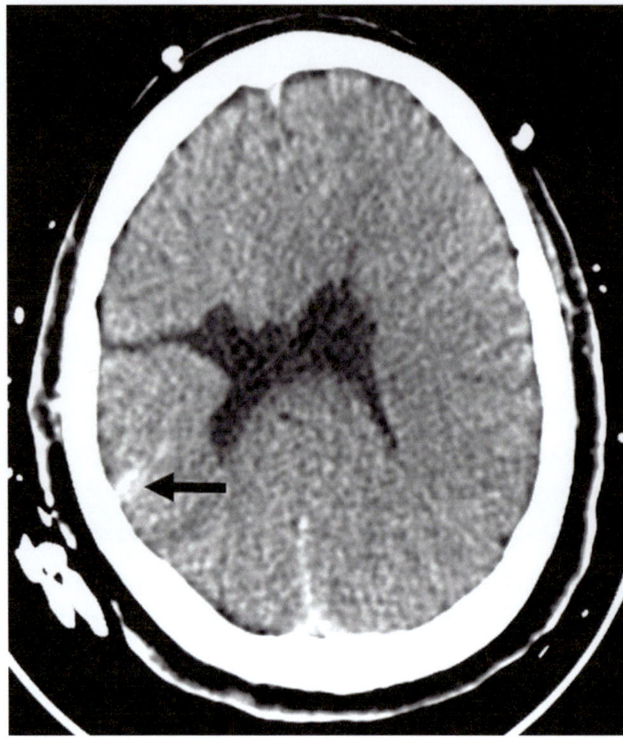

Fig. 23.10 CT axial plane at a level that is slightly inferior to Fig. 23.9. The lateral ventricles are distorted with abnormal continuity on the right with the subarachnoid space. The hyperdensity on the right (arrow) is artifact produced by EEG electrodes on the scalp. The cerebral density is normal bilaterally

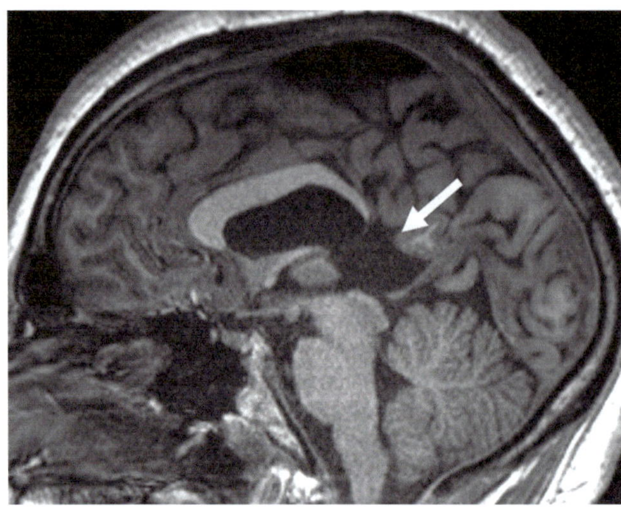

Fig. 23.11 MRI sagittal T1 sequence at a midline level. Dysgenesis of the splenium of the corpus callosum (arrow) is evident, as can occur with the absence of the septum pellucidum. The subarachnoid space at the superior convexity is abnormally enlarged

24 Lissencephaly

Clinical History

The first recognized seizure occurred at age 6 months with the occurrence of multiple infantile spasms during one night. Each spasm was manifested by sudden bilateral arm flexion, fist clenching, torso flexion, reddening of the face, and the appearance of being dazed. Treatment began at this time, but seizure control was not achieved despite corticosteroids and multiple anti-seizure medications. However, seizure control improved with intermittent periods of seizure freedom over the following years.

EEG and CT scan were obtained at the time of epilepsy onset. The EEG identified hypsarrhythmia with abnormal diffuse slowing and multifocal, independent spike discharges that were most prominent in the central regions and right temporal region. The CT identified a smooth cerebral surface with thickened cortex consistent with lissencephaly, type 1. MRI was then obtained, and it confirmed the diagnosis of lissencephaly, type 1, with identification of a smooth cerebral surface, pachygyria, and abnormal signal intensity within the white matter. Striated signal was present in the periventricular regions. No other abnormality was evident.

The identified epilepsy risk factor was Miller-Dieker syndrome with chromosomal screening identifying loss of the short arm of chromosome 17. Neurological examination was abnormal due to developmental delay that preceded the onset of epilepsy. At 6 months, rolling over and sitting had not been achieved, and there was no interest in toys. At age 5 years, there was no verbal ability, cooperation, reaching for objects, or walking. Plagiocephaly with a prominent forehead was evident on physical examination at age 7 months.

The history and evaluation indicate infantile spasms that are related to a diffuse cerebral malformation and generalized cerebral dysfunction. Medication-resistant seizures that do not demonstrate focal features, and diffuse intellectual disability are consistent with the diffuse, bilateral structural abnormality.

J. M. Stern, N. Salamon, *Imaging of Epilepsy*, https://doi.org/10.1007/978-3-030-86672-3_24

Imaging

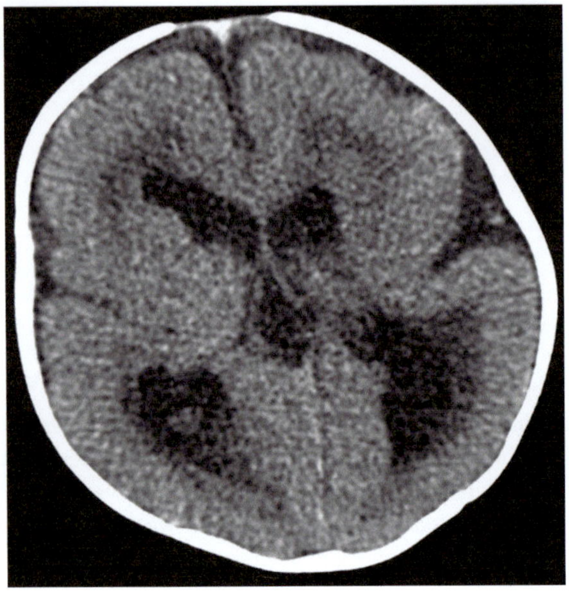

Fig. 24.1 CT axial plane at an atrium of the lateral ventricles level. The CT was obtained at age 6 months. Sulcation is not present other than the presence of the Sylvian fissures, which are simple oblique indentations. This maturational state would be normal for 16 to 17 weeks of gestation. Other findings are the thickened cortex and enlarged lateral and third ventricles. At this level, the smooth surface with two indentations and enlarged ventricles give the characteristic appearance of the number 8. The calcifications typical of a TORCH infection are not present

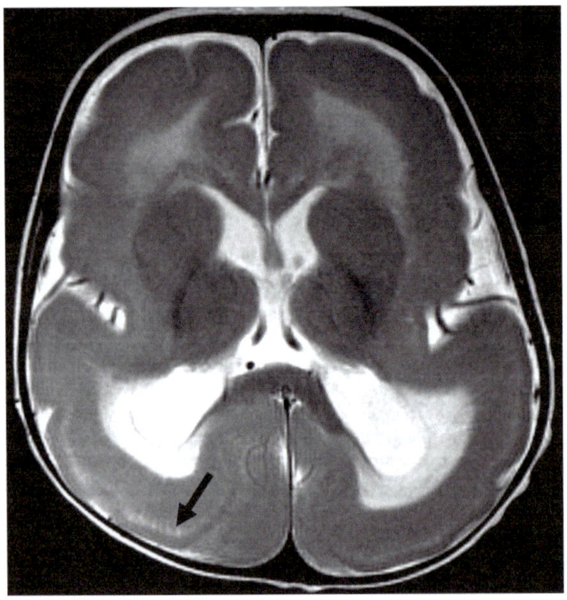

Fig. 24.2 MRI axial T2 sequence at a similar level as the CT in Fig. 24.1. The MRI was obtained at age 6 months, 1 week after the CT. The entirety of the cerebral surface is smooth with abnormally thickened cortex. The Sylvian fissures are atypical with an oblique orientation angled posteriorly. Corresponding to this, the insulae are evident anterior to the Sylvian fissures and along the cerebral surface that is coplanar to the frontal lobes. Subcortical, band heterotopic gray matter also is present, as is evident across bilateral temporal and occipital lobes (arrow)

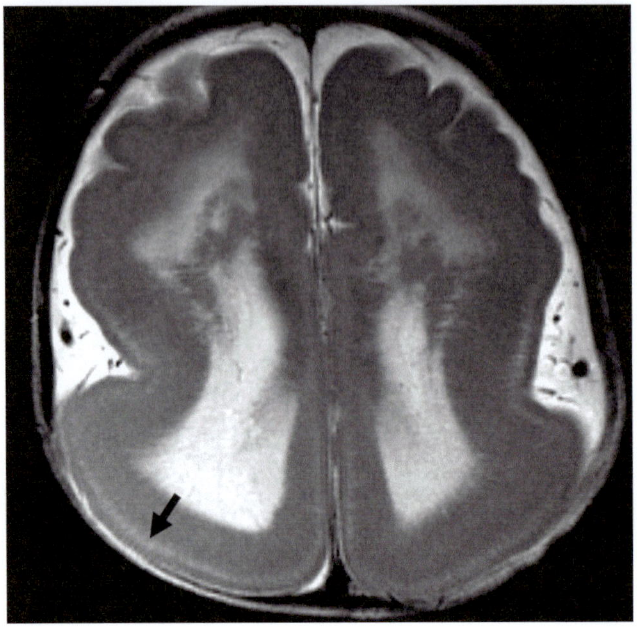

Fig. 24.3 MRI axial T2 sequence at a high ventricle level. The thickened cortex is present throughout the cerebrum with circumferential band heterotopia (arrow) across the posterior half bilaterally, including the parietal and posterior frontal lobes. The characteristic number 8 shape is less pronounced but still evident

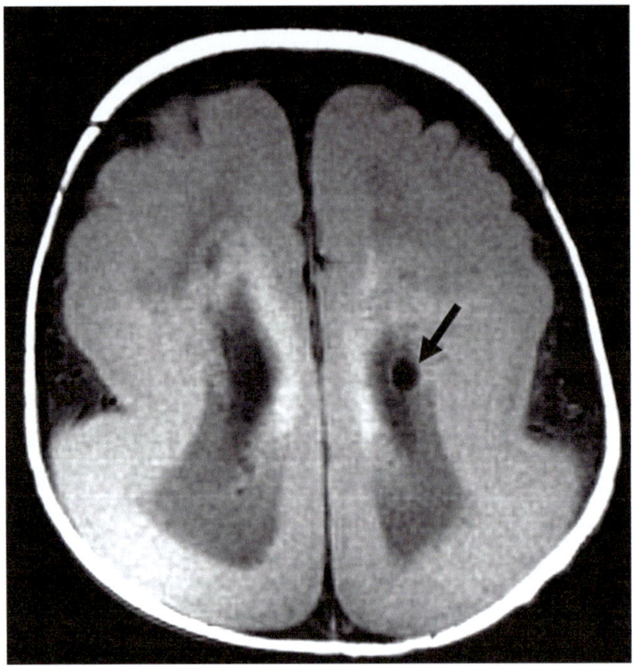

Fig. 24.4 MRI axial T1 sequence at a high ventricle level that is similar to Fig. 24.3. With the T1 sequence, the thickened cortex is visible, but the subcortical band heterotopia are not. Minor indentation is present across the anterior left frontal lobe, but it is not sufficiently deep to be normal sulcation. A connatal cyst is present lateral to the left lateral ventricle (arrow) and is a normal variant

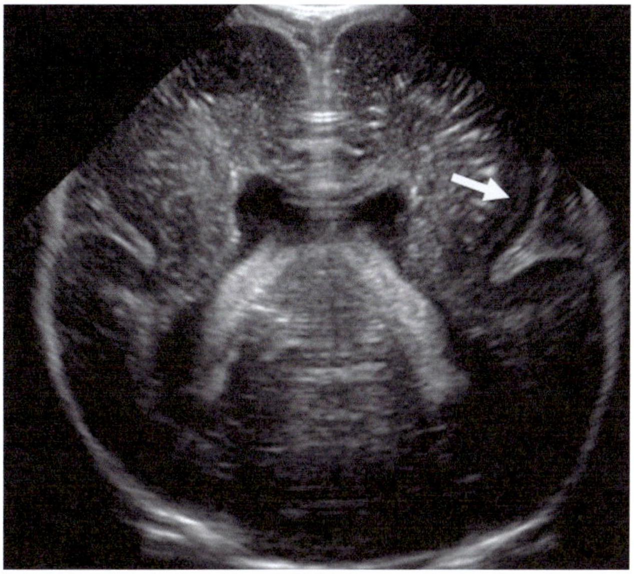

Fig. 24.5 Ultrasound coronal orientation at an atrium of the lateral ventricle level. The ultrasound was obtained at age 6 months, 1 week before the CT, to evaluate for hydrocephalus. Smooth cerebral surfaces are evident along with the obliquely oriented Sylvian fissures bilaterally. Subcortical band heterotopia are present bilaterally, and are more clearly seen on the left (arrow)

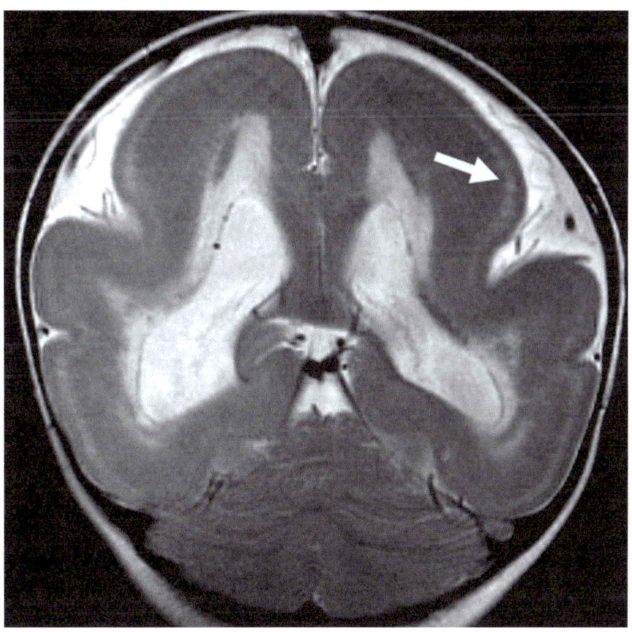

Fig. 24.6 MRI coronal T2 sequence at an atrium level that is similar to Fig. 24.5. The smooth cerebral surface with thickened cortex is evident. The subcortical band heterotopia is visible bilaterally, including frontal (arrow) and temporal lobes. The periventricular signal is normal white matter. The cerebellum also is normal

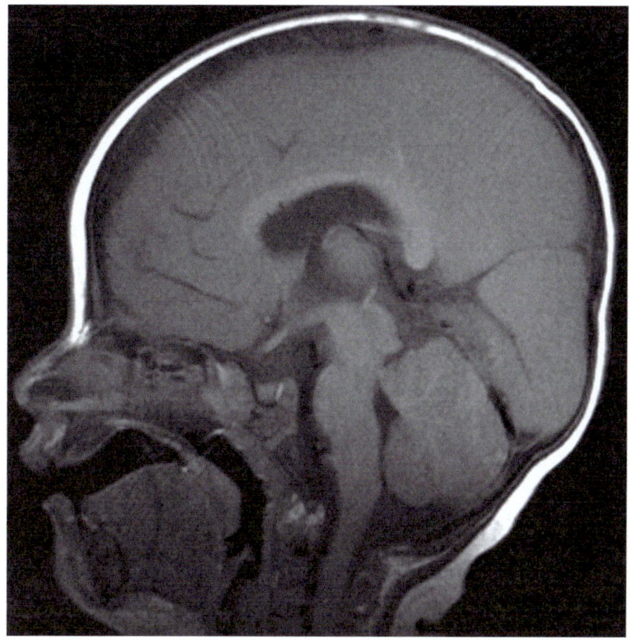

Fig. 24.7 MRI sagittal T1 sequence at a midline level. The abnormal, smooth cerebral surface is evident anteriorly and posteriorly. Contrasting to the uniform signal, the parietal-occipital fissure, calcarine fissure, and anterior cingulate sulcus are present and normal. The corpus callosum and posterior fossa also are normal

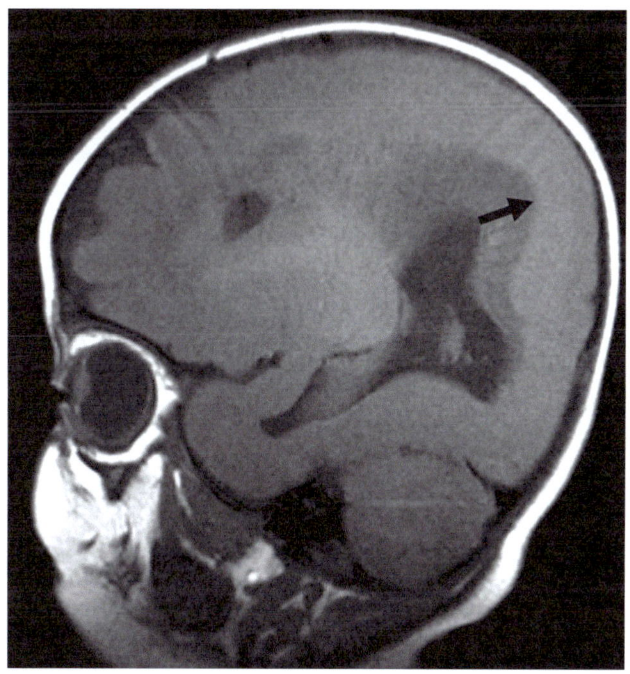

Fig. 24.8 MRI sagittal T1 sequence at a left atrium of the lateral ventricles level. The parietal and occipital cortical surfaces are smooth with an agyric appearance. The cortex in this region is thickened with narrowing of its underlying white matter, which is clearly differentiated at the junction (arrow). The anterior frontal lobe has minor indentations that are insufficient to be normal sulcation. The connatal cyst normal variant is evident in the frontal lobe periventricular region

Hemimegalencephaly

25

Clinical History

The first recognized seizure occurred during the immediate postpartum period. Neonatal intensive care was subsequently provided for infantile spasms that were manifested as bilateral, rapid eyelid fluttering with lip smacking and flexion of the four limbs. MRI at age 3 days identified left total hemimegalencephaly, involving left frontal, temporal, parietal, occipital cortex and left cerebellum. The right hemisphere was normal. Multiple anti-seizure medications were tried without seizure control. MRI at 3 months provided further evidence of polymicrogyria across the left temporal, occipital, and basal forebrain regions.

A left hemispherotomy was performed at age 4 months. Histopathological examination identified widespread polymicrogyria and multifocal regions of neuronal crowding and dyslamination with dysmorphic neurons in the cortex. Heterotopic neurons were present in the cortex and subcortical white matter. No additional infantile spasms occurred over the following few months and normal developmental milestones were achieved.

A new habitual seizure first occurred at age 10 months and was manifested as a sudden rightward gaze that sometimes also included head turning to the right. The seizure duration was 5 seconds, and the frequency was twice daily. Initially, this seizure was subtle, but it became more obvious over the following year when it began to include gagging. Video-EEG monitoring identified an epileptiform correlate to the episodes over the left frontal lobe. At approximately age 2 years, the seizure frequency had reached several daily, and the developmental delay was evident as no verbal ability. Motor function was compromised with a left hand limited to a pincer grasp, right hand lacking fine motor function, and walking requiring the use of orthotics.

At age 3 years, a left anatomic hemispherectomy was performed. Histopathological examination identified disorganized cortical architecture with neuronal crowding, cytomegaly, and dysmorphism. Band and nodular heterotopia were present in the white matter. Since the hemispherectomy, the previously occurring seizures have not recurred. Cognitive function is impaired with occasional attending to others, a nonverbal interaction, and autism-like behaviors. Video-EEG monitoring at age 6 years identified diffuse attenuation over the left hemisphere and abnormally slow background activity due to excessive theta and delta activity and a posterior dominant rhythm of 8 Hz. No interictal epileptiform abnormalities were present. Epileptiform abnormality was not present during the autism-like behaviors.

The history and evaluation indicate infantile spasms that are related to an extensive, hemispheric cerebral malformation. The achievement of developmental milestones after the hemispherotomy at age 4 months produced seizure control supports the understanding that the seizures were the immediate cause of the developmental delay. That is, generalized seizures due to a unilateral malformation resulted in generalized cerebral dysfunction. The potential of the seizures to impede neurologic development was further supported by the developmental delay that followed the recurrence of the seizures and their worsening at age 2 years.

J. M. Stern, N. Salamon, *Imaging of Epilepsy*, https://doi.org/10.1007/978-3-030-86672-3_25

Imaging

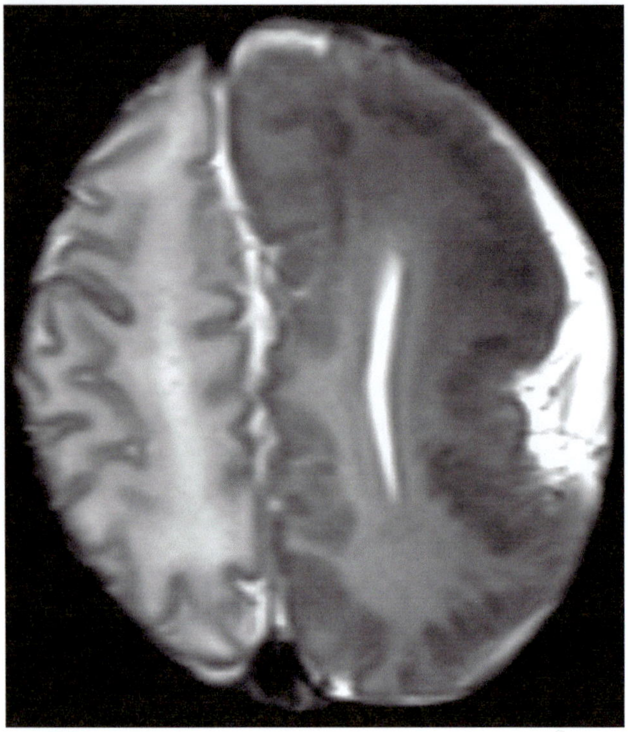

Fig. 25.1 MRI axial T2 sequence at a high lateral ventricle level obtained at age 3 days. The entire left cerebral hemisphere is larger than right with cortical sulci that are abnormally formed and indicate pachygyria. The left hemisphere's white matter is abnormally hypointense, indicating diffuse hypomyelination. The Sylvian fissure and central sulcus are abnormally oriented, producing an abnormal indentation along the left lateral surface

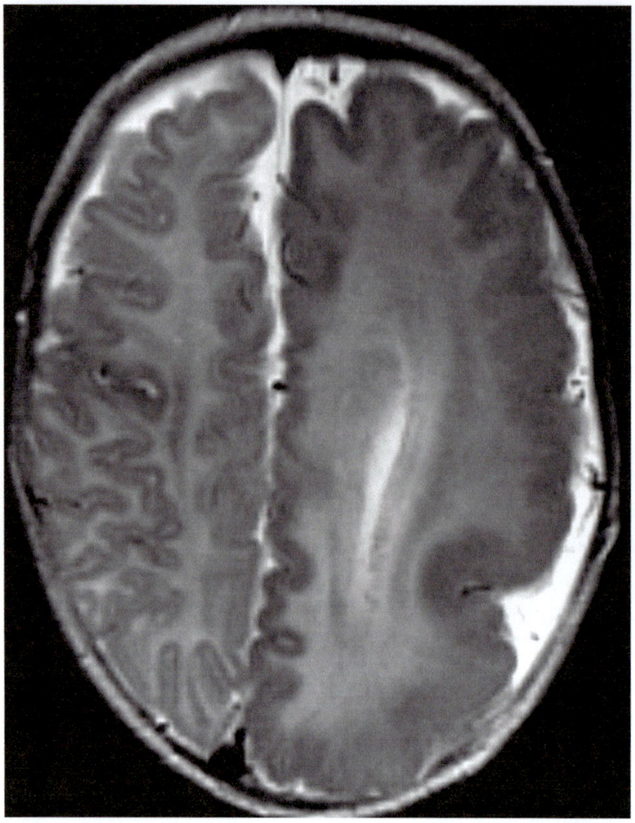

Fig. 25.2 MRI axial T2 sequence at a high lateral ventricle level that is slightly inferior to Fig. 25.1. The image was obtained at age 3 months. The entire left hemisphere is enlarged with resultant displacement of the superior sagittal sinus to the right of midline. Sulcation is evident across the left frontal lobe, but the lateral and posterior aspects of the left hemisphere have abnormal sulcation with pachygyria. A double cortex is lateral to the left lateral ventricle. The right hemisphere is normal with a region of normal hypointensity within the centrum semiovale that is developmentally normal myelination of the cortical spinal tract

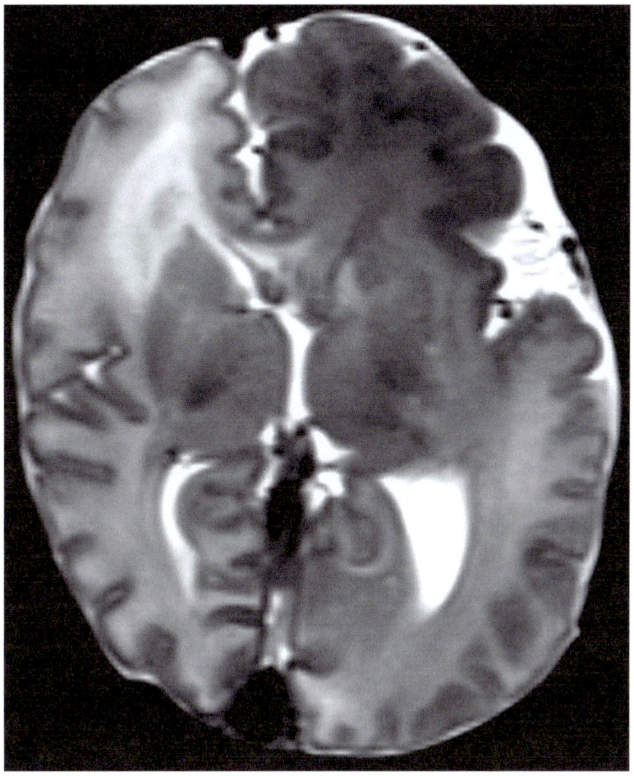

Fig. 25.3 MRI axial T2 sequence at a basal ganglia and thalamus level obtained at age 3 days. The left hemisphere is enlarged with a prominently enlarged atrium of the left lateral ventricle, as is characteristic of hemimegalencephaly. The frontal horn of the left lateral ventricle is slit and abnormally smaller, which also characteristic of hemimegalencephaly. This is due to adjacent fibers that are aberrantly enlarged and encroach on the ventricle. The thalamus and basal ganglia also are abnormally formed and enlarged. Sulcation is evident along the left hemisphere's lateral and posterior regions at this level. An enlarged and dysplastic vein is present in the left Sylvian fissure

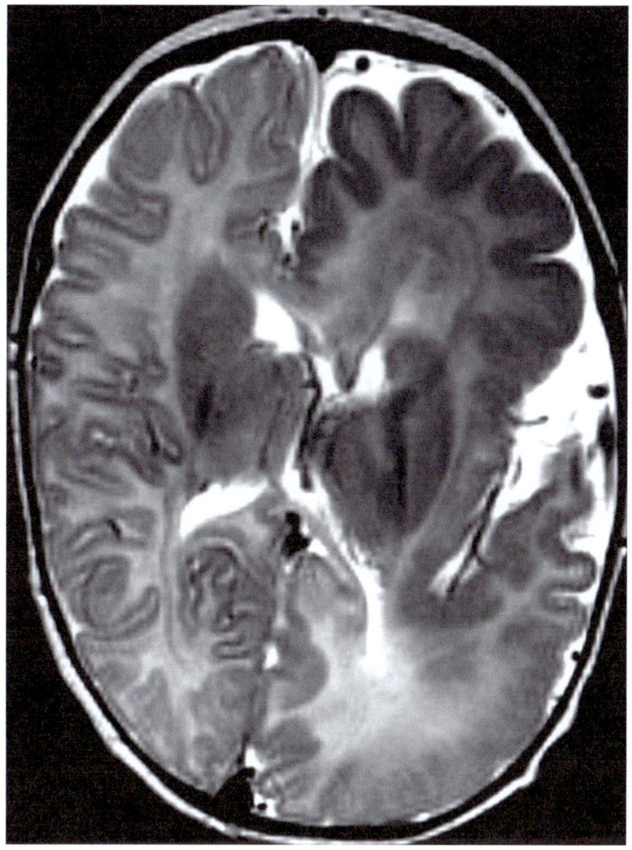

Fig. 25.4 MRI axial T2 sequence at a basal ganglia and thalamus level that is similar to Fig. 25.3 but obtained at age 3 months. The anterior and posterior limbs of the left internal capsule have abnormal hypermyelination, as is evident when compared to the right hemisphere's internal capsule. The internal capsule's anterior limb usually is not myelinated until age 7–8 months. The right hemisphere's internal capsule is normal for age with myelination only in a portion of the posterior limb. The genu of the corpus callosum is asymmetric and larger on the left. The left frontal lobe has clear gray-white differentiation and a double cortex. In contrast, the left temporal-occipital cortex has a blurred junction with pachygyria

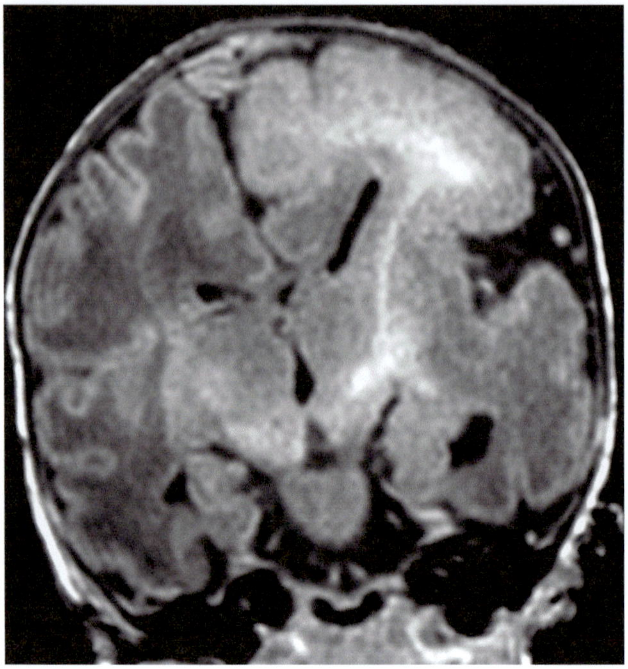

Fig. 25.5 MRI coronal T1 sequence at a hippocampal body level obtained at age 3 days. The left corticospinal tract is hyperintense and prominent because of its abnormal, partial myelination. The left frontal white matter also is hyperintense due to the abnormal myelination and contrasts with the right hemisphere's normal myelination. The slit-like deformation of the left frontal horn is related to the enlarged left frontal lobe, as is evident in Fig. 25.3. The left lateral ventricle's temporal horn also is enlarged

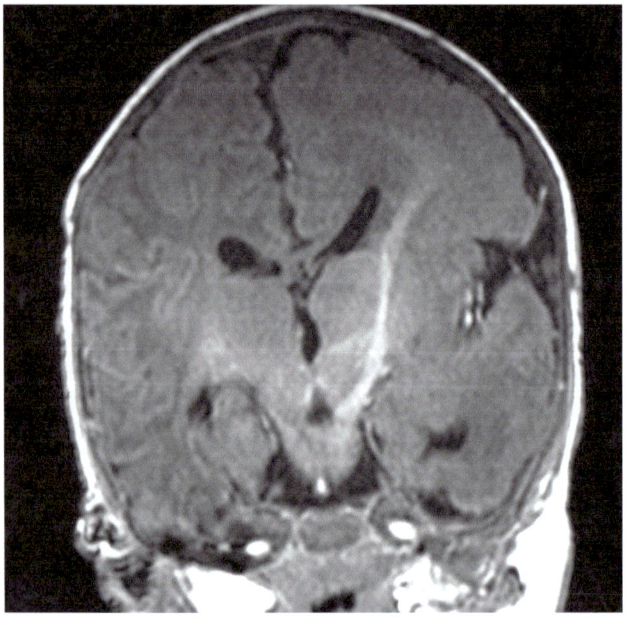

Fig. 25.6 MRI coronal T1 sequence at a thalamus level that is slightly posterior to Fig. 25.5. The image was obtained at age 3 months. The left corticospinal tract myelination is more matured, as is evident in the hyperintense signal. In comparison, a subtle corticospinal tract is present in the right hemisphere. The right hemisphere's white matter is less hypointense compared to age 3 days in Fig. 25.5, which is due to normal myelination with development

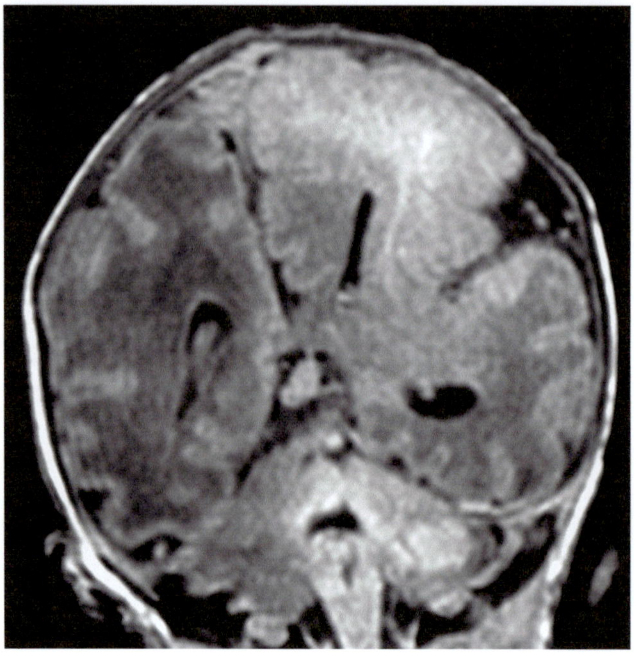

Fig. 25.7 MRI coronal T1 sequence at a splenium of the corpus callosum level that is more posterior to Fig. 25.6. The image was obtained at age 3 days. The parietal lobe is abnormal due to hypermyelination, as is evident in the hyperintense white matter. The left cerebral surface is abnormal with an abnormally deep Sylvian fissure that contains abnormal veins. The left cerebellum also demonstrates the hypermyelination

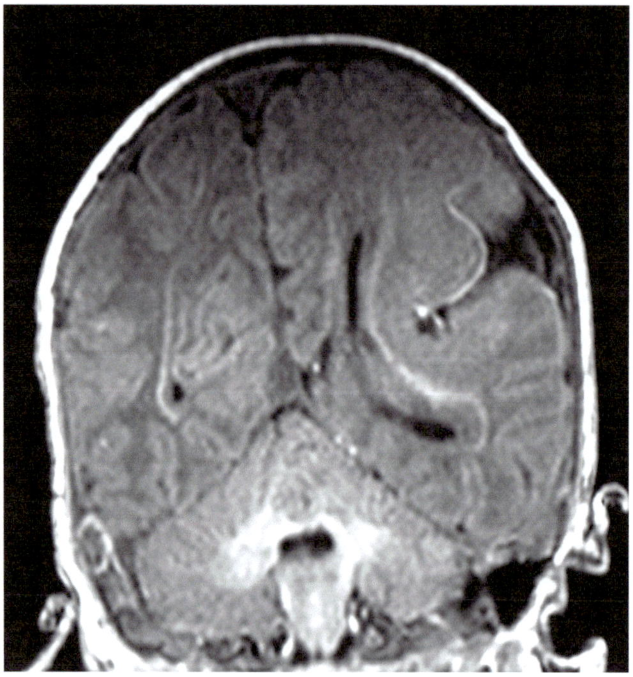

Fig. 25.8 MRI coronal T1 sequence at an occipital horn level that is slightly posterior to Fig. 25.7. The image was obtained at age 3 months. The left cerebrum is abnormally enlarged with an asymmetrically smaller left cerebellum at this level. However, other levels demonstrate that the left cerebellar hemisphere is enlarged overall, and this level is misleading regarding its size. The left-sided optic radiations are thicker and more hyperintense than on the right. The abnormally deep Sylvian fissure is evident

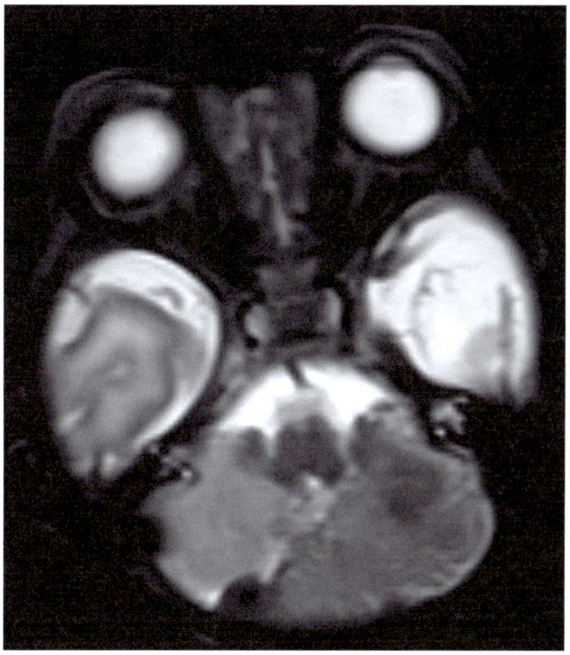

Fig. 25.9 MRI axial T2 sequence at a cerebellum level obtained at age 3 days. The cerebellum is asymmetric in size and signal with the left cerebellum demonstrating more advanced maturity and dysplastic cerebellar cortex, as is evident in the hypointensity. The brainstem is normally myelinated. The left temporal lobe is not visible because the malformation produces a truncation of this lobe

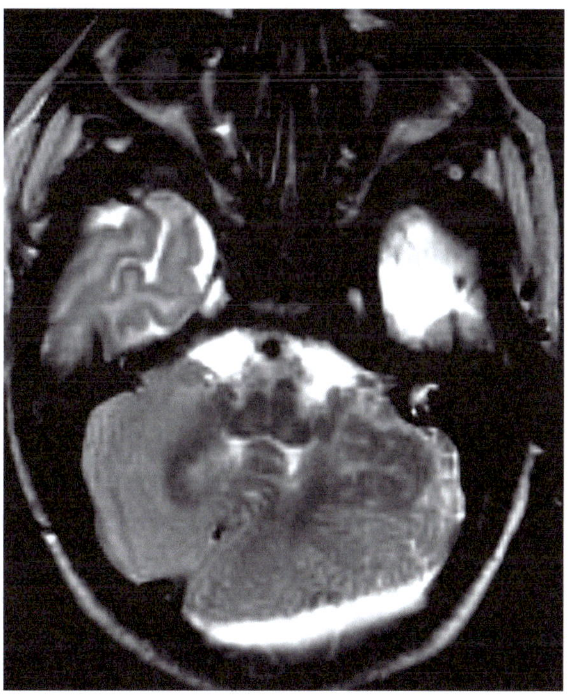

Fig. 25.10 MRI axial T2 sequence at a cerebellum level that is similar to Fig. 25.9. The image was obtained at age 3 months. The left cerebellar hemisphere and the left medulla are abnormally enlarged, and the anterior cerebellum includes a region of hypointensity, indicating abnormal gray matter. The left temporal lobe is not visible because of the malformation and a subsequent empty middle cranial fossa

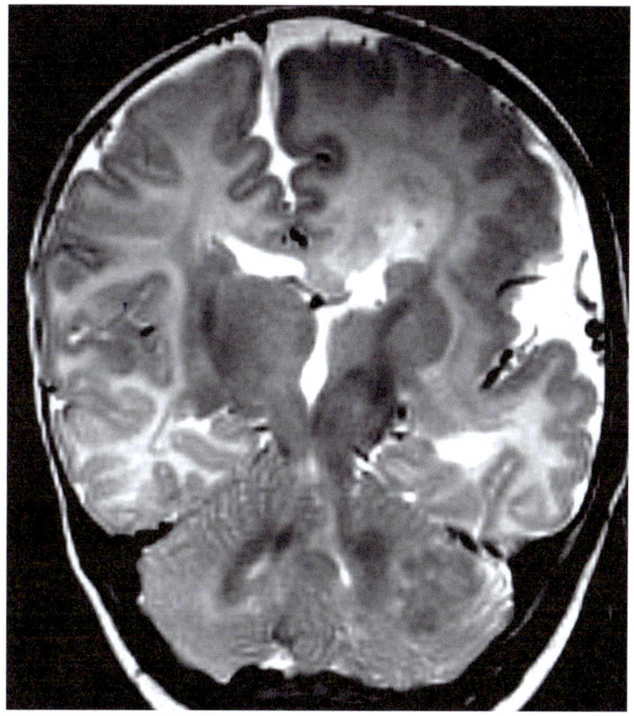

Fig. 25.11 MRI coronal T2 sequence at a hippocampus body level at age 3 months. The asymmetric cerebellum is evident with an enlarged left hemisphere with heterotopic gray matter. Hyperintensity indicating asymmetric myelination is evident in the left superior cerebellar peduncle and the immediately superior left cerebral peduncle

26 Hemimegalencephaly of the Cerebrum

Clinical History

The first recognized seizure occurred at age 3 days as an episode of right gaze deviation with drooling and bilateral upper and lower extremity extension with stiffening. An evaluation at that time was reported to identify a right cerebral malformation.

The next seizure occurred at about age 20 days and differed in its manifestation with left-sided twitching that recurred every few minutes with an increase during transitions into sleep. At age 2 months, the seizure manifestation reverted to the bilateral extension with stiffening, and chronic treatment was then initiated. Over the following 2 years, the habitual seizure manifestation was an epileptic spasm that included right gaze deviation and twitching of the left eyelid, left hand, and left foot with a duration of a few seconds. During this time, treatment included multiple anti-seizure medications with a seizure frequency of several daily.

Examination was abnormal with evidence of Proteus syndrome with right hemihypertrophy, mild left hemiparesis, and developmental delay. At age 3 years, the patient was able to stand, crawl, and understand speech but was unable to speak or walk.

Interictal EEG depicted diffuse, high-amplitude, abnormal slowing with frequent, brief generalized attenuations. Frequent, multifocal epileptiform discharges were frequent on the right and occasional on the left. Video-EEG monitoring recorded nearly continuous left-sided twitching and runs of the right-sided epileptiform discharges. With a reduction to anti-seizure medications, a left tonic seizure occurred.

MRI identified right cerebral hemimegalencephaly and a normal left hemisphere. PET identified heterogeneous metabolic activity across the right cerebral hemisphere.

The history and evaluation indicate infantile spasms with diagnostic testing identifying EEG hypsarrhythmia and right cerebral hemimegalencephaly. In addition to the spasms, focal motor seizures occurred on the left, and the EEG indicated asymmetrically greater epileptiform abnormality on the right, which furthers the relevance of the right cerebral hemimegalencephaly.

A right-sided hemispherectomy was performed at age 3 years, and the histopathological examination identified cortical dysplasia, type I, dystrophic calcification, and nodular and linear heterotopia in subcortical white matter. No seizures have occurred for 6 years since surgery and anti-seizure medications have been discontinued. Neurologic function includes speech, left-hand weakness, and unassisted ambulation.

J. M. Stern, N. Salamon, *Imaging of Epilepsy*, https://doi.org/10.1007/978-3-030-86672-3_26

Imaging

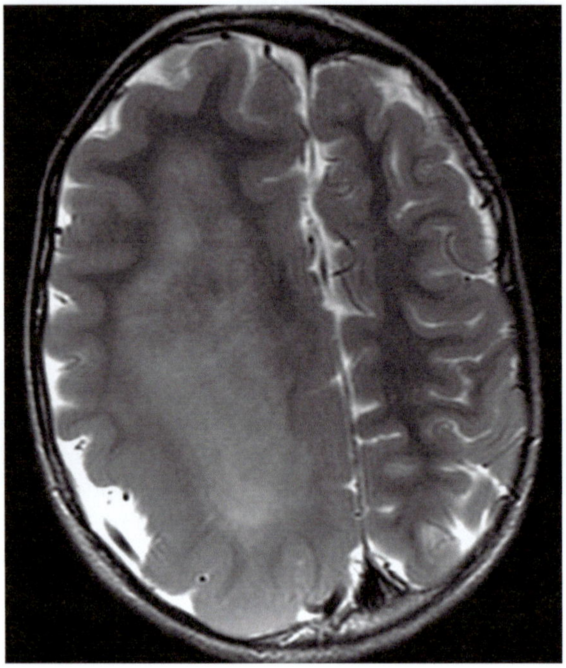

Fig. 26.1 MRI axial T2 sequence at a centrum semi-ovale level. The right hemisphere is markedly enlarged and has abnormal sulcation. Its abnormalities also include white matter hypomyelination, as indicated by abnormally increased signal and a thickening of the posterior cortical ribbon. The left hemisphere is normal

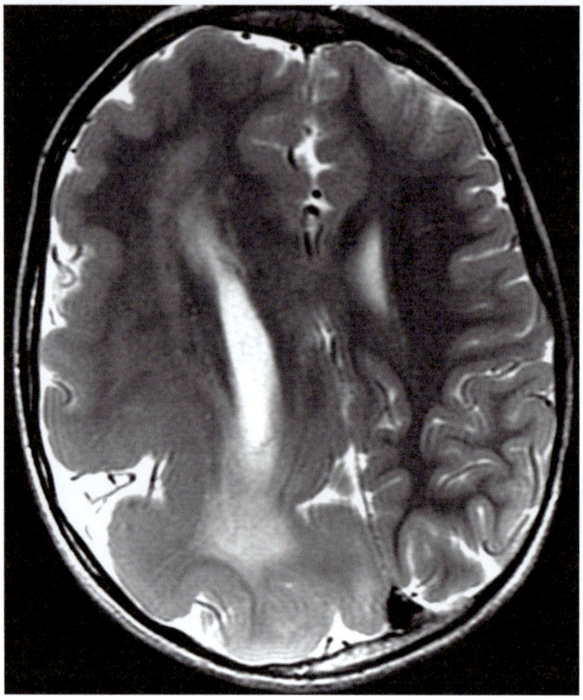

Fig. 26.3 MRI axial T2 sequence at a lateral ventricle level. The right lateral ventricle is abnormally enlarged with abnormal sulcation that is most prominent posteriorly. Hyperintensity due to hypomyelination is evident in the right parietal white matter and present to a lesser extent in the right frontal white matter. The right-sided cleft is an enlarged, posteriorly displaced Sylvian fissure

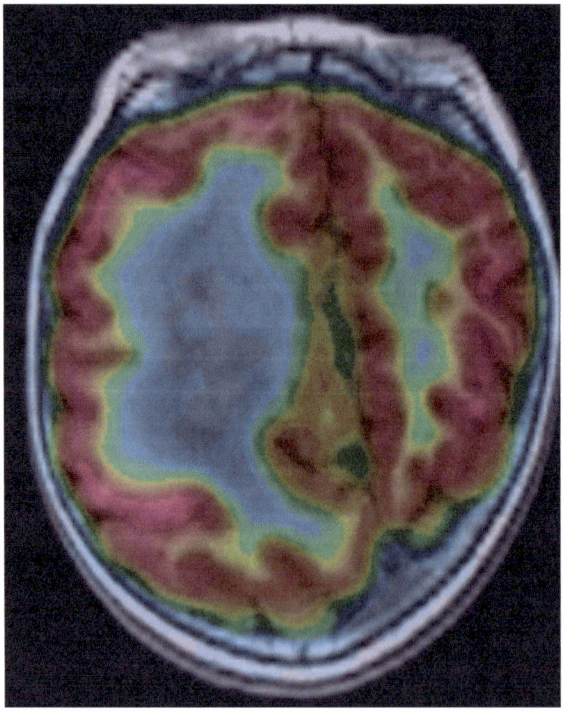

Fig. 26.2 PET-MRI co-registration with color-scale FDG tracer in an axial plane at a similar centrum semi-ovale similar level as Fig. 26.1. The right hemisphere is abnormally enlarged with hypometabolism of the medial posterior aspect, as compared to the left hemisphere. Subtly decreased metabolism is evident in the right hemisphere's white matter

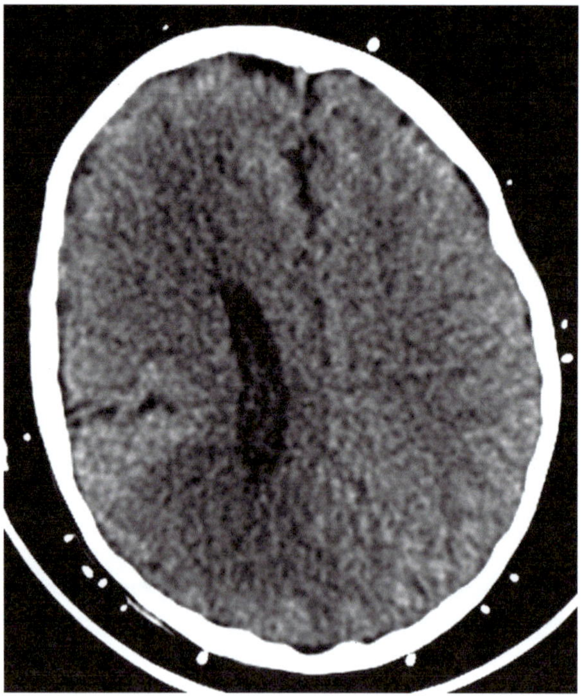

Fig. 26.4 CT in an axial plane at a lateral ventricular level that is between Figs. 26.1 and 26.3. An asymmetrically enlarged right hemispheres is present with associated enlargement of the right lateral ventricle. The left ventricle is not visible in this image. Subtle hyperdensity due to gray matter abnormality surrounds the right-sided cleft at the posterior Sylvian fissure. The multiple artifacts surrounding the skull are due to EEG electrodes

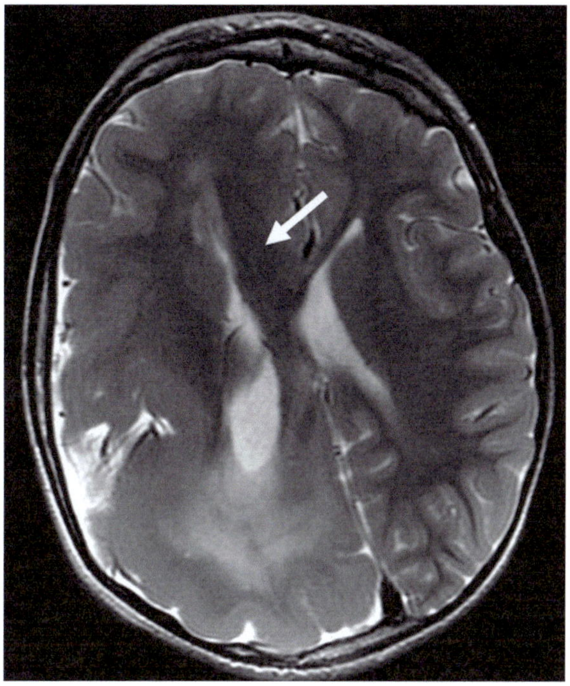

Fig. 26.5 MRI axial T2 sequence at a lateral ventricular level that is inferior to Fig. 26.3. The lateral ventricles are asymmetric in size and shape with thickened, aberrant fibers in the right medial frontal lobe along the lateral ventricle (arrow). Prominent abnormality is present in the posterior, right hemisphere, including hypomyelination, thickened cortex, and a cleft with dysplasia and enlarged vessels

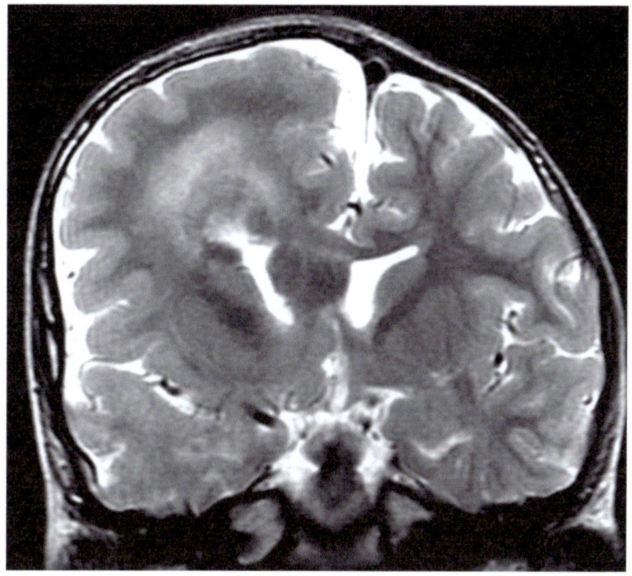

Fig. 26.7 MRI coronal T2 sequence at an anterior commissure level. A thick, bundle of aberrant fibers is present between the frontal horns with bulging of the fibers below the corpus callosum into the right lateral horn. The corpus callosum is asymmetric with thickening and abnormal signal on the right. The abnormal signal continues into the frontal and temporal lobes' white matter with hyperintensity indicating hypomyelination. Gray matter abnormality is evident in the abnormal sulcation across the frontal and temporal cortical surfaces. The left hemisphere is normal

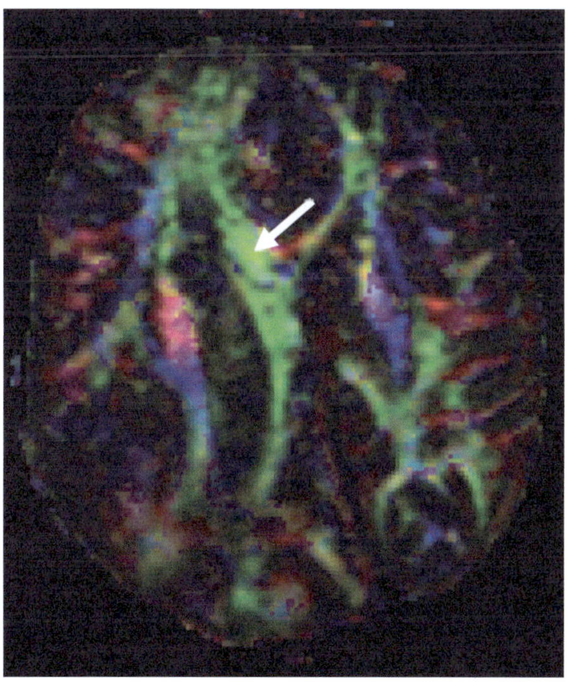

Fig. 26.6 MRI with axial diffusion tensor imaging at a lateral ventricle level similar to Fig. 26.5. A thickened fiber tract with an anterior to posterior orientation is evident medial to the right lateral ventricle (arrow). The fibers within this tract interrupt the anterior corpus callosum, which is identified by the red, left-right oriented fibers immediately posterior to the arrow. Overall, the right hemisphere's fiber tracts are thickened in the frontal lobe and reduced in the parietal lobe. The left hemisphere's fiber tracts are normal

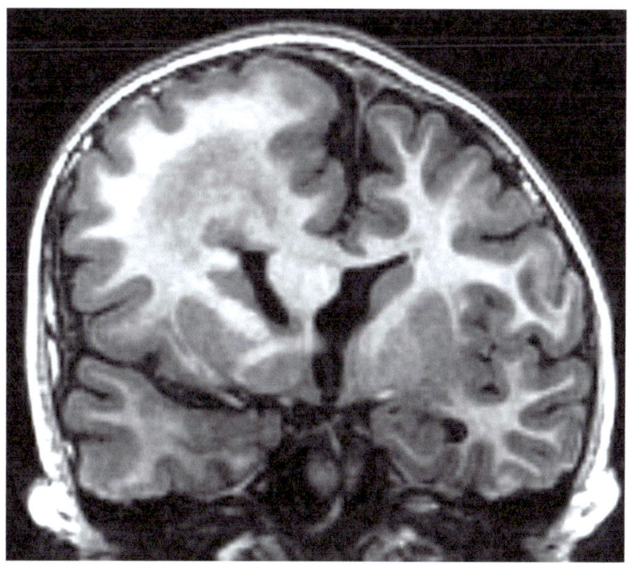

Fig. 26.8 MRI coronal T1 sequence at the same anterior commissure level as Fig. 26.7. A thickened bundle of fibers is present between the frontal horns of the lateral ventricles inferior to the corpus callosum. Hypointensity within the right frontal lobe white matter indicates abnormal hypomyelination. This is less evident but also present in the right temporal lobe white matter

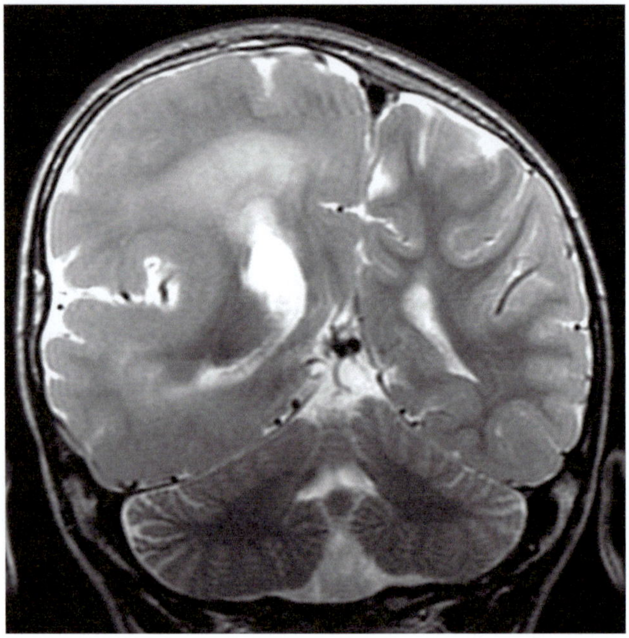

Fig. 26.9 MRI coronal T2 sequence at an atrium of the lateral ventricle level. Diffuse hypointensity due to hypomyelination is present throughout the parietal and occipital lobes. The protrusion of lower signal tissue into the right ventricle is the normal posterior thalamus. The right-sided deep cleft is a malformation of the Sylvian fissure. The cerebellum and left hemisphere are normal

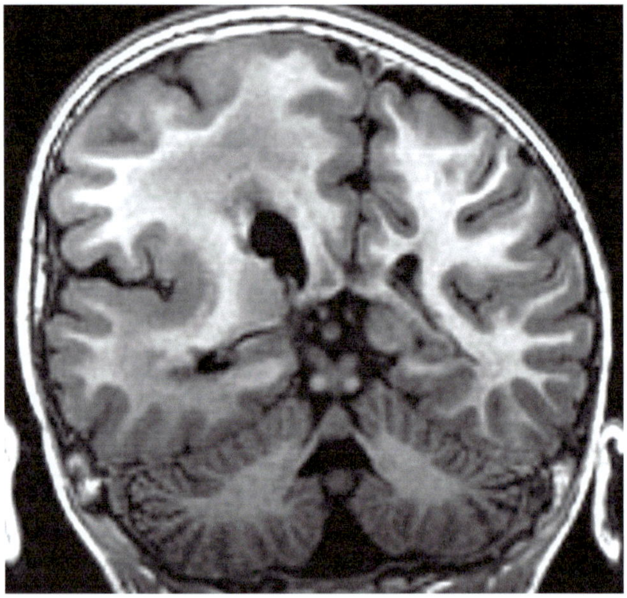

Fig. 26.10 MRI coronal T1 sequence at the same atrium of the lateral ventricle level as Fig. 26.9. A deep cleft is surrounded by abnormally thickened cortex in right posterior Sylvian fissure. The surrounding frontal and temporal lobe white matter is hypomyelinated, and the right lateral ventricle is enlarged. The cerebellum and bilateral superior and inferior colliculi are normal

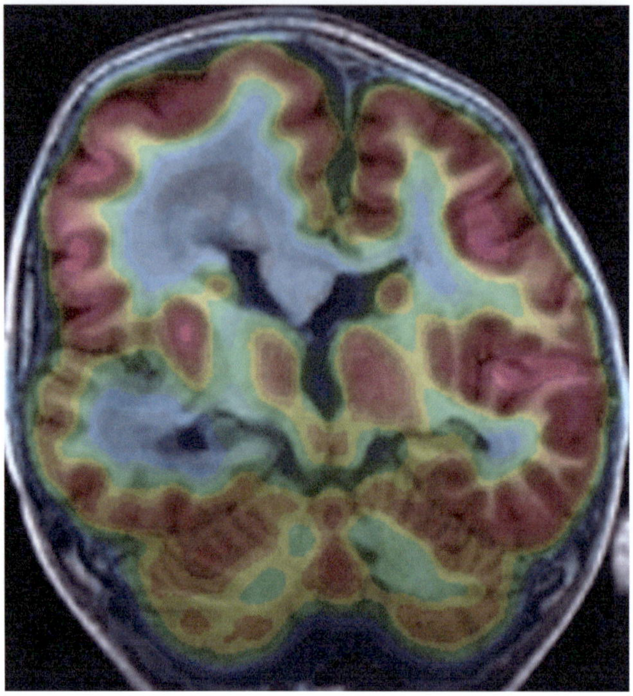

Fig. 26.11 PET-MRI co-registration with color-scale FDG in a coronal plane at a hippocampal body and thalamus level that differs from the MRI image plane angle. The right thalamus and right temporal lobe are asymmetrically hypometabolic. The white matter within the right frontal and temporal lobes also are hypometabolic. Metabolism is normal in the bilateral frontal lobe cortex and the cerebellum

27 Encephalocele

Clinical History

The first seizures occurred at age 7 years as behavioral arrests that each lasted about 10 seconds and recurred several times daily. Over the following months, the seizures changed to include an aura of a vertiginous spinning experience followed by behavioral arrest with subsequent lip smacking, grunting, manual automatisms, and then rocking for a total seizure duration of 30 to 60 seconds. Progression to bilateral tonic-clonic movements sometimes occurred, but this was uncommon. Postictal aphasia and fatigue were present for 5–10 minutes. With treatment, seizures occurred two to eight times monthly with either one seizure or a cluster of seizures occurring once weekly. Treatment included multiple antiseizure medications without sustained seizure control.

An epilepsy risk factor was not present in the history, and neurological development was normal. The patient performed well in school and was active in sports. Neuropsychological testing identified normal verbal and nonverbal memory and mild deficits of expressive language and reading.

Interictal EEG depicted frequent sharp wave epileptiform discharges over the left anterior temporal region. Video-EEG monitoring identified focal seizures manifested by the aura followed by grunting sounds and chewing automatisms with restless movements of the arms and repositioning of the body. Ictal EEG's seizure onset was over the anterior left temporal lobe with evolution over the left temporal region.

MRI identified a prominent left middle cranial fossa skull base arachnoid cyst with protrusion of the left anterior-mesial temporal cortex into the skull base defect. No associated gliosis or edema was present. PET identified moderately decreased left anterior temporal lobe metabolism.

The history and evaluation indicate left anterior temporal lobe epilepsy, as was supported by the focal seizures that typically do not progress to tonic-clonic and localization evident with interictal and ictal EEG, MRI, and PET. However, the seizures' features suggest neocortical abnormality more than limbic with their high frequency at the onset of epilepsy, the true vertigo as an aura (as compared to nonspecific lightheadedness), the normal episodic memory function, and the presence of language deficits.

A left anterior temporal lobe resection was performed at age 13 years with electrocorticographic guidance that identified epileptiform abnormality confined to the cortex adjacent to the encephalocele. Repair with skull closure also was performed. Because of the normal episodic memory function, the resection did not extend to include the left hippocampus. Seizure freedom has been present for the 15 months since the operation.

J. M. Stern, N. Salamon, *Imaging of Epilepsy*, https://doi.org/10.1007/978-3-030-86672-3_27

Imaging

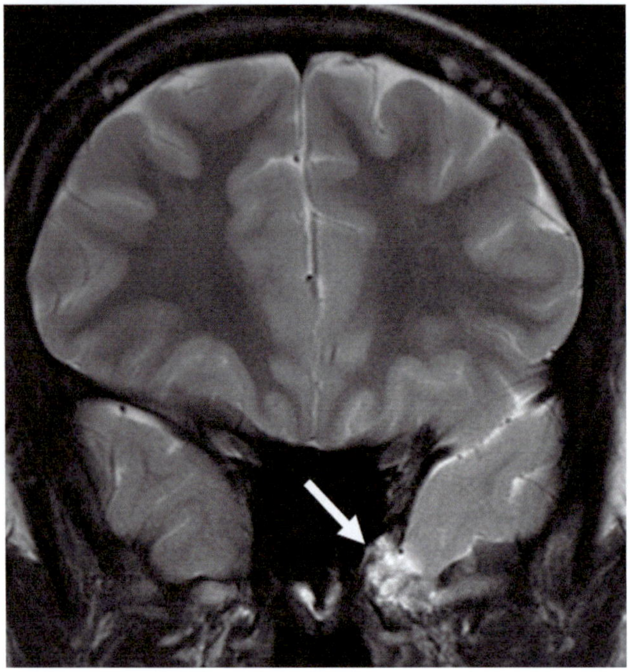

Fig. 27.1 MRI coronal T2 sequence at a temporal pole level. A defect of the dura and bone is evident medial to the left temporal pole with herniation of the temporal pole into the resultant space (arrow). The gray-white junction of the non-herniated left temporal pole is blurred. The right temporal lobe is normal

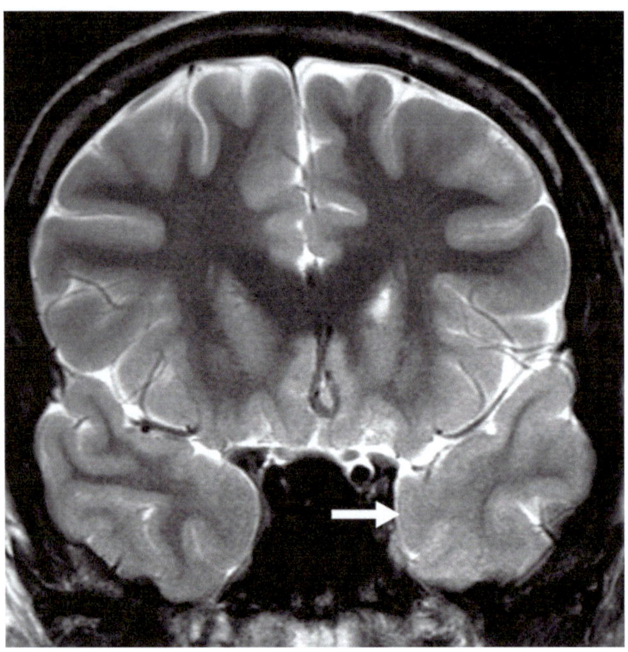

Fig. 27.2 MRI coronal T2 sequence at a temporal pole level posterior to Fig. 27.1. The dural defect is not present at this level, but the gray-white junction of the mesial temporal lobe is blurred (arrow). However, the gray-white junction is clearer across the left lateral temporal lobe. The right temporal lobe is normal, including the gray-white differentiation

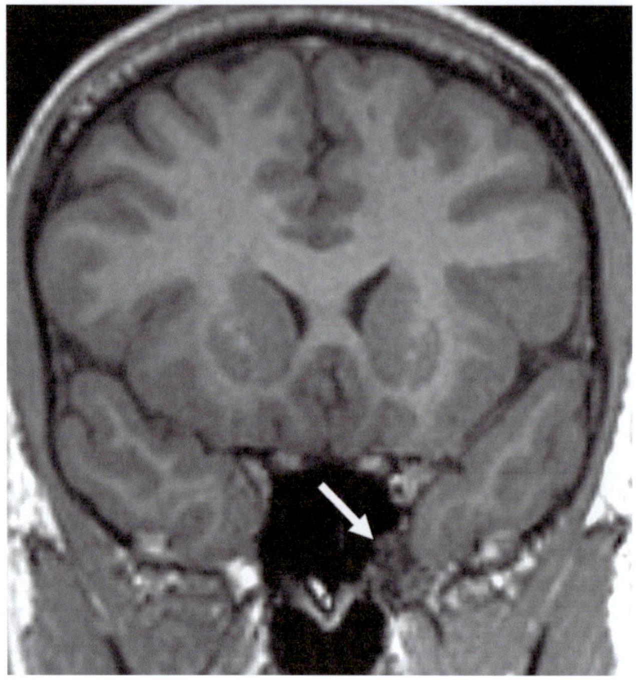

Fig. 27.3 MRI coronal T1 sequence at a temporal pole level between Figs. 27.1 and 27.2. A defect of the dura and bone is evident medial to the left temporal pole with herniation of the temporal pole into the resultant space (arrow). The gray-white junction is subtly blurred across the mesial temporal lobe, but the abnormality is not as clearly evident as with the T2 sequence

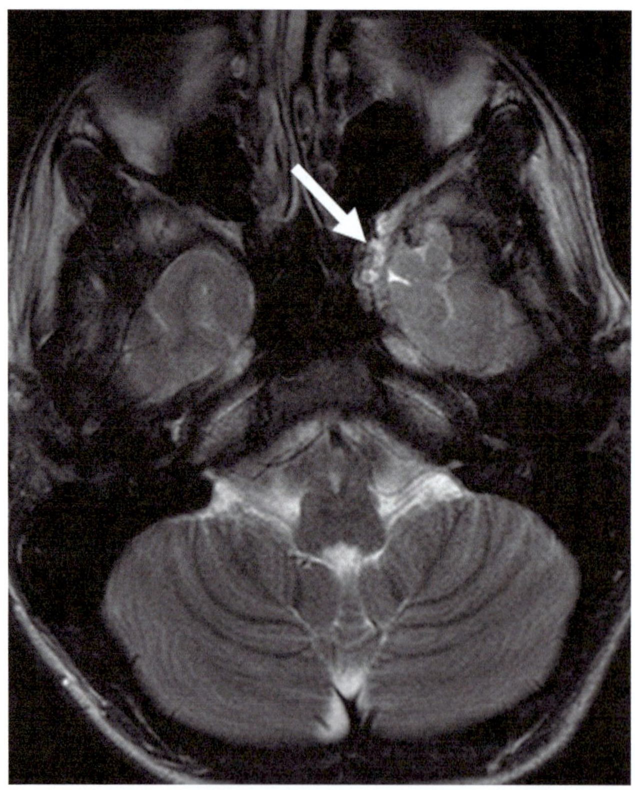

Fig. 27.4 MRI axial T2 sequence at a ponto-medullary junction level. The left mesial temporal lobe is herniated with projection through a dural and bone defect toward the sphenoid sinus. At this level, the gray-white junction is poorly visible, so its differentiation is difficult to assess. A clear gray-white junction is visible on the right

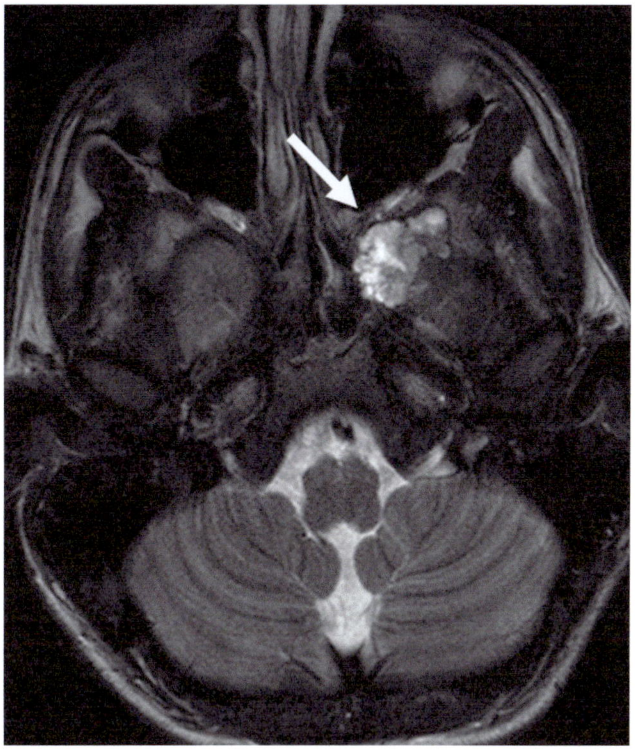

Fig. 27.5 MRI axial T2 sequence at a level slightly inferior to Fig. 27.4. The herniated temporal lobe tissue (arrow) has a complex contour with surrounding cerebrospinal fluid (CSF) that produces an appearance of overall increased signal. The posterior wall of the maxillary sinus is intact

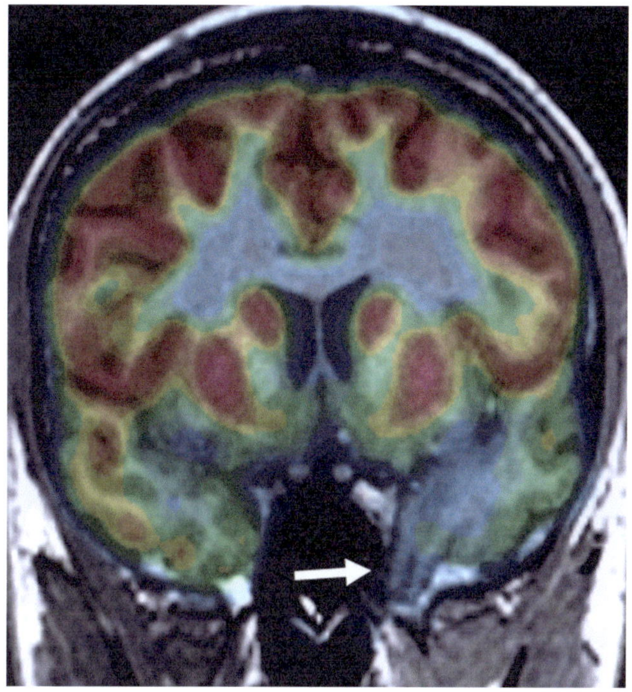

Fig. 27.7 PET-MRI co-registration with color-scale FDG tracer in a coronal plane at a temporal pole level. Herniation of the left mesial temporal lobe is evident as markedly hypometabolic tissue. However, the hypometabolism extends across the temporal pole with reduced metabolism along the non-herniated medial aspect and also the lateral aspect, as compared to the right temporal pole. The basal ganglia and frontal lobes are normal

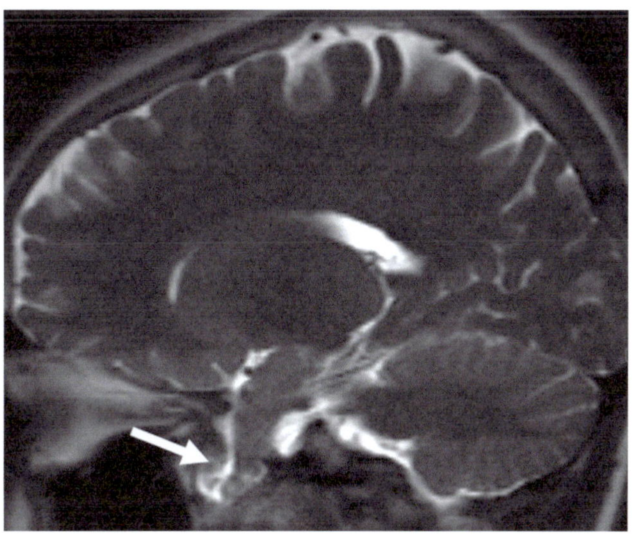

Fig. 27.6 MRI sagittal T2 sequence at a left hippocampus level. A bony defect is evident because of the CSF signal that surrounds herniating temporal lobe tissue into the middle cranial fossa (arrow). The circular CSF signal posterior to the herniation is a normal Meckel's cave

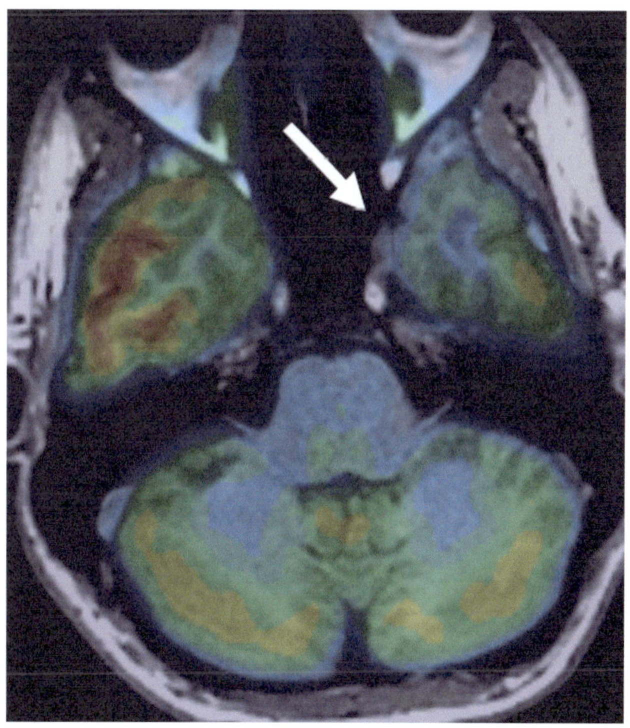

Fig. 27.8 PET-MRI co-registration with color-scale FDG tracer in an axial plane at a ponto-medullary junction level. The left temporal lobe is hypometabolic with marked hypometabolism of the mesial aspect (arrow) and the lateral aspect. The herniation is superior to this level and not visible in this image

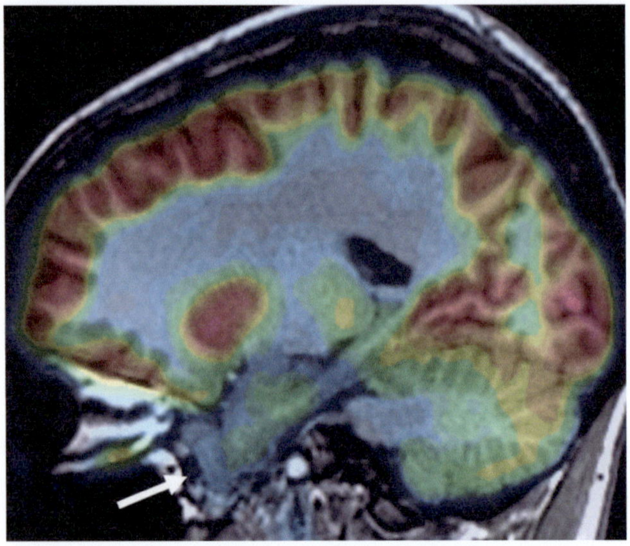

Fig. 27.9 PET-MRI co-registration with color-scale FDG tracer in a sagittal plane at a left hippocampus level. Herniated temporal pole tissue is anterior to the temporal lobe (arrow) with hypometabolism of the herniated tissue and the non-herniated temporal pole. The remaining tissue at this level is normal

28 Encephalocele After Surgical Repair

Clinical History

The first recognized seizure occurred at age 19 years as a tonic-clonic convulsion. An evaluation at that time identified a left temporal lobe encephalocele, which was surgically repaired within weeks of the seizure, and anti-seizure medications were then discontinued. Several months later, a second tonic-clonic seizure occurred, and anti-seizure medication was restarted.

The habitual seizures were identified after the second tonic-clonic seizure and retrospectively believed to have begun at about age 16 years. These seizures manifested as a déjà vu experience with a stereotyped abdominal or thoracic sensation. Sometimes, an experience of being "zoned out" accompanied this for several seconds. Postictally, a left periorbital headache was present for hours. Prior to treatment, the seizures occurred as often as several times a day and seizure freedom lasted up to 1 month. After the encephalocele repair and restarting anti-seizure medications, the seizures were as often as three monthly and as infrequent as none for 2 months. Treatment included multiple anti-seizure medications.

The epilepsy risk factor was the encephalocele. Neurological examination was normal. Medical history was significant only for migraine.

Interictal EEG both before and after the encephalocele surgery depicted left temporal lobe epileptiform discharges with a broad field. Video-EEG monitoring recorded focal seizures manifested as unresponsiveness and oral automatisms that sometimes progressed with versive rightward turning to bilateral tonic-clonic convulsions. Ictal EEG's seizure on set was over the left anterior temporal lobe.

MRI identified the left anterior temporal encephalocele repair with tissue abnormality in the adjacent left temporal pole. The mesial temporal lobes were normal. PET identified left temporal pole hypometabolism with normal metabolism of both hippocampi. MEG identified epileptiform dipoles in the left anterior temporal region.

The history and evaluation indicate left temporal lobe epilepsy with a limbic aura, limbic ictal behavior, and evidence of the left-sided lateralization in the asymmetric motor features and the imaging. However, the evaluation did not identify a concordant memory deficit or hippocampal imaging abnormality. An intracarotid amobarbital test identified left hemispheric dominance for language, poor recall after left hemispheric injection, and good recall after right hemispheric injection. As such, the left mesial temporal structures demonstrated intact function.

A left anterior temporal pole resection with sparing of the hippocampus was performed with the understanding that seizure control likelihood may be reduced, but inclusion of the hippocampus would introduce an unacceptable risk of a memory deficit. Histopathological examination identified gliosis and no other abnormality. No seizures or auras occurred for 2.5 years after surgery, including about 1 year without anti-seizure medications. Seizures then recurred with a manifestation and frequency that was similar to before surgery. Treatment was restarted with seizure control improvement, but the follow-up time is not sufficient to provide an assessment of sustained seizure control.

J. M. Stern, N. Salamon, *Imaging of Epilepsy*, https://doi.org/10.1007/978-3-030-86672-3_28

Imaging

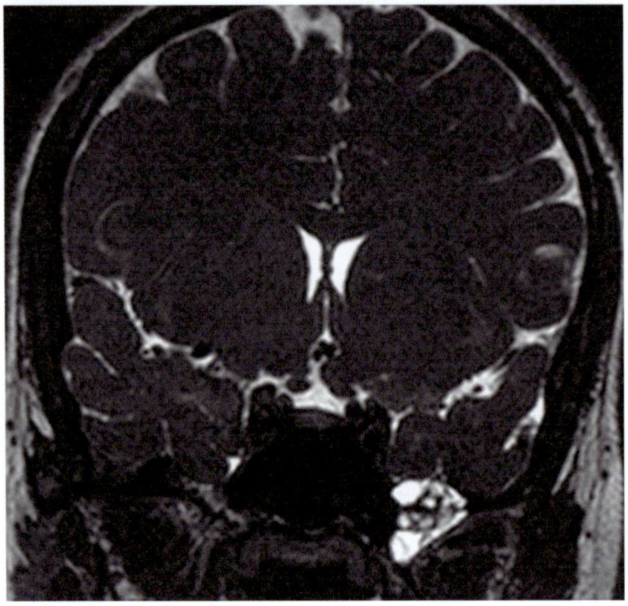

Fig. 28.1 MRI coronal T2 sequence at a temporal pole level. An encephalocele is evident as multi-septated, herniated tissue protruding through a bone and dural defect in the floor of the left middle cranial fossa

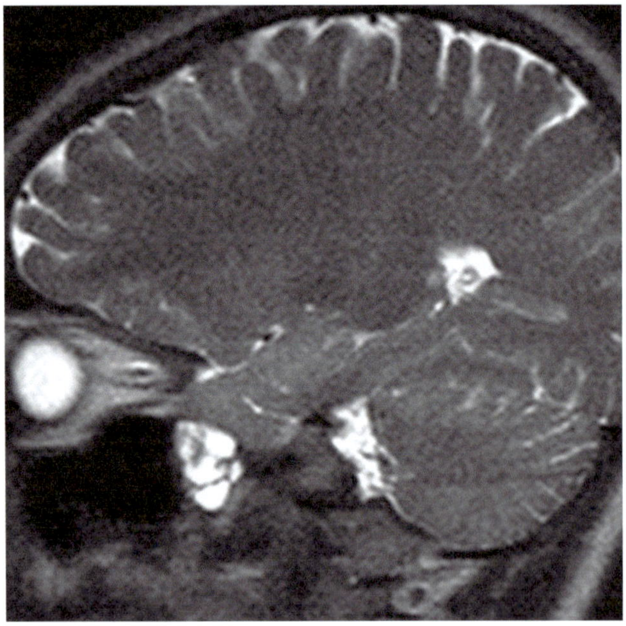

Fig. 28.2 MRI sagittal T2 sequence at a left hippocampus level. A multi-lobulated encephalocele with high signal due to cerebrospinal fluid (CSF) is evident anteroinferiorly to the left temporal lobe. No other abnormality is evident

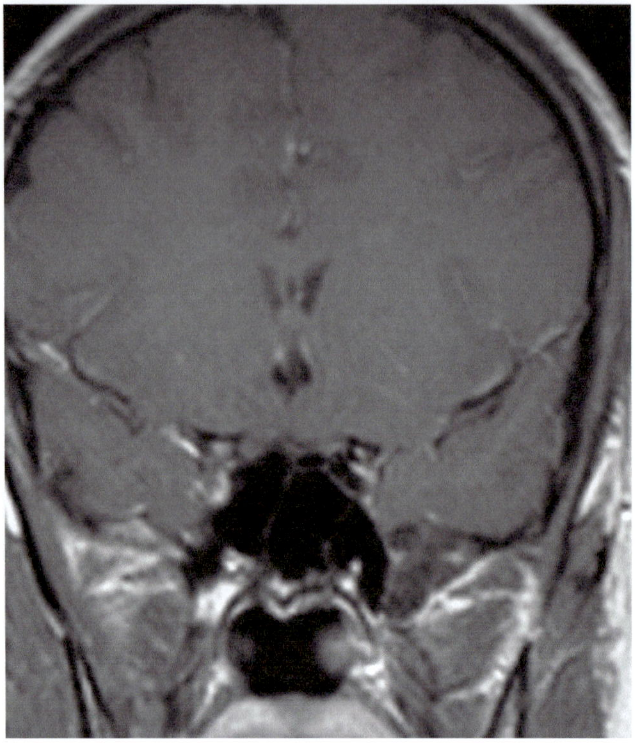

Fig. 28.3 MRI coronal T1 sequence after administration of contrast at a temporal pole level. Enhancement is evident in septated, herniated tissue, which is consistent with a left temporal pole encephalocele. The remaining temporal lobe is normal and not demonstrating abnormal enhancement

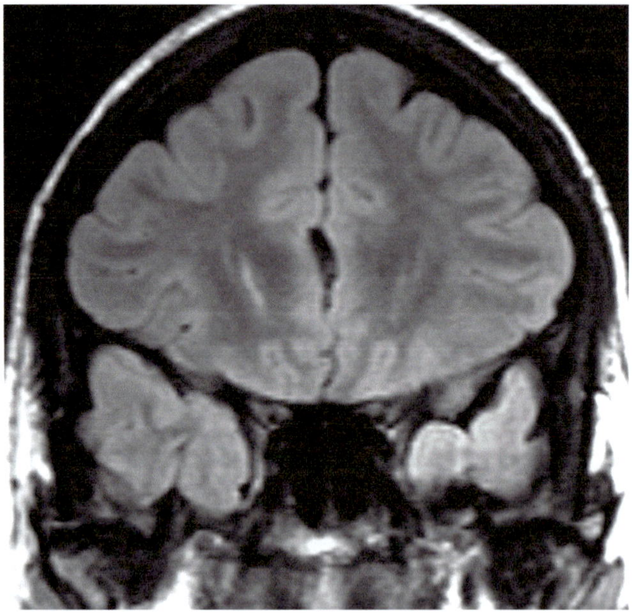

Fig. 28.4 MRI coronal FLAIR sequence at a temporal pole level after surgical repair of an encephalocele. Increased signal is evident across the left temporal pole with blurred gray-white differentiation. The right temporal lobe is normal and provides a useful comparison of signal and gray-white differentiation

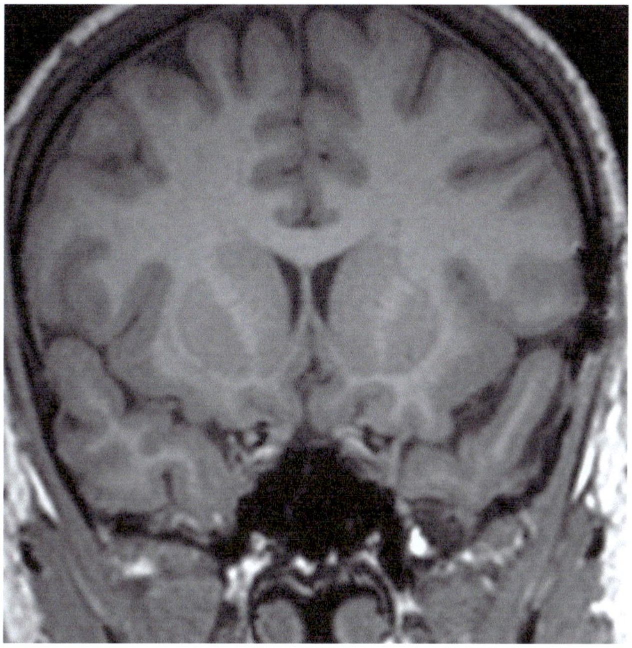

Fig. 28.5 MRI coronal T1 sequence at a temporal pole level posterior to Fig. 28.4 after surgical repair of an encephalocele. Craniotomy related to the encephalocele repair is evident along the lateral, inferior left frontal lobe. The herniated tissue was resected, and the remaining left temporal lobe has no evident abnormality. The hyperintensity immediately inferior to the bone defect is due to fatty tissue that was placed as part of a prior surgical treatment for the herniation

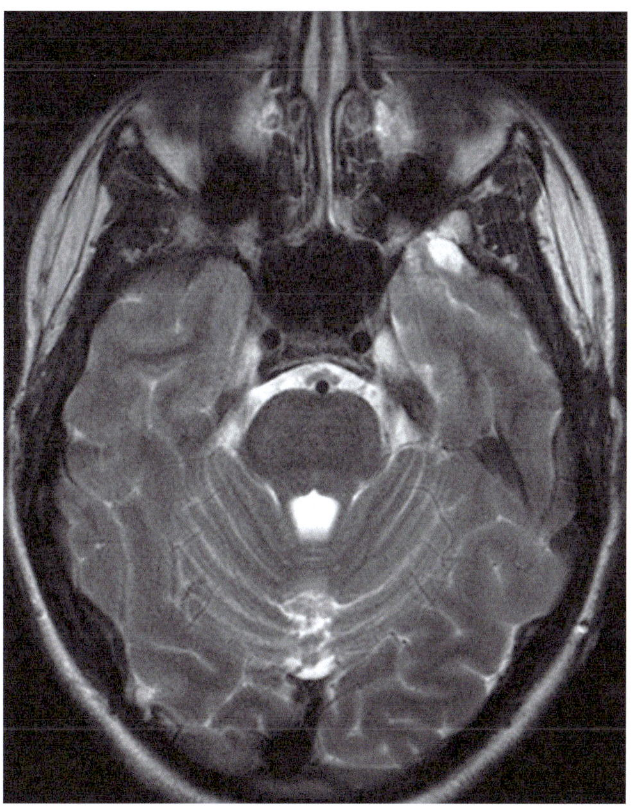

Fig. 28.6 MRI axial T2 sequence at a pons level after surgical repair of an encephalocele. Encephalomalacia is evident in the anterior portion of the left temporal pole, as is visible as an oval of hyperintensity due to CSF. Gray-white differentiation is poorly visible, so determination junction blurring is not reliable

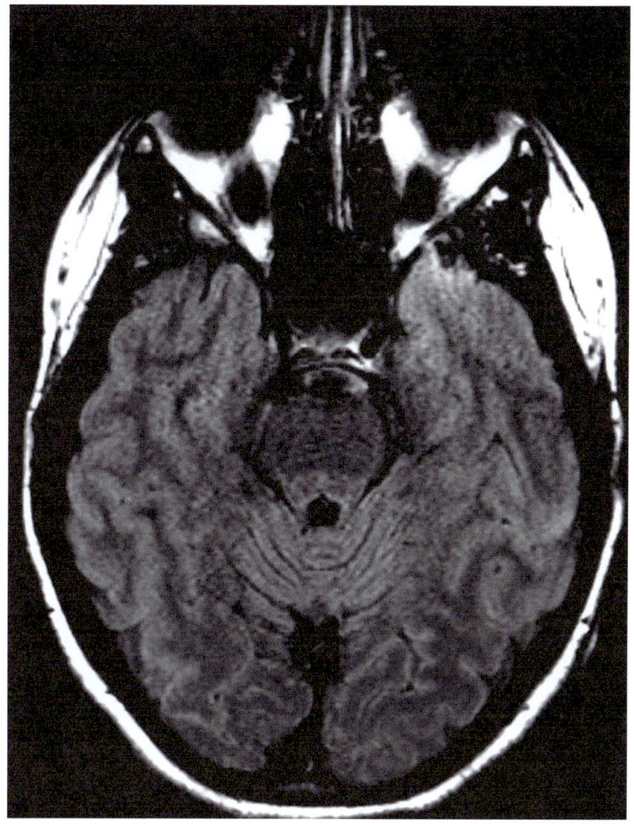

Fig. 28.7 MRI axial FLAIR sequence at a pons level that is the same as Fig. 28.6. Abnormally increased signal is evident at the left temporal pole with a region of encephalomalacia and a circle of hypointensity due to a CSF space. The signal abnormality is consistent with gliosis or dysplasia

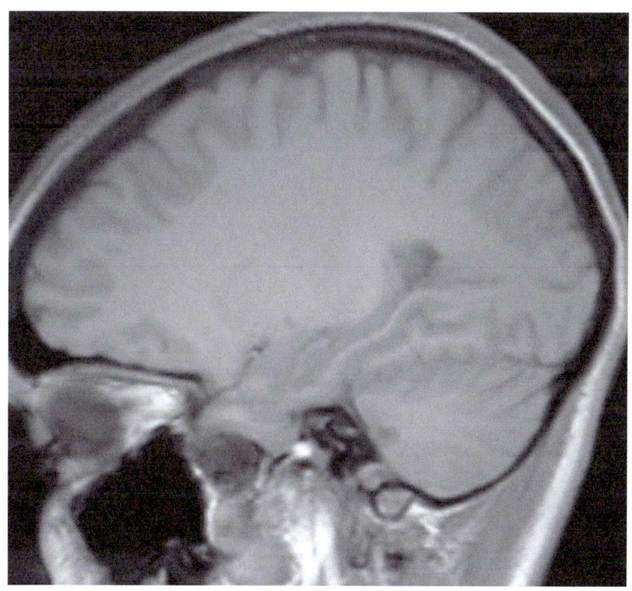

Fig. 28.8 MRI sagittal T1 sequence at a left hippocampus level after surgical repair of an encephalocele. A circular hypointense region is present anteroinferiorly to the anterior temporal lobe. It is smaller than the abnormality prior to the herniated tissue resection. This level is lateral to the fatty tissue evident in Fig. 28.5

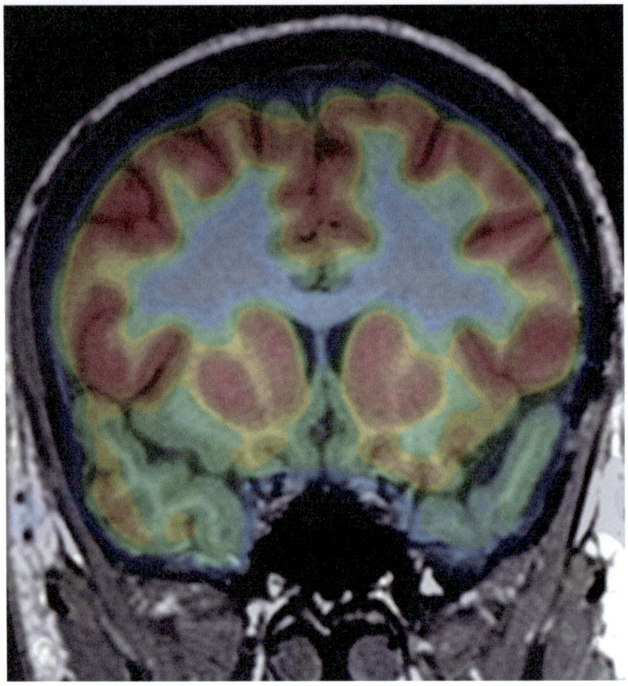

Fig. 28.9 PET-MRI co-registration with color-scale FDG in a coronal plane at the same temporal pole level as Fig. 28.5. Left temporal pole hypometabolism is evident. The triangle of hyperintensity inferior to the left temporal pole is the MRI depiction of fatty tissue that was placed below the prior encephalomalacia. The basal ganglia, frontal lobes, and right temporal lobe are normal

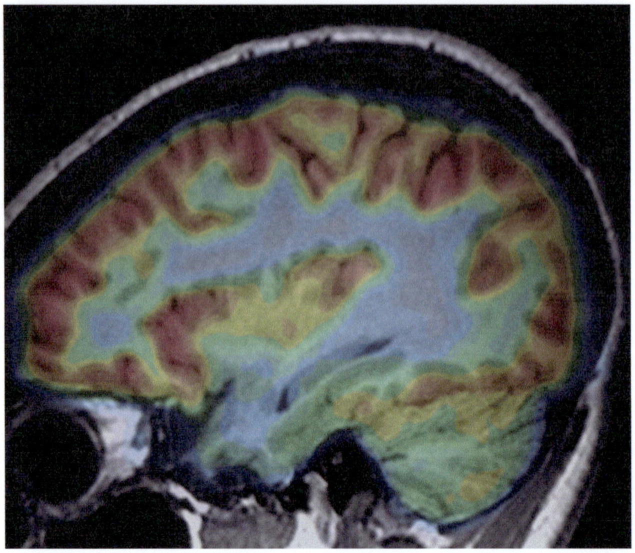

Fig. 28.11 PET-MRI co-registration with color-scale FDG in a sagittal plane at a left hippocampus level. Abnormal contour of the left temporal pole is due to the encephalocele and its surgical repair. The anterior and inferior temporal lobe is abnormally hypometabolic

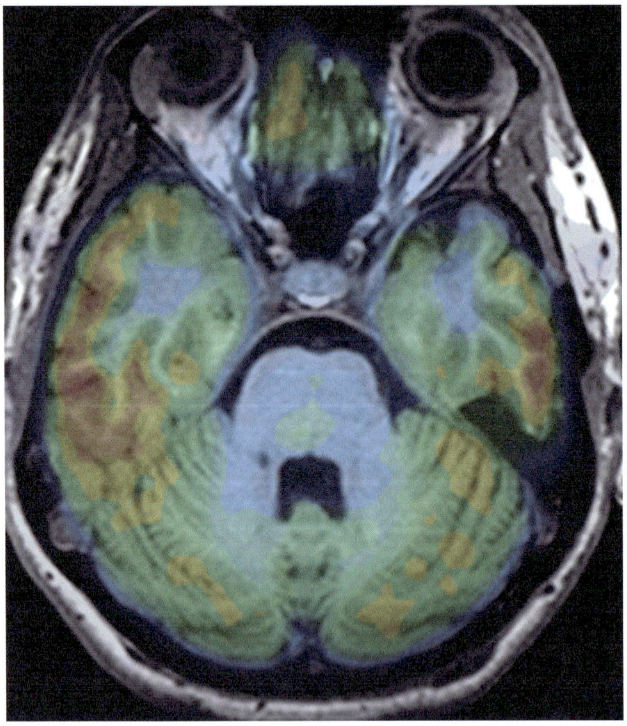

Fig. 28.10 PET-MRI co-registration with color-scale FDG in an axial plane at a mid-pons level. The left temporal lobe is hypometabolic across the pole and the mesial aspect. The left lateral temporal lobe and the right temporal lobe are normal

Part III

Trauma

Traumatic brain injury
Brain injury
Brain trauma
Encephalomalacia
Cerebral contusion

CT scans are readily used during the evaluation of acute traumatic brain injury because of their depiction of bone provides sensitivity to detection of skull fractures and the hyperdense appearance of a retracted blood clot provides sensitivity for acute hemorrhage. Although an intracerebral hemorrhage and a skull fracture are two risk factors for post-traumatic epilepsy, MRI is the preferred imaging modality after the acute time period. MRI provides sensitive visualization of chronic hemorrhage and gliosis. Gradient echo sequences imaging (GRE) or susceptibility-weighted sequences imaging (SWI) are particularly well-suited to detect hemosiderin staining that can indicate epileptogenic tissue. MRI's superiority also includes the anatomic detail and tissue characteristics of FLAIR and T2-weighted images for identification of encephalomalacia and gliosis. Beyond conventional structural imaging, diffusion tensor imaging (DTI) demonstrates fiber directionality, which provides an additional means to identify disrupted tissue. The visual qualitative assessment of the color map DTI is a straightforward way to visualize the gross asymmetry of the cerebrum's white matter fiber tracts. More subtle changes may be identified with the apparent diffusion coefficient (ADC) map and fraction anisotropy map (FA).

Key References

Brody DL, MacDonald CL, Shimony JS. Current and future diagnostic tools for traumatic brain injury: CT, conventional MRI, and diffusion tensor imaging. Handb Clin Neurol. 2015;127:267–75.

Diaz-Arrastia R, Agostini MA, Madden MJ, Van Ness PC. Posttraumatic epilepsy: the endophenotypes of a human model of epileptogenesis. Epilepsia. 2009;50(Suppl. 2):14–20.

Douglas DB, Muldermans JL, Wintermark M. Neuroimaging of brain trauma. Curr Opin Neurol. 2018;31:362–70.

Messori A, Polonara G, Carle F, Gesuita R, Salvolini. Predicting posttraumatic epilepsy with MRI: prospective longitudinal morphologic study in adults. Epilepsia. 2005;56:1472–81.

Temporal Lobe Trauma

29

Clinical History

The first recognized seizure occurred at age 18 years as a bilateral tonic-clonic seizure without an aura or warning.

The habitual seizures had a 30-minute prodromal warning that is described as being spacey without a change in awareness or focal neurological abnormality. The prodrome was followed by a brief aura of an indescribable sense of an imminent seizure along with a need to drink water. A focal seizure with impaired awareness followed either the aura or the prodrome, and the ictal behavior of this seizure included a wide-eyed stare with oral automatisms. Typically, the impaired awareness duration was between 1 and 3 minutes. Some prodromes and auras proceeded to a bilateral tonic-clonic seizure without the initial focal seizure. After bilateral tonic-clonic seizures, a left-sided Todd's paralysis was sometimes present for 15 to 20 minutes. Treatment included multiple anti-seizure medications without seizure freedom. The seizure frequency was one seizure or cluster of multiple seizures every 6 weeks.

The epilepsy risk factor was significant head trauma that occurred at age 17 years in a motor vehicle accident. The injury produced a coma that lasted 4 weeks.

Neurological examination demonstrated an incomplete left homonymous hemianopsia that resulted from the head trauma. The remainder of the exam, including motor and sensory function, was normal.

Interictal EEG depicted diffuse abnormal slowing that is greater on the right side. MRI identified extensive encephalomalacia of the right temporal lobe and inferior-lateral basal ganglia. The right hippocampus and amygdala had significant atrophy and signal abnormality.

The history and evaluation indicate right temporal lobe epilepsy that involves both limbic and neocortical features. The limbic aspects are the aura and focal seizures with impaired awareness and automatisms. Involvement of the neocortex is evident in the Todd's paralysis, which is unusual in mesial temporal lobe epilepsy, and indicates right neocortical involvement that extends beyond the temporal lobe. The imaging supports the right temporal lobe localization; however, a discrete region amenable to surgical treatment is not evident. The epileptic abnormality may include the right temporal and possibly adjacent neocortical regions, as can occur with epilepsy due to traumatic brain injury.

J. M. Stern, N. Salamon, *Imaging of Epilepsy*, https://doi.org/10.1007/978-3-030-86672-3_29

Imaging

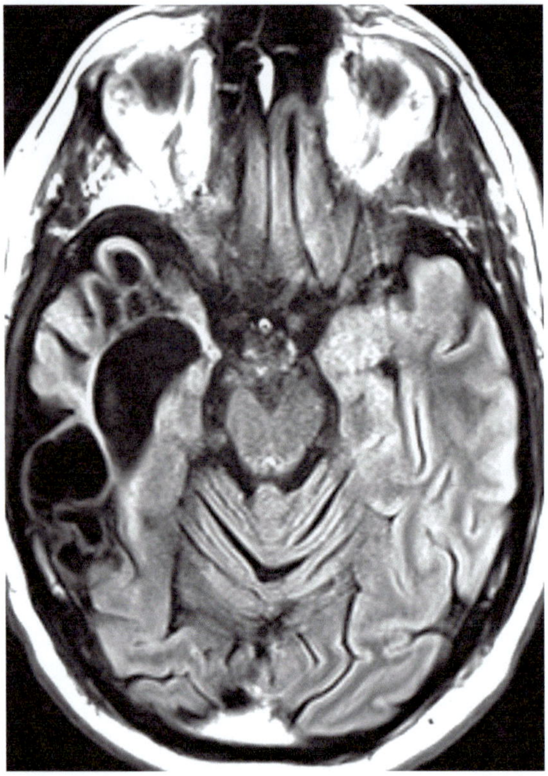

Fig. 29.1 MRI with axial FLAIR sequence at the temporal lobe level. Foci of encephalomalacia involving the right middle temporal gyrus and temporal pole are evident along with ex-vacuo enlargement of the right temporal horn of the lateral ventricle. High FLAIR signal suggests gliosis in the right periventricular white matter

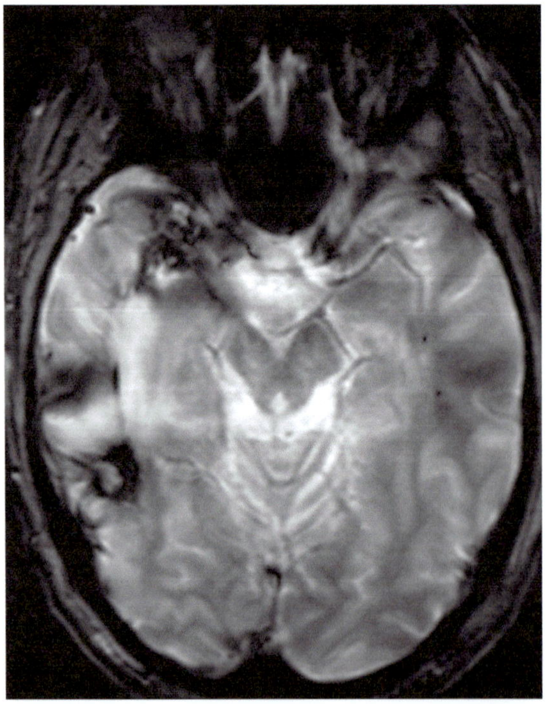

Fig. 29.2 MRI with axial gradient echo sequence at a temporal lobe level similar to Fig. 29.1. Susceptibility artifact indicates microhemorrhages in the right temporal lobe adjacent to the cystic encephalomalacia cavities. This is consistent with trauma

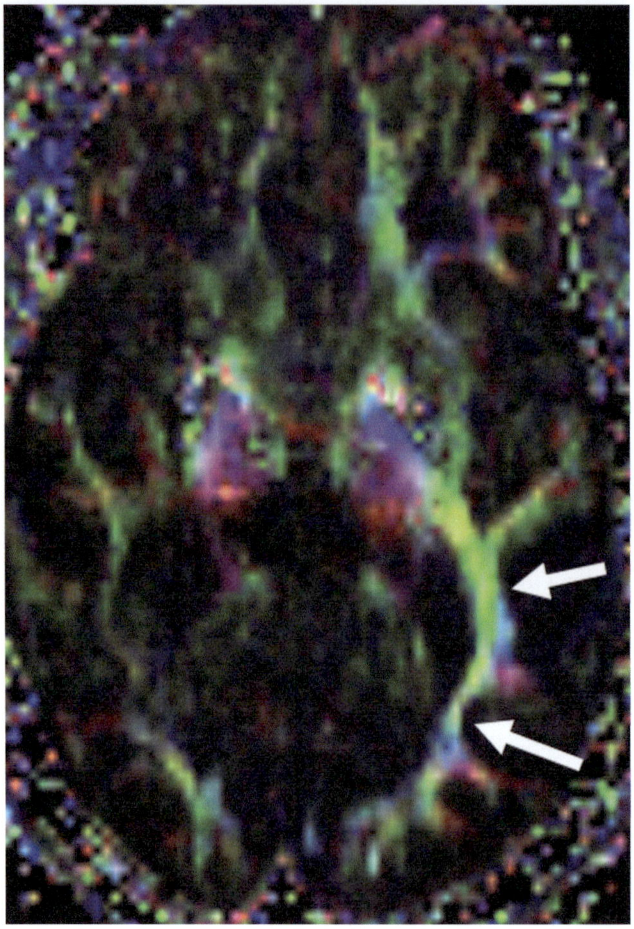

Fig. 29.3 MRI with axial diffusion tensor imaging at a temporal lobe level superior to Figs. 29.1 and 29.2. Color map imaging shows asymmetric optic radiations with decreased right-sided fibers. The left optic radiation (arrows) has anterior to posterior oriented (green) fibers evident. The findings are consistent with the left homonymous hemianopsia but do not necessarily indicate visual field loss

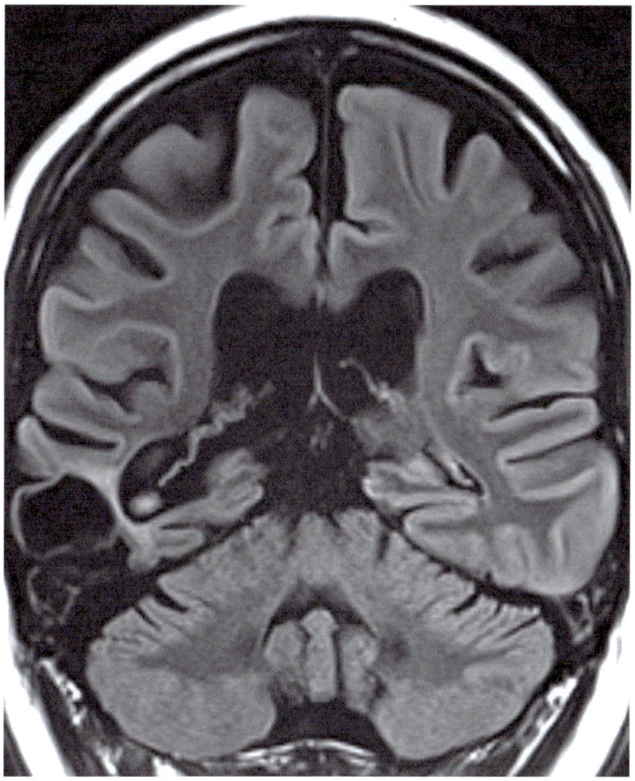

Fig. 29.4 MRI with coronal FLAIR sequence at a posterior temporal lobe level. Foci of encephalomalacia correspond to the abnormalities in Fig. 29.1. The hippocampi are small because of the posterior level, and the left temporal lobe is otherwise normal

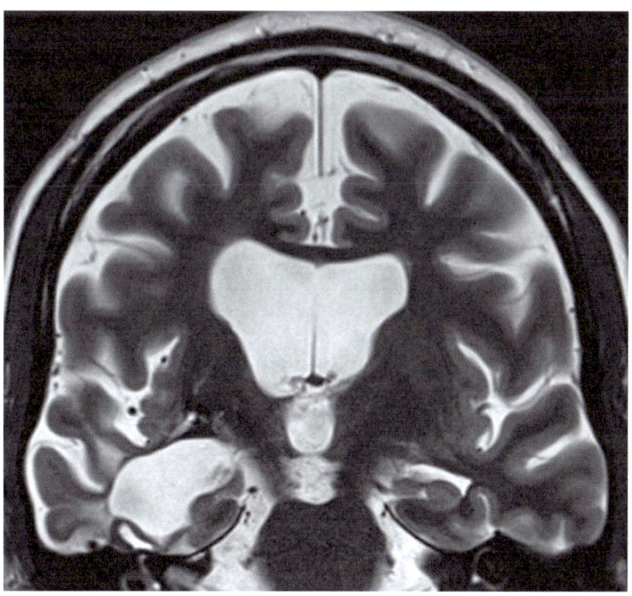

Fig. 29.5 MRI with coronal T2 sequence at an anterior temporal lobe level. The right temporal horn is markedly dilated. The right temporal lobe white matter has abnormal hyperintensity and is partly lost. The lateral ventricles also are asymmetric due to enlargement on the right side, which indicates right frontal lobe injury

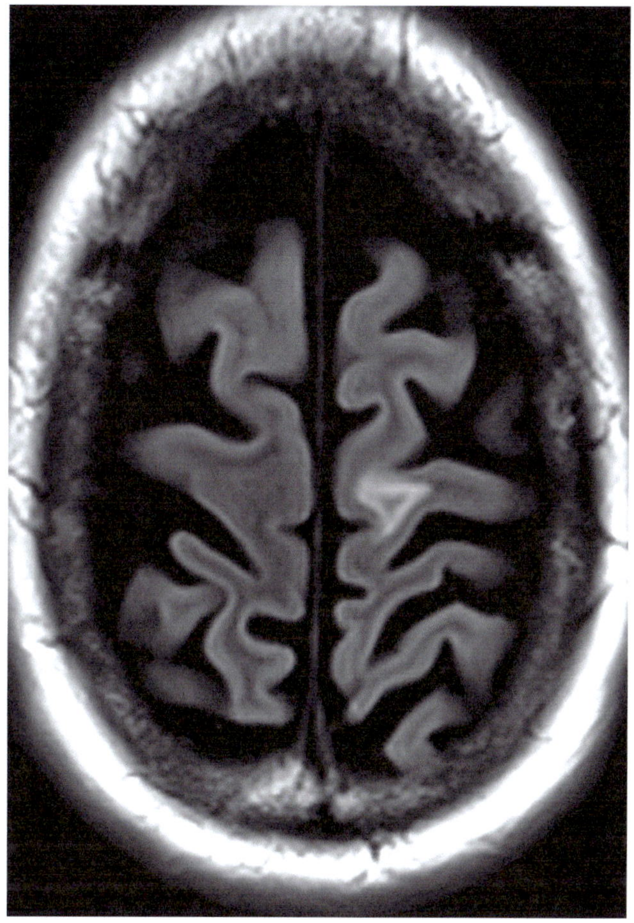

Fig. 29.6 MRI with axial FLAIR sequence at a superior convexity level. A triangular signal abnormality is present between the left superior frontal gyrus and precentral gyrus. This is likely due to a countercoup injury that occurred at the time of the right-sided head trauma. The finding is subclinical

30 Frontal Lobe Trauma

Clinical History

The first recognized seizure occurred at age 61 years as a bilateral tonic-clonic seizure during a hospitalization after severe traumatic brain injury.

The habitual seizures were bilateral tonic-clonic without lateralizing features and no longer followed an aura. Some seizures soon after the onset of epilepsy followed a sense of nonspecific light-headedness. Treatment included multiple anti-seizure medications with a seizure frequency of one monthly.

The epilepsy risk factor was significant head trauma that occurred when in a collision with a car while riding a bicycle, and the injury produced a coma that lasted several weeks. Evaluation at presentation identified a skull fracture with bilateral subdural hematomas and an intraparenchymal hematoma.

Neurological examination demonstrated a left abducens palsy. Mentation was normal during routine, neurological examination, but cognitive deficits of executive dysfunction and irritability produced disability.

Interictal EEG depicted abnormal right temporal slowing. Head CT identified enlarged ventricles. MRI identified hippocampal atrophy and focal encephalomalacia within the right superior and middle frontal gyri. Diffuse hemosiderin staining was evident along the surface of the right hemisphere.

The history and evaluation indicate focal epilepsy with seizures that quickly propagate across bilateral neocortex, as may occur after bilateral neocortical injury. The prior aura of light-headedness is not indicative of a discrete localization as it may occur with a diffuse seizure onset, so it is not contributory to the seizure localization. The loss of this aura may reflect the current seizures propagate quickly and with insufficient time for the aura to be experienced. Although the more severe imaging abnormality is asymmetric, the bilateral hippocampal and frontal lobe atrophy and the cognitive deficits support bilateral cerebral dysfunction and the possibility of bihemispheric contribution to the epilepsy, even if the seizures are focal. Essentially, the imaging findings may not fully represent the extent of the injury.

J. M. Stern, N. Salamon, *Imaging of Epilepsy*, https://doi.org/10.1007/978-3-030-86672-3_30

Imaging

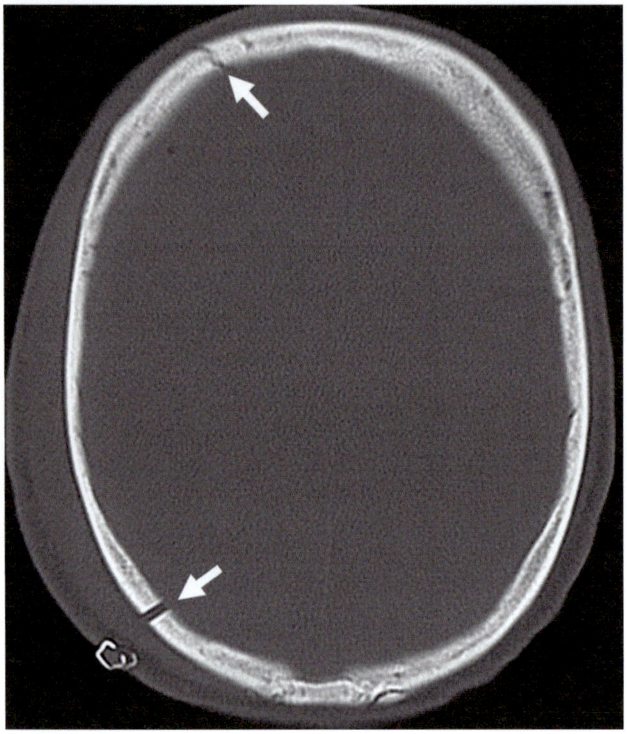

Fig. 30.1 CT scan with bone windows at a centrum semi-ovale level obtained at the time of the trauma. A skull fracture (anterior arrow) is evident as a jagged defect in the right frontal bone. Craniotomy (posterior arrow) is evident as a straight gap in the right parietal bone with an overlying surgical staple

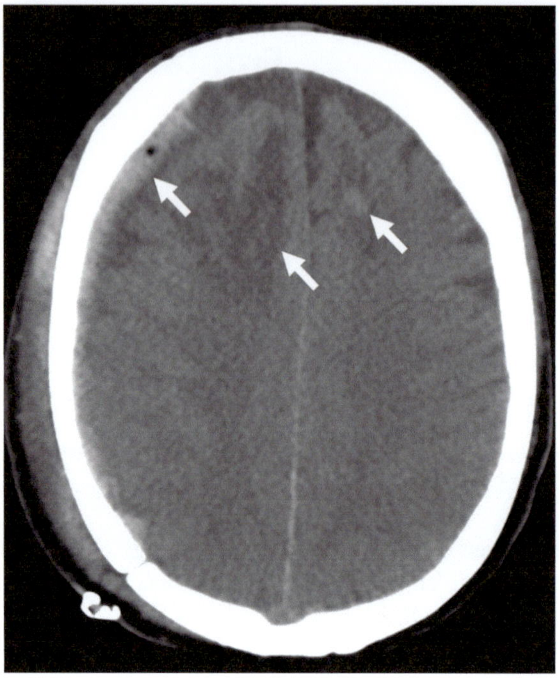

Fig. 30.2 CT scan with soft tissue windows at the same level as Fig. 30.1, also obtained at the time of the trauma. A right-sided, frontal subdural hematoma (right frontal lateral arrow) is present with displacement of the right frontal lobe and air bubble within the hematoma. Low density is present in the right superior frontal gyrus (right frontal midline arrow) and represents a cerebral contusion. A smaller region of low density is present in the left frontal lobe indicates contralateral contusion and is accompanied by a region of higher density indicating hemorrhage (left frontal arrow)

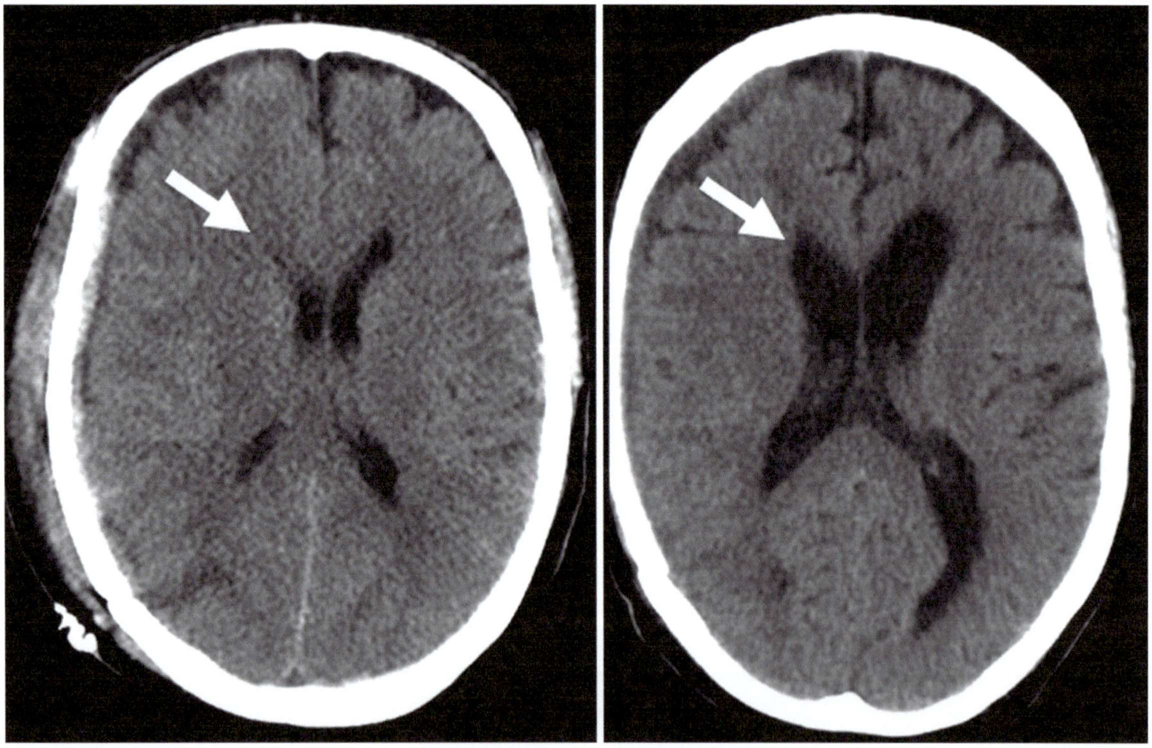

Fig. 30.3 CT scans with soft tissue windows at a ventricular level. The left figure was obtained at the time of trauma, and the right figure is 2 months later. The earlier CT scan demonstrates diffuse cerebral edema and soft tissue swelling along the scalp on the right side. The later CT demonstrates enlargement of the lateral ventricles. The arrows indicate a region of white matter loss

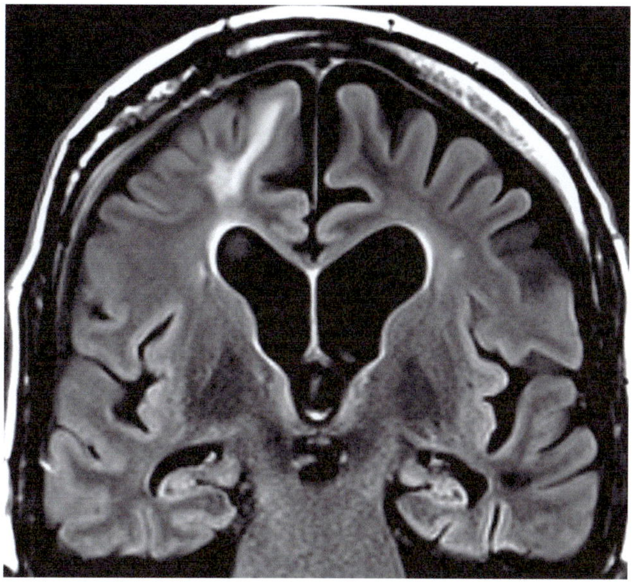

Fig. 30.4 MRI with coronal FLAIR sequence at a mid-temporal lobe level obtained 1.5 years after the trauma. Atrophy of bilateral frontal and temporal lobes is present with ventricular enlargement. High signal within the right superior and middle frontal gyri indicates additional subcortical injury. Bilateral hippocampal atrophy also is present

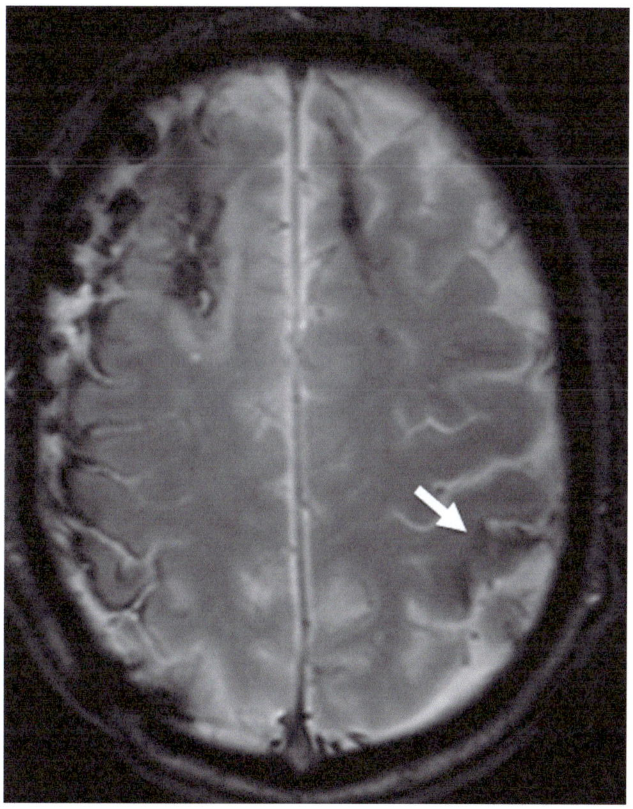

Fig. 30.5 MRI with axial gradient echo sequence at the high convexity level obtained 1.5 years after the trauma. Linear susceptibility artifact indicating microhemorrhages is present in bilateral frontal lobes with a larger extent on the right. Susceptibility artifact is present along the surface of the right convexity. Additional susceptibility artifact within the left anterior parietal lobe (arrow) indicates a countercoup injury

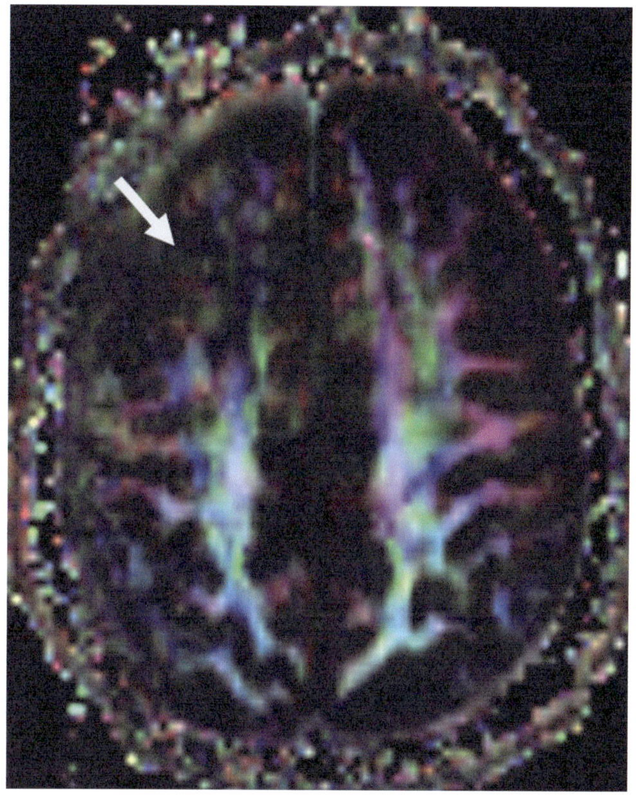

Fig. 30.6 MRI with axial diffusion tensor imaging at the high convexity level obtained 1.5 years after the trauma. Color map imaging depicts asymmetric white matter integrity with disruption of right frontal white matter direction integrity (arrow)

31 Bilateral Cerebral Trauma

Clinical History

The first recognized seizure occurred at age 19 years as a bilateral tonic-clonic seizure.

The habitual seizures manifested as stereotyped, abnormal sensations across the hands and mouth with progression to right arm shaking and then bilateral tonic-clonic movements with a duration of typically 2–3 minutes. None of the seizures were limited to either auras in isolation or impairment of awareness without bilateral motor activity. Treatment included multiple anti-seizure medications without seizure freedom, but months may separate the seizures. The seizure frequency was six yearly.

The epilepsy risk factor was traumatic brain injury that occurred at age 18 years due to a motor vehicle collision. The injury was compounded by a cerebral sinus thrombosis with bifrontal venous infarction due to an inflammatory reaction to the replaced skull after a therapeutic craniectomy.

Neurological examination was abnormal due to concentration difficulty. Additional post-traumatic deficits were evident in the history of episodes of anger and violence. Neuropsychological testing identified impairments in verbal memory and executive function.

Interictal EEG depicted abnormal, generalized slowing and epileptiform sharp waves over the right frontal-central region with less frequent epileptiform discharges over the superior frontal midline and left frontal-central region. Video-EEG monitoring recorded focal seizures that progressed to bilateral tonic-clonic. The ictal EEG's seizure onset was anterior, parasagittal, rhythmic slowing.

MRI obtained 2 years after the trauma identified encephalomalacia of the anterior frontal lobes that was more severe on the left and involved both cortex and white matter. Postoperative changes and left inferior frontal encephalomalacia were related to a hematoma evacuation. The hippocampal signals were normal, but the left hippocampal head was abnormally smaller than the right. PET identified bilateral frontal hypometabolism.

The history and evaluation indicate frontal lobe epilepsy with a non-localizing aura that quickly and consistently progresses to asymmetric motor activity that suggests a left-sided cerebral lateralization. The ictal EEG and both the midline and left frontal-central interictal discharges are consistent with a superior or anterior frontal lobe onset but do not provide lateralizing information within the expanse of the left frontal lobe. The right-sided interictal EEG abnormality does not preclude the possibility of left-sided onset, but it furthers the concern for a bilateral frontal lobe abnormality, which the imaging also identifics. Because of the broad extent of the potentially epileptogenic zone, resective surgical treatment was not performed.

J. M. Stern, N. Salamon, *Imaging of Epilepsy*, https://doi.org/10.1007/978-3-030-86672-3_31

Imaging

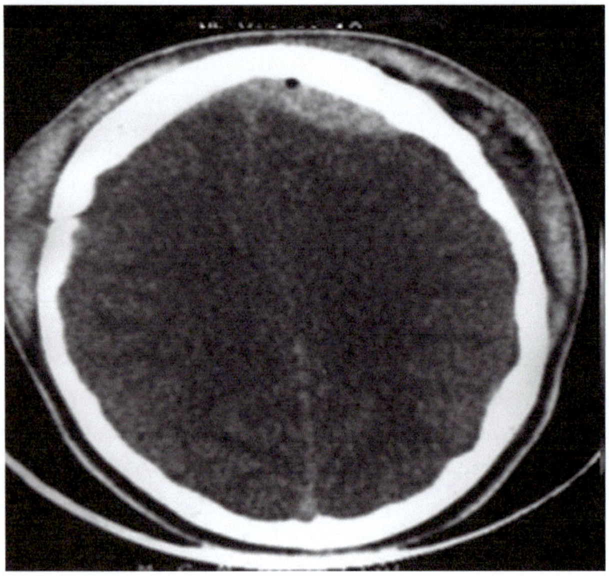

Fig. 31.1 CT scan with soft tissue windows at a centrum semi-ovale level obtained at the time of trauma. A left frontal hematoma with a small collection of air is displacing the left frontal lobe. Cortical sulci are effaced; however, the differentiation of the gray matter and white matter indicates that cerebral edema is not necessarily present. Severe scalp hematomas are present bilaterally. A right frontal skull fracture also is present

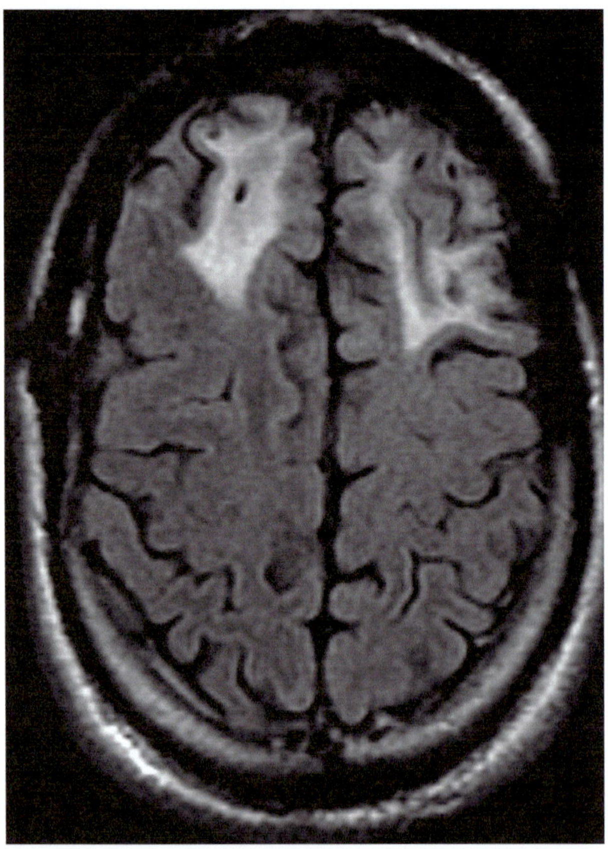

Fig. 31.2 MRI axial FLAIR sequence at a high convexity level obtained 2 years after the trauma. Bilateral frontal subcortical white matter high signal is evident and consistent with post-traumatic gliosis

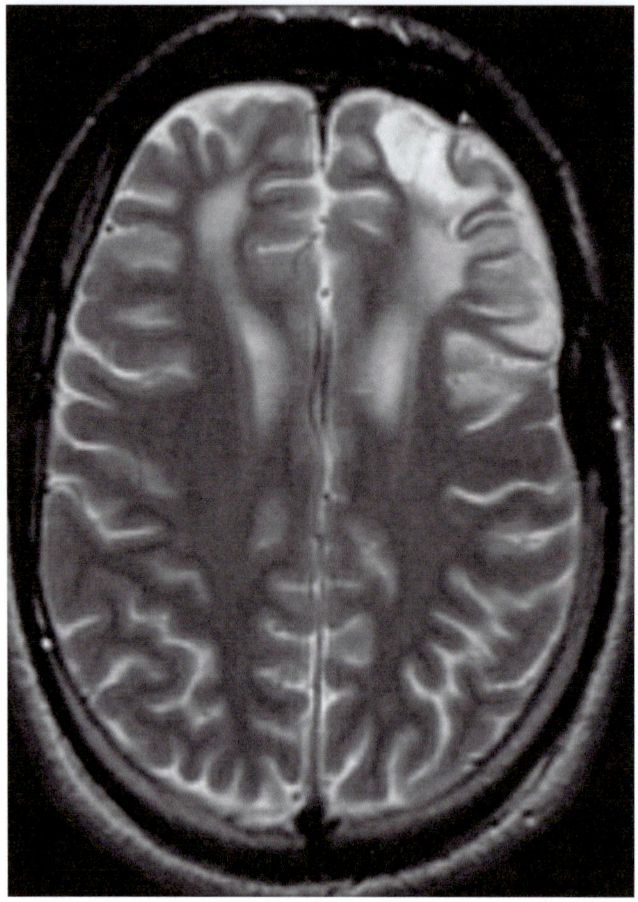

Fig. 31.3 MRI axial T2 sequence at a centrum semi-ovale level that is slightly inferior to Fig. 31.2. Subcortical signal abnormality is evident as inferior continuation of the finding in Fig. 31.2, but asymmetry is evident with left frontal pole encephalomalacia

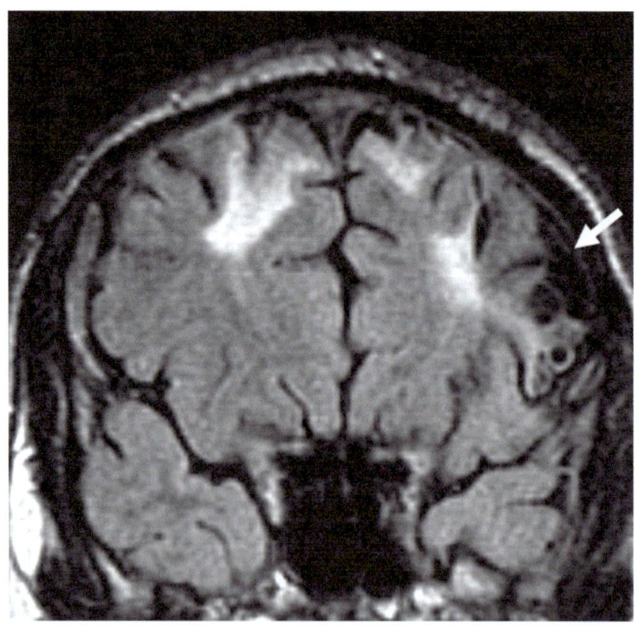

Fig. 31.4 MRI coronal FLAIR sequence at an anterior temporal level. Left lateral frontal encephalomalacia is present with low signal intensity cavity (arrow) in the left inferior frontal gyrus. Surgical changes related to a prior hematoma are present across the left lateral temporal lobe

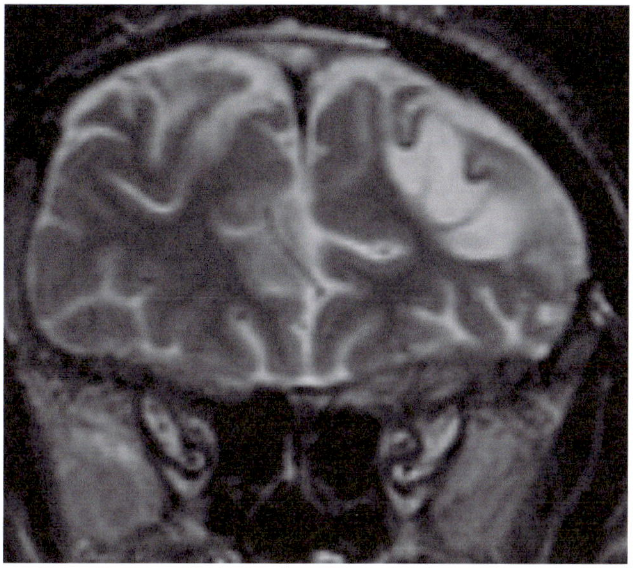

Fig. 31.5 MRI coronal T2 sequence at an anterior frontal level that is slightly anterior to the level in Fig. 31.4. A cavity produced by a prior hematoma is evident in the left frontal lobe. The orbital frontal regions are normal

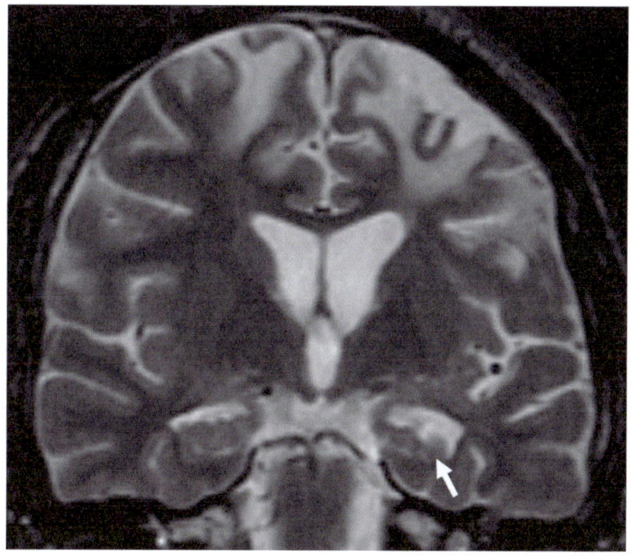

Fig. 31.6 MRI coronal T2 sequence at a hippocampal head level. Post-traumatic bilateral frontal gliosis with encephalomalacia is evident with greater encephalomalacia of the left superior and middle frontal gyri. Atrophy of the left hippocampus (arrow) also is evident. The temporal lobes are otherwise normal

Multilobar Cerebral Trauma

32

Clinical History

The first recognized seizure occurred at age 20 years after a traumatic brain injury. The details of this seizure are not known, and seizure freedom was present for 6 years until a nocturnal bilateral tonic-clonic seizure occurred.

The habitual seizures began soon after the second seizure and manifested as a wide-eyed, blank stare with oral automatisms, wandering, and sometimes also leftward head turning. The seizure duration was less than 1 minute. Treatment has included multiple anti-seizure medications with seizure frequency of three monthly.

The epilepsy risk factor was traumatic brain injury that was caused by falling from a moving motor vehicle. The fall produced a subdural hematoma that became an abscess.

Neurological examination was normal. Neuropsychological testing identified impairments in attention, concentration, recent memory, attention, executive function, and naming.

Interictal EEG depicted frequent epileptiform spike and slow-wave complexes that sometimes occurred in runs across the left side. Video-EEG monitoring recorded focal seizures manifested as leftward head turning prior to becoming bilateral tonic-clonic. A left-sided Todd's paralysis was present postictally. Ictal EEG's seizure onset was bilateral epileptiform discharges followed by generalized slowing and attenuation except for one seizure that had broad right-sided epileptiform fast activity leading into the generalized slowing and attenuation.

MRI identified extensive injury to the right frontal lobe and lesser injury to bilateral gyrus rectus orbitofrontal regions. PET identified diffuse hypometabolism with greater photopenia within the right frontal lobe.

The history and evaluation indicate the possibility of focal epilepsy with seizures that arise within the limbic system and then progress into the right cerebral neocortex, as manifested by the impairment of awareness with automatisms and then asymmetric motor activity with a left postictal paralysis. The one seizure with right-sided ictal onset on EEG and the extensive right frontal lobe injury support this localization. However, more than one localization may be present, as suggested by EEG's interictal epileptiform runs across the left side. A second localization within the left inferior frontal region may also be present, as supported by the left-sided runs of epileptiform abnormality. This localization may be related to the seizures that are limited to staring and wandering and the bilateral EEG ictal onsets if propagation is into the anterior or medial frontal lobe. Essentially, the severity of the trauma and the subsequent infection raise the possibility of more than one epileptogenic region.

J. M. Stern, N. Salamon, *Imaging of Epilepsy*, https://doi.org/10.1007/978-3-030-86672-3_32

Imaging

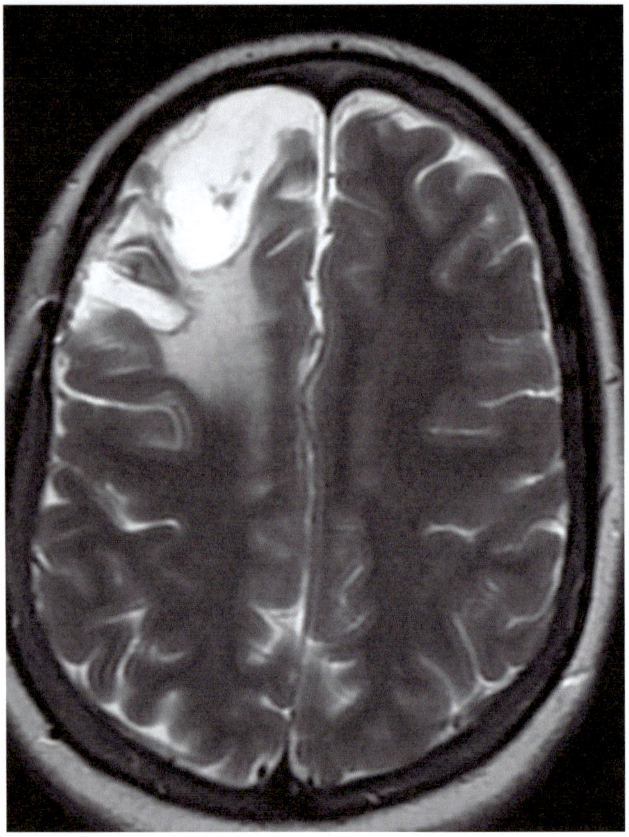

Fig. 32.1 MRI axial T2 sequence at a centrum semi-ovale level. A large right anterior, superior frontal gyrus region of tissue loss has produced a cavity surrounded by white matter gliosis. A smaller cavity is present laterally, in the right inferior frontal gyrus

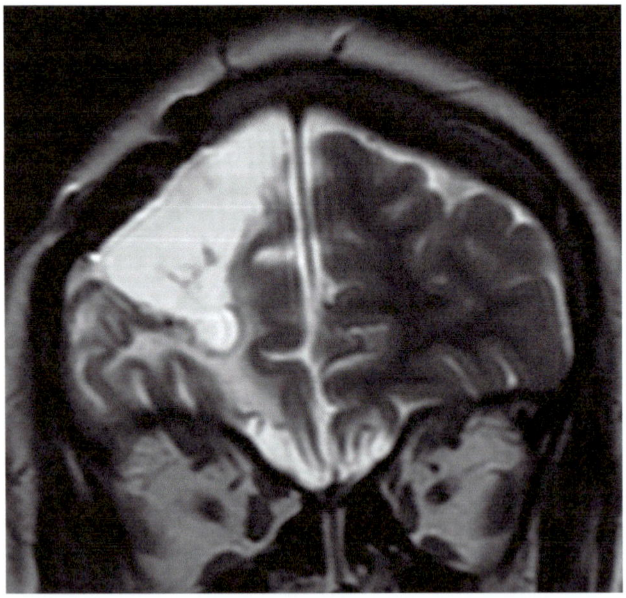

Fig. 32.2 MRI coronal T2 sequence at an anterior frontal level. The large region of right anterior frontal encephalomalacia is evident along with encephalomalacia of bilateral gyri recti and right orbital frontal regions. White matter signal abnormality indicating gliosis is present throughout the anterior right frontal lobe

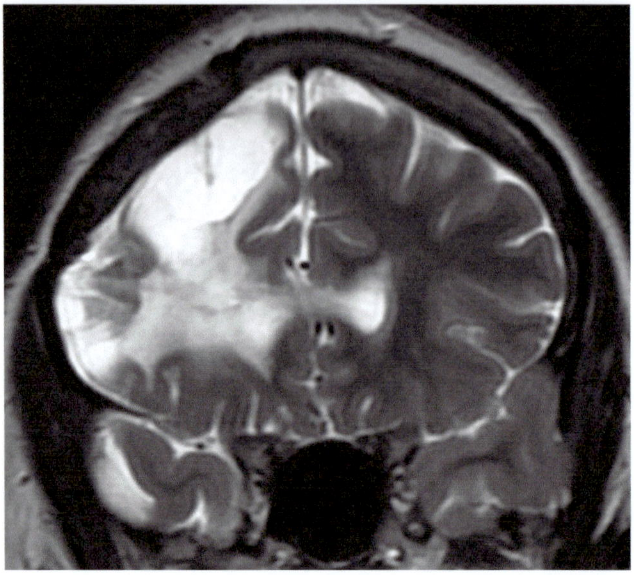

Fig. 32.3 MRI coronal T2 sequence at an anterior temporal level that is posterior to Fig. 32.2. The right frontal encephalomalacia is evident in the superior and lateral frontal lobe with extension of the white matter signal abnormality to include the corpus callosum. The lateral temporal lobes are asymmetric with minor encephalomalacia on the right

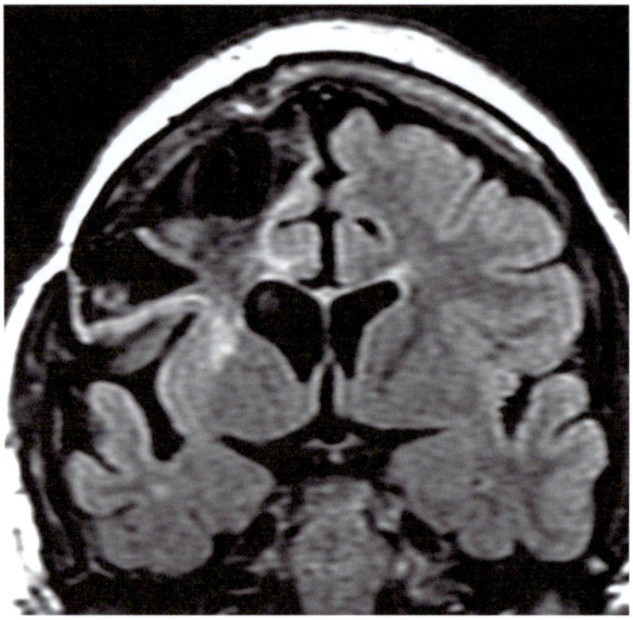

Fig. 32.4 MRI coronal FLAIR sequence at an amygdalar level. Extensive right frontal lobe encephalomalacia is evident with tissue loss along the cortical surface, abnormally low intensity signal in the residual tissue, and enlargement of the right lateral ventricle. Abnormally high intensity signal is evident in medial right frontal lobe and indicates gliosis. The right Sylvian fissure is dilated, and right superior temporal gyrus is atrophic with minor gliosis in the white matter

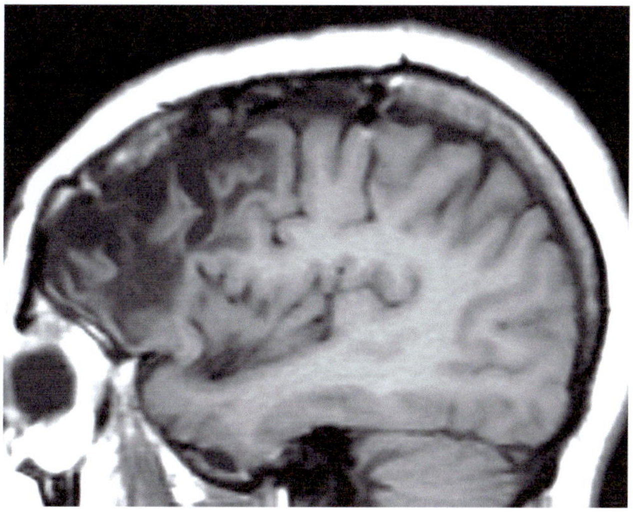

Fig. 32.5 MRI T1 sequence in right sagittal plane at an insular level. The anterior to posterior extent and multiple cavities of encephalomalacia of the frontal injury are evident in the low intensity signal across the anterior, mid, and orbitofrontal regions. The temporal lobe is normal

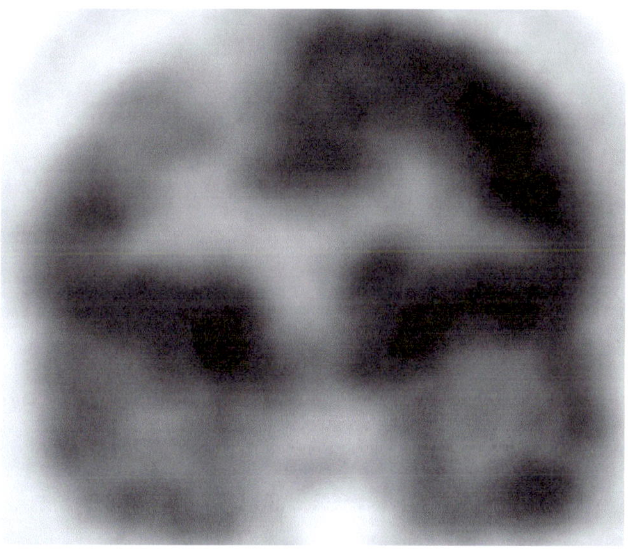

Fig. 32.6 PET with grayscale FDG tracer in the coronal plane at an anterior temporal level. Hypometabolism is evident in the right superior frontal lobe, including a smaller region of ametabolism related to complete tissue loss in the superior frontal gyrus. Less severe hypometabolism in the right temporal lobe is evident in the inferior and lateral aspects, when compared to the left temporal lobe

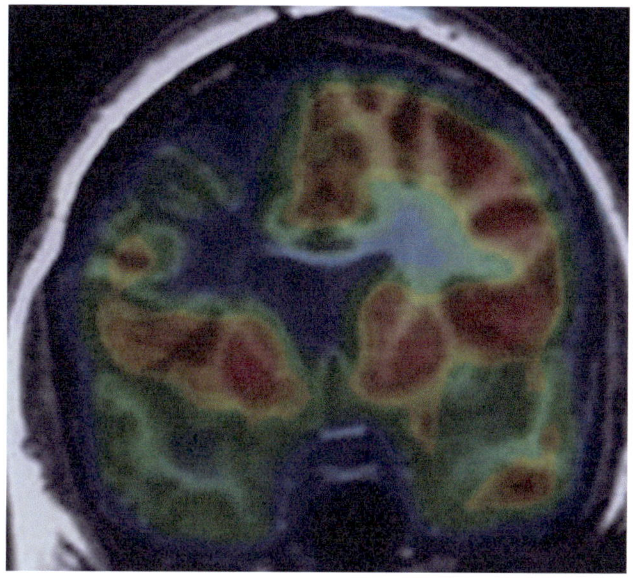

Fig. 32.7 PET-MRI co-registration with color-scale FDG tracer in the coronal plane at an anterior temporal level. Ametabolism of the right superior frontal gyrus and co-localized tissue loss are evident. The abnormal gyral structure along the lateral right frontal lobe is evident along with co-registered hypometabolism. The right temporal lobe is structurally normal with hypometabolism that is evident when compared to the left temporal lobe

Part IV
Infection and Inflammation

Brain infection
Brain inflammation
Herpes simplex virus encephalitis
Viral encephalitis
Neurocysticercosis
Limbic encephalitis
Autoimmune encephalitis
Autoimmune encephalopathy
Autoimmune epilepsy
Anti-GAD encephalitis
Anti-NMDA receptor encephalitis
Anti-VGKC complex encephalitis
Hashimoto encephalopathy
Steroid responsive encephalopathy associated with autoimmune thyroiditis
Rasmussen encephalitis
Herpes Encephalitis

Herpes simplex encephalitis's radiologic presentation differs according to age with neonates presenting with ischemia and both children and adults presenting with encephalitis. The encephalitis presentation appears as hyperintense T2 and FLAIR signal in the limbic regions, including the mesial temporal lobe, orbital frontal lobe, cingulate gyrus, and thalamus. Restricted diffusion can be evident with diffusion weighted imaging. Infection is evident as increased perfusion within the temporal lobe and abnormal leptomeningeal contrast enhancement.

Neurocysticercosis

Cerebral neurocysticercosis relates to infection by Taenia solium with consequent larvae within the brain's parenchyma. The larval lesions are divided into 4 stages that differ in their imaging and clinical features.

1. Vesicular: Viable parasite with an intact larval membrane and therefore less host reaction.
2. Colloidal: Turbid fluid within the cyst with surrounding edema because the parasite has died and the membrane has leaked. This is the most symptomatic stage.
3. Granular nodular: Edema has decreased as the cyst retracts but enhancement persists.
4. Nodular calcified: End-stage, quiescent, calcified cyst remnant is evident without edema.

MRI typically demonstrates round cystic lesions with contrast enhancing of the central core (scolex) and the periphery. Surrounding edema is evident in the colloid phase, and calcification is evident in the end-stage. When related to epilepsy, hippocampal sclerosis also may be present.

Autoimmune encephalitides

Glutamic acid decarboxylase (GAD) 65 autoimmune encephalitis produces hyperintense T2 and FLAIR signal in the limbic system, including the insula and temporal lobes with especially prominent hyperintensity in the mesial temporal lobes. Contrast enhancement rarely occurs.

Voltage gated potassium channel autoimmune limbic encephalitis produces hyperintense T2 and FLAIR signal in the temporal lobes with prominent mesial temporal lobe signal during an acute phase that is followed by hippocampal atrophy. Extra-temporal signal changes are rare. Contrast enhancement of the leptomeninges or cortex may be present.

NMDA receptor autoimmune encephalitis produces hyperintense T2 and FLAIR signal in the temporal lobes with greater abnormality in the mesial temporal lobes. Signal abnormality also may be evident in the frontal lobes, basal ganglia, insula, brainstem, and thalamus. DWI restriction abnormality of the temporal lobes or other areas of affected cortex is often present along with leptomeningeal or cortical contrast enhancement. PET may demonstrate abnormal cortical surface or basal ganglia hypermetabolism in the acute phase. Cerebral atrophy with more marked hippocampal atrophy is evident after the acute phase.

Hashimoto Encephalopathy / Steroid-Responsive Encephalopathy associated with Autoimmune Thyroiditis (SREAT)

Dural enhancement is evident along with nonspecific white matter abnormalities that have increased T2 and FLAIR signal. DWI can demonstrate restricted diffusion that is similar to ischemia.

Rasmussen Encephalitis

Rasmussen encephalitis produces a progressive, chronic abnormality of one cerebral hemisphere with an onset that is most often in middle childhood. In the early phase, MRI demonstrates high T2 and FLAIR signal in the perisylvian or limbic system white matter. Abnormal contrast enhancement is not present. PET during this phase demonstrates hypometabolism at the margins of the MRI abnormality.

In the late phase, hemispheric atrophy is evident and usually demonstrates greater atrophy within the perisylvian region, but a region of marked atrophy can be anywhere in the affected hemisphere. Associated caudate or putamen T2 and FLAIR hyperintensity and atrophy is usually present. The contralateral cerebellum also may have atrophy because of diaschisis. Abnormal contrast enhancement is not present, which is unchanged from the early phase. PET depicts hypometabolism across the affected hemisphere.

Key References

Bacchi S, Franke K, Wewegama D, et al. Magnetic resonance imaging and positron emission tomography in anti-NMDA receptor encephalitis: a systematic review. J Clin Neurosci. 2018;52:54–9.

Castillo P, Woodruff B, Caselli R, et al Steroid responsive encephalopathy associated with autoimmune thyroiditis. Arch Neurol. 2006;63:197–202.

Chiapparini L, Granata T, Farina L, et al. Diagnostic imaging in 13 cases of Rasmussen's encephalitis: can early MRI suggest the diagnosis? Neuroradiol. 2003;45:171–83.

Jayaraman K, Rangasami R, Chandrasekharan A. Magnetic resonance imaging findings in viral encephalitis: a pictorial essay. J Neurosci Rural Pract. 2018;9:556–60.

Kelley BP, Patel SC, Marin HL, et al. Autoimmune encephalitis: pathophysiology imaging review of an overlooked diagnosis. Am J Neuroradiol. 2017;38:1070–8.

Venkat B, Aggarwal N, Makhalik S, Sood R. A comprehensive review of imaging findings in human cysticercosis Japan J Radiol. 2016;34:241–57.

Acute Herpes Encephalitis

33

Clinical History

The first seizure was convulsive and required emergency medical care with administration of an intranasal benzodiazepine. No additional seizures were evident during transportation by ambulance to an emergency department. During the hospital evaluation, recurrent seizures with impaired awareness, tachycardia, and left gaze deviation occurred, so an intravenous benzodiazepine was administered. The seizures resolved, and the patient then became agitated and confused with mostly incomprehensible speech. An anti-seizure medication was started with a loading dose and continued as maintenance treatment along with treatment for bacterial meningitis and herpes simplex virus encephalitis.

The emergency department evaluation results included normal vital signs, normal CT of the head, normal serum chemistry and blood cell count panel, abnormal cerebrospinal fluid (CSF) due to elevated white blood cells of 121 per mm^3, protein of 57 mg/d, and herpes simplex virus, type 1 DNA. Interictal EEG depicted left hemispheric slowing and left frontal and temporal epileptiform discharges.

Seizures recurred 2 days later as status epilepticus, and treatment was escalated to anesthesia with intubation. EEG after anesthetization depicted bifrontal slowing with asymmetrically decreased faster frequencies across the left hemisphere and left frontal-central epileptiform discharges with recurrences every 5–10 seconds.

Seizure control was subsequently achieved, and successful extubation was performed 7 days after intubation. Neurological examination at that time identified alertness and attentiveness but poor cooperation and a verbalized refusal to answer questions. Mentation improved over the following days to a cooperative state but with poor orientation. Intermittent agitation and combativeness continued for the next few days and then resolved.

Nine days after presentation with acute herpes encephalitis, MRI identified abnormal signal within the left temporal pole, mesial temporal structures with extension to the hippocampal tail, subcallosal gyrus, and posterior gyrus rectus. Leptomeningeal enhancement was present.

The history and evaluation indicate acute herpes encephalitis with focal seizures of impaired awareness that also progressed to bilateral tonic-clonic convulsions. The EEG depicted asymmetric periodic discharges with features that are consistent with herpes encephalitis and the lateralization of the MRI abnormality. Antiviral treatment was given, and anti-seizure treatment was initially successful. Although seizure control was not maintained and escalating treatment for status epilepticus was necessary, seizure control was again successful. As of the last clinical encounter, which was 9 months after the hospital discharge, seizure freedom was present.

J. M. Stern, N. Salamon, *Imaging of Epilepsy*, https://doi.org/10.1007/978-3-030-86672-3_33

Imaging

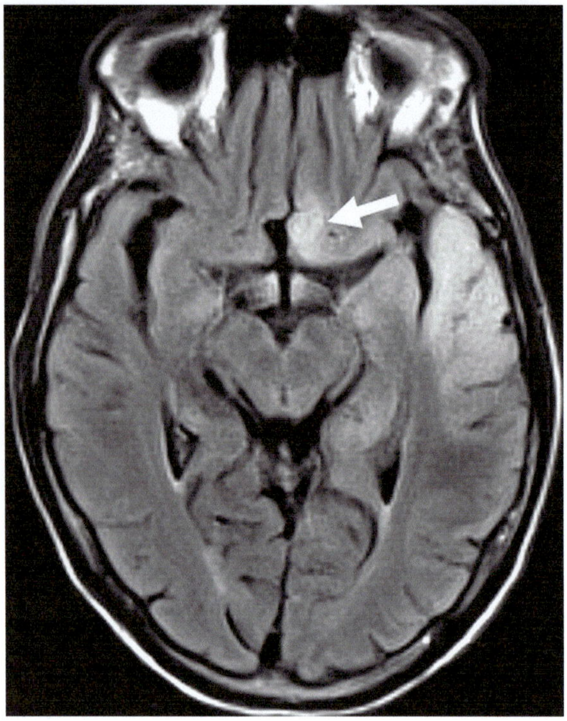

Fig. 33.1 MRI axial FLAIR sequence at a hippocampus level. Hyperintensity is evident in the left gyrus rectus (arrow), left orbitofrontal lobe, and across the left anterior temporal lobe's mesial and lateral aspects. The signal abnormality involves both gray and white matter. No volume loss is present. The right hemisphere is normal

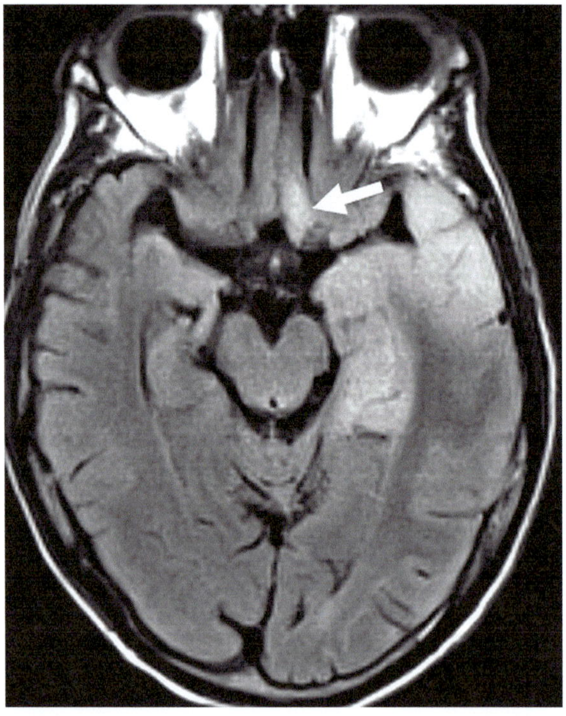

Fig. 33.2 MRI axial FLAIR sequence at an amygdala level that is slightly inferior to Fig. 33.1. Hyperintensity is evident in the left gyrus rectus (arrow), amygdala, hippocampus, temporal pole, and lateral temporal lobe. The right hemisphere is normal

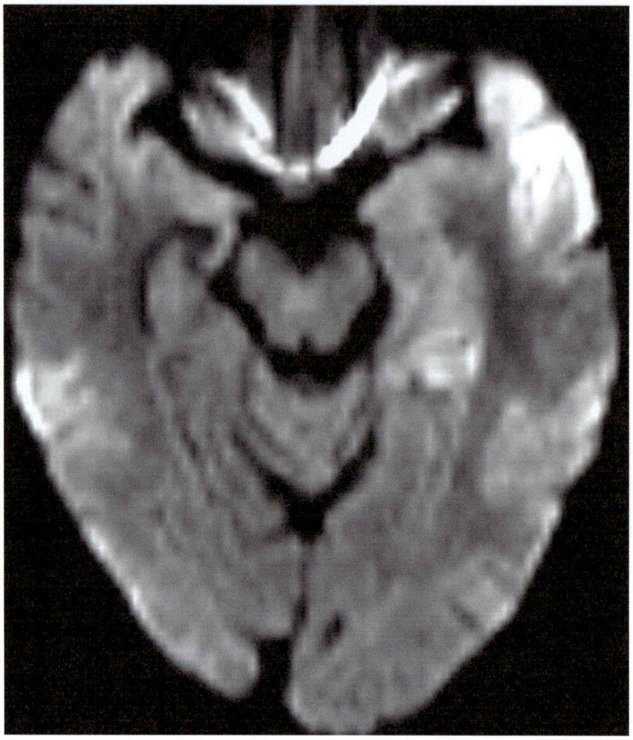

Fig. 33.3 MRI axial DWI sequence at the same amygdala level as Fig. 33.2. Restricted diffusion is evident across the anterior left temporal lobe. The left hippocampus and amygdala are hyperintense due to T2 signal shine through

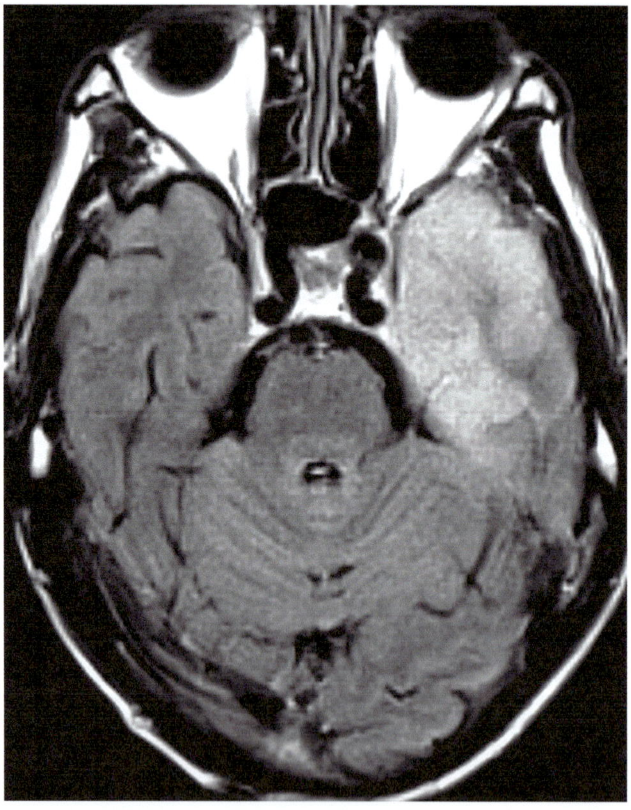

Fig. 33.4 MRI axial FLAIR sequence at a pons level. Marked hyperintensity of the left temporal pole is evident. The left temporal pole's sulci are effaced, indicating edema. The right temporal pole's sulci and tissue signal are normal

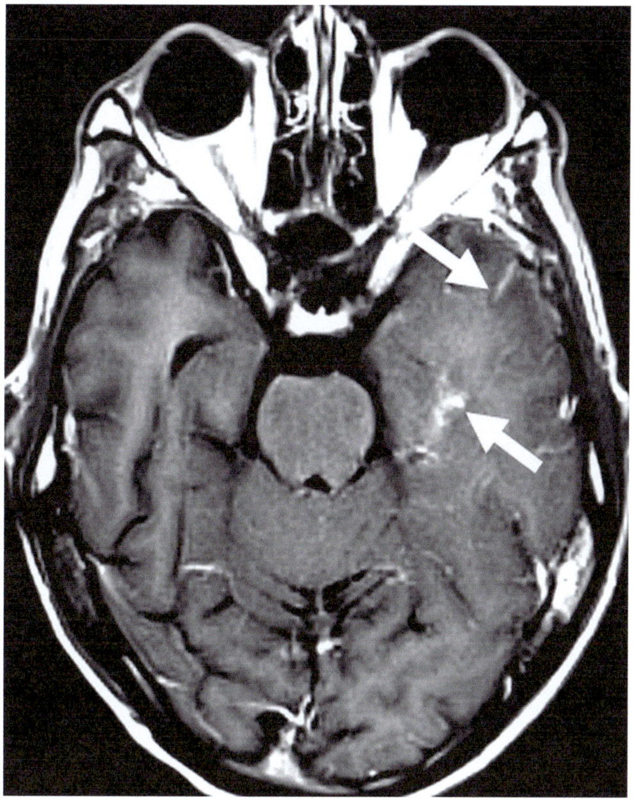

Fig. 33.5 MRI axial T1 sequence after contrast administration at a pons level that is the same as Fig. 33.3. The left temporal pole is edematous with effacement of the sulci and loss of the gray-white differentiation. Enhancement is evident within the sulci (arrows)

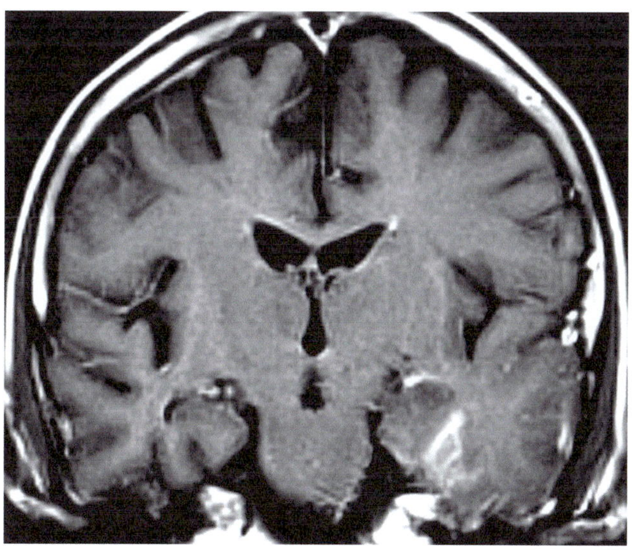

Fig. 33.6 MRI coronal T1 sequence after contrast administration at a hippocampal body level. The left temporal lobe is edematous with blurring of the gray-white junction. Contrast enhancement is evident along the temporal lobe's sulci, with the collateral sulcus most markedly hyperintense. The hyperintensity in the left temporal horn is due to the contrast-enhanced choroid plexus and similar to the homotopic, right-sided choroid plexus

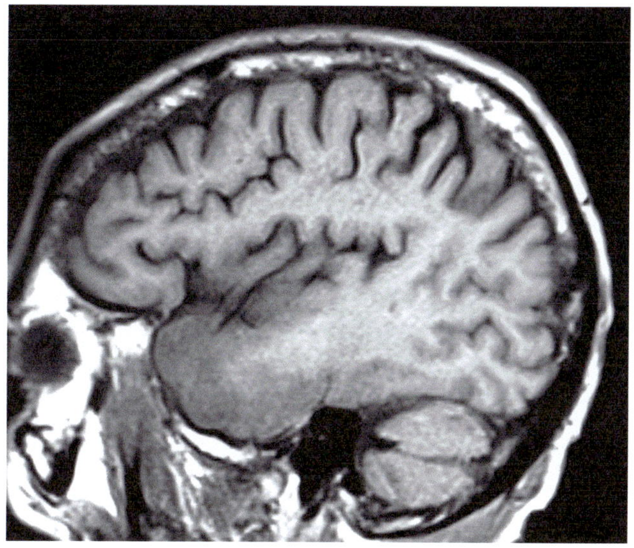

Fig. 33.7 MRI sagittal T1 sequence at a left insula level. The temporal lobe is edematous, and gray-white differentiation is lost at the temporal pole and the inferior temporal surface

34 Remote Herpes Encephalitis

Clinical History

The first recognized seizure occurred at age 40 years while traveling in a remote region and were identified by impaired interactions. An evaluation at that time identified seizures, cerebral edema, and acute herpes encephalitis.

The habitual seizures first occurred later and during a 1.5-year period of rehabilitation. These seizures manifested as an out-of-body experience described as a sense that his body is not his own. The auras progressed to focal seizures with impaired awareness and sometimes bilateral tonic-clonic convulsions. Treatment included multiple anti-seizure medications with incomplete seizure control, but the seizure frequency could be estimated because of memory impairment. Based on ancillary information, the frequency was estimated to be two to three annually.

The only epilepsy risk factor was herpes encephalitis.

Neurological examination was abnormal because of dysphasia and poor memory. Comprehension was limited to one-step instructions. Speech was tangential and had paraphasic errors. Naming and repetition were intact during routine testing, but neuropsychological testing identified deficits in confrontational naming along with nonverbal memory, dividing attention, and planning. The recent medical history also included depression and behavioral disinhibition.

A 72-hour ambulatory EEG depicted left-sided abnormal slowing without epileptiform abnormality.

MRI obtained 8 years after the acute herpes encephalitis identified encephalomalacia of the left temporal lobe and anterior cingulate gyrus with marked left hippocampal atrophy. Abnormal signal is present in the left frontal and temporal white matter. Contrast administration did not produce abnormal enhancement.

The seizure manifestation is consistent with a limbic epileptogenic zone, but propagation into the limbic system from an injured region of neocortex is a reasonable alternative localization. The out-of-body experience cannot be localized with certainty but may be related to propagation to the parietal lobe. Overall, the herpes infection produced a region of potential epileptogenesis within and beyond the left mesial temporal lobe. Additional diagnostic testing or treatment was declined by the patient.

J. M. Stern, N. Salamon, *Imaging of Epilepsy*, https://doi.org/10.1007/978-3-030-86672-3_34

Imaging

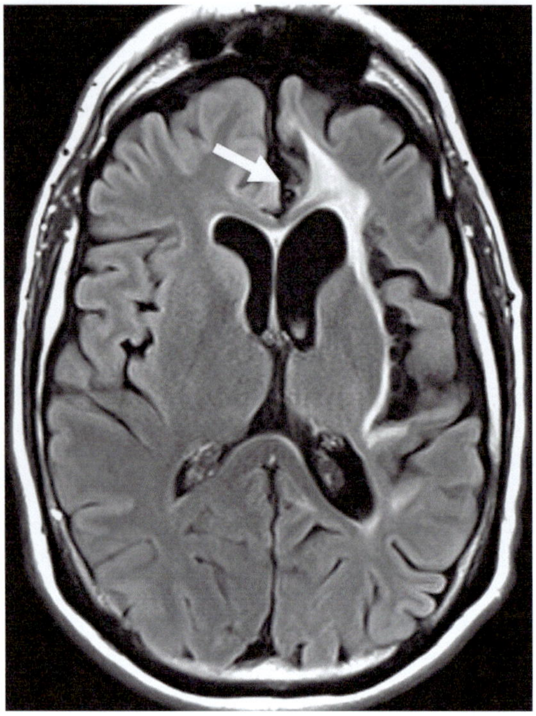

Fig. 34.1 MRI axial FLAIR sequence at a basal ganglia level. Atrophy and encephalomalacia are evident across the left anterior cingulate gyrus (arrow) and the left insula. Hyperintensity of the left frontal lobe white matter, external capsule, and left parietal operculum represents associated gliosis. The left lateral ventricle is enlarged due to left hemispheric volume loss

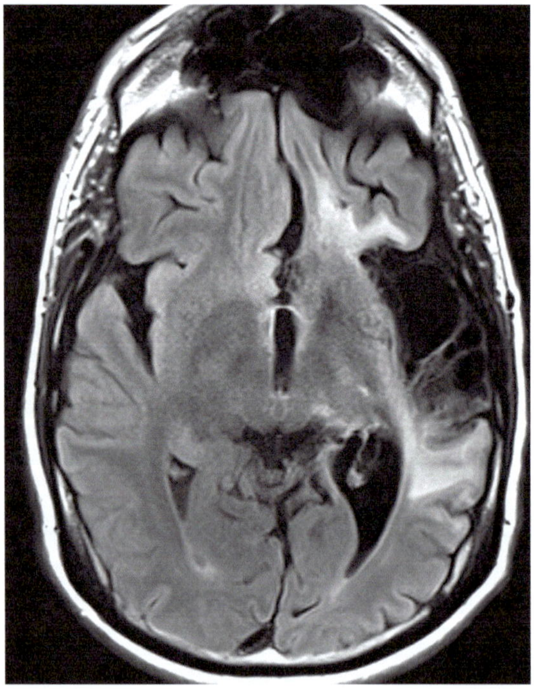

Fig. 34.2 MRI axial FLAIR sequence at an anterior and posterior commissure level. Atrophy and encephalomalacia are evident across the left insula and superior temporal gyrus. Hyperintensity indicating gliosis is present in the left orbitofrontal white matter, lateral temporal white matter, and external capsule. The atrium of the left lateral ventricle is enlarged due to left temporal lobe atrophy

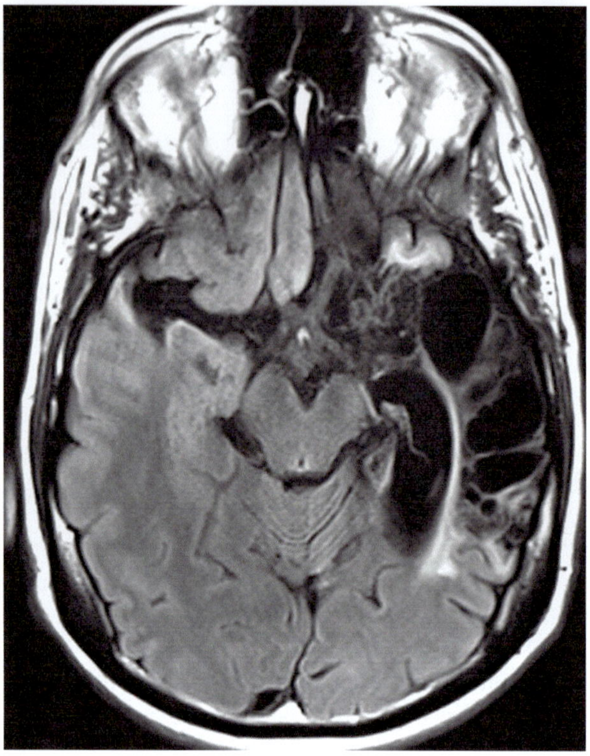

Fig. 34.3 MRI axial FLAIR sequence at an optic chiasm level. Marked encephalomalacia is evident across the left middle temporal gyrus and amygdala. A remnant of the left orbitofrontal gyrus is visible with hyperintense white matter. At this level, the left gyrus rectus is minimally visible, and the left hippocampus is not visible. The enlarged ventricle is due to temporal lobe atrophy

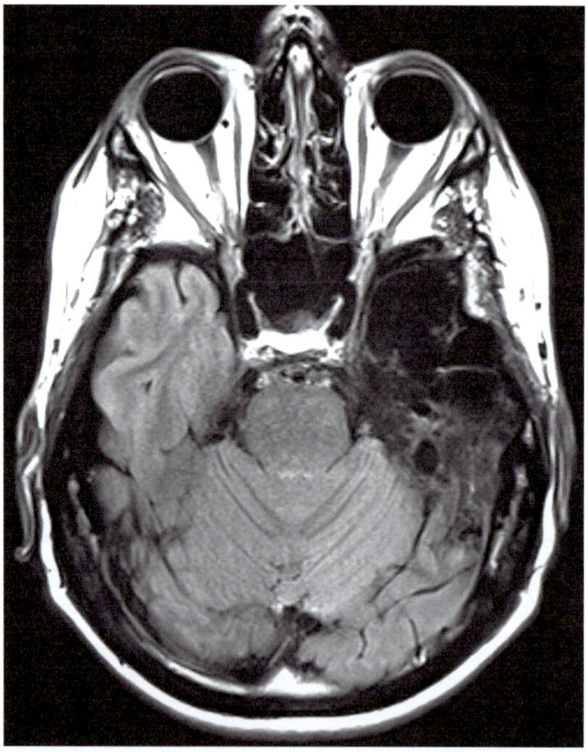

Fig. 34.4 MRI axial FLAIR sequence at a pons level. The left temporal pole has marked tissue loss, and its inferior-lateral aspect demonstrates encephalomalacia extending to the fusiform gyrus

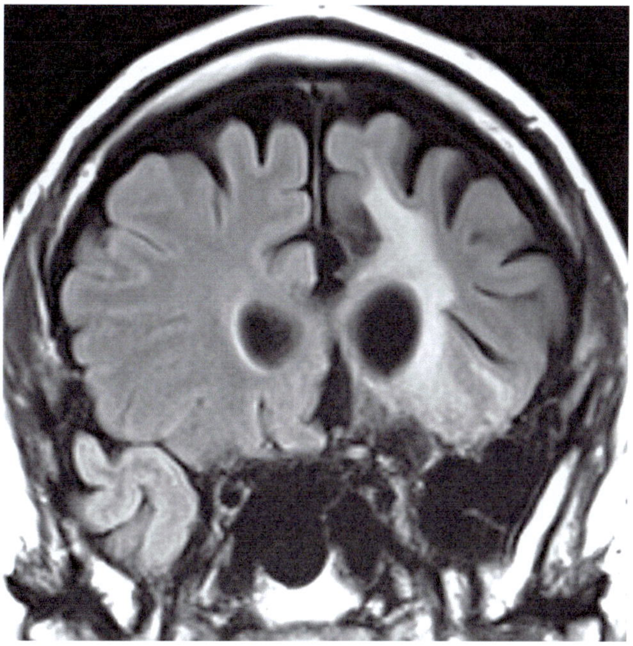

Fig. 34.5 MRI coronal FLAIR sequence at a temporal pole level. Marked tissue loss of the left temporal pole is evident. Less marked encephalomalacia is evident across the left orbitofrontal cortex, gyrus rectus, and cingulate gyrus. The left lateral ventricle is asymmetrically enlarged, and the surrounding white matter is abnormally hyperintense. The left frontal lobe is atrophic with sulci that are asymmetrically more prominent than the right frontal lobe's homotopic sulci

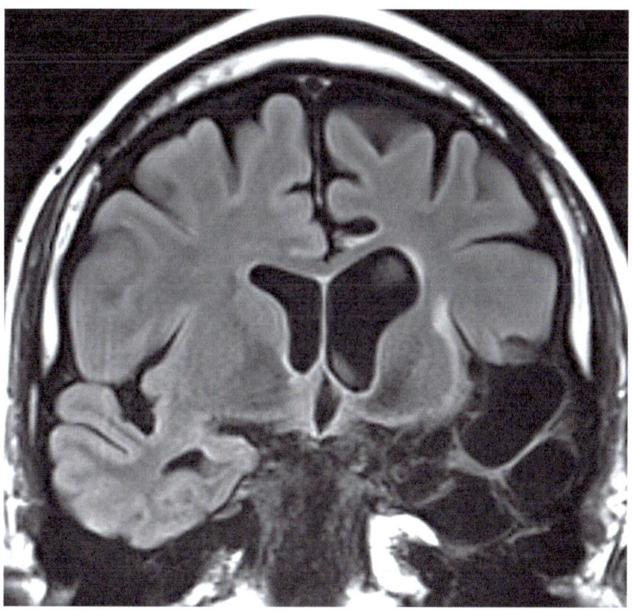

Fig. 34.6 MRI coronal FLAIR sequence at a hippocampal head level. Marked encephalomalacia and atrophy of the left temporal lobe is evident and extends to include the left insula and anterior cingulate gyrus. Hyperintensity of the external capsule indicates gliosis. The left lateral ventricle is asymmetrically enlarged, and the third ventricle is deformed because of the left hemispheric atrophy

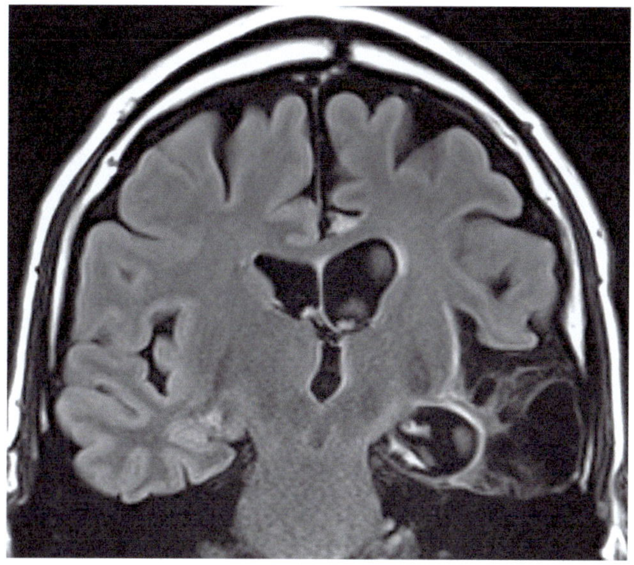

Fig. 34.7 MRI coronal FLAIR sequence at a hippocampal body level. Marked encephalomalacia and atrophy extends across the entire left temporal lobe, including the hippocampus, which produces marked enlargement of the temporal horn of the lateral ventricle. The atrophy extends to include the left hemisphere, as is evident in the asymmetrically enlarged left lateral ventricle and deformed third ventricle. Hyperintensity within the insula and anterior cingulate gyrus is due to gliosis. The right hemisphere is normal

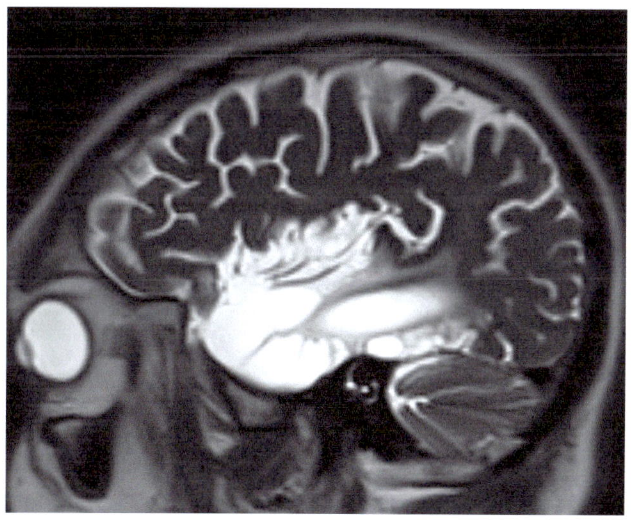

Fig. 34.8 MRI sagittal T2 sequence at a left insula level. Marked atrophy and encephalomalacia of the left temporal lobe are present with an enlarged horn of the lateral ventricle. The insula also has encephalomalacia

Acute Neurocysticercosis

35

Clinical History

The first recognized seizure occurred on the day of presentation and followed 10 minutes of left-sided headache with tingling across the distal right upper extremity. It was witnessed as a loss of consciousness with bilateral convulsive movements. The experience of the left-sided headache and the right-sided tingling had never previously occurred.

Two additional bilateral tonic-clonic seizures occurred during the transportation to an emergency department by ambulance. Upon arrival at the hospital, the patient was unresponsive, and treatment was escalated to include multiple intravenous anti-seizure medications, anesthesia, and intubation.

Emergent diagnostic testing included CT, MRI, and EEG. CT identified small hyperdense and hypodense lesions without edema. MRI identified multiple lesions, some of which were contrast enhancing, and one in the left temporal-parietal junction had surrounding edema. EEG was obtained after anesthesia and intubation, and it depicted diffuse slowing in the theta frequency range and no epileptiform abnormalities.

Based on the diagnostic testing indicating neurocysticercosis, antiparasitic and corticosteroid medications were given. Seizure control was achieved, and the patient was discharged from the hospital with anti-seizure medication treatment. Seizure freedom was present for 1 year when a bilateral tonic-clonic seizure occurred without an aura.

The epilepsy risk factor was neurocysticercosis. The patient lived in a neurocysticercosis endemic country from birth through youth and has lived in the United States for about 15 years.

Neurological examination was abnormal with right-sided weakness that persisted for at least 1 month after the seizure. Medical history included no additional relevant findings.

The history and evaluation indicate focal seizures in the context of acute neurocysticercosis with a history of chronic neurocysticercosis. The seizures' initial somatosensory features and progression to become bilateral tonic-clonic are potentially consistent with the neocortical lesion surrounded by edema. As such, treatment was considered to be related to an acute infection, so it included anti-seizure medications, antiparasitic medications, and corticosteroids. The anatomic origin of the seizure that occurred 1 year later is not clear and may be related to remote changes from the lesion that produced the status epilepticus but also may be related to one of the other chronic neurocysticercosis lesions.

J. M. Stern, N. Salamon, *Imaging of Epilepsy*, https://doi.org/10.1007/978-3-030-86672-3_35

Imaging

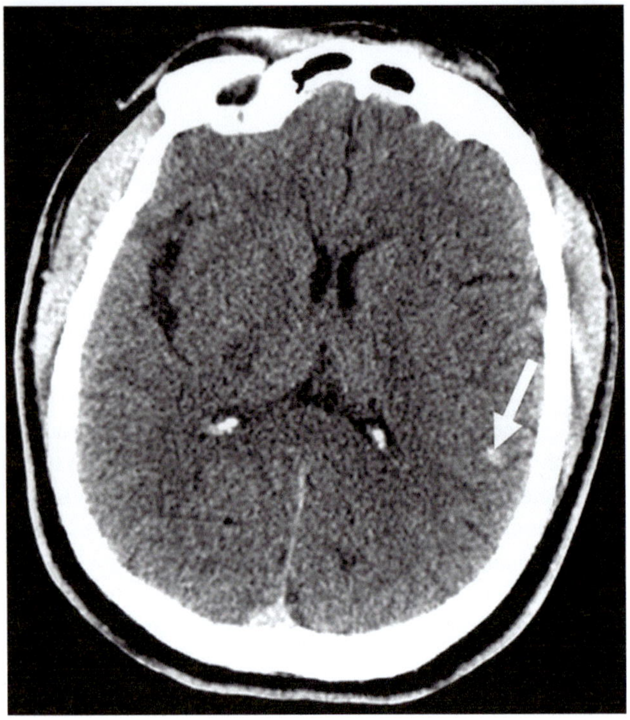

Fig. 35.1 CT axial plane at a basal ganglia level. A round calcification (arrow) is evident in the left supramarginal gyrus. Edema is not evident. No other abnormality is present

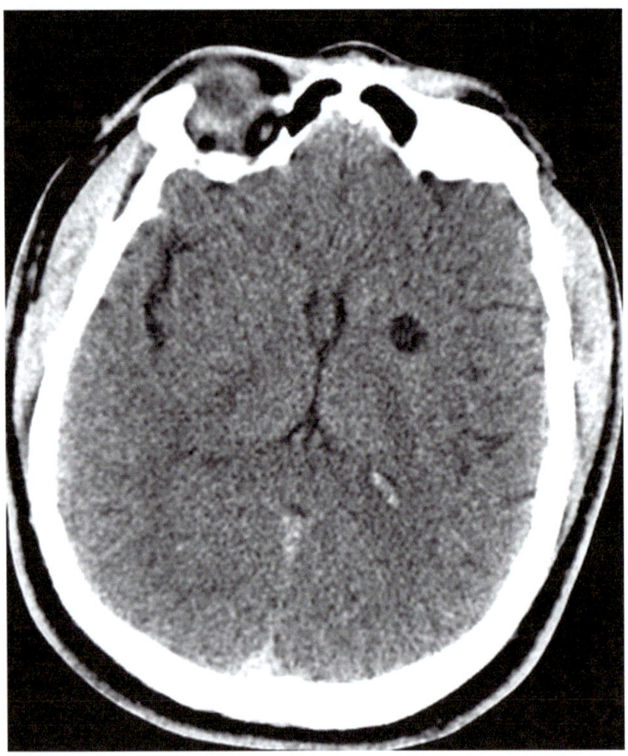

Fig. 35.2 CT axial plane at a basal ganglia level slightly inferior to Fig. 35.1. A round hypodense lesion is present in the left basal ganglia. The internal density is similar to cerebrospinal fluid (CSF), and a faint increase in density is evident in the central portion. No calcification or edema is present

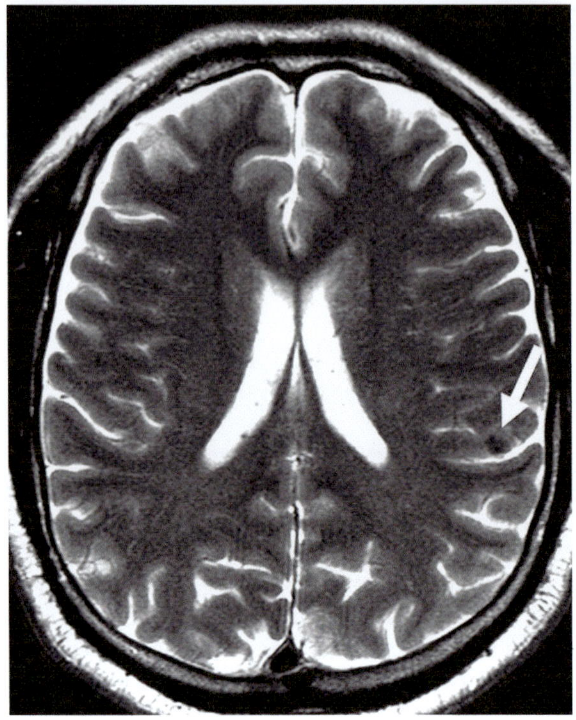

Fig. 35.3 MRI axial T2 sequence at a lateral ventricle level and slightly superior to Fig. 35.1. A round hypointense lesion (arrow) is evident and corresponds to the calcification in Fig. 35.1. The image confirms the lack of edema around the lesion

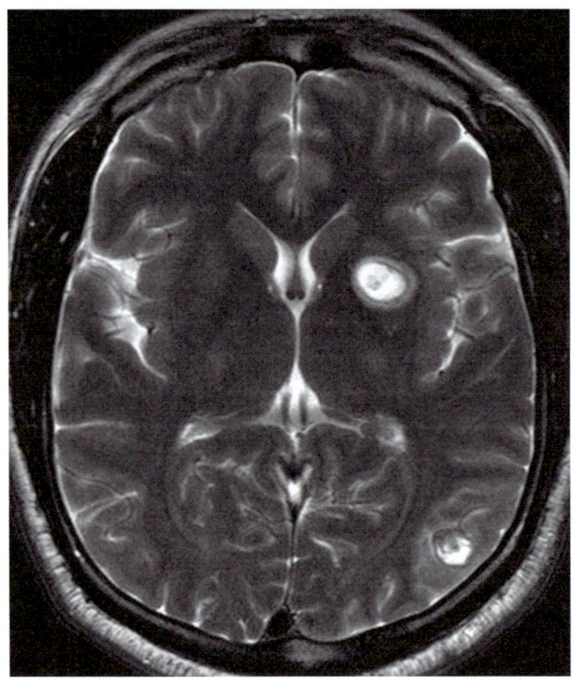

Fig. 35.4 MRI axial T2 sequence at a basal ganglia level similar to Fig. 35.2. The left basal ganglia cyst includes a central hypointensity that suggests a scolex. The cyst also has a halo of surrounding edema. A second lesion is present in the left occipital cortex. Compared to the basal ganglia lesion, this lesion has a broader region of edema surrounding it, and the central hypointensity has a shape suggestive of a scolex

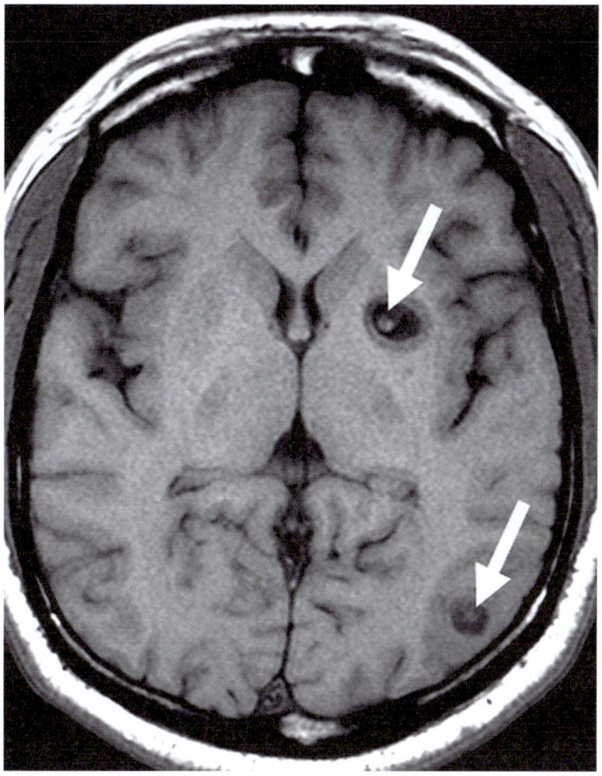

Fig. 35.5 MRI axial T1 sequence at the same basal ganglia level as Fig. 35.4. The arrows indicate a scolex in each of the two lesions that is more clearly present than with the T2 sequence. The surrounding edema is similar to Fig. 35.4

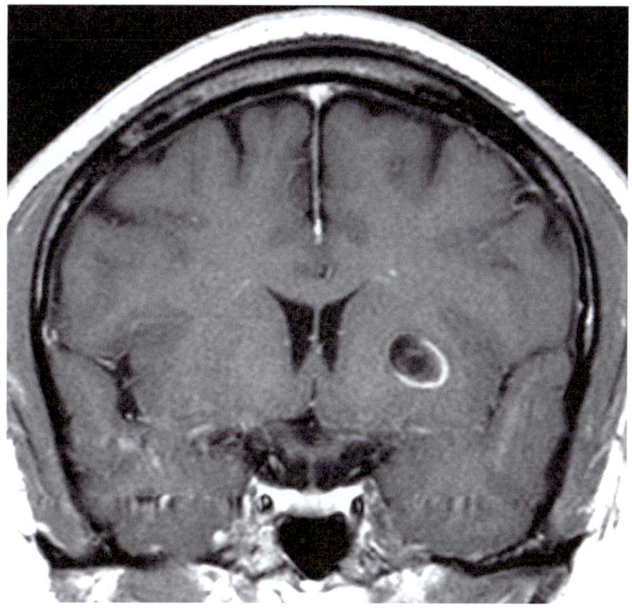

Fig. 35.7 MRI coronal T1 sequence after contrast administration at an amygdala level. The left basal ganglia lesion has incomplete enhancement of the surrounding periphery but is essentially similar to the enhancement evident with the axial images. A faint scolex is visible within the cyst

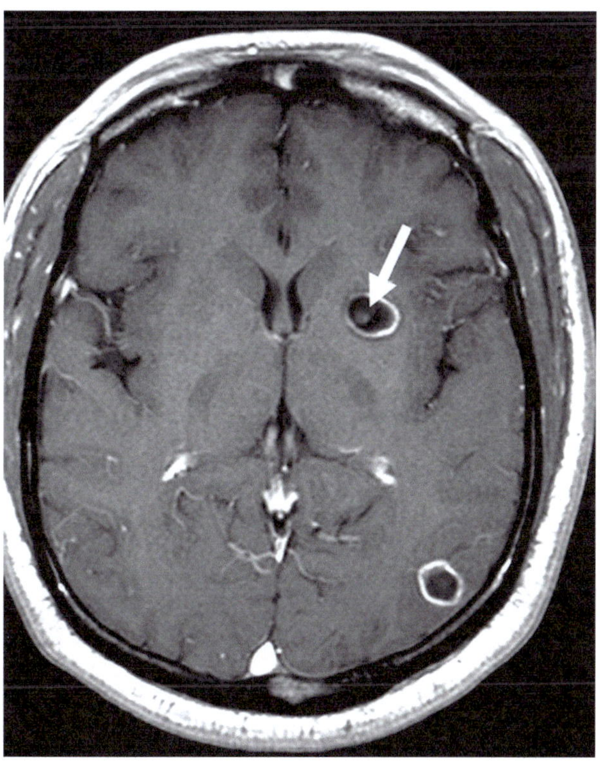

Fig. 35.6 MRI axial T1 sequence after contrast administration at the same basal ganglia level as Figs. 35.4 and 35.5. The two lesions each have ring enhancement of their peripheries. Enhancement is not present within the lesions and no other areas demonstrate abnormal enhancement

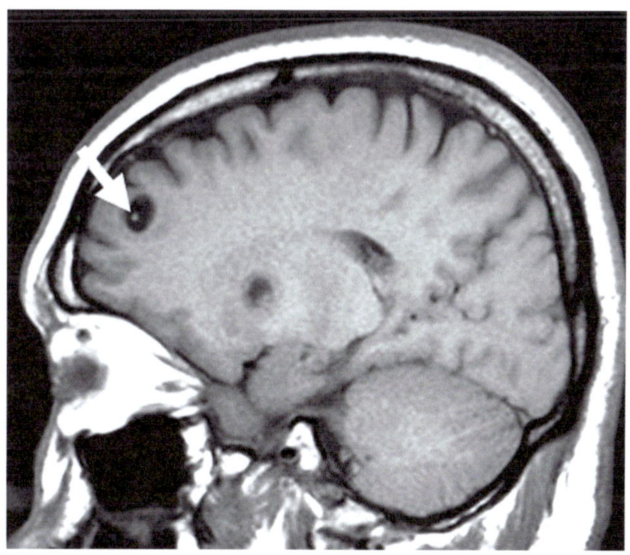

Fig. 35.8 MRI sagittal T1 sequence at a left amygdala level. A left, anterior frontal lobe lesion (arrow) is visible within a scolex within it. The basal ganglia lesion is visible as a less hypointense cyst

Remote Neurocysticercosis

36

Clinical History

The first recognized seizure occurred at about age 30 years as an episode of impaired awareness. However, the history included episodes of loss of consciousness during adolescence and episodes of unusual sleep movements during childhood that were retrospectively recognized as possibly seizures.

The habitual seizures manifested as an aura of an indescribable sense of seizure onset that lasted 5 seconds and was sometimes followed by a bilateral visual distortion described as a cartoonish transformation of whatever is being viewed that lasts about 20 seconds. Impaired awareness occasionally followed the aura, and this was accompanied by oral automatisms, restless movements of the arms, kicking, and wandering. The impairment lasted 1–2 minutes. Most seizures were auras in isolation, and progression to a bilateral tonic-clonic seizure did not occurred. Treatment included multiple anti-seizure medications with a monthly seizure frequency of 20 auras and three seizures with impaired awareness.

The epilepsy risk factor was neurocysticercosis that was diagnosed at age 48 years and not treated because of its late stage at the time of diagnosis.

Neurological examination was normal. Neuropsychological testing identified subtle visuospatial deficits.

Interictal EEG depicted occasional right anterior temporal epileptiform discharges. Video-EEG monitoring recorded auras and focal seizures that were consistent with the habitual seizures. Ictal EEG seizure onset was broad across the right temporal lobe for seizures with impaired awareness. No change was present during the auras in isolation.

CT of the head identified more than 20 calcified, neurocysticercosis lesions. MRI identified numerous, punctate calcifications and right hippocampal sclerosis. PET identified right temporal hypometabolism. MEG identified bilateral, independent temporal epileptiform dipoles with a greater number on the left.

The history and evaluation suggest right temporal lobe epilepsy based on the auras in isolation, focal seizures with automatisms that have not progressed to bilateral tonic-clonic, and both interictal and ictal EEG. However, the radiologic evaluation identified neuroeysticercosis with multiple lesions, which introduces the possibility that the ictal behavior and EEG are due to propagation into the limbic system. Although the auras of a cartoonish visual distortion may be limbic when considered as a derealization experience, they also may be localized to association neocortex within visual processing areas, so the auras further the possibility that the seizure manifestation and EEG are due to propagated abnormality.

Chronic neurocysticercosis can be associated with mesial temporal lobe epilepsy, possibly because of hippocampal injury during the acute phase of the neurocysticercosis, and such patients can benefit from an anterior temporal lobe resection. This patient had evidence of right mesial temporal lobe epilepsy, but the neuropsychological testing was not strongly supportive of right hippocampal system dysfunction. To better determine the risk of a memory deficit after an anterior temporal lobe resection, an intracarotid amobarbital test was performed. It identified left hemispheric dominance for language, intact episodic memory with a right-sided injection, and impaired recall with a left-sided injection. As such, right hippocampal system dysfunction was evident, which further supported candidacy for a right anterior-mesial temporal lobe resection.

Based on the evidence of right mesial temporal lobe epilepsy and no evidence of an epileptogenic neurocysticercal lesion, a right anterior-mesial temporal lobe resection was performed at age 64 years. Histopathological examination identified hippocampal sclerosis. No seizures or auras have occurred for the 4 years since surgery.

J. M. Stern, N. Salamon, *Imaging of Epilepsy*, https://doi.org/10.1007/978-3-030-86672-3_36

Imaging

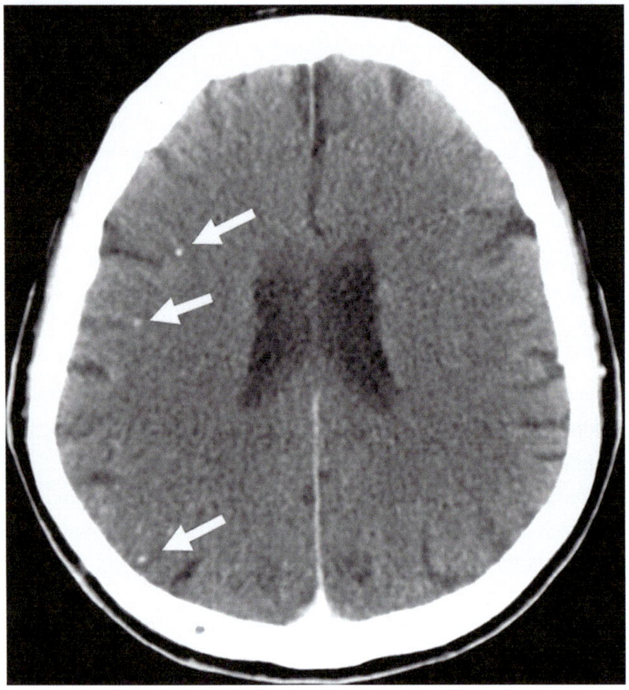

Fig. 36.1 CT axial plane at a lateral ventricle level. Multiple, small punctate foci of calcification are present in the right cerebral hemisphere. The three most prominent are indicated (arrows). The hemispheres are otherwise normal

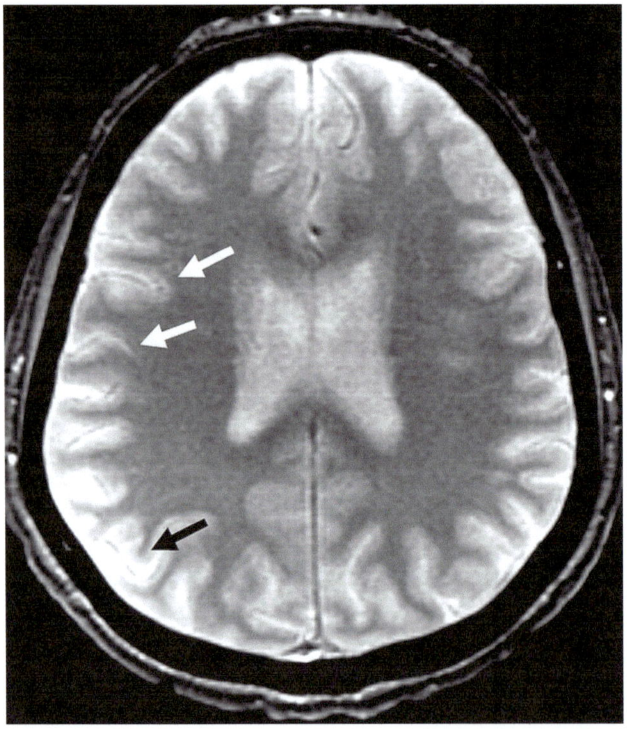

Fig. 36.2 MRI axial GRE sequence at the same lateral ventricle level as Fig. 36.1. The three more prominent calcifications identified with the CT are not visible, as indicated by the arrows that are aligned to the regions on the CT. The GRE sequence is the most sensitive sequence for calcifications, but small calcifications may still be invisible. No abnormality is evident

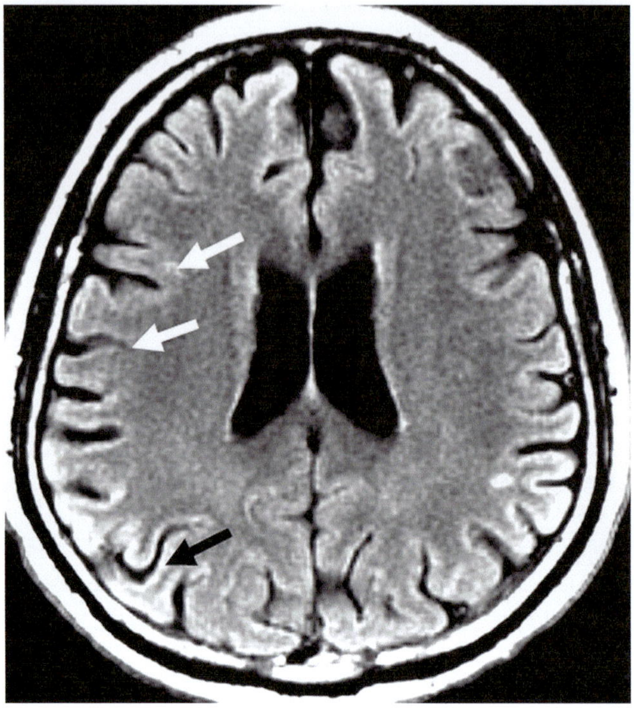

Fig. 36.3 MRI axial FLAIR sequence at the same lateral ventricle level as Figs. 36.1 and 36.2. No signal abnormality is present at the locations of the three calcifications identified by the CT (arrows). A small region of hyperintensity is present in the left parietal lobe at the supramarginal gyrus. This signal abnormality is nonspecific and may be tissue injury from neurocysticercosis

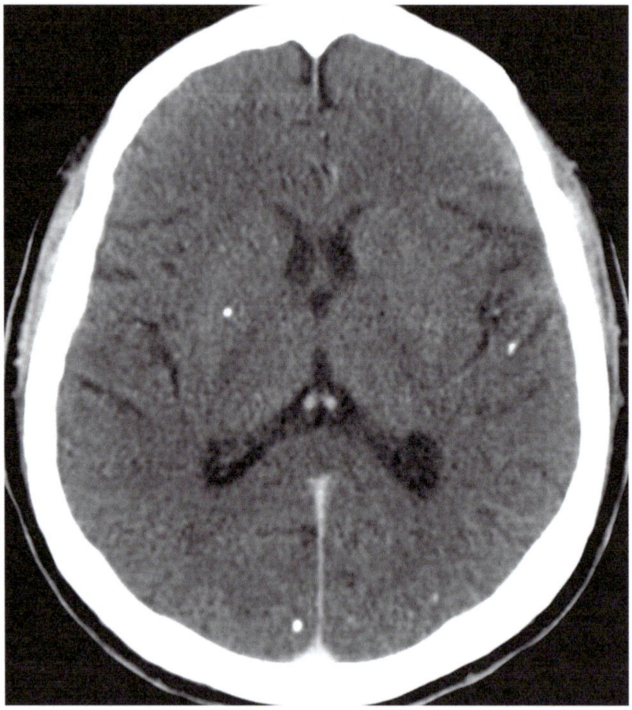

Fig. 36.4 CT axial plane at a basal ganglia level. Multiple punctate calcifications are evident in bilateral cerebral hemispheres, including the right putamen. The calcifications are similar to those evident on CT in Fig. 36.1. The image is otherwise normal

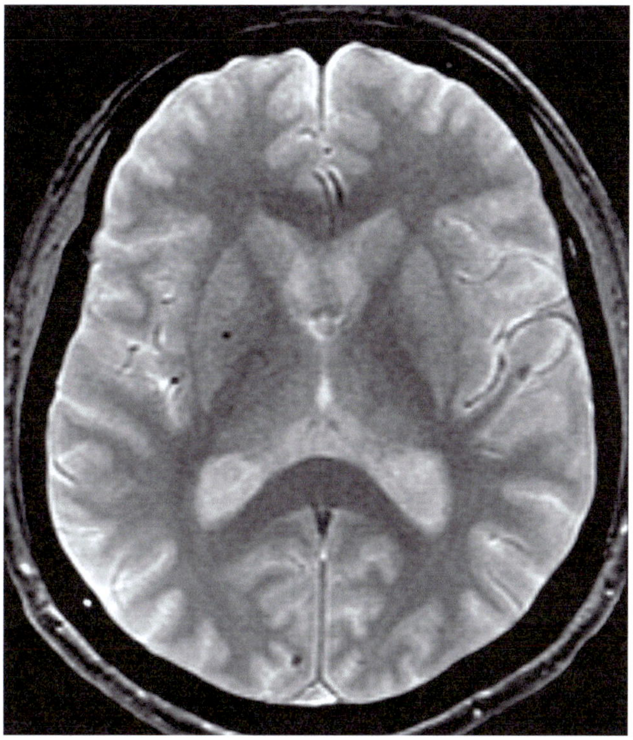

Fig. 36.5 MRI axial GRE sequence at the same basal ganglia level as Fig. 36.4. Multiple punctate hypointensities correspond to the calcifications evident in the CT. Although the calcifications are similar to the CT in Figs. 36.1 and 36.4, they are evident in this image but not in the Fig. 36.2's GRE image. Moreover, this image identifies additional, subtler hypointensities that correspond to subtle hyperdensities in Fig. 36.4, including two in the left occipital cortex and one in the left anterior cingulate gyrus

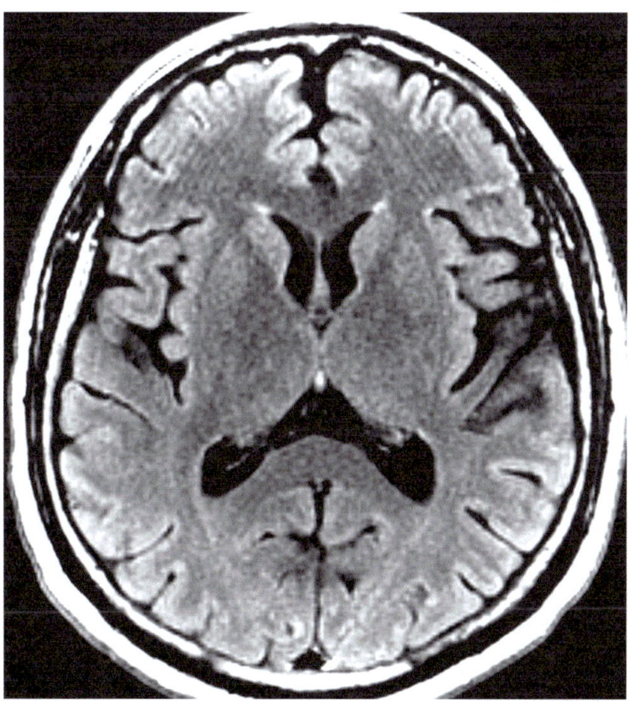

Fig. 36.6 MRI axial FLAIR sequence at a similar basal ganglia level as Figs. 36.4 and 36.5. The calcifications are not visible with this sequence. No abnormalities are evident

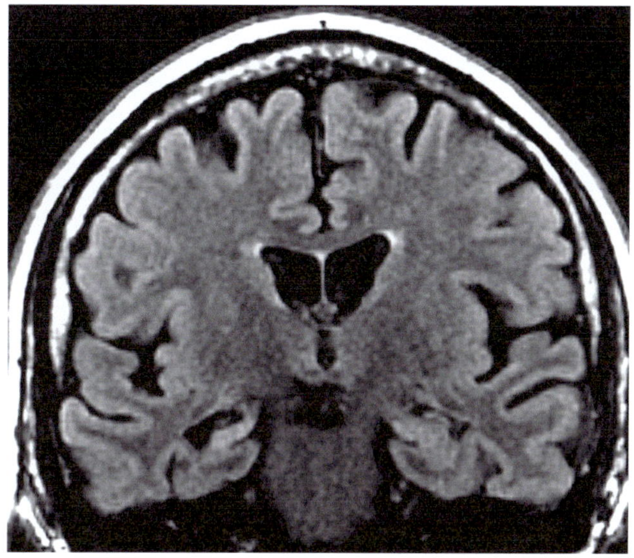

Fig. 36.7 MRI coronal FLAIR sequence at a hippocampal head level. The right hippocampus is hyperintense and atrophic, especially when compared to the left hippocampus. No other abnormality is present; however, the Sylvian fissures are mildly larger than expected

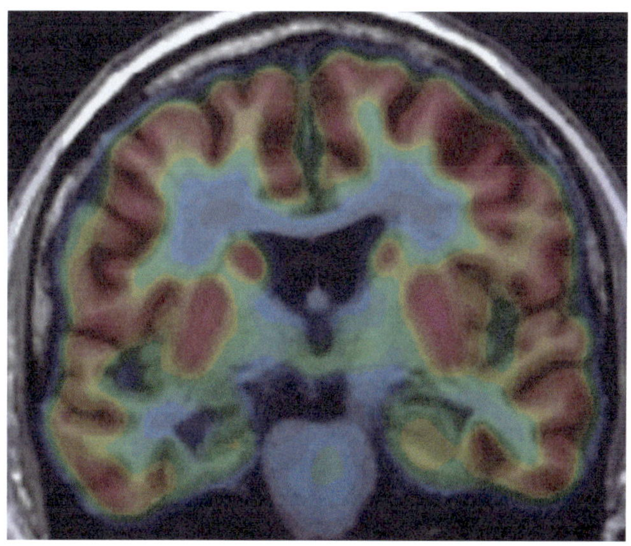

Fig. 36.8 PET-MRI co-registration in a coronal plane at the same hippocampal head level as Fig. 36.7. The right hippocampus and parahippocampal gyrus are hypometabolic. Metabolic signal is normal elsewhere, including the remainder of the right temporal lobe

GAD65 Autoimmune Limbic Encephalitis

37

Clinical History

The first recognized seizure occurred at age 47 years as a bilateral tonic-clonic convulsion. An evaluation at that time included an MRI that depicted abnormality indicating possible limbic encephalitis. In retrospect, memory problems began developing about 4 months before the MRI was obtained.

The habitual seizures manifesteded as confusion with possibly worsening of recent recall. The identification of the episodes was difficult for caregivers because of the interictal memory impairment, and none of the seizures included automatisms. A total of three tonic-clonic seizures occurred, and all were around the time of initial diagnosis and before treatment was initiated. Treatment included multiple anti-seizure medications without seizure freedom based on long-term EEG recordings to determine seizure control. These recordings established the subtle behavioral manifestations of the seizures and were necessary to determine seizure control.

The epilepsy risk factor was autoimmune limbic encephalitis due to GAD65 antibodies. At the time of presentation, the antibody test result was 134,000 U/mL (normal <0.5 U/mL).

Neurological examination identified memory deficits. Orientation was limited to circumstance, day of the week, and city. Month, year, and hospital name were not recalled. When queried after 5 minutes, three of four words given to remember were not recalled. Language, autobiographical memory, and concentration were intact. Medical history included diabetes, which was diagnosed at around the same time as limbic encephalitis, and a negative evaluation for occult malignancy.

Interictal EEG depicted bilateral temporal region abnormality with independently occurring slowing and epileptiform discharges. Video-EEG monitoring recorded numerous focal seizures with minimal or no behavioral change. The number of seizures within a day was so large that it was not counted. Ictal EEG's seizure onset was independently over the right and left anterior temporal regions.

MRI identified hyperintense FLAIR and T2 signal abnormality of bilateral hippocampi without volume loss or contrast enhancement. PET identified hypermetabolic signal in bilateral hippocampi and diffuse cerebral hypometabolism.

The history and evaluation indicate GAD65 limbic encephalitis with resultant memory deficits, focal seizures from bilateral mesial temporal lobes, and the associated diabetes. Initial treatment was a combination of anti-seizure medications and steroids and then intravenous immunoglobulin. This produced an improvement in the seizure control, as identified by video-EEG monitoring, and a minor improvement in memory function. Ongoing care has included immunosuppressant medications and has used video-EEG to assess the treatment response. Seizure control has been achieved, but memory deficits have produced disability.

J. M. Stern, N. Salamon, *Imaging of Epilepsy*, https://doi.org/10.1007/978-3-030-86672-3_37

Imaging

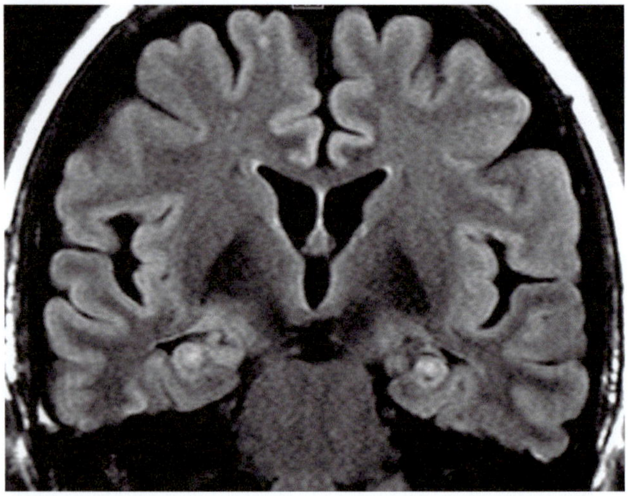

Fig. 37.1 MRI coronal FLAIR sequence at a body of the hippocampus level. The hippocampal signal is abnormally increased bilaterally, but the hippocampal volumes are normal and symmetric. The remainder of brain is normal

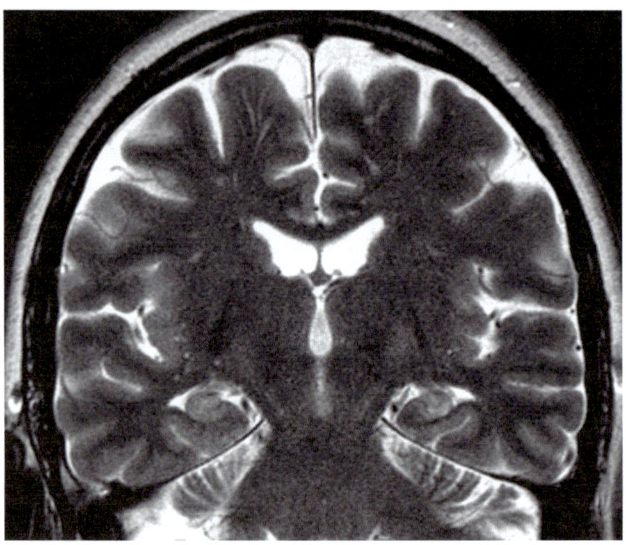

Fig. 37.2 MRI coronal T2 sequence at the same body of the hippocampus level as Fig. 37.1. Bilateral hippocampi have abnormally increased signal and normal volume and symmetry. No other abnormality is evident. The asymmetric signal in the left and right entorhinal cortices is normal and due to volume averaging

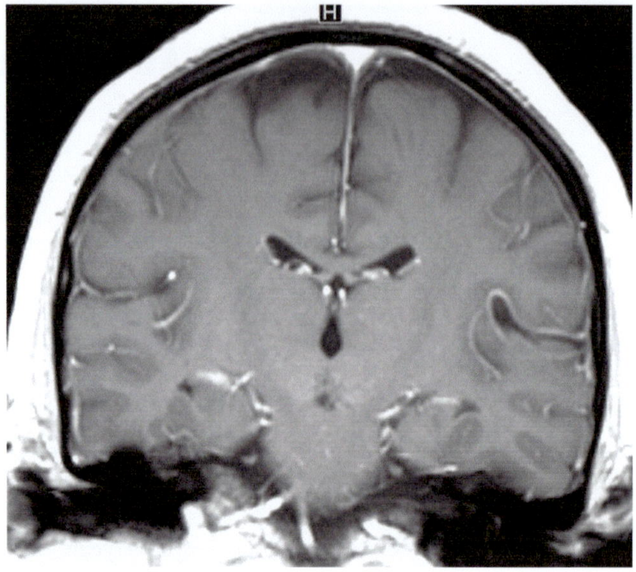

Fig. 37.3 MRI coronal T1 sequence with contrast at the same body of the hippocampus level as Figs. 37.1 and 37.2. No abnormal enhancement is present. Hyperintensity that is superior to both hippocampi is normal choroid plexus enhancement

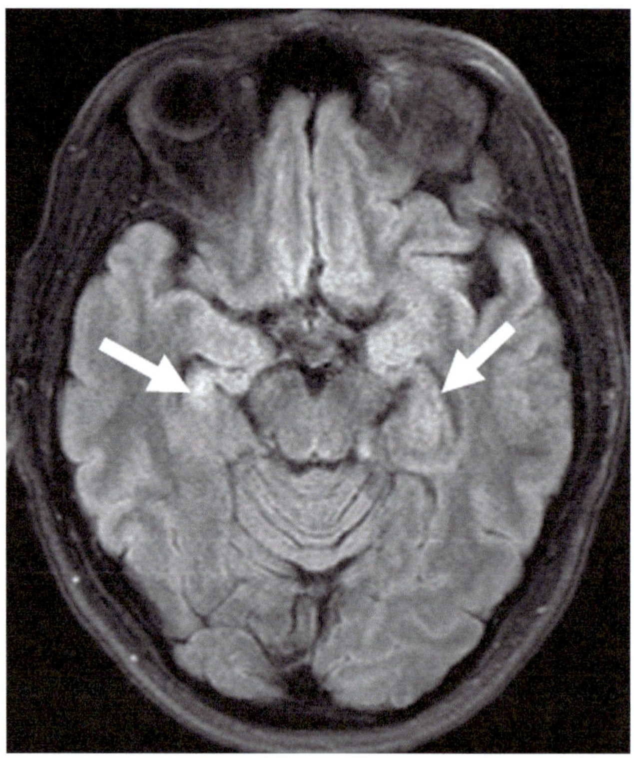

Fig. 37.4 MRI axial FLAIR sequence at a hippocampal head level. Abnormal hyperintensity is evident bilaterally in the heads of the hippocampi (arrows). The asymmetric distribution of the hippocampal hyperintensity is not abnormal

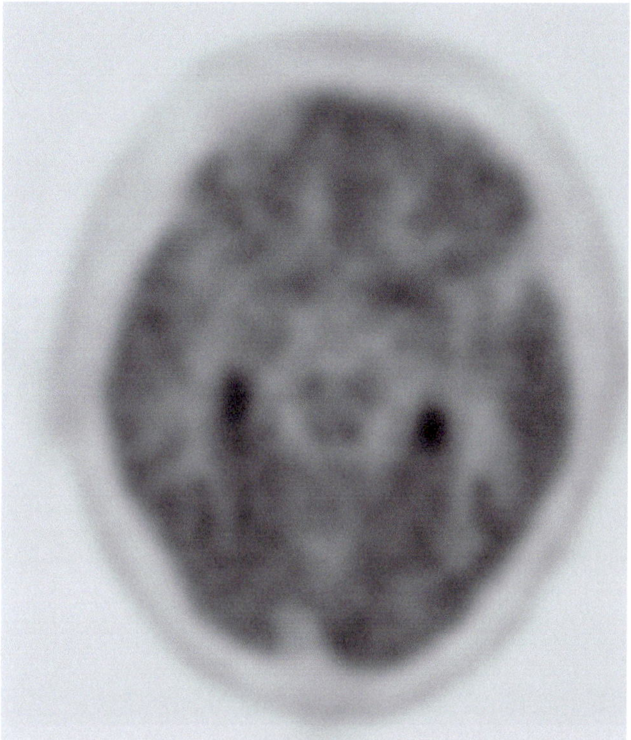

Fig. 37.5 PET grayscale FDG tracer in an axial plane at a hippocampus level. Abnormally increased glucose uptake is evident in bilateral hippocampal bodies and indicates hypermetabolism. The extra-hippocampal temporal lobes and other cortical ribbon have normal metabolic signal

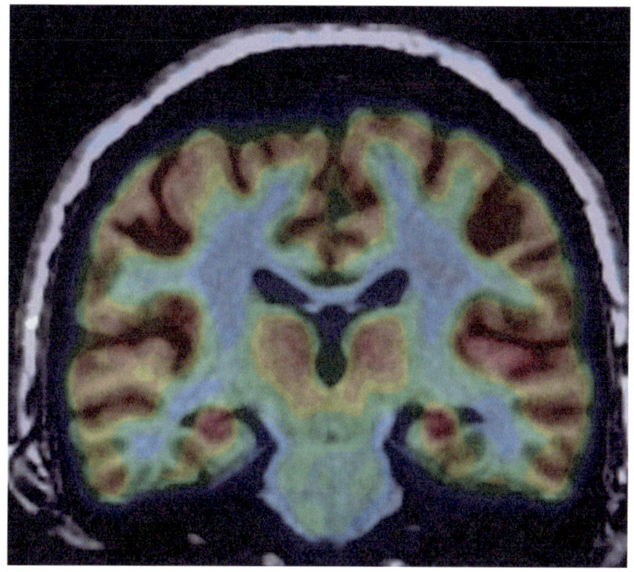

Fig. 37.7 PET-MRI co-registration with color-scale FDG tracer in a coronal plane at a hippocampal body level. Red signal in bilateral hippocampi corresponds to abnormal hypermetabolism. The regions of darker red in the bilateral central sulci and Sylvian fissures are due to cerebrospinal fluid (CSF) spaces overlapping with cortical ribbons to produce an artifactual darker signal that differs from the red signal within the hippocampi

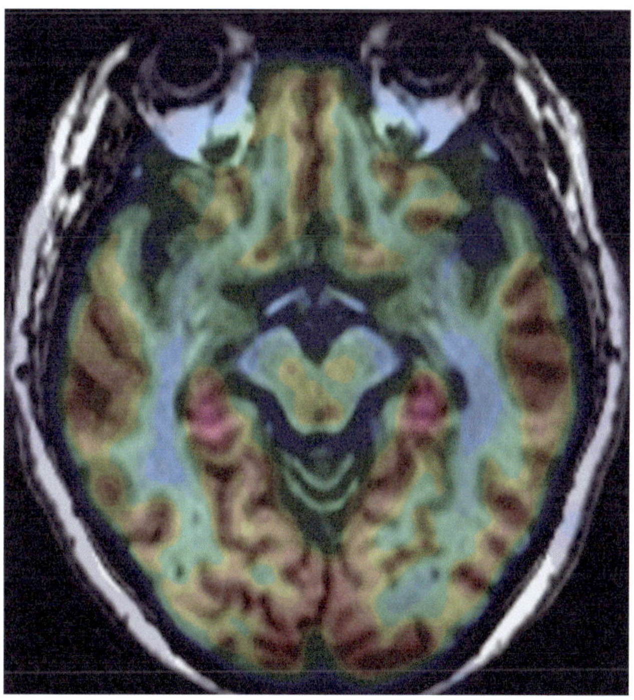

Fig. 37.6 PET-MRI co-registration with color-scale FDG tracer in an axial plane at the same hippocampus level as Fig. 37.5. The abnormally increased glucose uptake in the hippocampal bodies is evident with normal metabolism in the extra-hippocampal regions. The co-registration to MRI produces clearer anatomic detail and specificity to the hippocampi

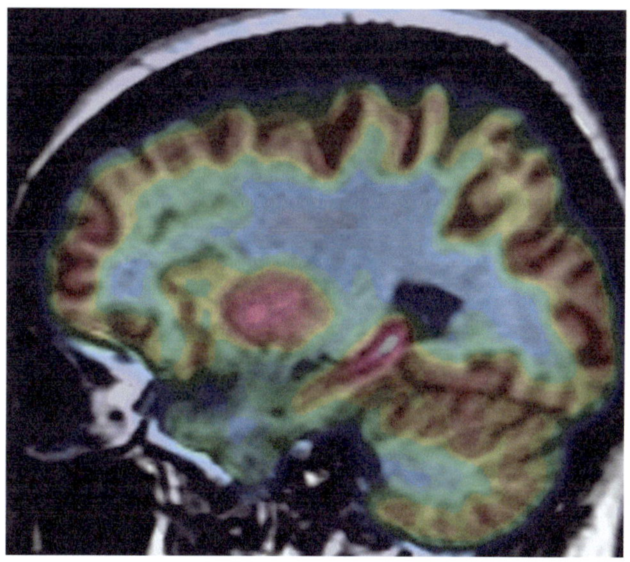

Fig. 37.8 PET-MRI co-registration with color-scale FDG tracer in a sagittal plane at a right hippocampal level. Increased glucose uptake is evident in the hippocampus from the body to the tail. The circular pink metabolic region that is superior-anterior to the hippocampus is normal basal ganglia glucose uptake

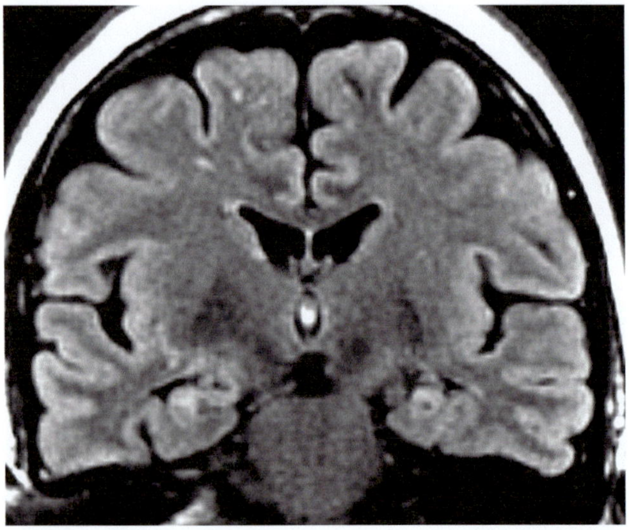

Fig. 37.9 MRI coronal FLAIR sequence at the same hippocampal body level as Fig. 37.1. This image was obtained 1 year after Fig. 37.1 Abnormal hyperintense FLAIR signal is evident in bilateral hippocampi. A minor amount of hippocampal atrophy is present bilaterally. The temporal lobes are otherwise normal and not atrophic

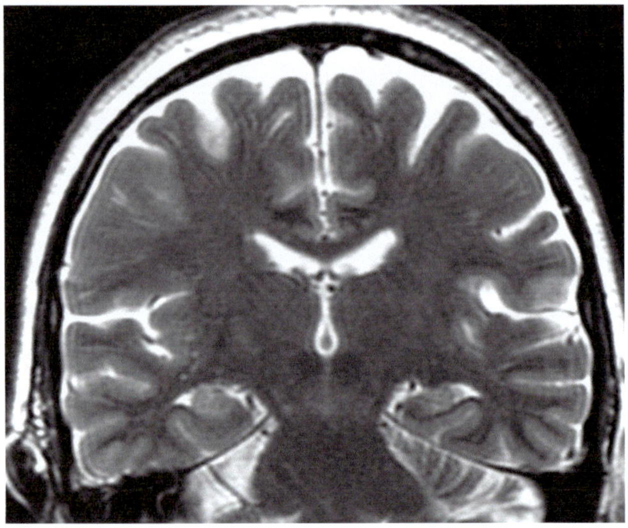

Fig. 37.10 MRI coronal T2 sequence at the same hippocampal level as Fig. 37.9 and obtained during the same scan as Fig. 37.9. Abnormal hyperintensity is evident in bilateral hippocampi. The T2 sequence's greater anatomic detail allows identification of the left hippocampus' asymmetric volume loss

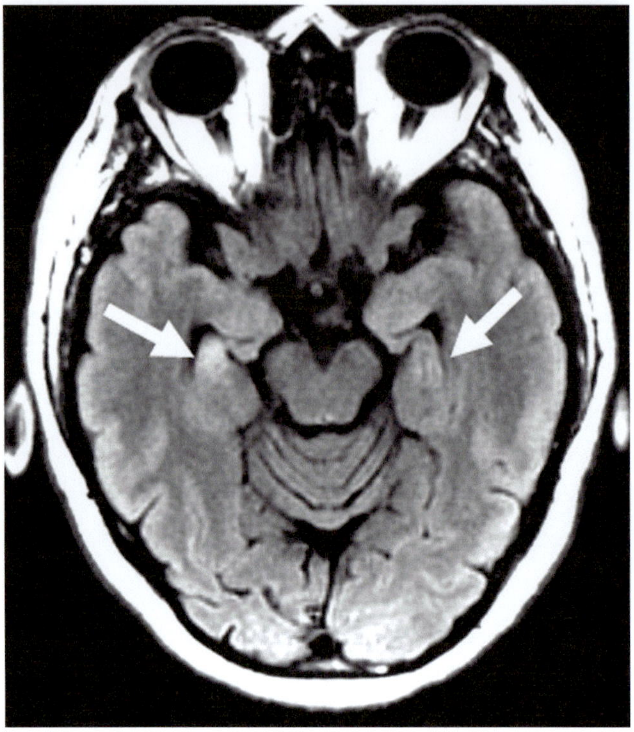

Fig. 37.11 MRI axial FLAIR sequence at a hippocampal body level. Abnormal hyperintensity and volume loss is evident in bilateral hippocampi (arrows). The volume loss has produced an increase in the temporal horns of the lateral ventricles

Voltage Gated Potassium Channel Autoimmune Limbic Encephalitis

38

Clinical History

The first recognized seizure occurred at age 38 years as an episode of slowed responsiveness that resolved over hours. The episode was sufficiently abnormal that evaluation included EEG and MRI. Based on the testing, epilepsy was diagnosed, and treatment was started. A similar seizure occurred about a week later, and the treatment dose was increased. Because of the EEG and MRI findings, a PET scan was obtained around this time.

After another week, sustained impaired awareness developed, and nonconvulsive status epilepticus was diagnosed based on emergent EEG. The EEG initially depicted bifrontal slowing to the delta frequency range and then gradually changed over days to depict left-sided periodic discharges. MRI was repeated and identified FLAIR hyperintensity of the left hippocampus and caudate nucleus. Because of concern for limbic encephalitis, serum and cerebrospinal fluid (CSF) analyses were performed. The serum identified antibodies to the voltage-gated potassium channel (VGKC) complex. Treatment with anti-seizure medications, steroids, and intravenous immunoglobulin successfully treated the status epilepticus. EEG at that time depicted mild, generalized, abnormal slowing.

The habitual seizures after the episode of status epilepticus manifested as dystonic posturing of the left hand and arm with leftward gaze deviation. This sometimes progressed to falling, but some seizures produced a fall without the dystonic posturing. An aura was never reported. Initial treatment included multiple anti-seizure medications with a seizure frequency of between one hourly and four daily. With immunotherapy, the VGKC complex antibody titer normalized, and seizure control improved to seizure freedom.

The epilepsy risk factor is autoimmune limbic encephalitis due to VGKC complex antibodies. Upon presentation, the antibody testing result was 737 to 934 pmol/L (negative <450 pmol/L and positive >650 pmol/L). With immunotherapy, the result decreased to 19 pmol/L.

Neurological examination identified memory and concentrations deficits that developed with the VGKC complex limbic encephalitis and possibly increased in the context of the worsening encephalitis with development of the status epilepticus. Myokymia (indicating VGKC associated Morvan's syndrome) and neuromyotonia (indicating VGKC-associated Isaacs' syndrome) were not present. With seizure control and immunotherapy, memory and concentration improved and no longer was disabling. Medical history includes a negative evaluation for occult malignancy at the time of the autoimmune encephalitis diagnosis.

During the recovery, video-EEG monitoring was obtained to determine the seizure control. It recorded episodes of behavioral arrest and confusion without the motor aspects of the habitual seizures, and EEG of these episodes was normal. As such, the episodes are not clearly seizures and may instead be related to the cognitive consequences of the encephalitis. The episodes subsequently resolved, and a 72-hour ambulatory EEG after recovery was normal.

The history and evaluation indicate focal seizures due to autoimmune encephalitis. The improvement in cognition and seizure control corresponds to the anti-inflammatory treatment, which the laboratory testing showed as highly successful.

J. M. Stern, N. Salamon, *Imaging of Epilepsy*, https://doi.org/10.1007/978-3-030-86672-3_38

Imaging

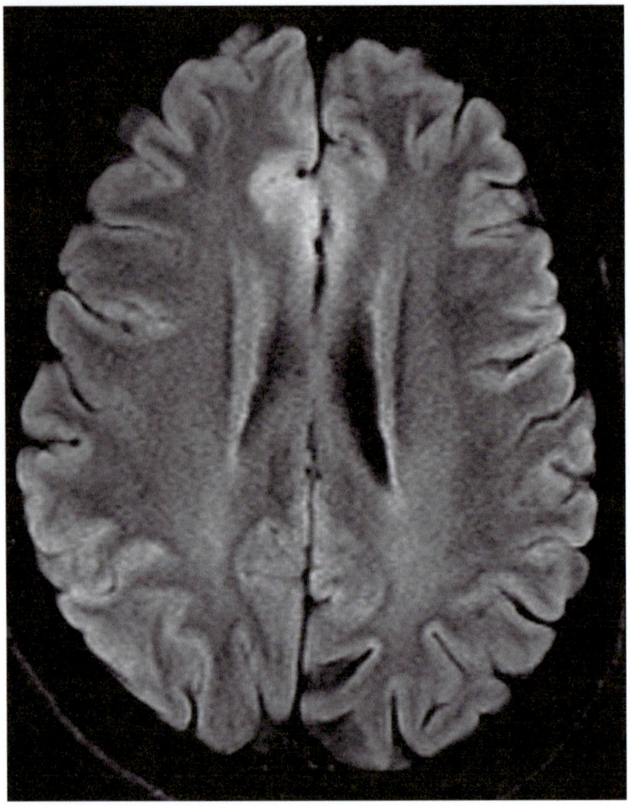

Fig. 38.1 MRI axial FLAIR sequence at a lateral ventricle level. MRI in Figs. 38.1 to 38.5 was obtained at initial presentation. Abnormal hyperintensity is evident in the right anterior cingulate gyrus. The remaining brain is normal

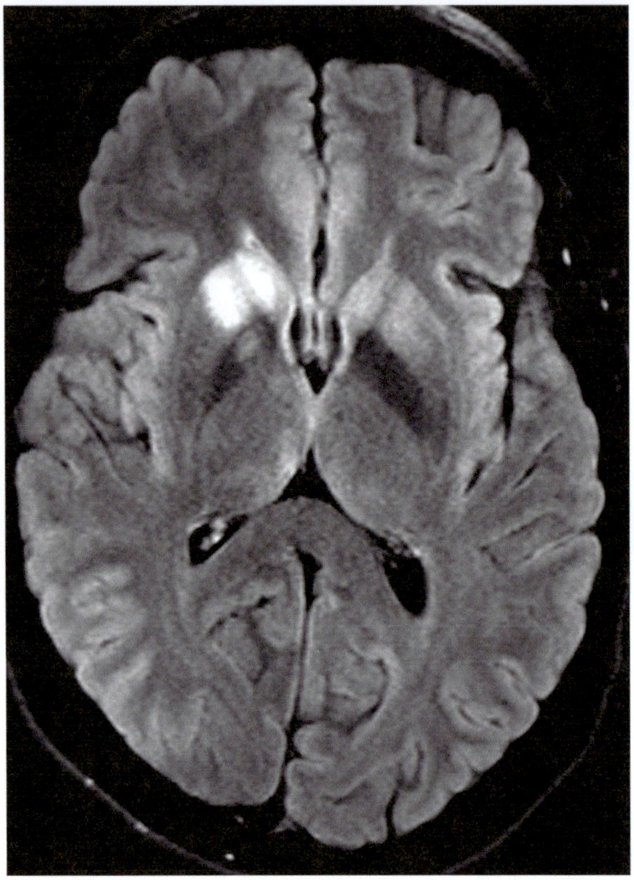

Fig. 38.2 MRI axial FLAIR sequence at a basal ganglia level. The right caudate nucleus head and the right anterior putamen are abnormally hyperintense. Asymmetric hyperintensity is evident within the right globus pallidus and the medial aspect of right thalamus. The cingulate gyrus is hyperintense bilaterally with asymmetrically greater hyperintensity on the right. The insulae are normal and symmetric. The increased signal of right parietal-occipital cortex is artifactual and due to magnetic field inhomogeneity

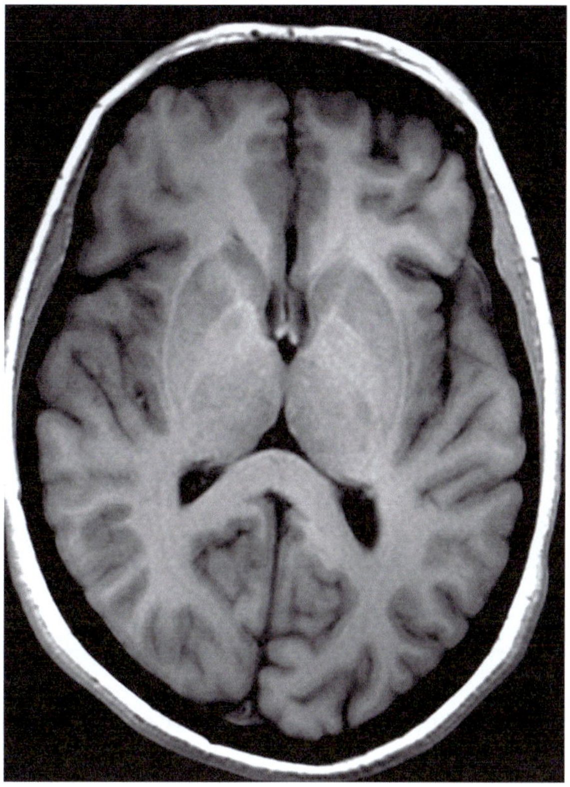

Fig. 38.3 MRI axial T1 sequence at the same basal ganglia level as Fig. 38.2. Subtle increased signal is evident within the right caudate head and anterior putamen. The remainder of the brain is normal

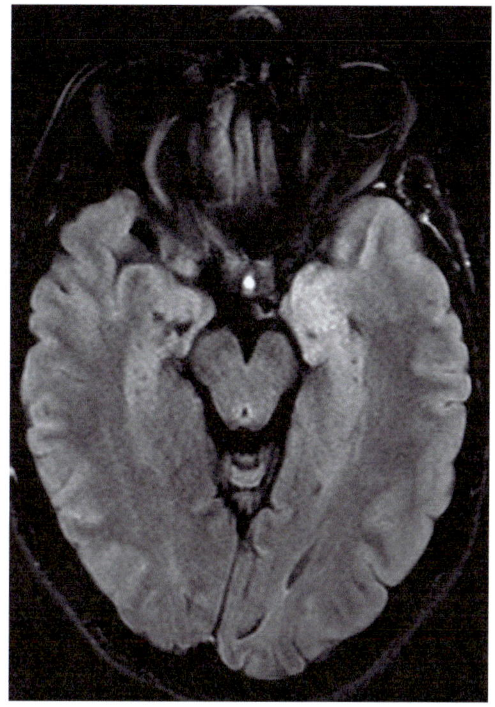

Fig. 38.5 MRI axial FLAIR sequence at an amygdala level. The left amygdala and left hippocampal head are abnormally hyperintense. The remaining left temporal lobe and the right temporal lobe are normal

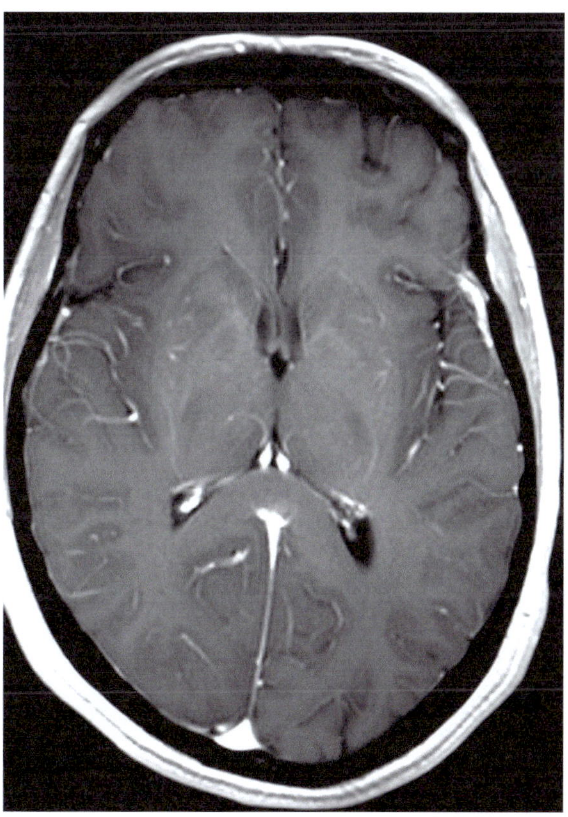

Fig. 38.4 MRI axial T1 sequence after contrast administration at the same basal ganglia level as Fig. 38.2. No abnormal contrast enhancement is present

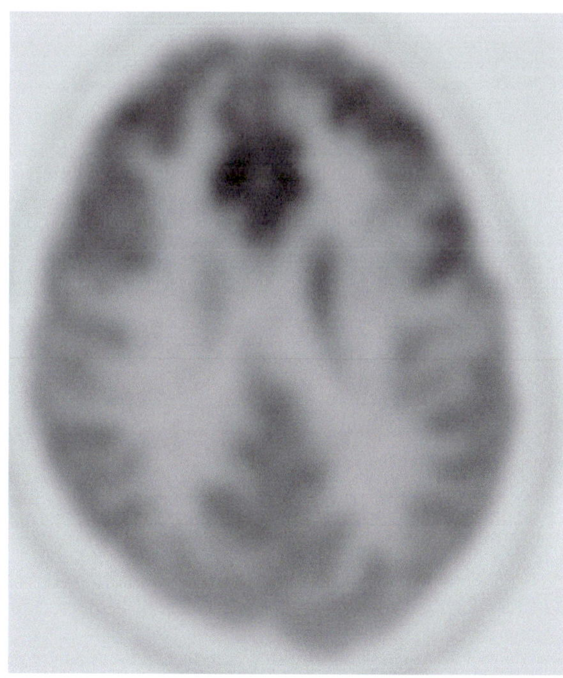

Fig. 38.6 PET with grayscale FDG in an axial plane at a lateral ventricle level superior to Fig. 38.1. PET was obtained 9 days after presentation and the initial MRI. Abnormally increased uptake is evident in bilateral anterior cingulate gyri. The remaining cortex is normal. The scattered regions of increased signal are due to gyral anatomy

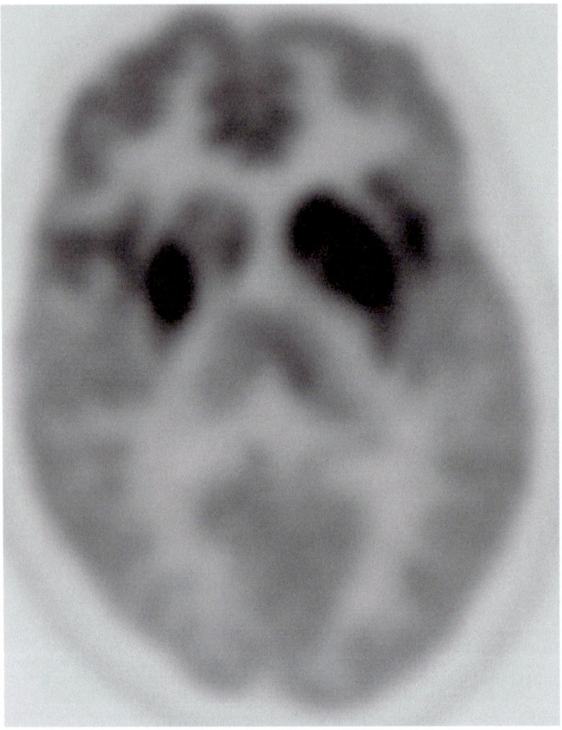

Fig. 38.7 PET with grayscale FDG in an axial plane at a basal ganglia level similar to Figs. 38.2, 38.3, and 38.4. Abnormally increased uptake is evident in bilateral insulae and putamina. The caudate nuclei heads also have bilaterally increased uptake, but the left caudate head has asymmetrically greater uptake than right. Subtle, asymmetric, increased uptake is present in the left medial thalamus

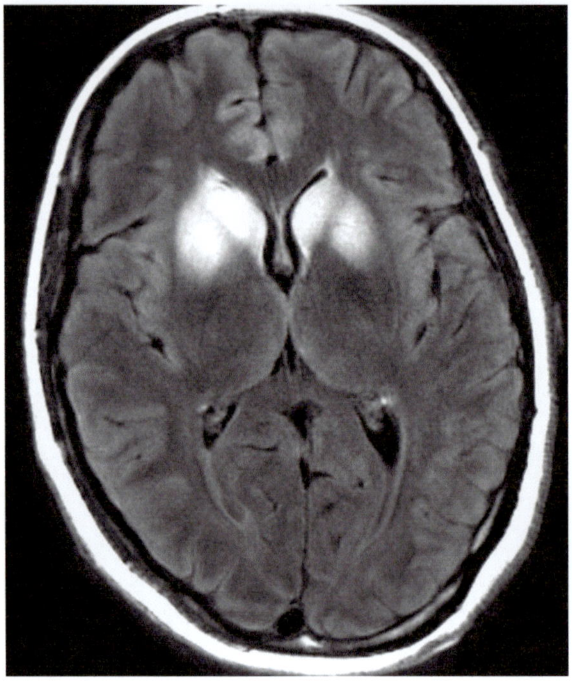

Fig. 38.9 MRI axial FLAIR sequence at a basal ganglia level similar to Fig. 38.2. This MRI, which is in Figs. 38.9 to 38.10, was obtained 17 days after initial presentation and at the time of presentation with nonconvulsive status epilepticus. Bilateral increased signal is evident in the caudate heads and anterior putamina and is still asymmetrically greater on right. The anterior cingulate cortex abnormality is less evident. The insulae are normal

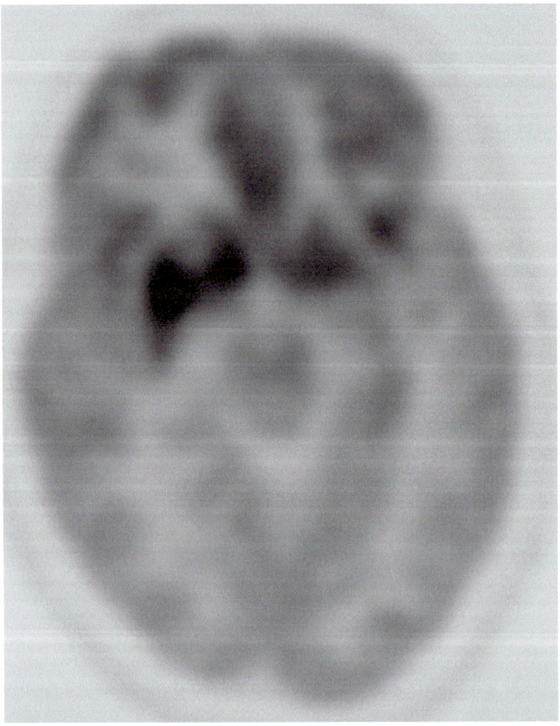

Fig. 38.8 PET with grayscale FDG in an axial plane at a basal ganglia level slightly inferior to Fig. 38.7. Abnormally increased update is evident in bilateral caudate nuclei and putamina, but the right basal ganglia update is asymmetrically greater. Abnormally increased update also is evident in the left insula and bilateral anterior cingulate gyri

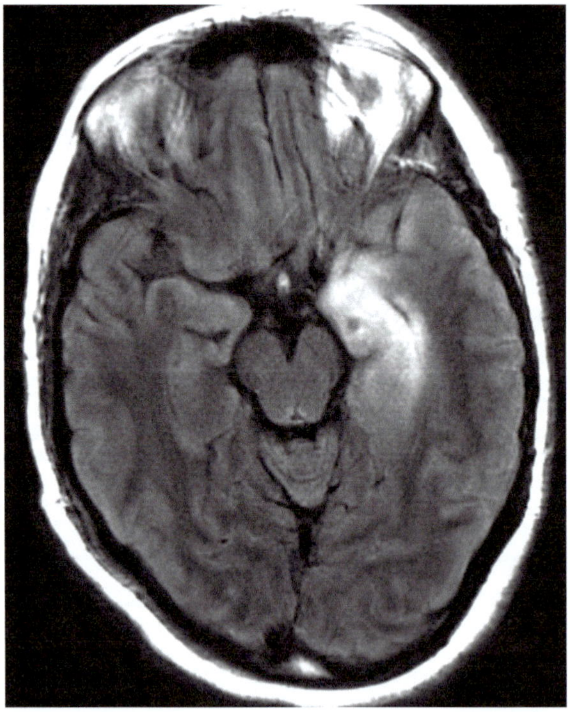

Fig. 38.10 MRI axial FLAIR sequence at an amygdala level slightly superior to Fig. 38.5. A further increase in signal is evident in the left amygdala with extension into the left hippocampus and parahippocampal gyrus. The left temporal pole and lateral temporal lobe are normal along with the remaining cerebral cortex bilaterally

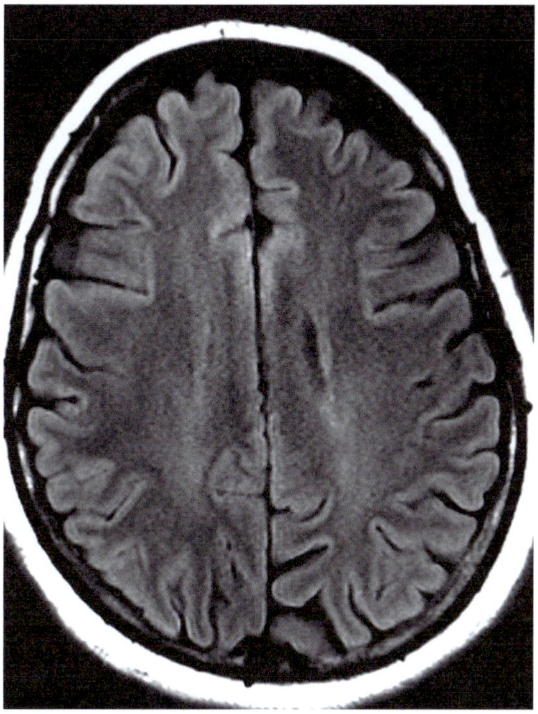

Fig. 38.11 MRI axial FLAIR sequence at a lateral ventricle level superior to Fig. 38.1. This MRI, which is in Figs. 38.11 to 38.17, was obtained 15 months after initial presentation. The anterior cingulate gyrus signal has decreased and is now normal. The remaining brain also is normal

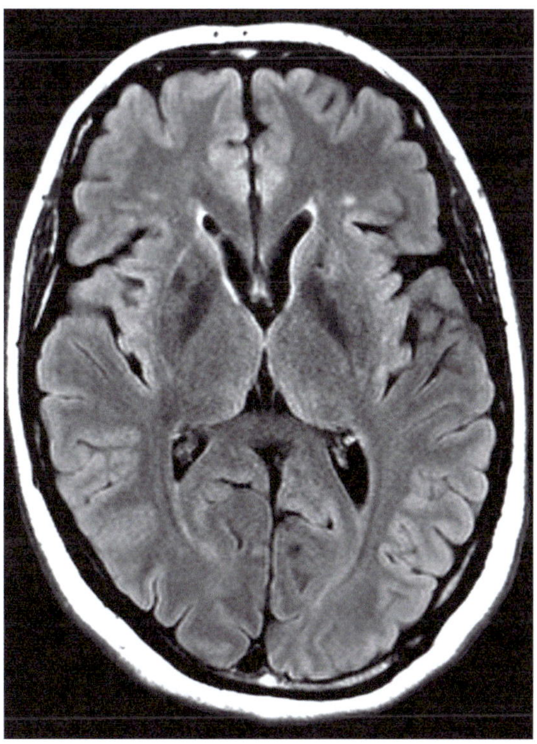

Fig. 38.12 MRI axial FLAIR sequence at a basal ganglia level similar to Figs. 38.2 and 38.9. The abnormally increased signal has resolved bilaterally. The frontal horns of the lateral ventricles are slightly increased, demonstrating resolution of the edema. The basal ganglia demonstrate minor volume loss. Minor, abnormally increased signal is evident in bilateral anterior cingulate gyri

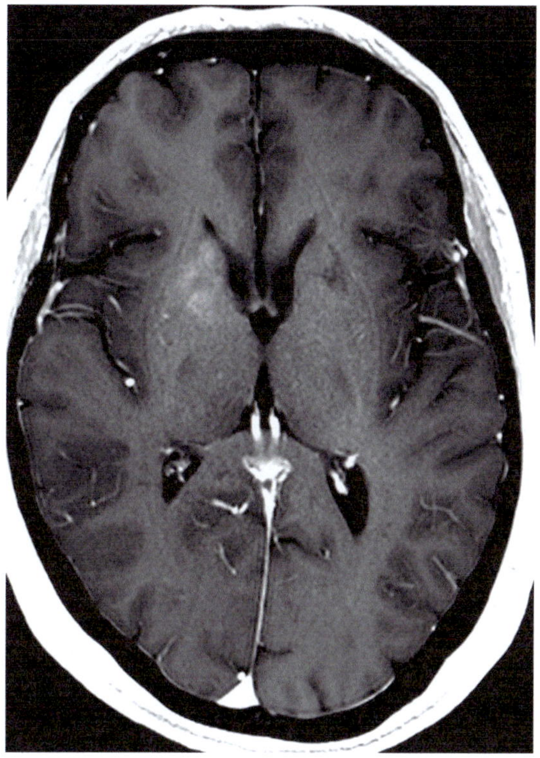

Fig. 38.13 MRI axial T1 sequence at a basal ganglia level after contrast administration. Abnormal contrast enhancement is evident in the right caudate head, right anterior putamen, and right globus pallidus. No other abnormality is present

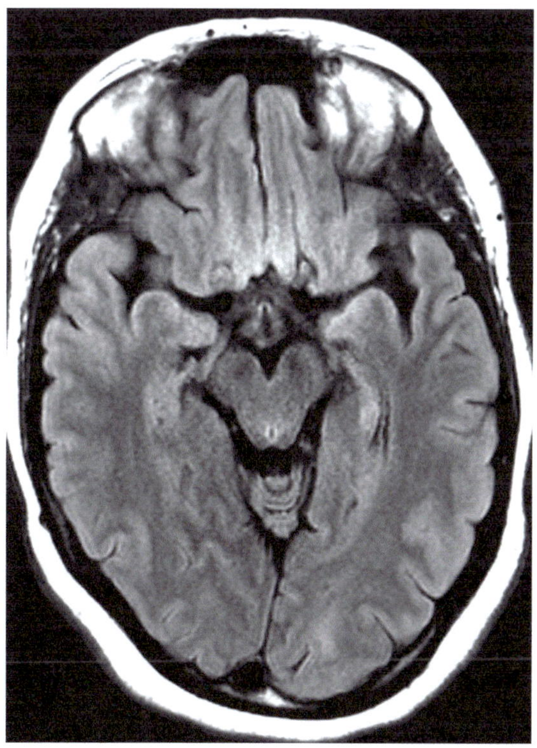

Fig. 38.14 MRI axial FLAIR sequence at an amygdala level similar to Fig. 38.5. The signal abnormality of the right amygdala hippocampus and parahippocampal gyrus has resolved. The hyperintensity in the posterior gyrus rectus is normal and due to skull base artifact

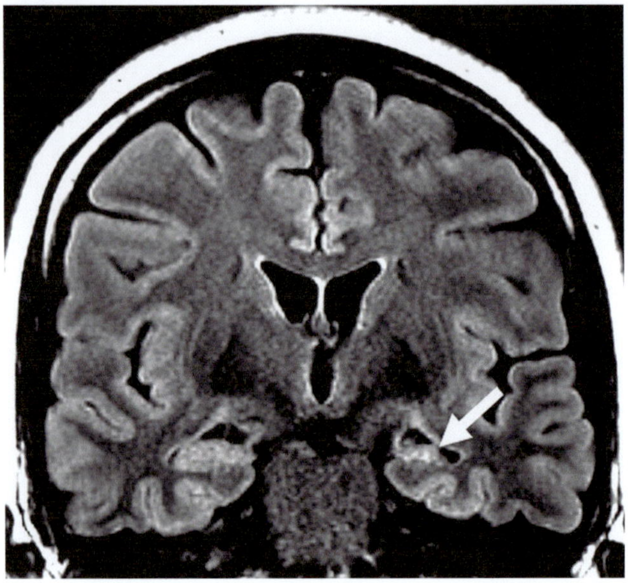

Fig. 38.15 MRI coronal FLAIR sequence at a hippocampal head level. The left hippocampus is asymmetrically atrophic, but its internal signal is symmetric (arrow). The remainder of left temporal lobe is normal

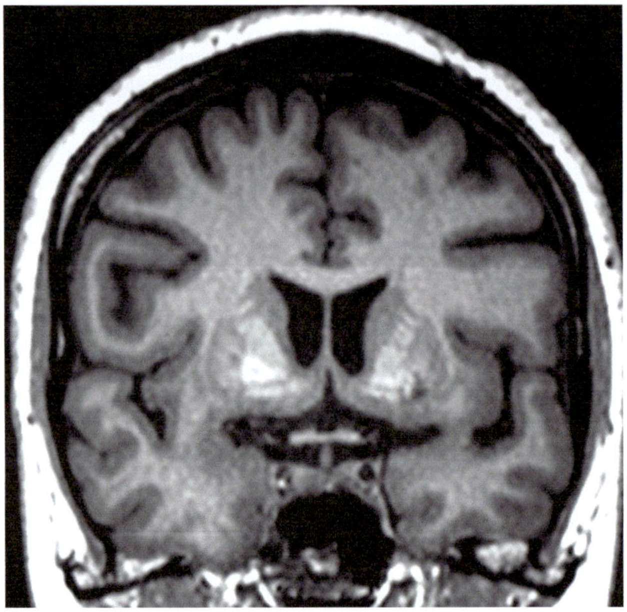

Fig. 38.16 MRI coronal T1 sequence at an amygdala level. Abnormally increased signal is bilaterally evident in the globus pallidus and reflects post-inflammatory changes. The caudate nuclei are normal and symmetric

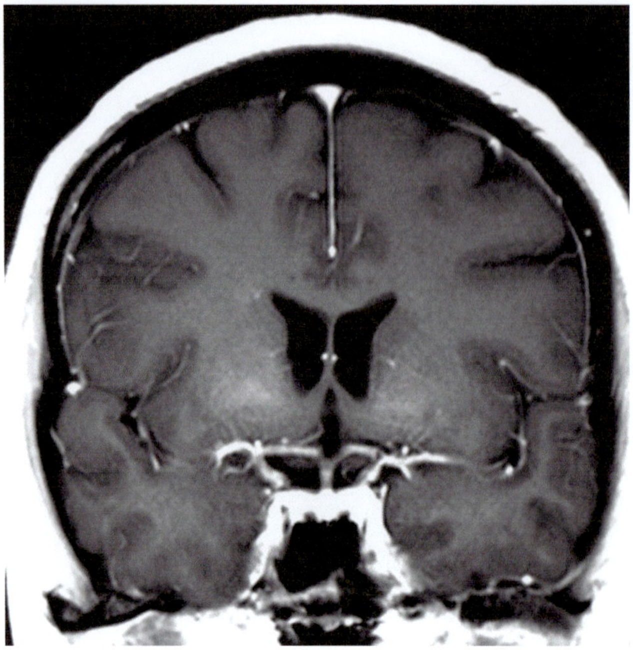

Fig. 38.17 MRI coronal T1 sequence after contrast administration at the same level, amygdala level, as Fig. 38.16. Subtle increased signal is evident bilaterally in the globus pallidus, but it is not enhancing. The increased signal also is evident without contrast administration in Fig. 38.16. No abnormal enhancement is present

NMDA Receptor Autoimmune Encephalitis

39

Clinical History

The first recognized seizures occurred at age 12 years and 2 weeks after an illness with fever, sore throat, and dysphagia. The seizures manifested as orofacial dyspraxia and right body hyperesthesia that was followed by repeated tonic contractions of the right face with hypersalivation and body turning to the right. Each seizure lasted minutes and then recurred several minutes later. After presentation to an emergency department, right-sided clonic status epilepticus was diagnosed.

Emergent care was provided in an intensive care unit and included anesthesia and intubation. MRI identified evidence of inflammation within the left operculum, and seizure control was achieved with a combination of an anti-seizure medications and intravenous immunoglobulin. After 4 days, improvement allowed reduction of the sedation and extubation. When awake, orofacial dyskinesias, slurred speech, and repeated contractions of the right hand returned, and these gradually resolved over the subsequent week as mentation also returned to normal. Seizure freedom continued after discharge home with continuation of the anti-seizure medication. After 1.5 years, the medication was discontinued.

At age 15 years, which was approximately 1 year after anti-seizure medication discontinuation, a second episode of status epilepticus occurred. This also followed an illness with fever and sore throat; however, it differed by being manifested as a loss of right-sided vision followed by unresponsiveness to voice and then progressing to the previously occurring right-sided clonus. Urgent, medical care was obtained, and the evaluation included brain MRI that again identified abnormality of the left operculum. Cerebrospinal fluid (CSF) analysis had normal results for protein, glucose, cells, oligoclonal bands, and PCR testing for infectious agents. An anti-seizure medication was started, and the clonus resolved within several days. The overall recovery was slow with the right-sided visual field deficit lasting about 3 weeks and a more gradual resolution of problems with language, articulation, decreased verbal output, intermittent mutism, and episodes of childlike behavior.

The habitual seizures first occurred after the second episode of status epilepticus and were manifested as episodic impaired awareness and interaction without motor features or a preceding aura. Status epilepticus has not recurred. The illness with fever and sore throat, the abnormal speech, dyskinesias, and childlike behavior also have not recurred.

Because the second anti-seizure medication did not produce seizure freedom, the patient was referred to an epilepsy center where additional diagnostic testing was performed. Detailed mental status testing and neurological examination were normal at this time. An interictal EEG recorded frequent bursts of generalized slowing and no epileptiform abnormality. An MRI identified improvement with resolution of the left opercular abnormality but residual left hippocampal sclerosis, and FDG-PET depicted asymmetrically greater hypometabolic abnormality of the left more than right mesial temporal lobe. CSF analysis provided a more specific diagnosis with identification of antibodies to the NMDA receptor. No other abnormality was present, including evidence of infection or other auto-immune antibodies. A total body PET, obtained to evaluate for occult malignancy, was normal.

A third anti-seizure medication was added to the treatment at the time of the testing, and seizure freedom was achieved, so the three-medication regimen was continued. A 24-hour EEG after 1 year and a routine EEG after another 2 years were both normal. Cognitive function, MRI, PET, and a 72-hour EEG 4 years later also are normal.

The history and seizures are consistent with NMDA receptor autoimmune encephalitis based on a presentation with frequent, focal, medication-resistant seizures and also speech dysfunction, dyskinesias, and psychiatrically abnormal behavior. Ultimately, the identification of NMDA receptor antibodies in CSF confirmed the diagnosis, and the imaging identification of limbic system abnormality was supportive of the diagnosis. Notably, the imaging abnormality

J. M. Stern, N. Salamon, *Imaging of Epilepsy*, https://doi.org/10.1007/978-3-030-86672-3_39

lateralization was concordant with the right-body motor and sensory seizures. For this patient, the autoimmune illness was postinfectious and, as is typical for children with NMDA receptor autoimmune encephalitis, not associated with a teratoma or another tumor. The long-term outcome for this patient has been excellent, which may be related to the early immunosuppressive treatment.

Imaging

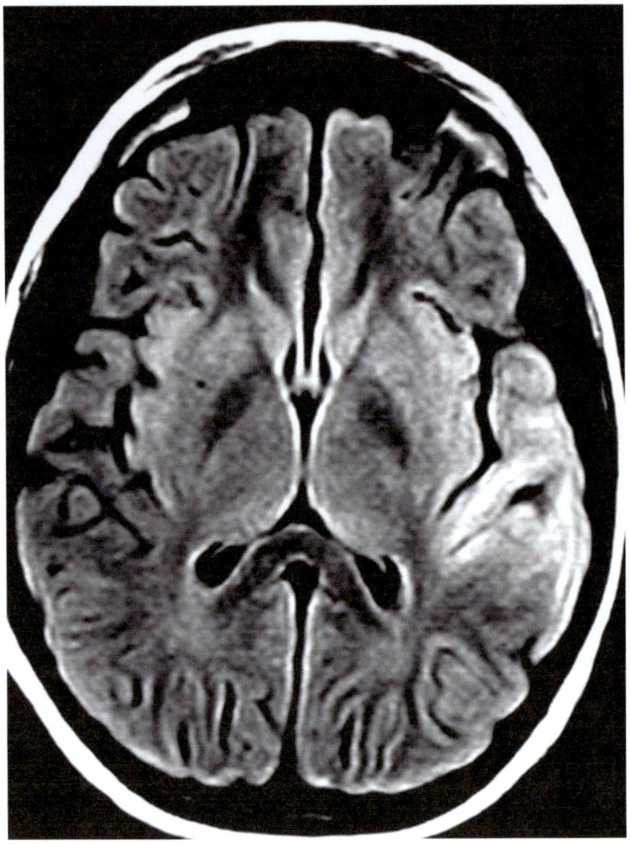

Fig. 39.1 MRI axial FLAIR sequence at a basal ganglia level. The image was obtained at the time of initial presentation. Abnormally increased signal is evident in the left insula and left superior temporal gyrus. Subtle, increased signal also is evident in the medial left thalamus and left orbitofrontal cortex. The cingulate gyri are normal bilaterally

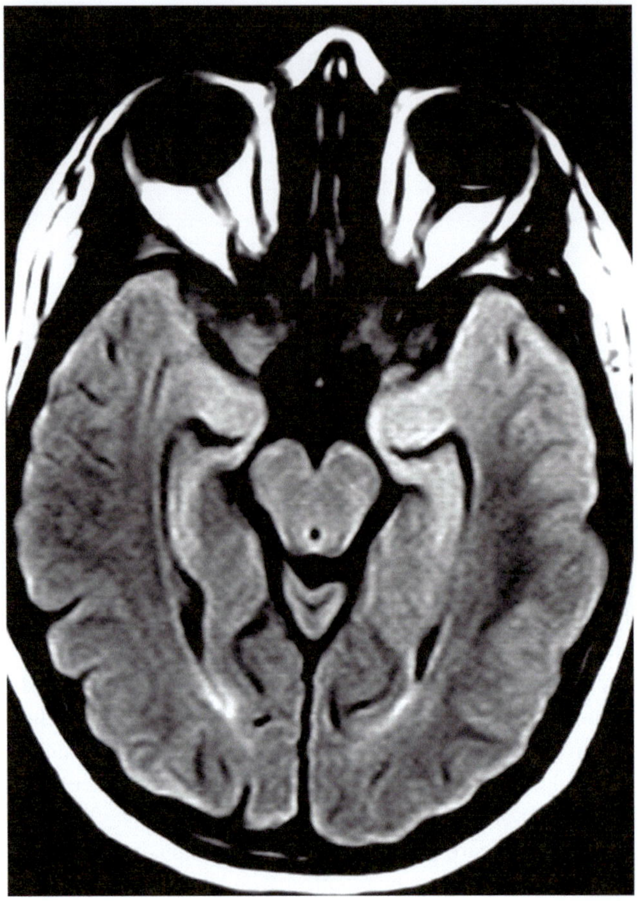

Fig. 39.2 MRI axial FLAIR sequence at an amygdala level. The image was obtained at the time of initial presentation. Abnormally increased signal is evident in bilateral amygdalae and hippocampi, but the left is worse and has extension of the increased signal to the temporal pole

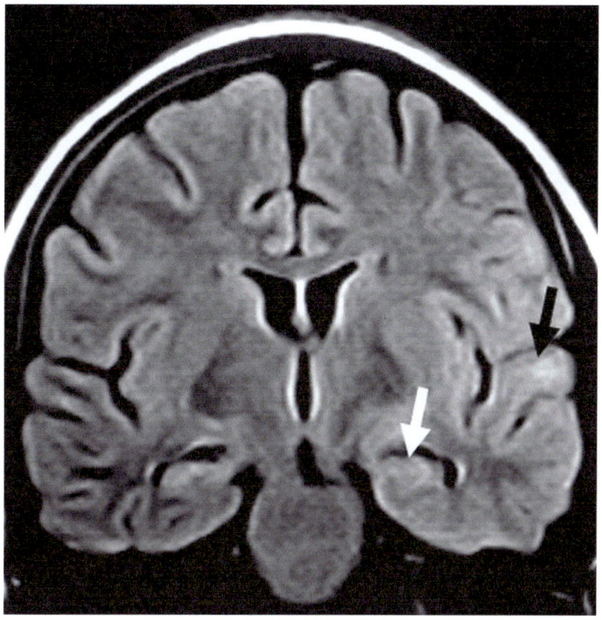

Fig. 39.3 MRI coronal FLAIR sequence at a hippocampal head level. The image was obtained at the time of initial presentation. Bilateral hippocampi have abnormally increased signal, but the signal is asymmetrically greater in extent on the left (white arrow). Abnormally increased signal also is evident in the left superior temporal gyrus (black arrow). When compared to the right side, the left middle temporal gyrus, left insula, and left operculum also are hyperintense. The remainder of the left front and temporal lobes is normal

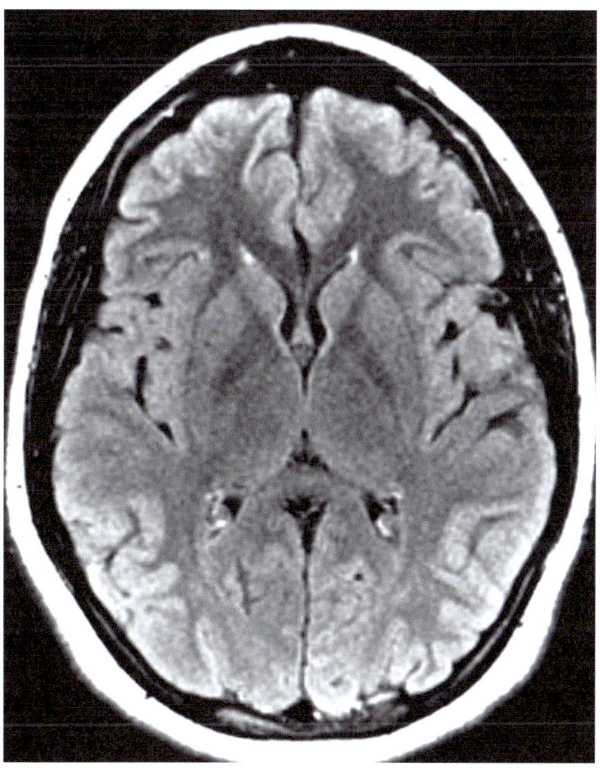

Fig. 39.4 MRI axial FLAIR sequence at a basal ganglia level. The image was obtained 3 years after Fig. 39.1 and at the time of the second episode of status epilepticus. The superior temporal gyrus signal abnormality has resolved. The insula and thalamus are now normal with resolution of all prior signal abnormality

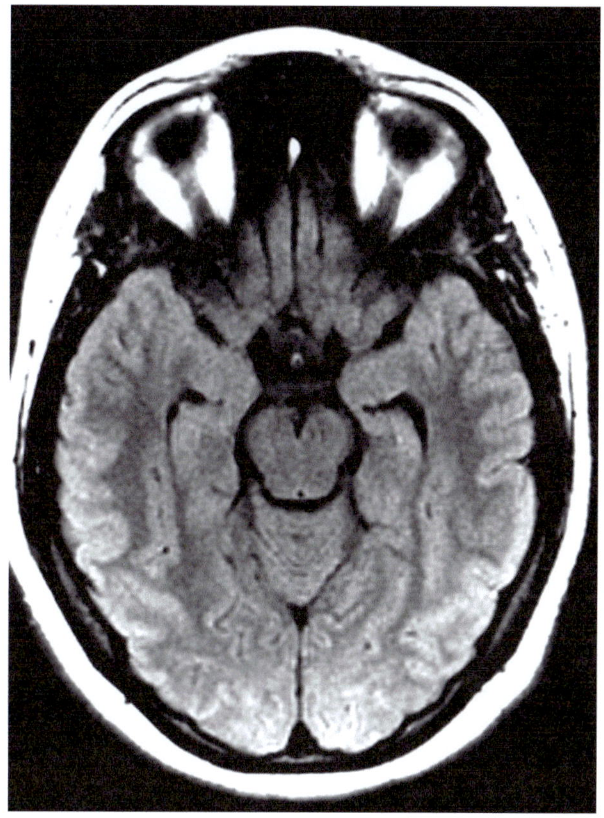

Fig. 39.5 MRI axial FLAIR sequence at an amygdala level similar to Fig. 39.2. The image was obtained 3 years after Fig. 39.2. The signal intensity is normal throughout the amygdalae and hippocampi. The temporal horn of the left lateral ventricle is asymmetrically enlarged due to left hippocampal atrophy. The remainder of the brain is normal

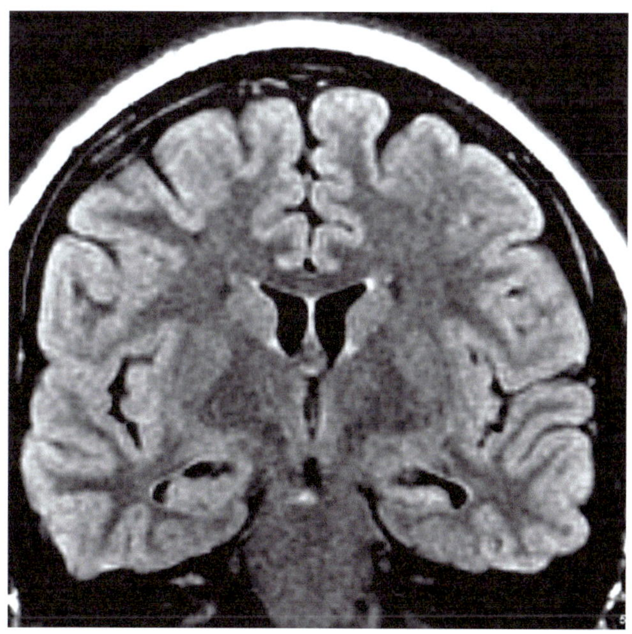

Fig. 39.6 MRI coronal FLAIR sequence at the hippocampal head level in Fig. 39.3. The image was obtained 3 years after Fig. 39.3. Left hippocampal atrophy is evident along with abnormally increased signal, which is consistent with left hippocampal sclerosis. The left superior temporal gyrus and operculum are normal. The hyperintensity at cerebral aqueduct is normal CSF pulsation artifact

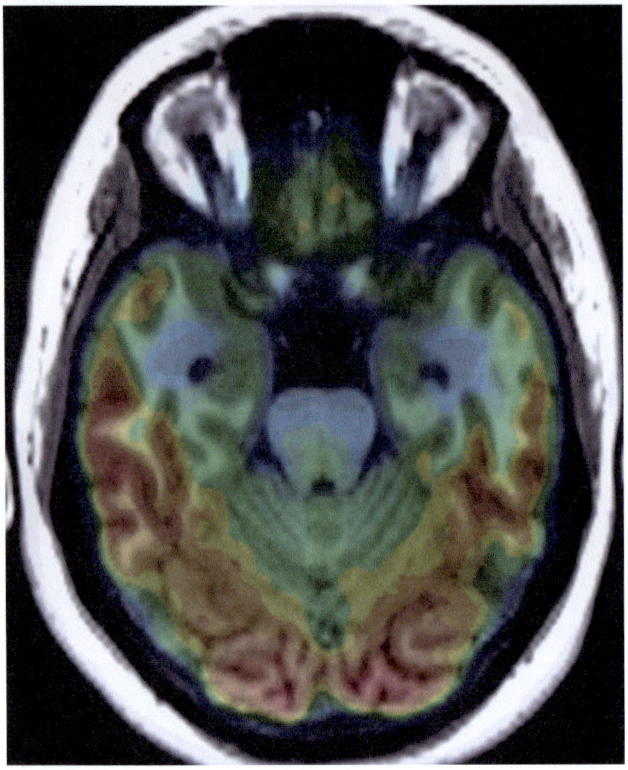

Fig. 39.7 PET-MRI co-registration with color-scale FDG tracer in an axial plane at an amygdala level similar to Figs. 39.2 and 39.5. The PET was obtained at the time of the later MRI. Bilateral anterior-mesial temporal hypometabolism is evident

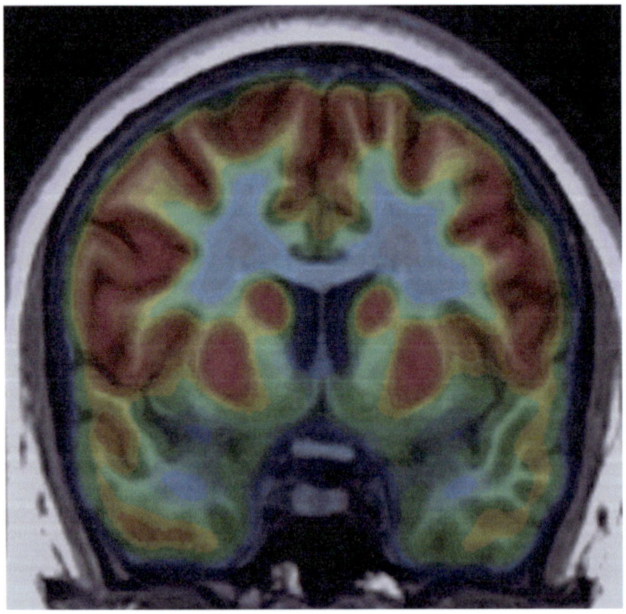

Fig. 39.8 PET-MRI co-registration with color-scale FDG tracer in a coronal plane at temporal pole level. Bilateral temporal hypometabolism is evident with greater prominence on the left and more prominent along the inferior and lateral surfaces. No other asymmetry or abnormality is present

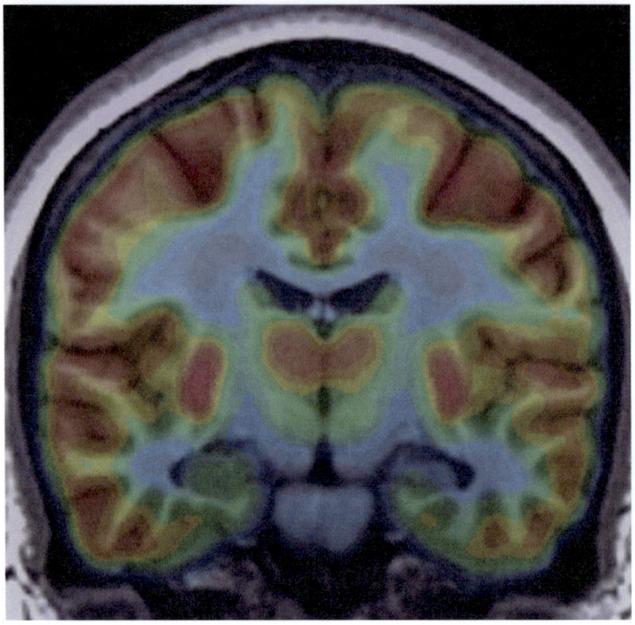

Fig. 39.9 PET-MRI co-registration with color-scale FDG tracer in a coronal plane at a hippocampal head level. Asymmetrically greater hypometabolism of the left hippocampus is evident with blue signal in the left hippocampus, which also is atrophic. The diminished warmer colors along the inferior and lateral surfaces of the left temporal lobe are further evidence of left temporal hypometabolism. The left thalamus also is asymmetrically hypometabolic. The opercula and insulae are normal and symmetric

40 Hashimoto Encephalopathy also Known as Steroid-Responsive Encephalopathy Associated with Autoimmune Thyroiditis (SREAT)

Clinical History

The first recognized seizure occurred between ages 20 and 30 years and was identified in retrospect years later, so the exact age and details were not recalled. Greater detail was known for the episodes that occurred after age 30 years that led to the diagnosis of epilepsy. These episodes were stereotyped with an aura of nonspecific dizziness and a generalized sensation of skin tightening followed by emotional distress and occasionally an olfactory hallucination of a burning aroma. Most auras occurred in isolation. When the auras preceded seizures with impaired awareness, they progressed to include a painful tightening in the neck that was followed by loss of consciousness and a bilateral tonic-clonic convulsion. While in the 30s, several tonic-clonic seizures occurred each year, and several episodes of status epilepticus occurred over the decade.

The most recent tonic-clonic seizure was at about age 40 years and occurred as convulsive status epilepticus. The subsequent postictal confusion lasted several days and included psychosis with hallucinations and paranoia. The evaluation during the postictal period included moderate diffuse abnormal slowing on EEG, thyroid peroxidase antibodies elevated to 214 IU/mL (normal < 2 IU/mL), and the MRI images in Figs. 40.1, 40.2, 40.3, 40.4, 40.5, 40.6, 40.7, and 40.8. Thyroglobulin antibody, serologic tests of thyroid function, and cerebrospinal fluid (CSF) studies for infectious and autoimmune causes were negative.

The habitual seizure over the past 15 years was not been associated with an aura and have been recognized only by discrete episodes of impaired memory or awareness. These sometimes were evident as repeated questioning without recall for several minutes. The occurrences have been sporadic with periods of years between episodes and then episodes of several in succession.

The only identified risk factor was a history of Hashimoto's thyroiditis. Thyroid disease was diagnosed at age 25 years as hyperthyroidism that later became hypothyroidism. A euthyroid state was achieved with hormone supplementation, and this was found to be present at the time of epilepsy presentation. At around the age thyroiditis developed, memory impairment, anxiety, and depression also developed. The anxiety and depression have markedly improved over the years, but memory impairment continues to be a problem.

The history and evaluation indicate focal seizures with limbic features suggestive of insula, olfactory cortex, and amygdala involvement. Based on a history of Hashimoto's thyroiditis, the elevated thyroid peroxidase antibodies at presentation, and the MRI findings, Hashimoto's encephalopathy was diagnosed, and this led to the addition of immunosuppression to the anti-seizure medication regimen. Within days of starting methylprednisolone, memory and concentration improved, and the psychosis resolved. Seizure freedom has been present for the past few years with a combination of anti-seizure medications, mycophenolate, and low-dose prednisone. Thyroid peroxidase antibodies have been at the borderline of normal during this time. Follow-up imaging also has demonstrated improvement.

J. M. Stern, N. Salamon, *Imaging of Epilepsy*, https://doi.org/10.1007/978-3-030-86672-3_40

Imaging

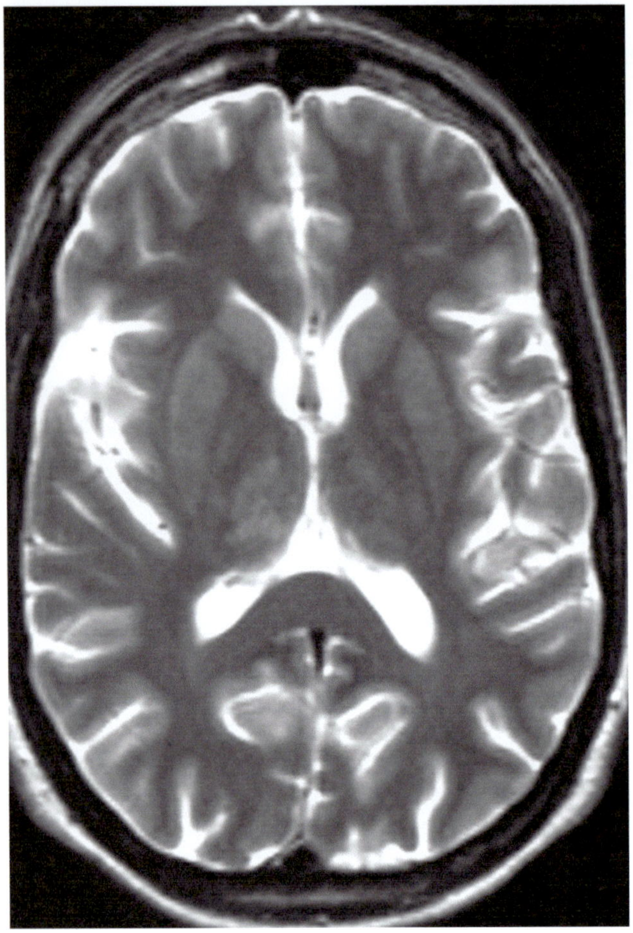

Fig. 40.1 MRI axial T2 sequence at a thalamus level. This image and the images in Figs. 40.2, 40.3, 40.4, 40.5, 40.6, 40.7, and 40.8 were obtained after status epilepticus at age 40 years. Patchy hyperintense signal is evident in the bilateral thalamus with greater abnormality on the right than on the left. The remainder of the brain is normal

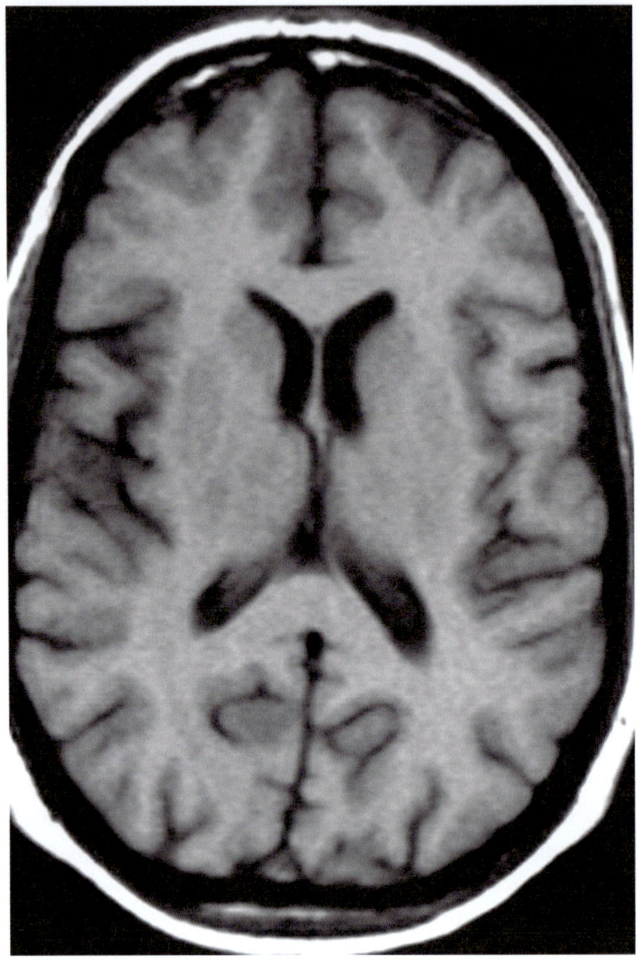

Fig. 40.2 MRI axial T1 sequence at a similar thalamus level as Fig. 40.1. A subtle hypointensity is evident in the right thalamus, and the abnormality less apparent than with the T2 sequence in Fig. 40.1. The left thalamus abnormality is not evident

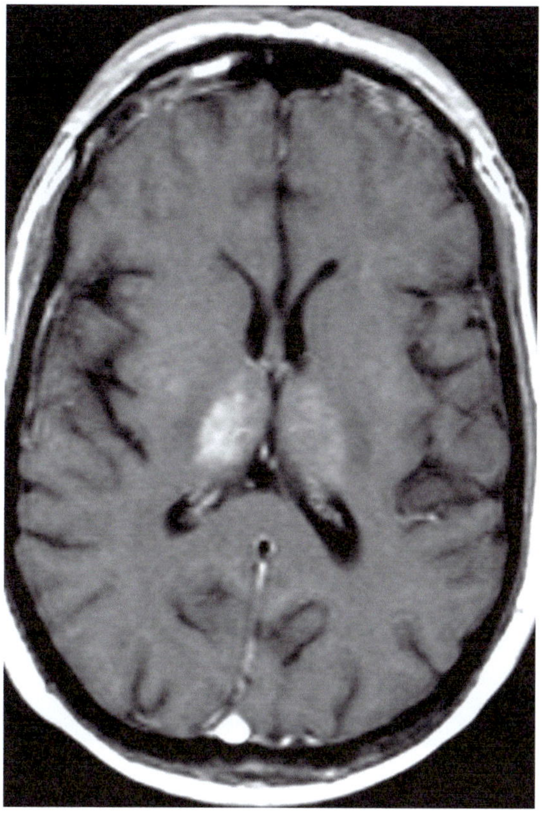

Fig. 40.3 MRI axial T1 sequence after contrast administration at the same thalamus level as Fig. 40.1. Diffuse enhancement of the thalamus is present bilaterally with greater enhancement on right. No other abnormal enhancement is present

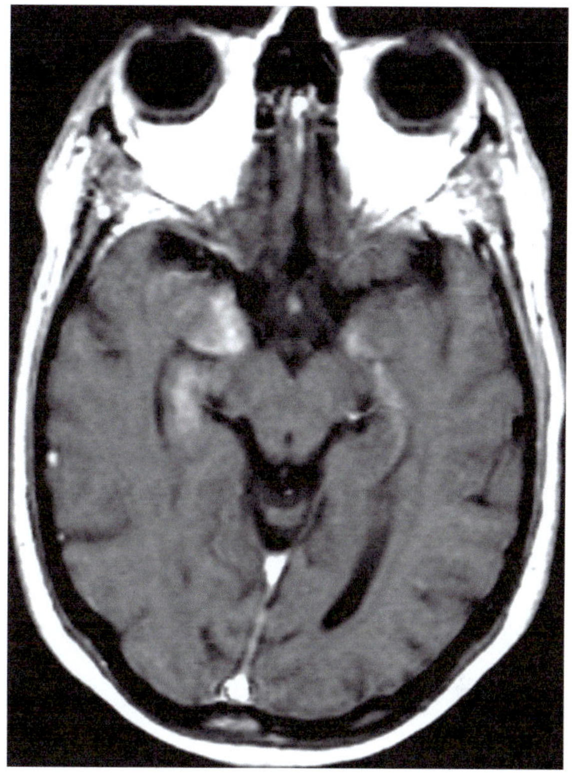

Fig. 40.5 MRI axial T1 sequence after contrast administration at a similar amygdala level as Fig. 40.4. Bilateral amygdalae demonstrate abnormal enhancement with the right having greater enhancement than the left. The head and body of the right hippocampus also has abnormal enhancement. The enhancement adjacent to the left hippocampus is normal choroid plexus

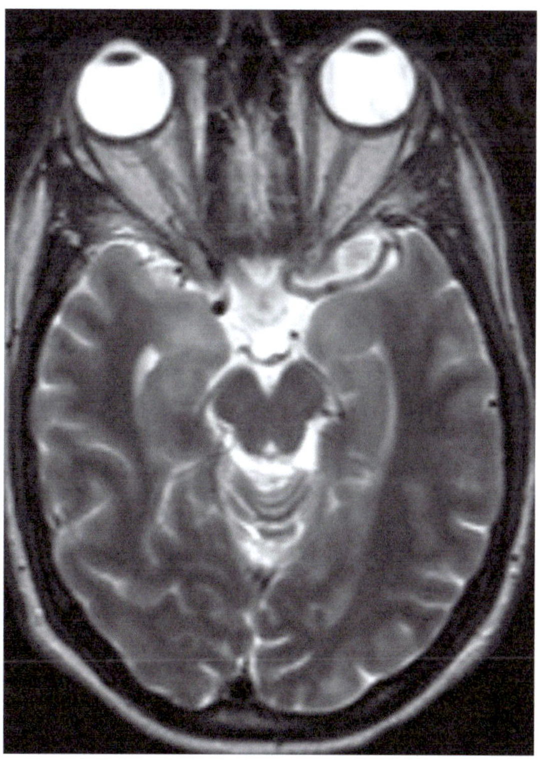

Fig. 40.4 MRI axial T2 sequence at an amygdala level. Abnormally increased signal is evident in the right amygdala and the head of the right hippocampus. The left amygdala and hippocampus are normal

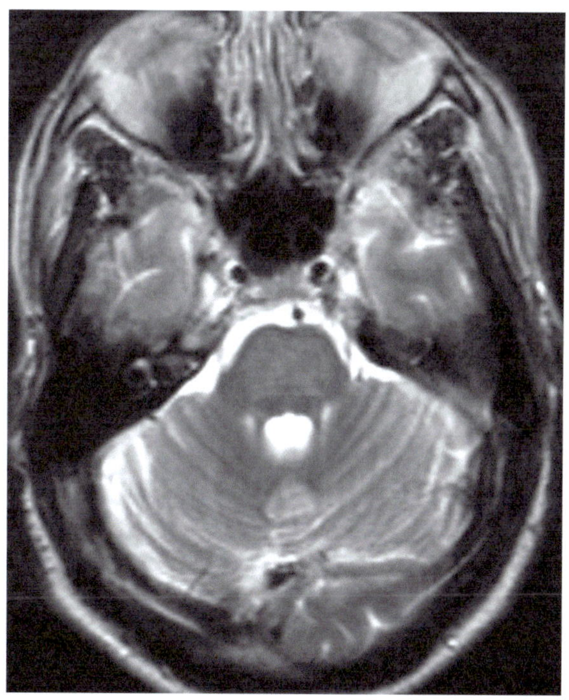

Fig. 40.6 MRI axial T2 sequence at a pons level. Diffuse hyperintense signal is present in the basis pontis. The diffuse distribution suggests a metabolic process more than infarction or neoplasm. The temporal poles and cerebellum are normal

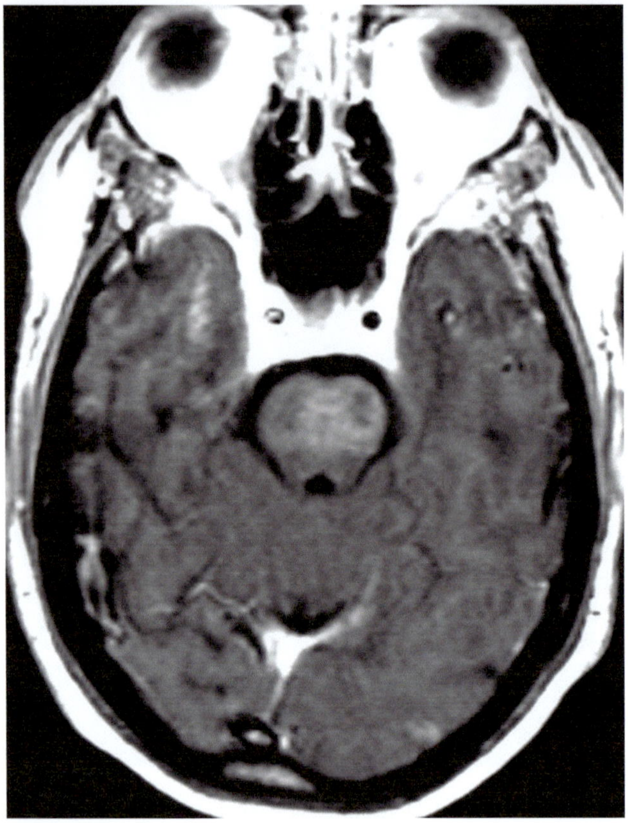

Fig. 40.7 MRI axial T1 sequence after contrast administration at a basis pontis level superior to Fig. 40.6. Diffuse enhancement of basis pontis is present, but it does not include the cortical spinal tracts. The linear hyperintensity within the anterior-medial right temporal lobe is pulsation artifact

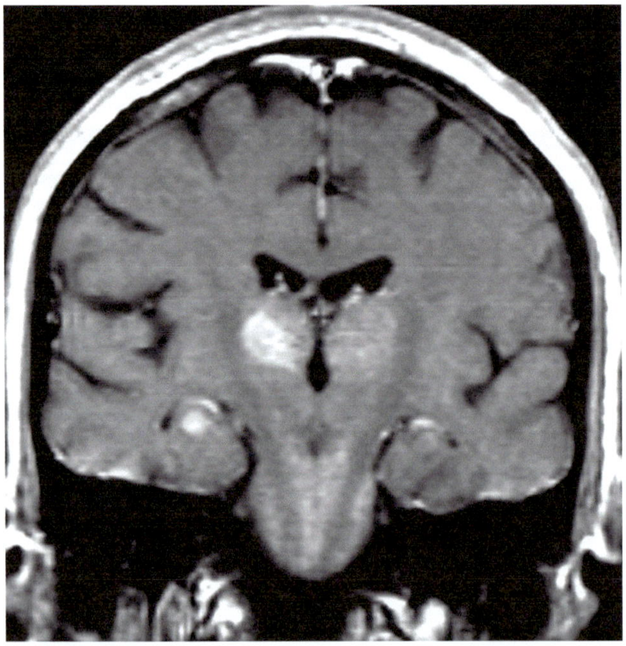

Fig. 40.8 MRI coronal T1 sequence after contrast administration at a thalamus level. The basis pontis has diffuse abnormal enhancement that spares the cortical spinal tracts. Enhancement also is present in the thalamus bilaterally, with the right thalamus demonstrating greater enhancement, and in the right hippocampal body

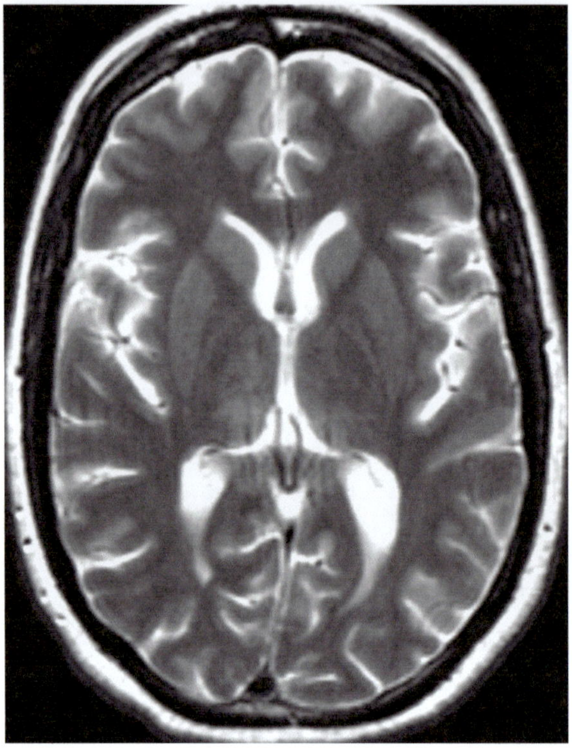

Fig. 40.9 MRI axial T2 sequence at a thalamus level similar to Fig. 40.1. The image was obtained 1 year after Fig. 40.1. The hyperintensity within the right thalamus has decreased slightly. The left thalamus' abnormal hyperintensity also has decreased, but a subtle abnormality remains evident

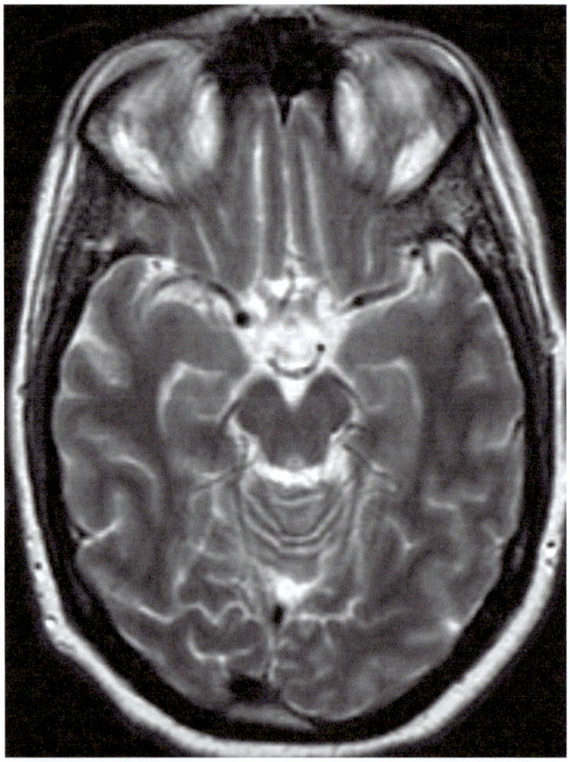

Fig. 40.10 MRI axial T2 sequence at an amygdala level similar to Fig. 40.4. The image was obtained 1 year after Fig. 40.4. Compared to Fig. 40.4, the abnormally increased signal within the right amygdala and hippocampus has decreased. The left amygdala and hippocampus remain normal

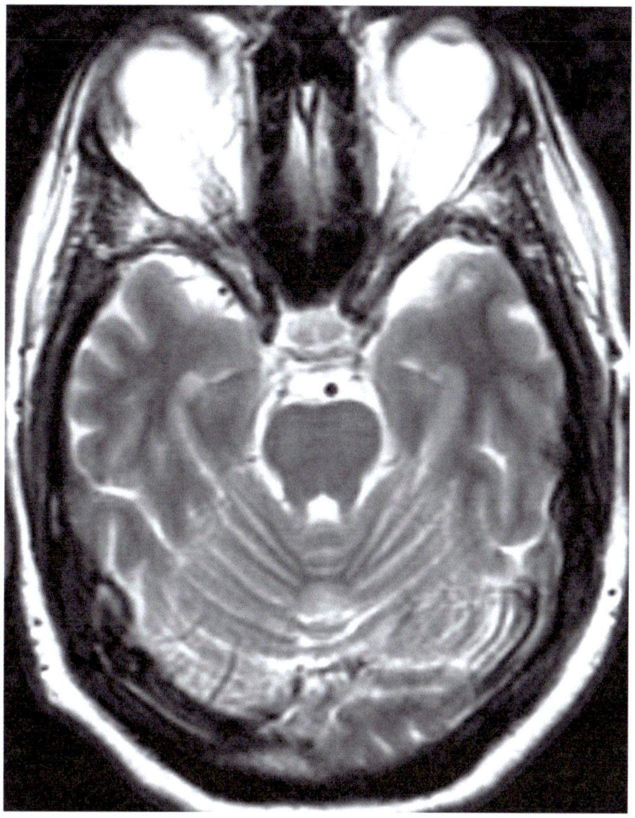

Fig. 40.11 MRI axial T2 sequence at a pons level similar to Fig. 40.6. The image was obtained 1 year after Fig. 40.6. The basis pontis signal has decreased and is now essentially normal

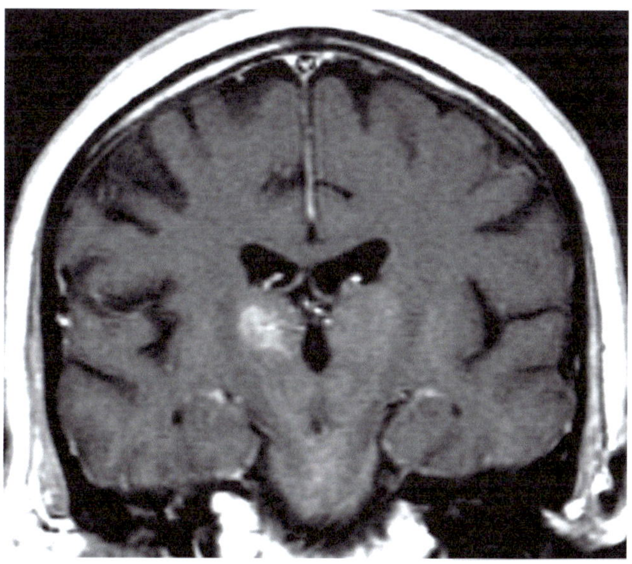

Fig. 40.12 MRI coronal T1 sequence after contrast administration at the same thalamus level as Fig. 40.8. The right thalamus enhancement has decreased in intensity and size. The abnormal enhancement of right hippocampus and left thalamus has resolved. Minor hyperintensity of the brainstem continues to be present

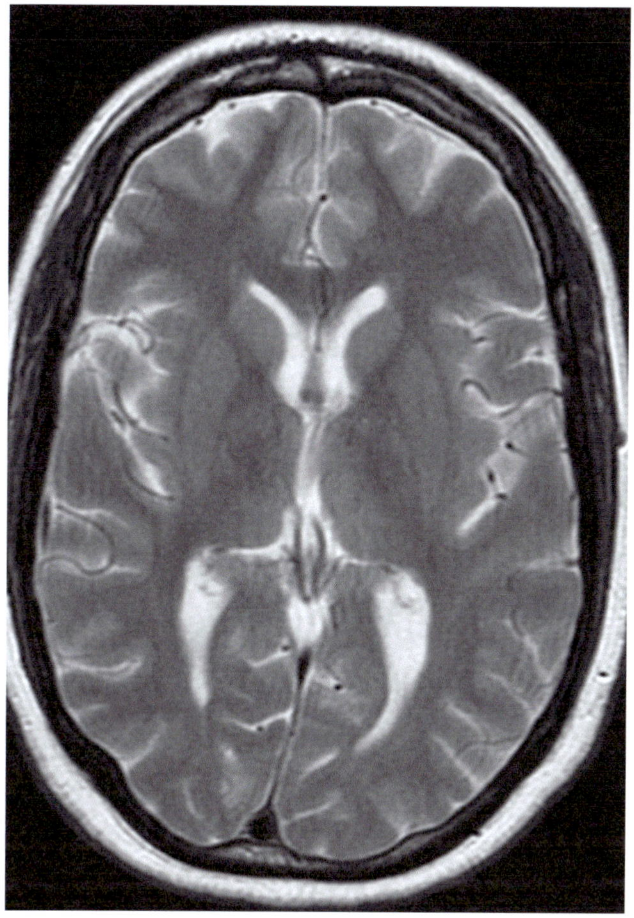

Fig. 40.13 MRI axial T2 sequence at a thalamus level similar to Figs. 40.9 and 40.1. The image was obtained 7 years after Fig. 40.9 and 8 years after Fig. 40.1. The thalamus signal is normal bilaterally. The remainder of the brain also is normal

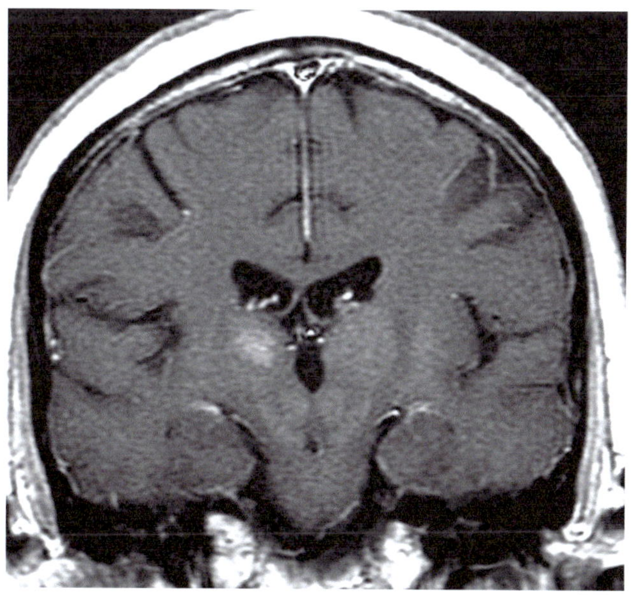

Fig. 40.14 MRI coronal T1 sequence after contrast administration at a thalamus level similar to Figs. 40.12 and 40.8. The image was obtained 7 years after Fig. 40.12 and 8 years after Fig. 40.8. The right thalamus enhancement is now smaller and residual. The brainstem enhancement has resolved, and the right hippocampus and left thalamus remain non-enhancing

Early Stage Rasmussen's Encephalitis

41

Clinical History

The first recognized seizure occurred at age 4 years as a cluster of episodes that included unresponsive staring, drooling, orofacial automatisms, and tonic contraction of the face to the left. The total duration was 5–10 minutes, and no postictal deficits were present. An evaluation at that time was normal, including MRI and routine cerebrospinal fluid (CSF) studies of cells, protein, and glucose.

The habitual seizures developed soon after the presenting seizures, and they were similar to the initial seizure but also included an abnormal sensation or sometimes pain across the left body. About half of the seizures were focal sensory, and the remaining included the motor features with impaired awareness. The seizures often occurred in clusters, and either individual seizures or clusters occurred several times monthly despite treatment that included multiple anti-seizure medications.

An epilepsy risk factor was not present.

Neurological examination identified minor asymmetric flattening of the left nasolabial fold, slight left pronator drift, left-hand clumsiness, a slight left-sided limp, and asymmetrically increased left deep tendon reflexes. The clumsiness and limp were noted by the parents to have developed a few months after the first seizure.

Medical history and childhood development were normal.

Interictal EEG depicted frequent multifocal right-sided epileptiform discharges that often occurred in long trains over the right central and temporal regions. Video-EEG monitoring recorded multiple focal seizures in the first 24 hours that were consistent with the habitual seizure. Ictal EEG's seizure onset was 1 Hz right frontal spike and slow-wave discharges.

MRI identified progressive abnormalities over months within the right cerebrum. Four months after the normal MRI, a right-sided subcortical signal abnormality was present. After another month, the abnormality had expanded and produced mass effect. FDG-PET identified a region of abnormal hypometabolism that co-localized with the MRI abnormality and had a region of hypermetabolism within it indicating ongoing epileptic abnormality.

The history and evaluation indicate right hemispheric epilepsia partialis continua with seizures manifested by sensory and motor features. The epilepsy was accompanied by an anatomically corresponding and progressive motor deficit. The combination of the seizures, motor deficit, and imaging abnormalities support the diagnosis of Rasmussen's encephalitis.

A right hemispherotomy was performed about 6 months after the epilepsy onset. Histopathological examination identified marked, patchy astrocytogliosis with significant neuron loss in a laminar pattern. Perivascular clusters of lymphoid cells, microglial nodules, and cortical spongiosis were present. The findings were interpreted as supporting the Rasmussen's encephalitis diagnosis. No seizures or auras have occurred for 4 years since surgery, including the recent 6 months without anti-seizure medications. School performance is normal, and the left hemiparesis does not prevent independent ambulation.

J. M. Stern, N. Salamon, *Imaging of Epilepsy*, https://doi.org/10.1007/978-3-030-86672-3_41

Imaging

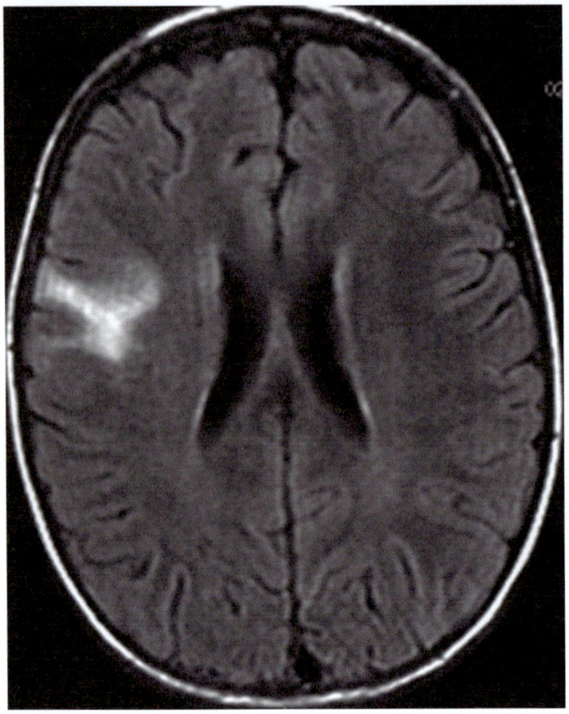

Fig. 41.1 MRI axial FLAIR sequence at a lateral ventricle level. This image and the image in Fig. 41.2 were obtained 4 months after the first seizure. Abnormally increased signal is evident in the subcortical white matter of the right precentral gyrus. No volume loss or mass effect is present

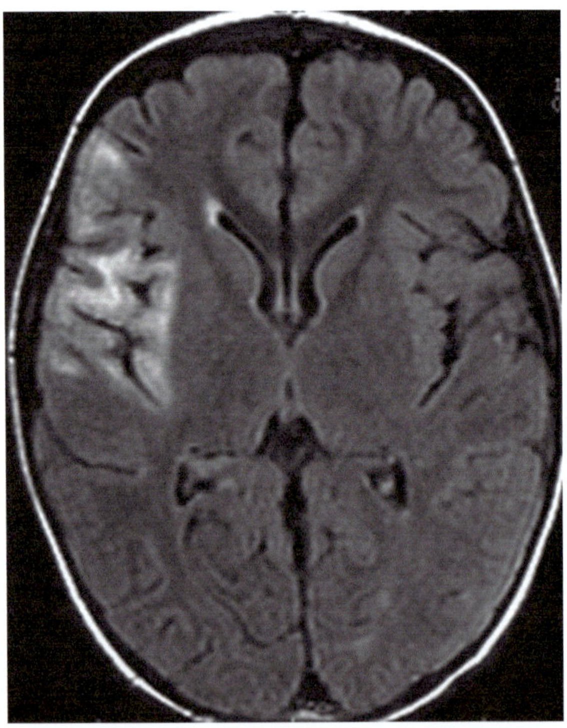

Fig. 41.2 MRI axial FLAIR sequence at an insula level. Abnormally increased signal is evident in the subcortical white matter of the right insula, right inferior frontal gyrus, and right operculum. No volume loss or mass effect is present. The remaining cerebrum is normal

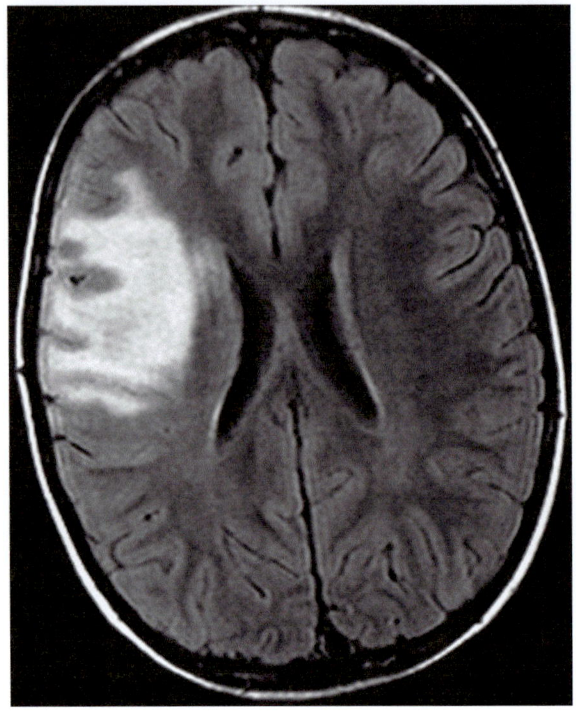

Fig. 41.3 MRI axial FLAIR sequence at the same lateral ventricle level as Fig. 41.1. This image and all subsequent images were obtained 1 month after Figs. 41.1 and 41.2. The abnormally increased signal in the right frontal lobe's subcortical white matter has expanded anteriorly and posteriorly and is now beyond the precentral gyrus. The abnormality now causes minor mass effect toward the right lateral ventricle, but the gray-white junction is visible, and there is no architectural distortion

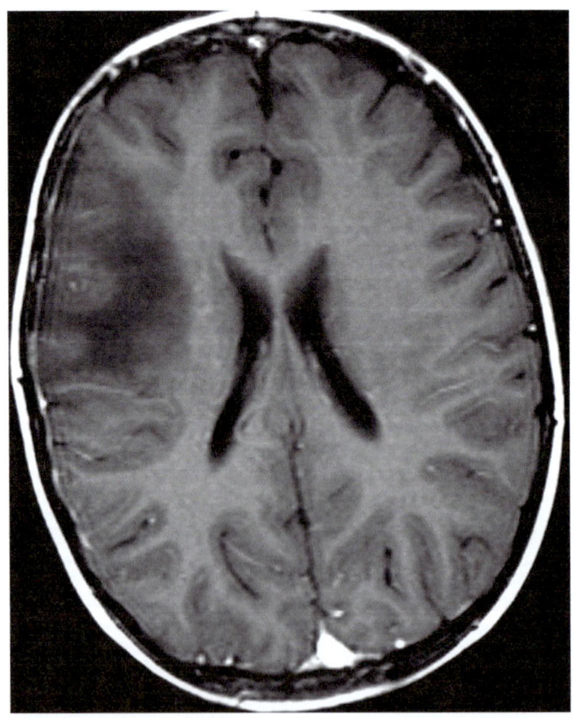

Fig. 41.4 MRI axial T1 sequence after contrast administration at the same lateral ventricle level as Fig. 41.3. The right frontal lobe subcortical white matter is hypointense and does not demonstrate abnormal enhancement. The overlying cortical sulci are effaced

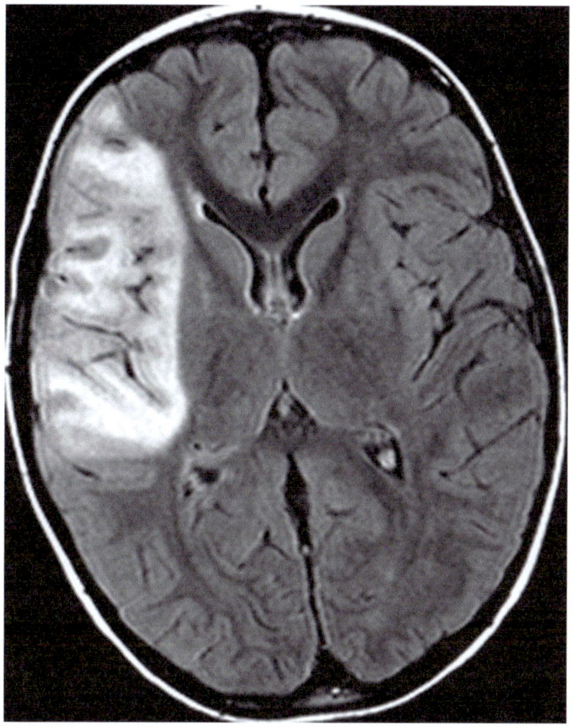

Fig. 41.5 MRI axial FLAIR sequence at the same insula level as Fig. 41.2. The hyperintense FLAIR signal abnormality now involves the entirety of the subcortical white matter around the right insula to the perisylvian regions, including the right inferior frontal gyrus, right operculum, and right superior temporal gyrus. Mild mass effect against the frontal horn of the right lateral ventricle is evident. There is no midline shift or volume loss. The gray-white junction is visible

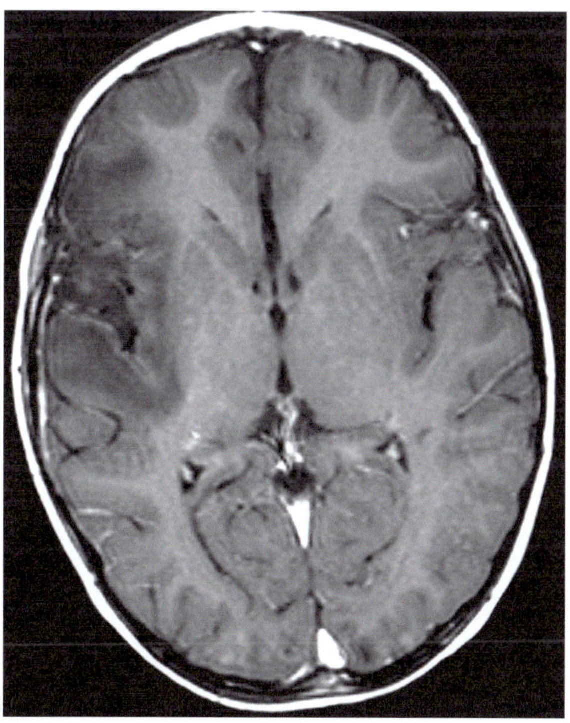

Fig. 41.6 MRI axial T1 sequence after contrast administration at an insula level similar to Fig. 41.5. The right perisylvian region subcortical white matter is hypointense and does not demonstrate abnormal enhancement. The overlying cortical sulci are effaced

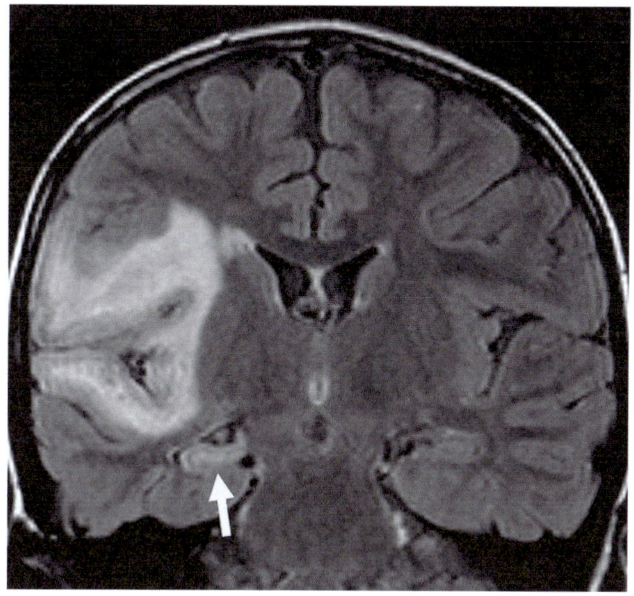

Fig. 41.7 MRI coronal FLAIR sequence at a hippocampal head level. Abnormal subcortical hyperintensity extends across the right perisylvian region and includes the right frontal operculum, right superior temporal gyrus, and the right external capsule. The right hippocampal head (arrow) is hyperintense but not atrophic

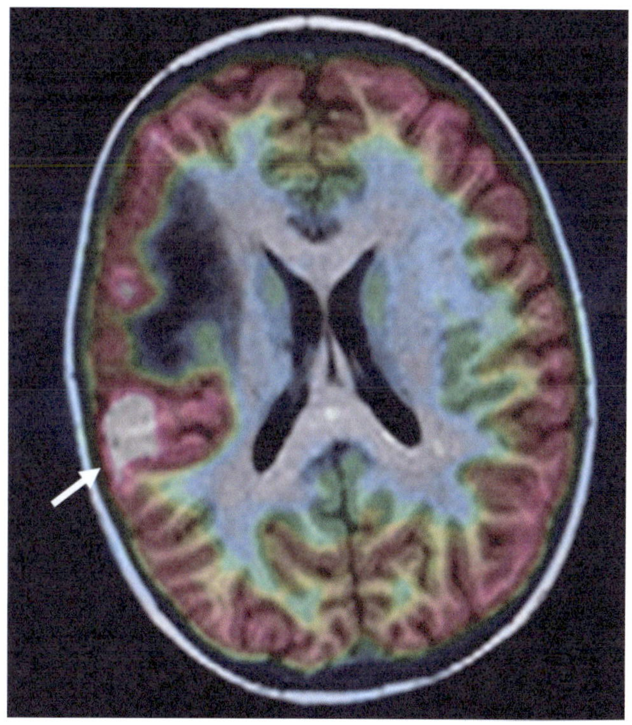

Fig. 41.8 PET-MRI co-registration with color-scale FDG tracer in an axial plane at the same lateral ventricle level as Fig. 41.3. An extensive right frontal subcortical hypometabolic region is present with a region of hypermetabolism (arrow) at its posterior margin. The hypermetabolism suggests the location of epileptic abnormality with ongoing seizure generation. The frontal cortex is not abnormally asymmetric

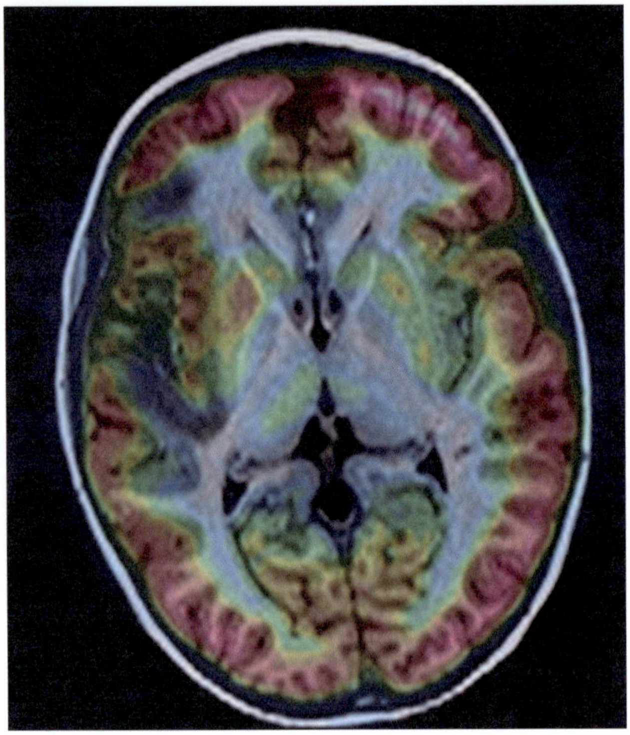

Fig. 41.9 PET-MRI co-registration with color-scale FDG tracer in an axial plane at the same insula level as Fig. 41.6. Asymmetric hypermetabolism is evident in the right basal ganglia and right insula, as relates to seizure generation. Asymmetric hypometabolism is evident in the peripheral portions of the perisylvian region, extending from the right inferior frontal gyrus to the right superior temporal gyrus

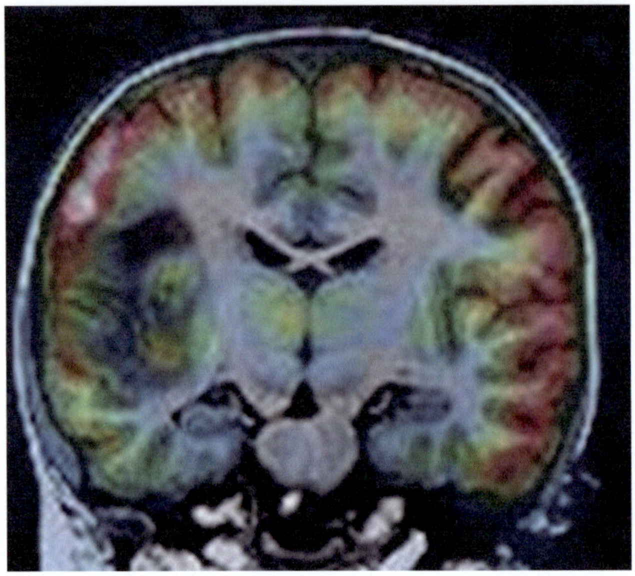

Fig. 41.10 PET-MRI co-registration with color-scale FDG tracer in a coronal plane at a hippocampal head level slightly anterior to Fig. 41.7. The inferior right parietal lobe is asymmetrically hypermetabolic, suggesting the location of epileptic abnormality and seizure generation. Hypometabolism is evident across the right temporal lobe, operculum, subcortical white matter, and external capsule

Late Stage Rasmussen's Encephalitis

42

Clinical History

The first recognized seizure occurred at age 6 years as a twitching of the right foot's toes. An evaluation at that time included an MRI that identified a small focus of gliosis in the left hemisphere. Seizures were not disabling after diagnosis, and the specific epilepsy diagnosis was not reached.

Over the subsequent 2 years, the habitual seizures changed to manifest as right lip or chin twitching for 15–45 seconds that sometimes was associated with staring and impaired awareness. Less commonly, the seizures progressed to a bilateral tonic-clonic convulsion that lasted 1 minute. With the change in seizure manifestation and the increased frequency, a reevaluation was undertaken, and this led to the diagnosis of Rasmussen's encephalitis. Treatment was then expanded to include immunosuppressive therapies. During this time, the seizure frequency varied from a few seizures within 1 day to one seizure every few days. Hemispheric epilepsy surgery was initially deferred because of concerns for the functional deficit and was then reconsidered after deterioration in seizure control with an emerging pattern of multiple bilateral tonic-clonic seizures every night.

An epilepsy risk factor was not present. Medical history and childhood development were normal.

Neurological examination identified a right hemiparesis with right-sided hyperreflexia. The hemiparesis was mild for much of the time after the onset of epilepsy and progressed over months prior to the surgical evaluation. Neuropsychological testing identified expressive language deficits.

Interictal EEG depicted decreased faster frequencies and increased slower frequencies across the left side with poorly formed vertex sharp waves and sleep spindles on the left. Video-EEG monitoring recorded focal seizures that occurred about 100 times daily and were manifested as behavioral arrest sometimes with right arm dystonic posturing. Ictal EEG's seizure onset was increased rhythmicity of slow activity across the left frontal-temporal region. Lateralized periodic discharges were present across the left posterior temporal region.

MRI identified progressive left hemispheric atrophy that involved both gray and white matter. The cortical ribbon remained intact. FDG-PET identified widespread and patchy abnormal hypometabolism. Functional MRI for language identified expressive language function in the left hemisphere and some receptive language function in right hemisphere.

The history and evaluation indicate left hemispheric seizures that progressed over 3 years from isolated focal seizures to epilepsia partialis continua and then to a presentation in bilateral convulsive status epilepticus. The epilepsy was accompanied by a similarly lateralized progressive motor and language deficit. With the imaging findings, the diagnosis of Rasmussen's encephalitis was reached.

A left hemispherotomy was performed soon after presentation in status epilepticus at age 9 years. Histopathological examination identified moderate lymphocyte infiltration of the perivascular spaces and rare microglial nodules, which was interpreted as suggestive of Rasmussen's encephalitis. No seizures have occurred for the 3 months since surgery. At this time, school performance was improved with increased cognitive focus, and motor function of the right hand included open and closing but not movements of individual fingers.

J. M. Stern, N. Salamon, *Imaging of Epilepsy*, https://doi.org/10.1007/978-3-030-86672-3_42

Imaging

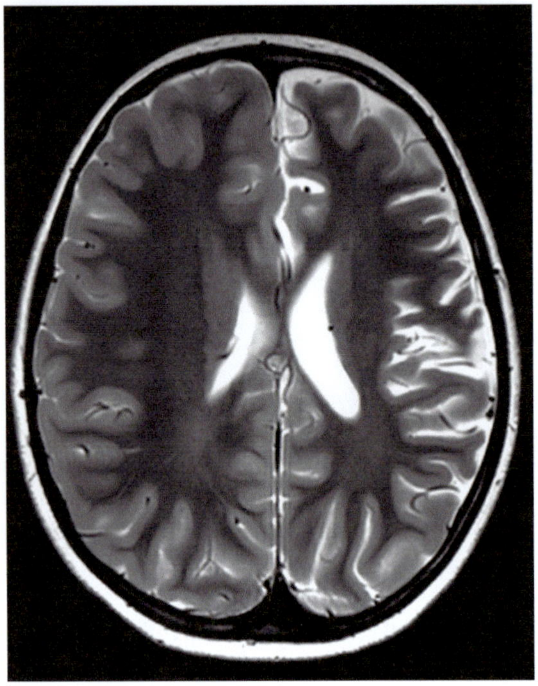

Fig. 42.1 MRI axial T2 sequence at a lateral ventricle level. This image and the images in Figs. 42.2 and 42.3 were obtained 1.5 years after the first seizure. Left hemispheric atrophy includes the left anterior cingulate gyrus, frontal lobe, operculum, and inferior parietal lobule. Volume loss involves both gray matter and white matter. Ex-vacuo enlargement of the right lateral ventricle is proportional to the cerebral tissue volume loss. The cortical ribbon is normal with normal gray-white differentiation. The right hemisphere is normal

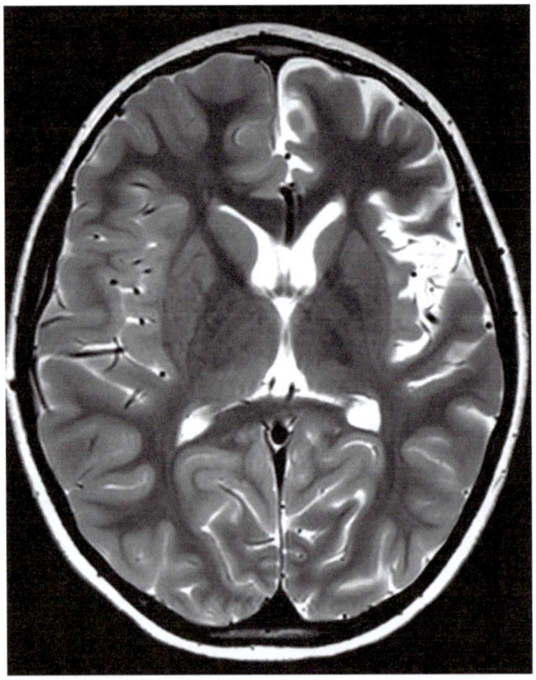

Fig. 42.2 MRI axial T2 sequence at a thalamus level. Left hemispheric atrophy includes the left anterior cingulate gyrus, frontal lobe, insula cortex, and superior temporal gyrus. The basal ganglia and thalamus are symmetric and normal. The right hemisphere is normal

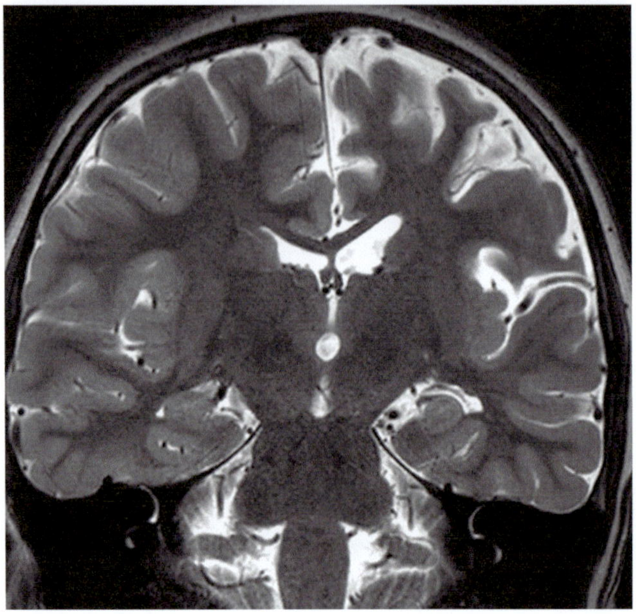

Fig. 42.3 MRI coronal T2 sequence at a hippocampal body level. Left hemispheric atrophy includes the left anterior cingulate gyrus, frontal lobe, operculum, and insula. Less prominently, it includes the left temporal lobe. The left lateral ventricle is enlarged in proportion to the cerebral tissue loss. The hippocampi, basal ganglia, and brainstem are symmetric and normal. The corpus callosum is normal, but it is deflected superiorly because of the ventricular enlargement

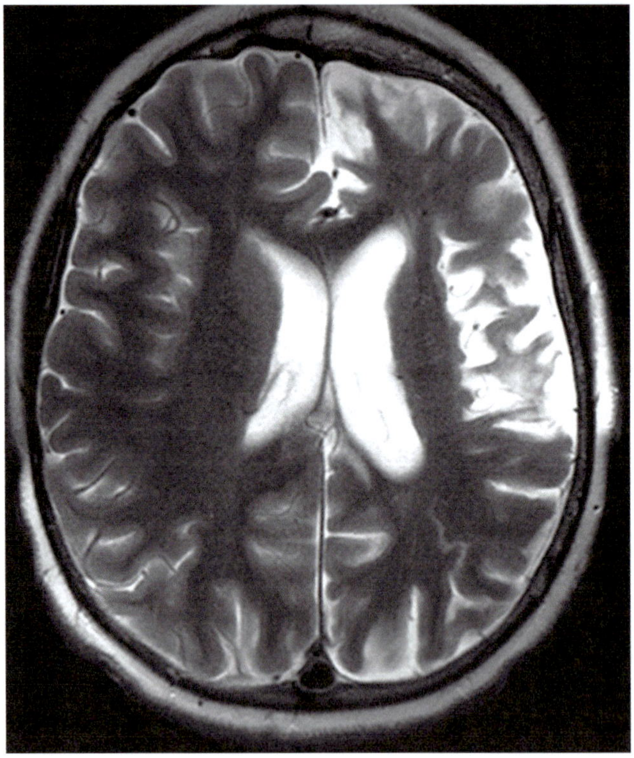

Fig. 42.4 MRI axial T2 sequence at a lateral ventricle level similar to Fig. 42.1. This image and all of the subsequent images were obtained just prior to hemispherotomy, which was 1.5 years after Figs. 42.1, 42.2, and 42.3. Additional atrophy of the left hemisphere is evident with significant atrophy of left frontal lobe, operculum, insula, and, to a lesser extent, the left parietal lobe. The left lateral ventricle has ex-vacuo enlargement. The corpus callosum and right hemisphere are normal

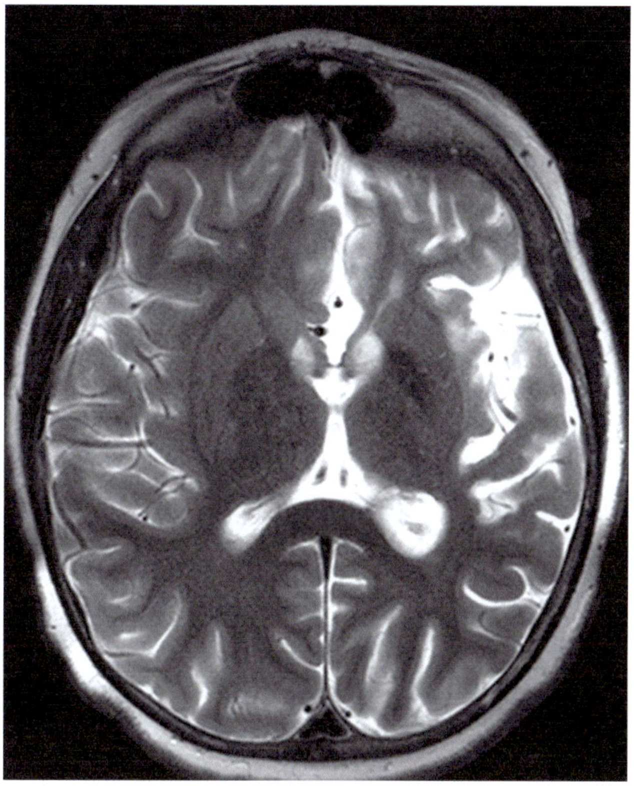

Fig. 42.5 MRI axial T2 sequence at a thalamus level similar to Fig. 42.2 but with a slightly different angle. Left hemispheric atrophy is evident with more marked atrophy of the left cingulate gyrus, frontal lobe, insula, and superior temporal gyrus. The basal ganglia and thalamus are symmetric and normal. The cortical ribbon is normal bilaterally. The right hemisphere is normal

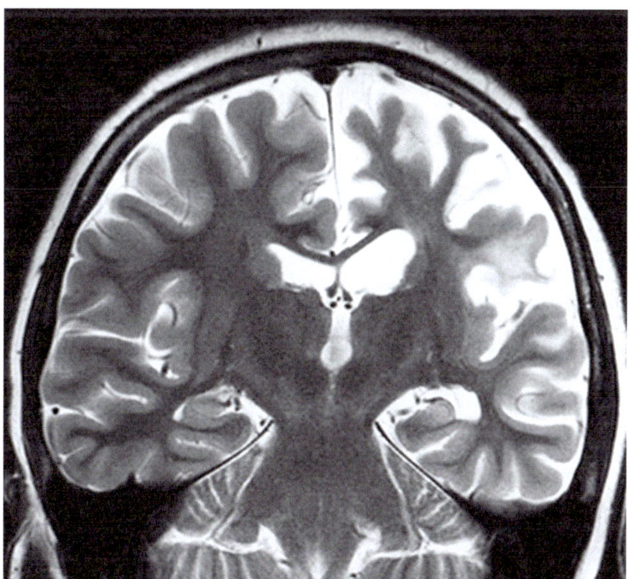

Fig. 42.6 MRI coronal T2 sequence at the same hippocampal body level as Fig. 42.3. The left hemispheric atrophy has progressed across the left cingulate gyrus, frontal lobe, operculum, and temporal lobe. The left hippocampus is now also included and also has slightly increased signal, which suggests the development of hippocampal sclerosis. The left lateral ventricle has concomitantly enlarged, and the left corpus callosum has thinned. The thalamus, brainstem, and cerebellum are symmetric and normal

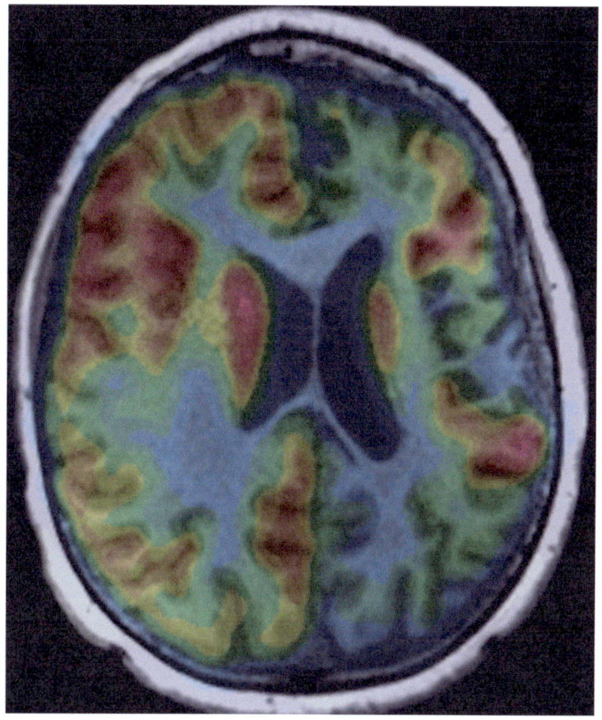

Fig. 42.7 PET-MRI co-registration with color-scale FDG in an axial plane at the same lateral ventricle level as Fig. 42.1. The left hemisphere has widespread hypometabolism that is more extensive than the hemispheric atrophy and patchy in its occurrence across the cortical surface. In addition to the cortical hypometabolism, the left caudate nucleus is asymmetrically hypometabolic

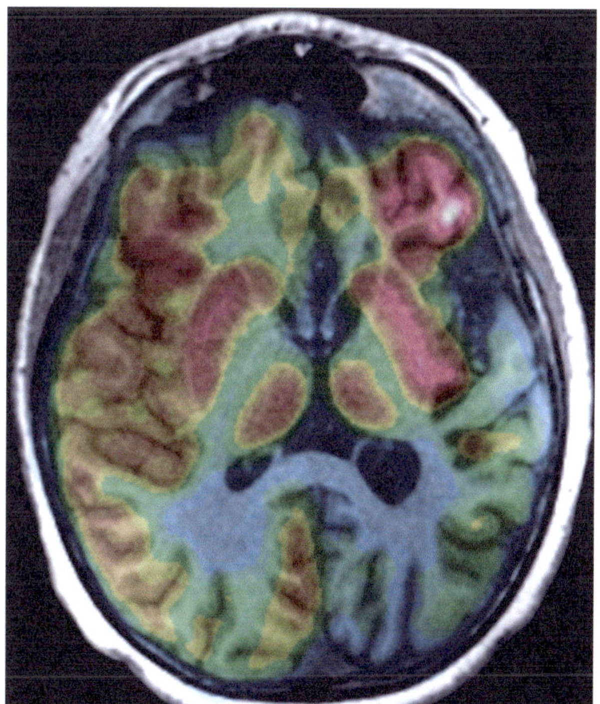

Fig. 42.8 PET-MRI co-registration with color-scale FDG in an axial plane at the same thalamus level as Fig. 42.2. Hypometabolism is evident across the left temporal and occipital lobes and is more extensive than the atrophy. Hypermetabolism is present within an atrophic portion of the left orbitofrontal region and indicates epileptic activity. The left putamen and thalamus are relatively symmetric and preserved

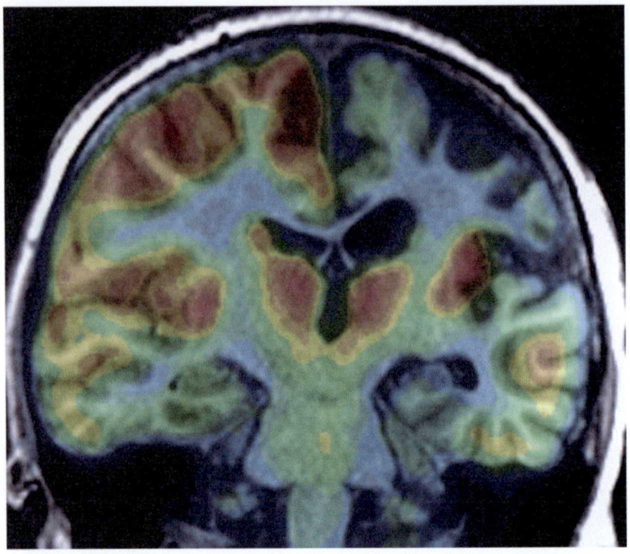

Fig. 42.9 PET-MRI co-registration with color-scale FDG tracer in a coronal plane at the same hippocampal body level as Fig. 42.3. Hypometabolism is evident across the left frontal lobe, operculum, and temporal lobe. The left hippocampus and left caudate are also asymmetrically hypometabolic. Hypermetabolism is present in the left insula

Part V
Vascular Abnormalities

Cerebro-vascular abnormality
Cavernous angioma
Cavernous malformation
Arteriovenous malformation
Ischemic infarction
Ischemic stroke
Cerebral hemorrhage
Porencephaly
Sturge-Weber syndrome

Vascular abnormalities related to epilepsy are ischemic or hemorrhagic injuries that may be due to either congenital or acquired abnormality. Among the major types of vascular malformations, cavernous malformations and arteriovenous malformations are most associated with epilepsy. Developmental venous anomaly is a more common finding that is less associated with epilepsy and is discussed in Section 8- Non-epileptogenic Findings.

Cavernous malformations

Cavernous malformations are a low flow abnormality that is well-circumscribed and mulberry-like in appearance with a sinusoidal vasculature and without intervening arteries, capillary beds, or veins. Because of chronic, minor hemorrhages, cavernous malformations are usually surrounded by hypointense T2 signal indicating hemosiderin staining. Gradient echo (GRE) and susceptibility weighted imaging (SWI) are especially sensitive for identifying cavernous malformations because of the hemosiderin deposition. MRI is superior to CT for detection and diagnosis, but CT can suggest the presence of a cavernous malformation through calcification producing faint hyperdensity. Between 70 and 90% of cavernous malformations are single malformations within the brain.

Arteriovenous malformations

Brain AVMs are abnormal connections between pial arteries and draining veins with the consequence of blood shunting through an abnormal, intervening network of vessels within the brain parenchyma. A true capillary bed is not present. The transition between artery and vein can be visible at a nidus with a tangle of surrounding vessels. This is evident as low T2 signal with contours that indicate the tangle. Hypointense T2 signal may surround part of the malformation because of prior hemorrhages and hemosiderin deposition.

Ischemic infarction

Ischemic infarction can be produced by a variety of mechanisms that may impact the relationship to epilepsy; however, the age at time of the infarction also has an impact on the epileptogenesis and epilepsy manifestation. In particular, the relationship to epilepsy is sensitive to the stage of brain development, so infarctions are considered according to whether they are prenatal, perinatal, or postnatal. Regardless of the age, the middle cerebral artery territory is a common localization for epileptogenic infarctions.

Porencephaly

Porencephaly is a hemispheric cystic cavity due to a prenatal hemispheric ischemic or hemorrhagic infarction. The appearance relates to the immature collateral circulation at the time of the infarction, and the cysts can be extensive with communication between the ventricle and subarachnoid space. Signal abnormality due to gliosis can be evident in the tissue adjacent to the porencephaly. More diffuse anoxic injury can accompany the infraction, so hippocampal sclerosis can be associated. Porencephalies can occur bilaterally.

Sturge-Weber syndrome

Leptomeningeal angiomatosis, which is termed Sturge-Weber syndrome (SWS), is a capillary malformation that appears to result from failure of the primitive cephalic venous plexus to regress. With MRI, focal atrophy and enhancement of the leptomeninges are evident. The most characteristic features of SWS are due to a poorly developed superficial cortical venous drainage system with engorgement of the venous outflow to the deep drainage system causing engorged leptomeningeal and pial vessels and consequential contrast enhancement. The choroid plexus is also enlarged and compensating cortical bone thickening is present on the atrophic side. When the age is younger than 6 months, hypermyelination can be present.

CT depicts hemispheric atrophy and calcification and, when younger than 6 months, white matter hyperdensity indicates hypermyelination. Although plain X-ray is not a technique of choice, it is possible to observe the classical gyriform cortical calcifications also known as the tram track appearance.

Key References

Geibprasert S, PongpechS, Jiarakongmun P, et al. Radiologic assessment of brain arteriovenous malformations: what clinicians need to know. Radiographics 2010;30:483–501.

Higueros E, Roe E, Granell E, Baselga E. Sturge-Weber syndrome: review. Actas Dermo-sifiliogr 2017;108:407–17.

Pasternak JF, Mantovani JF, Volpa JJ. Porencephaly from periventricular hemorrhage in a premature infarct. Am J Dis Child 1980;134:674–5.

Pinto AL, Chen L, Friedman R, et al. Sturge-Weber syndrome: brain magnetic resonance imaging and neuropathology findings. Pediatr Neurol. 2016;58:25–30.

Zafar A, Fiani B, Hadi H, et al. Cerebral vascular malformations and their imaging modalities. Neurol Sci. 2020;1–5.

Cavernous Malformation with Acute Hemorrhage

43

Clinical History

The first recognized seizures occurred in early childhood as auras in isolation. These originally were experienced as a visual memory with a sense of deja vu that would typically prompt futile attempts to remember the source of the image. By early adolescence, the auras changed to also include a warm, pleasant, rising sensation in the chest.

The habitual seizures of adulthood first developed later in adolescence. The auras changed to be unpleasant with a sense of cold or fear that usually progressed to a depersonalized, impaired state. During the impairment, behavior included nonsensical language, behavioral arrest with a blank stare, and then chewing movements. The seizure duration was several minutes, and recovery required several additional minutes. Bilateral tonic-clonic seizures did not occur. Because of the episodes of impairment, an evaluation was undertaken, and an EEG indicated a diagnosis of epilepsy. Treatment included multiple anti-seizure medications with a seizure frequency of two to three individual seizures or clusters of seizures weekly.

An epilepsy risk factor was not present until adulthood when a vascular malformation was identified.

Neurological examination was normal. Neuropsychological testing identified excellent overall performance, including excellent verbal and also visuospatial memory. Medical history included no relevant abnormality.

Interictal EEG depicted epileptiform spikes in the left anterior to middle temporal region. Video-EEG monitoring recorded focal seizures manifested as staring with fumbling automatisms of the left hand and dystonic posturing of the right hand. Ictal EEG's seizure onset was in the left anterior to middle temporal region.

MRI identified a left anterior temporal cavernous angioma with a diameter of 3 cm that bordered the hippocampus. PET identified a large hypometabolic region within the anterior left temporal lobe.

The history and evaluation indicate left temporal lobe epilepsy. The onset was in childhood with auras in isolation that had limbic features related to memory, suggesting the mesial temporal lobe. With adolescence, the seizures changed to include other limbic features of emotional and possibly autonomic experiences, suggesting involvement of the amygdala and insula. Presentation followed the development of seizures with impaired awareness that did not progress to convulsive motor features, which also suggests a limbic rather than neocortical epileptogenic abnormality.

The right-hand dystonic posturing and left temporal ictal EEG onset lateralize the seizures to the left anterior temporal lobe, which corresponds to the anterior left temporal lobe cavernous malformation. The evidence of recent and remote hemorrhages provides a possible explanation to the progressive changes to the seizures, but such seizure changes also can occur with mesial temporal lobe epilepsy without a progressive pathology. Remarkably, neuropsychological testing indicated that the adjacent hippocampal system was not compromised. As such, a memory deficit would be expected if a standard left anterior-mesial temporal lobe resection was performed. Because of this, a more limited resection was offered.

An anterior temporal lobe resection of the cavernous angioma and the surrounding tissue was performed with inclusion of the amygdala but not the hippocampus. Histopathological examination identified a cavernous hemangioma with a collection of dilated, tightly packed, variable, amuscular vessels without intervening neuroglial stroma. No seizures have occurred for 10 years since surgery, and anti-seizure medication treatment was discontinued more than 5 years ago.

J. M. Stern, N. Salamon, *Imaging of Epilepsy*, https://doi.org/10.1007/978-3-030-86672-3_43

Imaging

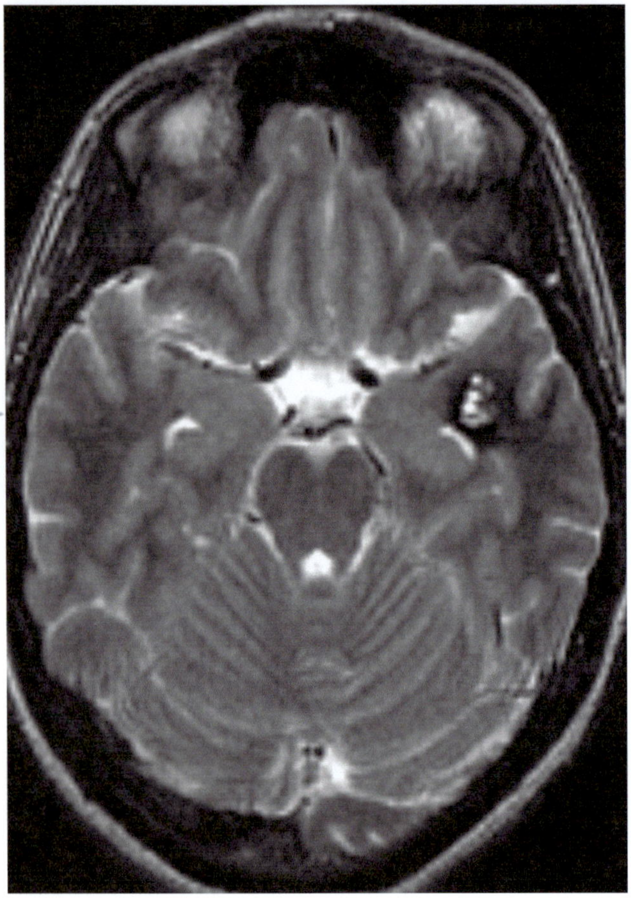

Fig. 43.1 MRI axial T2 sequence at an amygdala level. Mixed intensity signal abnormality is present in the left temporal lobe lateral to the amygdala. The lesion has multiple small hyperintensities that differ in brightness, indicating blood products from minor hemorrhages at differing ages. The hyperintensities are collectively surrounded by hypointensity due to hemosiderin staining. No edema is present. The mesial temporal structures are normal bilaterally

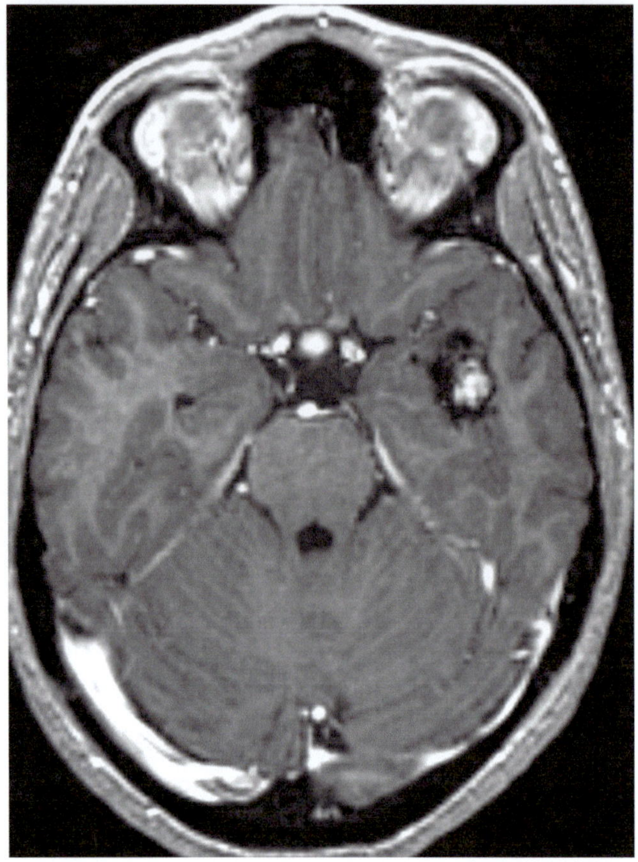

Fig. 43.2 MRI axial T1 sequence after contrast administration at the same amygdala level as Fig. 43.1. Mixed intensity signal abnormality is evident in the left temporal lobe with surrounding hypointensity due to hemosiderin staining. The abnormality is consistent with multiple minor hemorrhages at different times. No abnormal contrast enhancement is present, including no evidence of a developmental venous anomaly surrounding the cavernous malformation. No edema is present

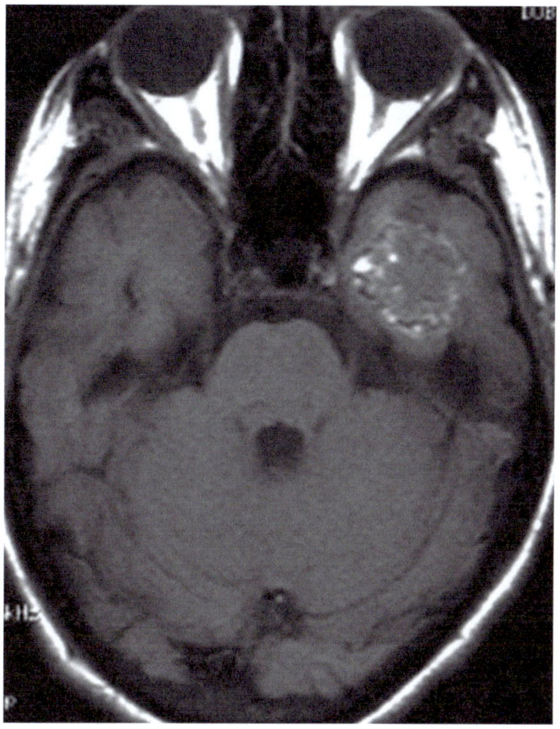

Fig. 43.3 MRI axial T1 sequence at an upper pons level. A large left temporal lobe abnormality is evident with speckled hyperintensities that are along the edge and not in the center or periphery. The hyperintensities indicate subacute hemorrhage. With this T1 sequence, acute hemorrhage is isointense and may be identified as acute if hyperintense with a T2 sequence, which is evident in Fig. 43.4

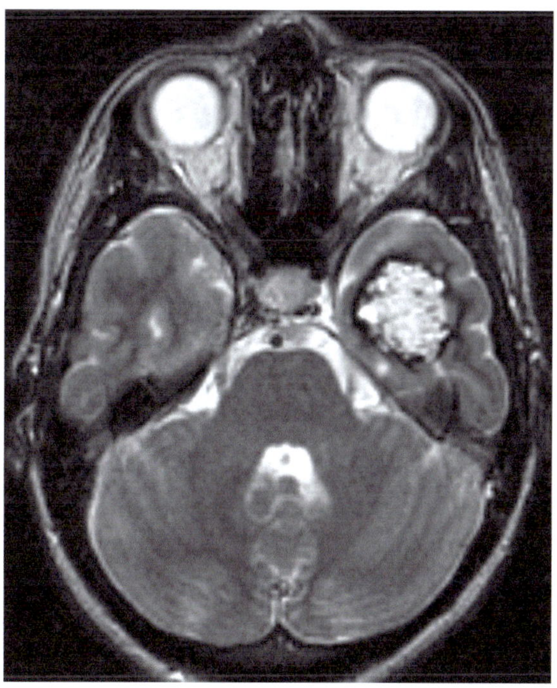

Fig. 43.4 MRI axial T2 sequence at a middle cerebellar peduncle level that is slightly inferior to Fig. 43.3. A large mixed intensity lesion with multiple compartments is evident in the left temporal lobe. The lesion's prominent hyperintensity corresponds to T1 isointensity in Fig. 43.3 and indicates acute hemorrhage. The surrounding hypointensity is hemosiderin staining. The lesion has no mass effect or surrounding edema. The remainder of the brain is normal

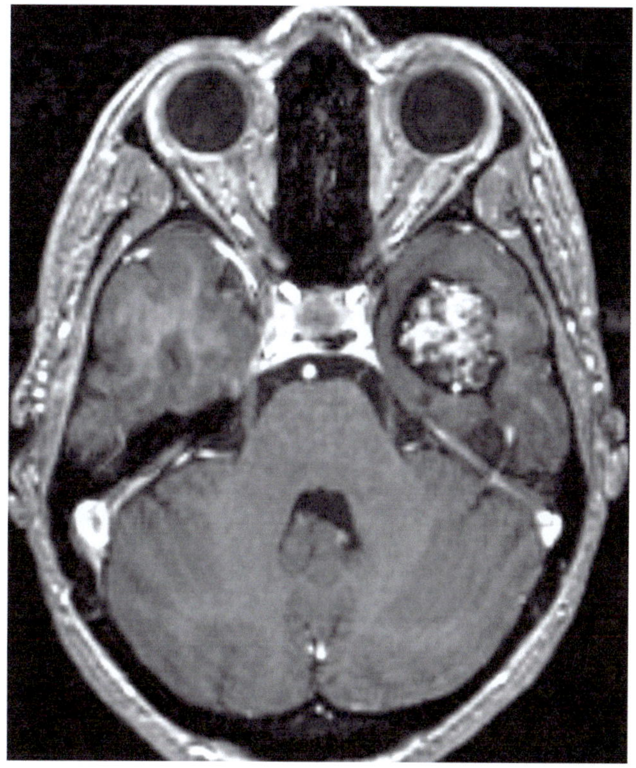

Fig. 43.5 MRI axial T1 sequence after contrast administration at the same middle cerebellar peduncle level as Fig. 43.4. A large left temporal lobe heterogeneous intensity lesion has surrounding hemosiderin staining hypointensity that is more extensive medially than laterally. No abnormal contrast enhancement or developmental venous anomaly is present. The lesion does not produce edema or mass effect

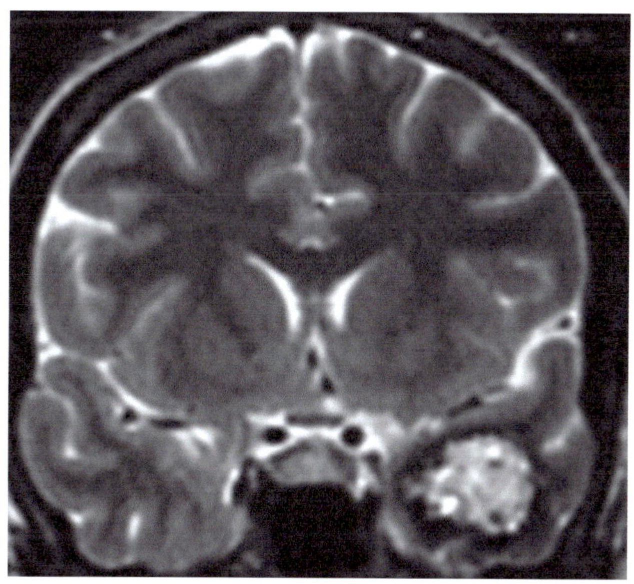

Fig. 43.6 MRI coronal T2 sequence at a temporal pole level. A mixed signal intensity lesion is evident in the left temporal lobe with a surrounding hypointense rim. No edema or mass effect is present. The remaining brain is normal

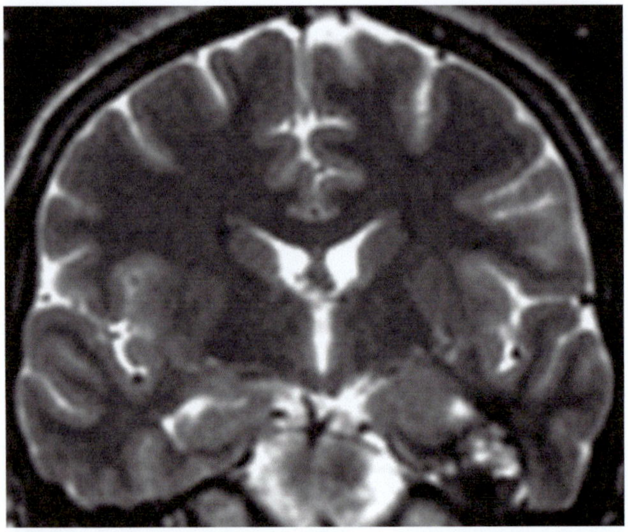

Fig. 43.7 MRI coronal T2 sequence at a hippocampal head level. The hemosiderin staining around the mixed intensity lesion extends into the left fusiform gyrus; however, the adjacent left amygdala is normal. Because of a turned head position, the hippocampus is visible on the right and it also is normal

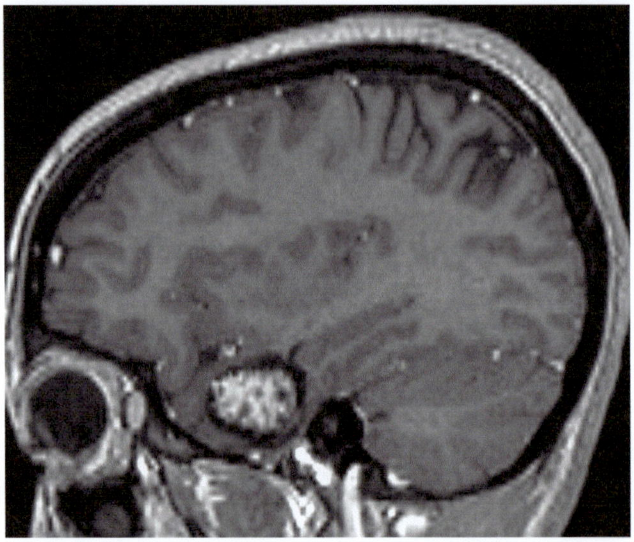

Fig. 43.8 MRI sagittal T1 sequence after contrast administration at a left hippocampus level. A mixed intensity lesion with surrounding hypointensity is located anterior of the head of the hippocampus. The lesion does not produce mass effect or edema. No abnormal contrast enhancement or developmental venous anomaly is present

44 Cavernous Malformation with Resolving Hemorrhage

Clinical History

The first recognized seizure occurred at age 30 years as episodic difficulty with word finding or reading. This was sometimes accompanied by an indescribable "weird" feeling. The episodes typically lasted 15–30 seconds and were not associated with an impairment in awareness, responsiveness, or memory. An evaluation at that time identified a vascular malformation of the anterior aspect of the left middle temporal gyrus.

Gradually over the subsequent years, the habitual seizures changed to become more impairing of language, eventually causing inability to communicate or understand, and to have a longer duration, now lasting 30 seconds to 2 minutes. No subjective experience of impairment was present, but family members observed that the more recent seizures included purposeless word repetition and amnesia. Postictally, nausea sometimes was present. Treatment included multiple anti-seizure medications with about two seizures each month that caused impaired awareness identified by witnesses. No seizures progressed to bilateral tonic-clonic convulsions.

The only epilepsy risk factor was the cerebral vascular malformation.

Neurological examination was normal. Neuropsychological testing identified high average to very superior results in verbal fluency, verbal memory, and verbal abstract reasoning. Medical history was not relevant to epilepsy.

Interictal EEG depicted occasional epileptiform spike and slow-wave complexes over the left anterior temporal lobe and rare left temporal slowing. Video-EEG monitoring recorded focal seizures manifested as behavioral arrest with impaired awareness. The ictal EEG's seizure onset was over the left middle temporal region.

MRI identified a 9-mm cavernous malformation in the anterior aspect of the left middle temporal gyrus. PET identified hypometabolism surrounding the left temporal cavernous malformation.

The history and evaluation indicate left temporal lobe epilepsy with seizures that originally manifested as aphasia and without evidence of additional impairment. As such, the likely localization was the lateral aspect of the language-dominant temporal lobe. This was supported by the EEG and imaging, which identified a left temporal lobe cavernous malformation that did not involve the mesial structures. Because of medication resistance and progression to seizures producing impairment, epilepsy surgery was offered with a surgical plan to spare the mesial temporal structures because of the evidence of intact function.

An extended resection of the cavernous malformation was performed, and histopathological examination identified a cavernous hemangioma. No seizures or auras have occurred for the 5 years since surgery. Anti-seizure medication regimen have been gradually reduced with currently one medication eliminated and the other at half of the presurgery dose.

J. M. Stern, N. Salamon, *Imaging of Epilepsy*, https://doi.org/10.1007/978-3-030-86672-3_44

Imaging

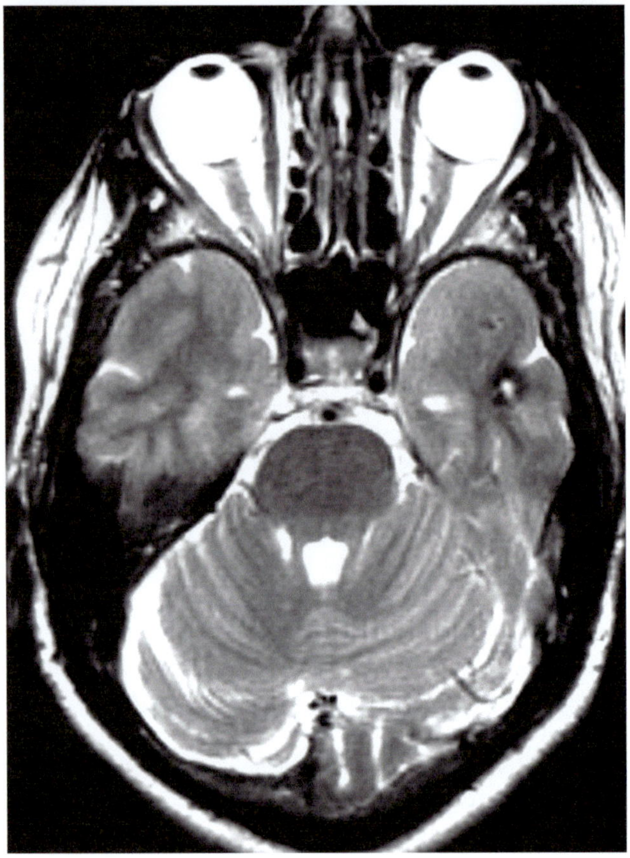

Fig. 44.1 MRI axial T2 sequence at a temporal pole level. A small round focus of hyperintensity with surrounding hypointensity is present in the left middle temporal gyrus. The surrounding hypointensity is due to hemosiderin staining. No edema is present, and the remaining brain is normal. The smaller hypointensity anterior to the abnormality is due to volume averaging of a vessel

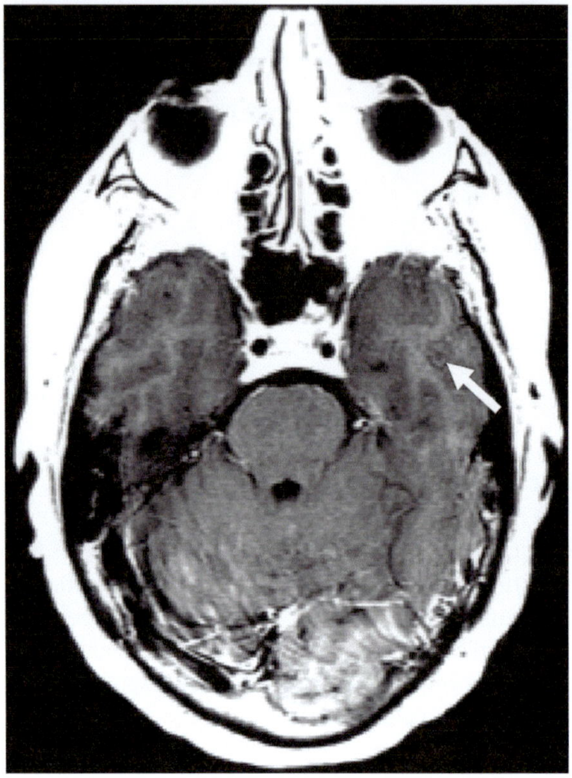

Fig. 44.2 MRI axial T1 sequence after contrast administration and at the same temporal pole level as Fig. 44.1. The lesion evident in Fig. 44.1 is subtle and does not demonstrate contrast enhancement (arrow). No abnormal enhancement or other abnormality is present

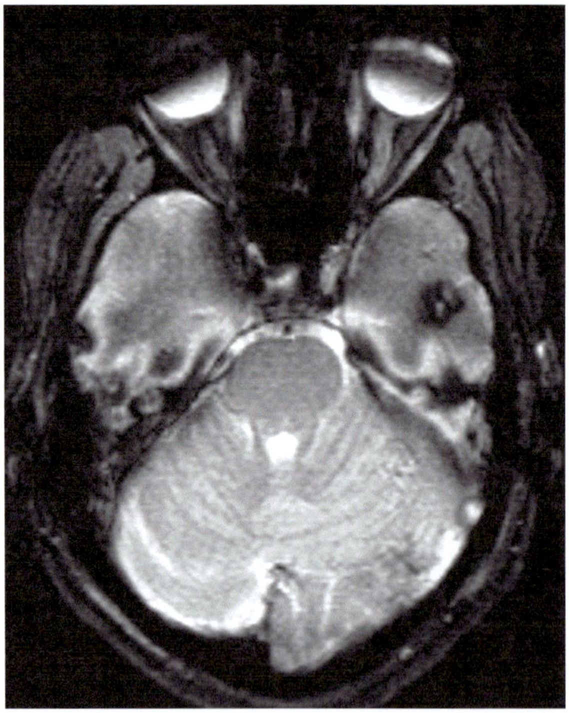

Fig. 44.3 MRI axial GRE sequence at the same temporal pole level as Figs. 44.1 and 44.2. The hypointensity surrounding the lesion extends beyond the borders of the cavernous malformation, as it is evident in Figs. 44.1 and 44.2. This extension into normal tissue is termed blooming artifact. Within the hypointensity, the regions of hyperintensity indicate resolving hemorrhage of indeterminate age

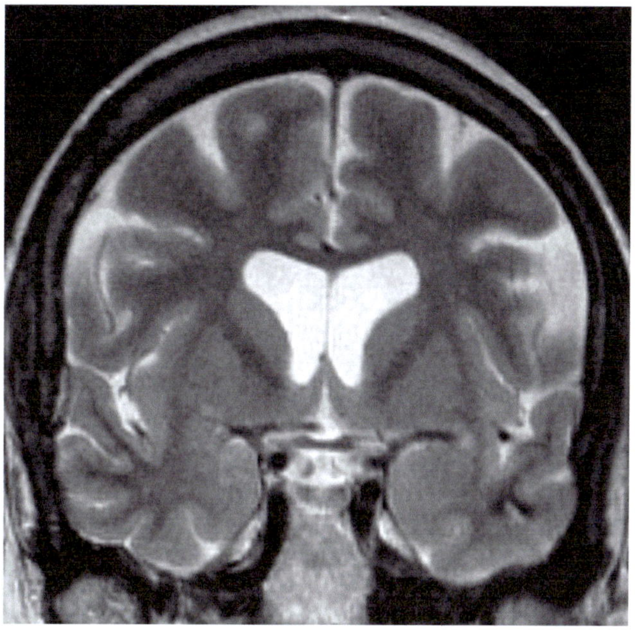

Fig. 44.4 MRI coronal T2 sequence at an amygdala level. The cavernous malformation is visible in the subcortical white matter of the left middle temporal gyrus as a linear hyperintensity with surrounding hypointensity. The overall appearance suggests resolving hemorrhage with minimal hyperintensity within the hemosiderin staining

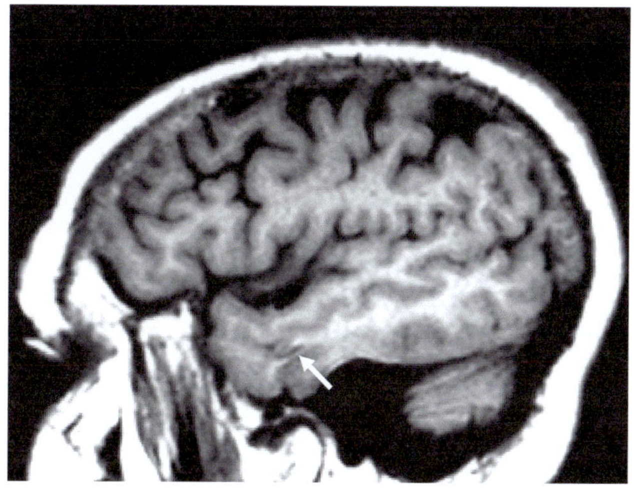

Fig. 44.6 MRI sagittal T1 sequence at a left Sylvian fissure level. A linear hypointensity (arrow) is subtle in the anterior, left middle temporal gyrus. The remaining brain is normal

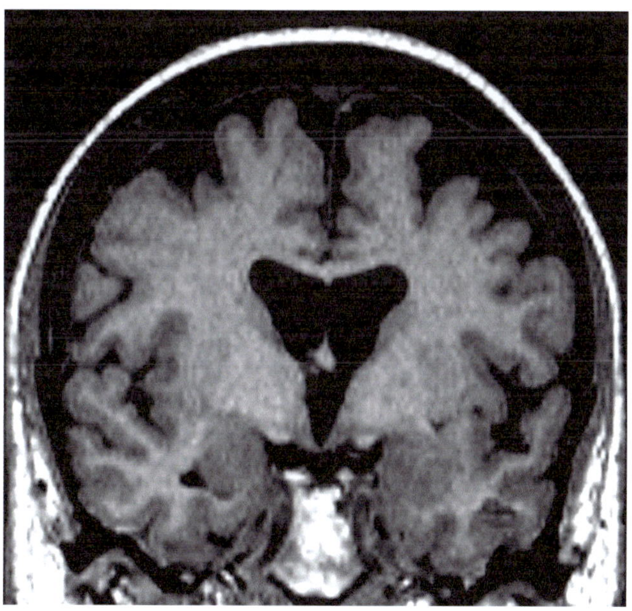

Fig. 44.5 MRI coronal T1 sequence at the same amygdala level as Fig. 44.4. A linear hypointensity is evident in the white matter of the left middle temporal gyrus. No abnormal hyperintensity is present. The remaining temporal lobe is normal and has well-preserved gray-white differentiation

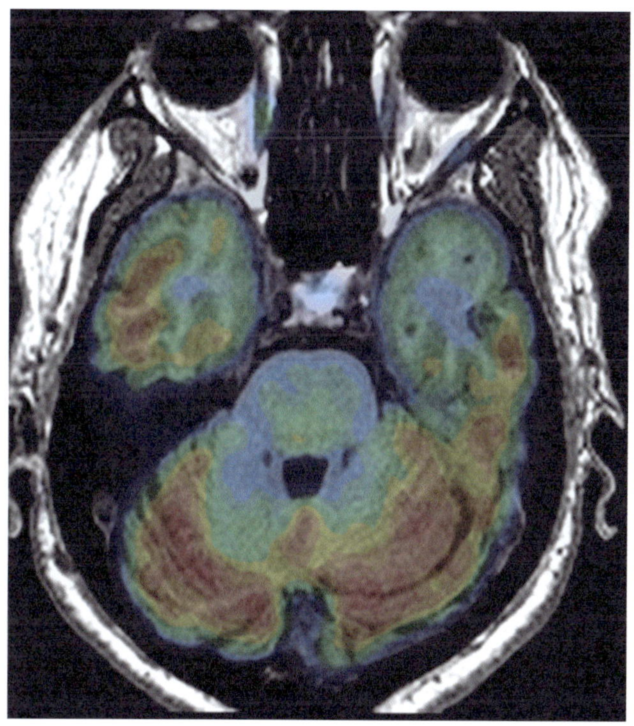

Fig. 44.7 PET-MRI co-registration with color-scale FDG tracer in an axial plane at the same temporal pole level as Fig. 44.1. Left temporal pole hypometabolism extends from the cavernous malformation to the surrounding region, including both mesial and lateral aspects of the anterior temporal lobe. The cavernous malformation is evident as a round, dark focus with a curvilinear hypointensity along the medial border because of the co-registered MRI. The right temporal lobe is normal

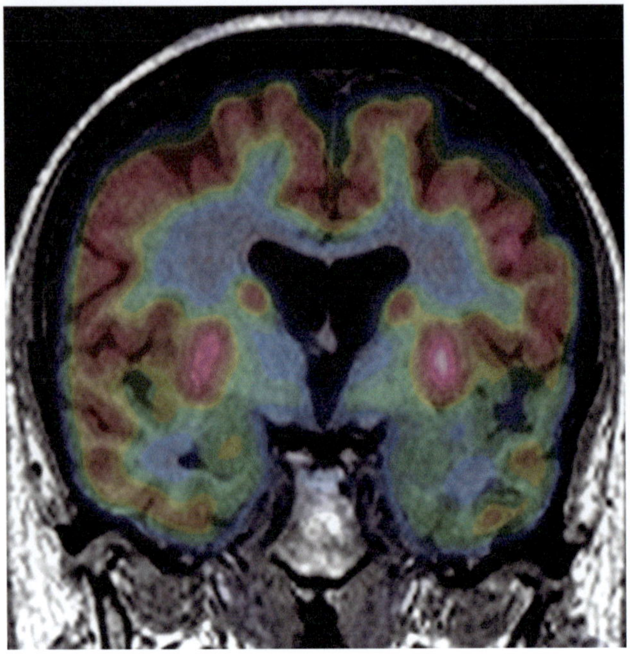

Fig. 44.8 PET-MRI co-registration with color-scale FDG tracer in a coronal plane at the same amygdala level as Fig. 44.4. The medial, inferior, and lateral left temporal lobe is hypometabolic. The cavernous malformation is evident in the left middle temporal gurus as an irregular, curvilinear region that is darker because of the co-registered MRI. The right temporal lobe is normal

Cavernous Malformation with Developmental Venous Anomaly

45

Clinical History

The first recognized seizure occurred at age 40 years as an experience of a full-body chill that was followed by generalized stiffening and loss of consciousness. In retrospect, the full-body chill experiences had occurred for about 1 year without recognition of their significance. About 3 months after the loss of consciousness, a chill episode occurred that progressed to dilated pupils, nonsensical speech, and manual automatisms with picking and wringing. The seizure lasted several minutes and was followed by 10 minutes of postictal confusion. An evaluation was not undertaken at that time.

The habitual seizures manifesteded as the aura of the full-body chill followed by impaired awareness with various purposeless behaviors. Treatment included multiple anti-seizure medications with a seizure frequency of about 12 monthly, including days that had more than one seizure. One additional seizure with generalized stiffening occurred, and the detailed description suggests that this was bilateral tonic-clonic.

An epilepsy risk factor was not present.

Neurological examination was normal. Medical history was not relevant to the epilepsy diagnosis.

Interictal EEG depicted occasional poorly formed epileptiform sharp waves over the right frontal-temporal region and rare poorly formed epileptiform sharp waves over the left temporal region. Video-EEG monitoring recorded focal seizures manifested as behavioral arrest with impaired awareness that progressed to fidgeting and then several minutes of postictal confusion. The ictal EEG's seizure onset was over the left temporal region when movement artifact was not obscuring.

MRI identified a 40-mm cavernous malformation within the body of the left hippocampus. PET identified hypometabolism of the left temporal pole. An intracarotid amobarbital test was performed and demonstrated candidacy for a left mesial temporal resection.

The history and evaluation indicate left mesial temporal lobe epilepsy. The presenting seizure as an aura in isolation manifested as a bilateral chill is not sufficiently specific for localization, but its regular occurrence in isolation suggests a limbic epileptogenic region. The subsequent development of focal seizures with impaired awareness that rarely progress to bilateral tonic-clonic convulsions is further evidence for a limbic epilepsy. Ultimately, the EEG and imaging provide evidence of left mesial temporal lobe epilepsy with hippocampal abnormality. The long-standing nature of the hippocampal structural abnormality is likely the basis for the right mesial temporal lobe's support for declarative memory, as identified during the intracarotid amobarbital test.

A left anterior-mesial temporal lobe resection was performed, and histopathological examination identified a cavernous malformation. No seizures occurred during the weeks following surgery, but long-term seizure control outcome is not known. Declarative memory performance was unchanged after the surgery.

J. M. Stern, N. Salamon, *Imaging of Epilepsy*, https://doi.org/10.1007/978-3-030-86672-3_45

Imaging

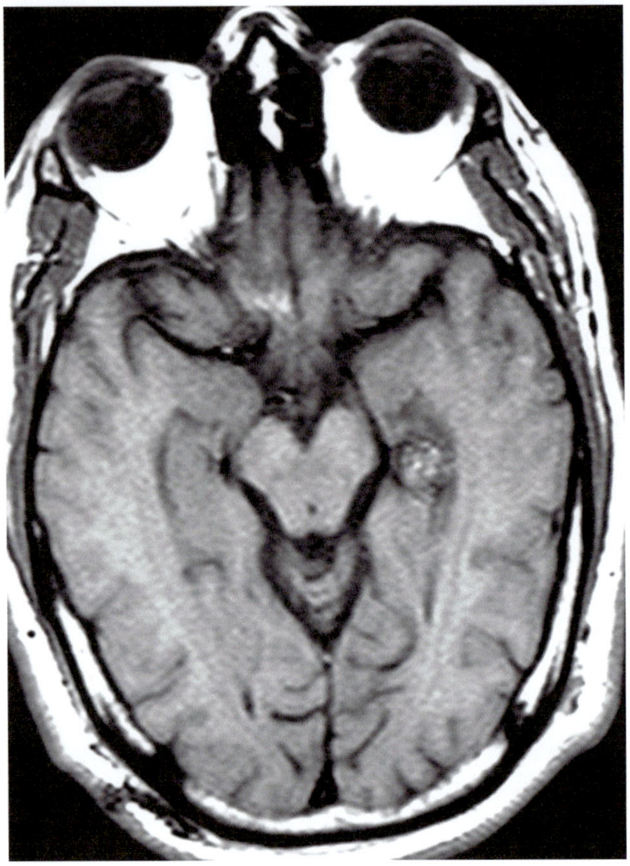

Fig. 45.1 MRI axial T1 sequence at a hippocampus body level. A round, mixed intensity lesion is evident in the body of the left hippocampus. No edema, mass effect, or ventricular enlargement is present. The heterogeneous signal intensity is due to minor hemorrhages of different ages, and the overall appearance suggests a cavernous malformation. The decreased signal immediately anterior to the lesion is normal and due to signal averaging with the temporal horn of the lateral ventricle

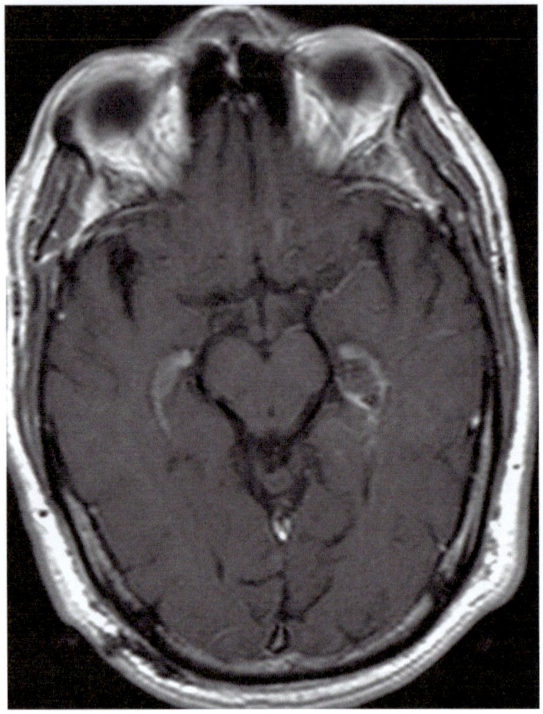

Fig. 45.2 MRI axial T1 sequence after contrast administration at the same hippocampus body level as Fig. 45.1. The linear contrast enhancement at the posterior margin of the cavernous malformation is produced by an associated developmental venous anomaly. No other abnormal contrast enhancement is present. The curved contrast enhancement anterior-lateral to the lesion is the choroid plexus of the lateral ventricle, and this enhancement is symmetric to a similarly enhancing region on the right

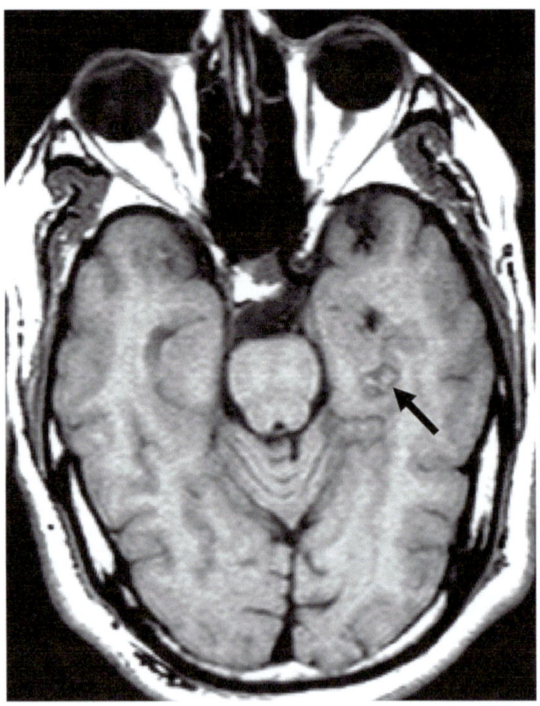

Fig. 45.3 MRI axial T1 sequence at a pons level and inferior to Figs. 45.1 and 45.2. The mixed signal lesion (arrow) is evident in the left temporal lobe, within the body of the left hippocampus and extending inferiorly to the parahippocampal gyrus. The hypointense oblong signal anterior to the lesion is normal and due to the temporal horn of the lateral ventricle

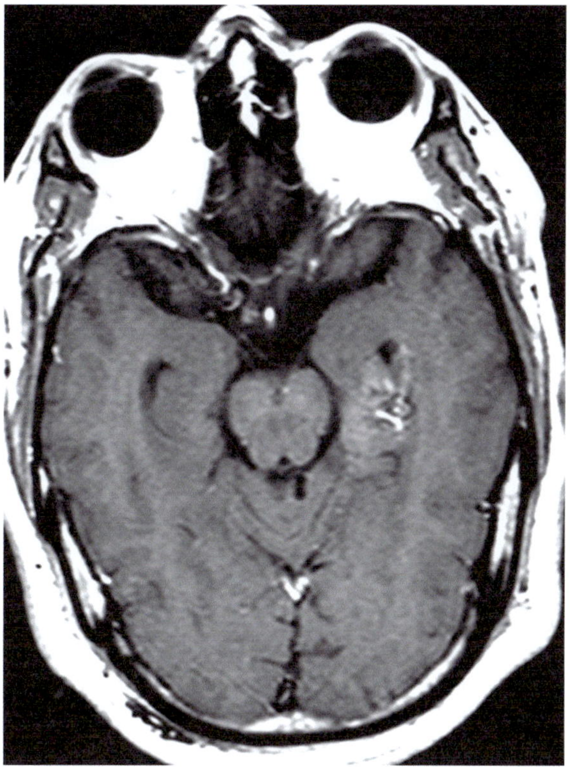

Fig. 45.4 MRI axial T1 sequence after contrast administration at the same pons level as Fig. 45.3. Linear contrast enhancement is evident along the posterior-medial aspect of the cavernous malformation and corresponds to a developmental venous anomaly. Heterogenous enhancement is present within the cavernous malformation. Hypointensity surrounds the lesion due to hemosiderin staining. Subtle enhancement is evident in the left mesial temporal lobe, medial and adjacent to the lesion. This is related to small vasculature leading to the developmental venous anomaly

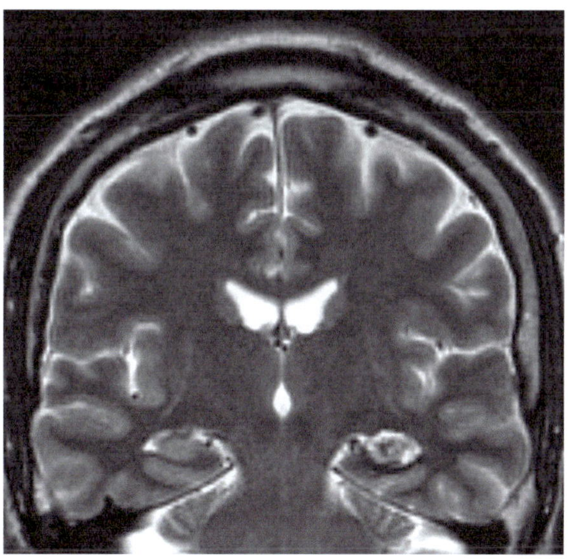

Fig. 45.5 MRI coronal T2 sequence at a hippocampal body level. Mixed intensity signal is evident within the region of the hippocampal body. Hypointensity is inferior to the hippocampal body and within the subiculum due to hemosiderin staining. No edema is present. The right hippocampus and temporal lobe and the remaining left temporal lobe are normal

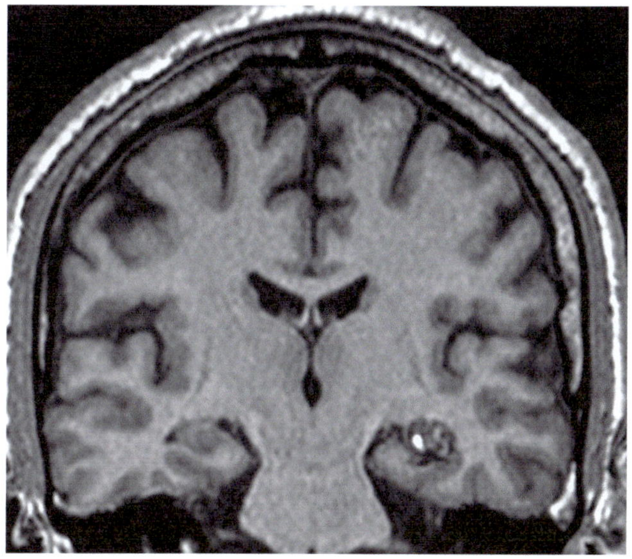

Fig. 45.6 MRI coronal T1 sequence at the same hippocampal body level as Fig. 45.5. A heterogenous intensity signal lesion is adjacent to the left hippocampal body. The medial aspect of the lesion has hyperintensity suggesting subacute hemorrhage. Inferior to the lesion, hypointensity corresponds to a chronic hemorrhage component of the lesion with hemosiderin staining

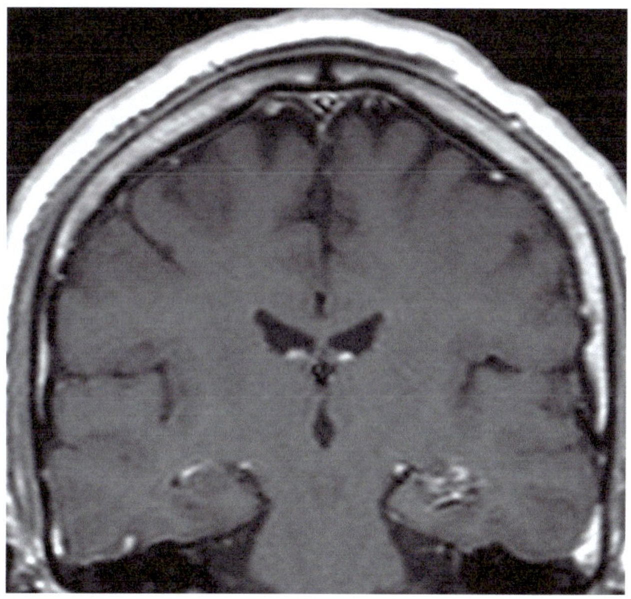

Fig. 45.7 MRI coronal T1 sequence after contrast administration at the same hippocampal body level as Figs. 45.5 and 45.6. The heterogenous signal intensity contrast enhancement of the left temporal lobe lesion is due to developmental venous anomaly that is along the lesion's superior aspect and also normal contrast enhancement within the choroid plexus along the lesion's superior-lateral aspect. Normal enhancement due to the choroid plexus is evident along the right hippocampus' superior-lateral aspect

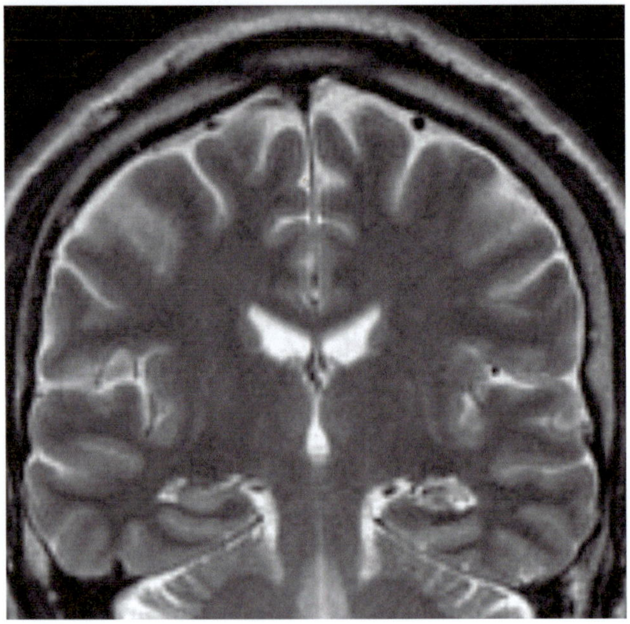

Fig. 45.8 MRI coronal T2 sequence at a thalamus level. The heterogenous signal lesion is within the region of the left hippocampus, and the left hippocampus is not evident. The left parahippocampal white matter is abnormally hypointense along the inferior border of the lesion, indicating hemosiderin. The right hippocampus is normal

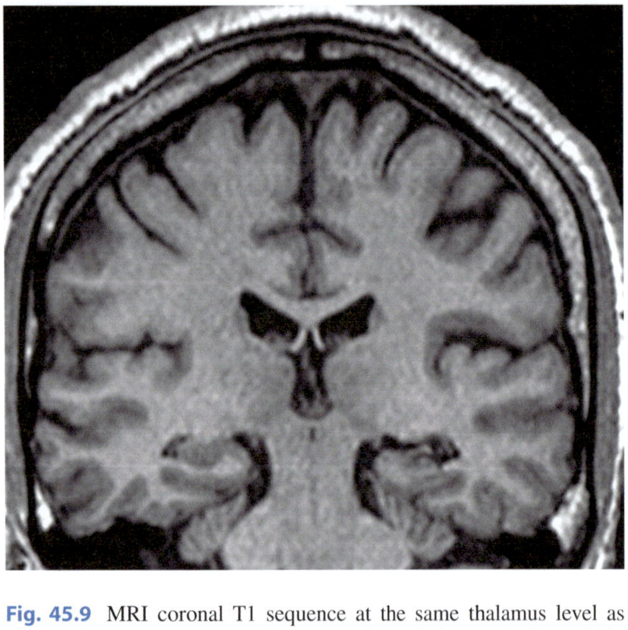

Fig. 45.9 MRI coronal T1 sequence at the same thalamus level as Fig. 45.8. The cavernous malformation is an isointense lesion within the region of the left hippocampus and choroid plexus that is evident because of its associated deformation of the left mesial temporal lobe. The right mesial temporal lobe and hippocampus are normal

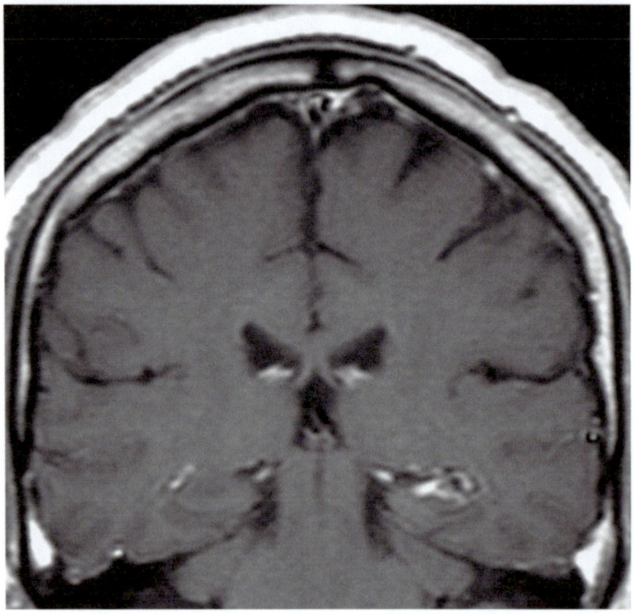

Fig. 45.10 MRI coronal T1 sequence after contrast administration at the same thalamus level as Fig. 45.9. The developmental venous anomaly is evident as an irregular, linear enhancement in the region of the left hippocampus and along the medial aspect of the lateral ventricle. The normal choroid plexus is evident laterally as a separate, linear enhancement that is similar to the left choroid plexus enhancement

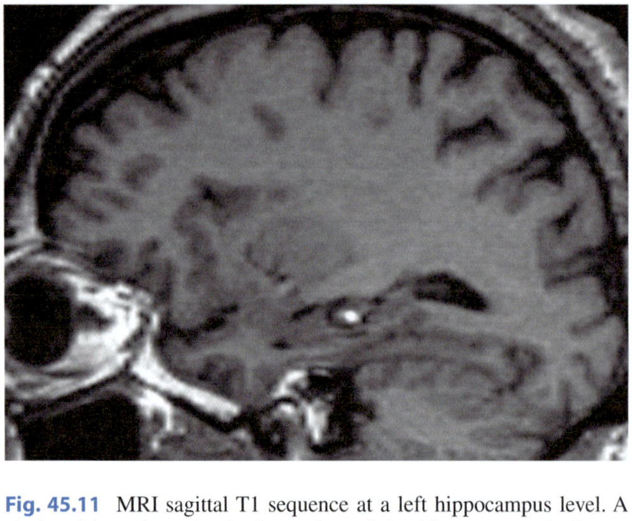

Fig. 45.11 MRI sagittal T1 sequence at a left hippocampus level. A circle of hyperintensity in the region of the hippocampus is due to remote hemorrhage within the cavernous malformation and is within surrounding hypointensity due to hemosiderin staining. The malformation is indenting the body of the hippocampus, causing a thinning of the hippocampus at the location of the indentation. The hippocampal head and visible tail are normal

46 Multiple Cavernous Malformations

Clinical History

The first recognized seizures occurred at age 45 years as episodes of being "spaced out." Each occurred without warning, lasted seconds, and then resolved with an immediate return to normal mentation. The episodes were initially identified by others, as the patient was not aware of their occurrences.

The habitual seizures were similar and noted to manifest as behavioral arrest with impaired awareness that lasted up to 30 seconds. None progressed to automatisms, posturing, or a tonic-clonic convulsion. Rarely, a "surreal" aura preceded a seizure and the same aura also occurred rarely without a subsequent, impairing seizure. Treatment included multiple anti-seizure medications with a seizure frequency of up to three seizures in a week and up to 3 weeks of seizure freedom.

An epilepsy risk factor was not present.

Neurological examination was normal. Neuropsychological testing identified difficulty with complex visual forms and nonverbal memory tasks. Medical history was otherwise normal.

Interictal EEG depicted occasional epileptiform spike discharges over the right anterior temporal and middle temporal regions. Video-EEG monitoring recorded focal seizures manifested as chewing and left or bilateral hand automatisms, a motionless or stiff right hand, and a right-hand postictal nose wipe. The ictal EEG's seizure onset was across the anterior right temporal lobe for five seizures and across the left anterior temporal lobe for one. The ictal behavior was the same for the two ictal EEG lateralizations.

MRI identified multiple cavernous malformations with a large malformation in the right inferior temporal lobe and others in the right middle temporal gyrus, right orbitofrontal lobe, and left temporal lobe white matter. PET identified bilateral anterior temporal hypometabolism. An intracarotid amobarbital test identified left-sided language dominance and dependence of the left side for declarative memory based on intact memory with a right-sided injection and amnesia with a left-sided injection.

The history and evaluation suggest right mesial temporal lobe epilepsy based on seizures with limbic behavioral features, anterior temporal ictal EEG onset, and a potentially epileptogenic lesion in the right temporal lobe. However, the evaluation is not straightforward as the history of rare and nonspecific auras, brief seizure durations, and immediate return to normal mentation can suggest a neocortical epilepsy. Moreover, the lateralization included evidence for left-sided epilepsy in the occurrence of right-hand posturing, one seizure with a left-sided ictal EEG onset, and PET evidence of bilateral anterior temporal hypometabolism. Nevertheless, the MRI, neuropsychological testing, and intracarotid amobarbital test indicate greater structural and functional abnormality within the right temporal lobe.

A resection of the right inferior temporal cavernous malformation with a partial hippocampectomy was performed, and histopathological examination identified a cavernous malformation with hemosiderin and calcification. The last follow-up visit was not sufficiently long since the surgery to determine the seizure-free outcome.

J. M. Stern, N. Salamon, *Imaging of Epilepsy*, https://doi.org/10.1007/978-3-030-86672-3_46

Imaging

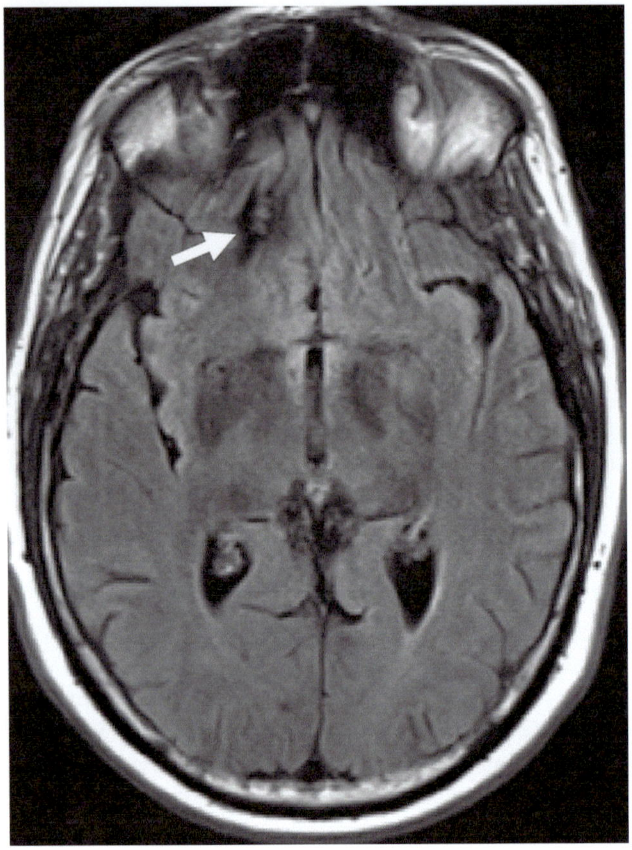

Fig. 46.1 MRI axial FLAIR sequence at a thalamus level. A cavernous malformation is evident as a multi-lobulated, isointense signal focus (arrow) in the right orbitofrontal lobe with surrounding hypointensity of hemosiderin staining. No edema or other abnormality is present

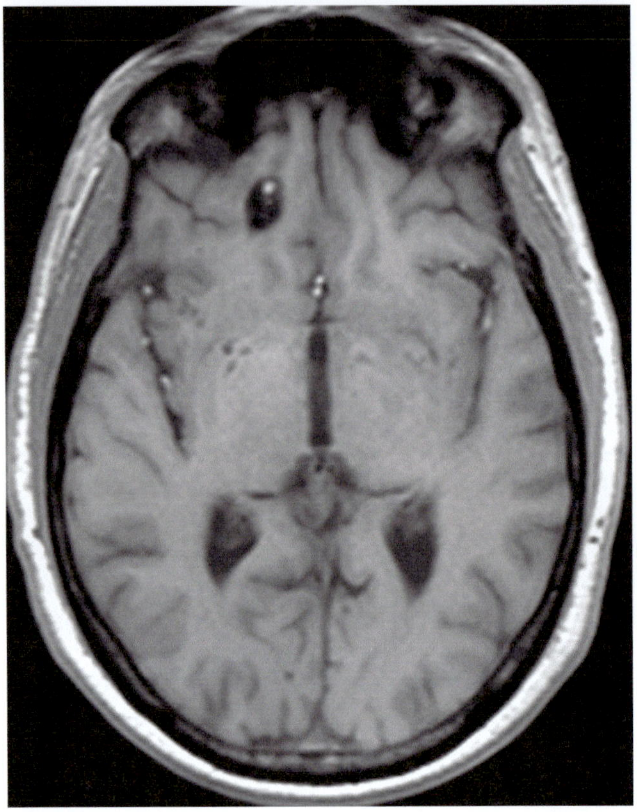

Fig. 46.2 MRI axial T1 sequence at the same thalamus level as Fig. 46.1. A cavernous malformation is evident as a round, hypointense focus in the right orbitofrontal lobe with an internal node of hyperintensity that indicates remote hemorrhage. The difference in shape compared to Fig. 46.1 is due to a slight difference in the angle of the level

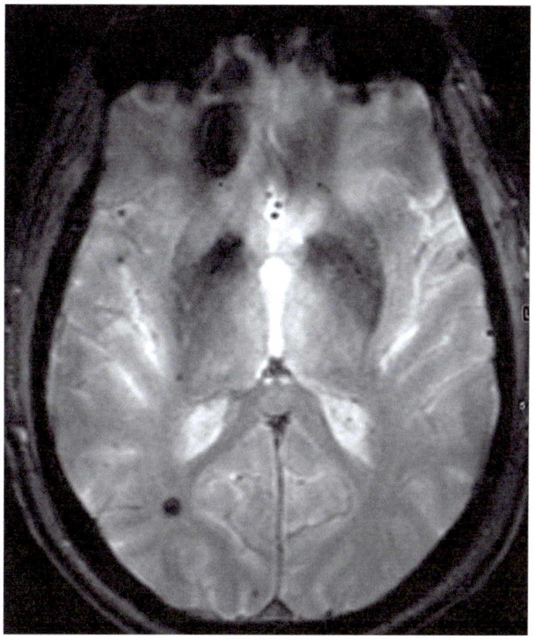

Fig. 46.3 MRI axial GRE sequence at a similar thalamus level as Figs. 46.1 and 46.2. The expansion of the hypointensity beyond the cavernous malformation's borders evident with T1 and FLAIR is due to blooming artifact. An additional hypointensity focus is evident in the right occipital lobe and is blooming artifact around a microhemorrhage from a cavernous malformation that is smaller and not visible on the T1 or FLAIR images. The small, punctate, bilateral hypointensities are normal blood vessels

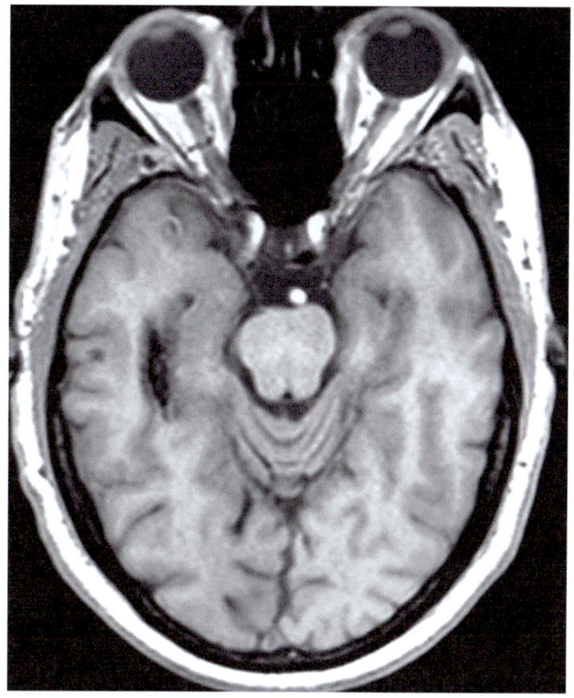

Fig. 46.5 MRI axial T1 sequence at the same hippocampal head level as Fig. 46.4. One cavernous malformation is an oblong, mixed signal intensity abnormality that is lateral to the right hippocampus. The abnormality's hypointensity is due to hemosiderin staining, and the faint hyperintensity is due to a subacute hemorrhage. A small hypointensity is lateral to the abnormality and is consistent to the second malformation in Fig. 46.4. No edema is present. Both hippocampi are normal

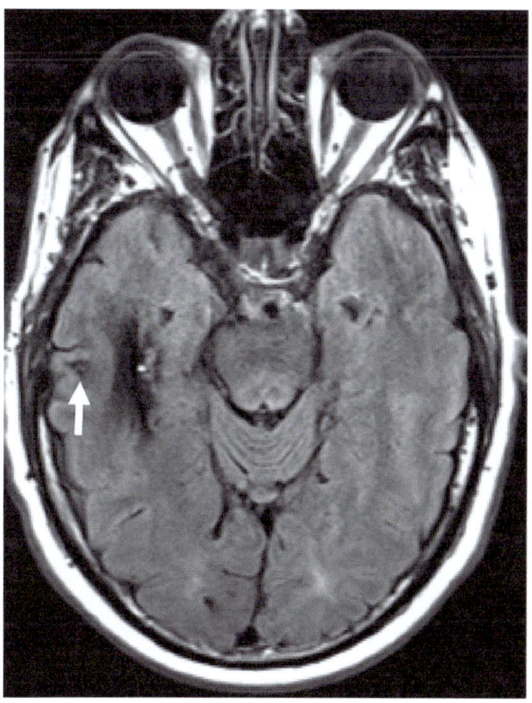

Fig. 46.4 MRI axial FLAIR sequence at a hippocampal head level. Two cavernous malformations are evident in this image. One is a linear, anterior to posterior hypointensity in the right temporal lobe's white matter, lateral to the hippocampal region. A small, round hyperintensity within the malformation's medial aspect is due to subacute hemorrhage. The other cavernous malformation is a triangular hypointensity (arrow) that is in the right middle temporal gyrus and lateral to the larger abnormality. Both hippocampi are normal

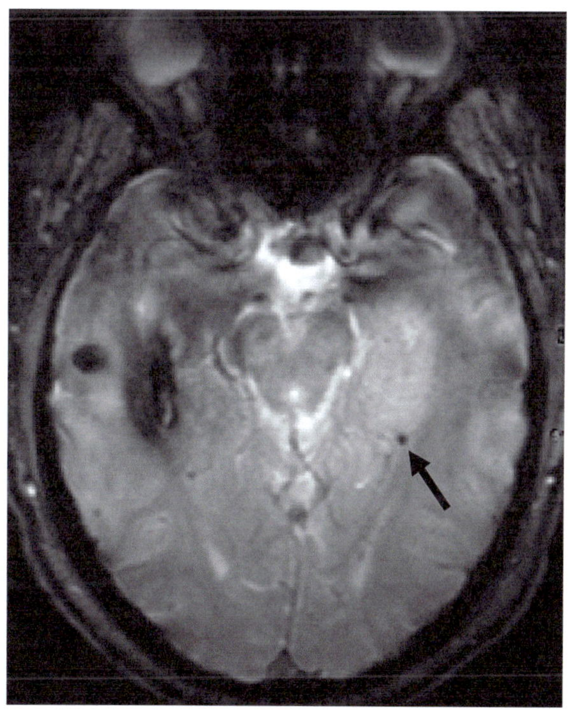

Fig. 46.6 MRI axial GRE sequence at the same hippocampal head level as Figs. 46.4 and 46.5. Large blooming artifact surrounds the left temporal white matter cavernous malformation, and a smaller blooming artifact surrounds the right middle temporal lesion. In addition, a small focus of hypointensity in the left temporal white matter (arrow) indicates another cavernous malformation. The faint, punctate hypointensities are normal blood vessels

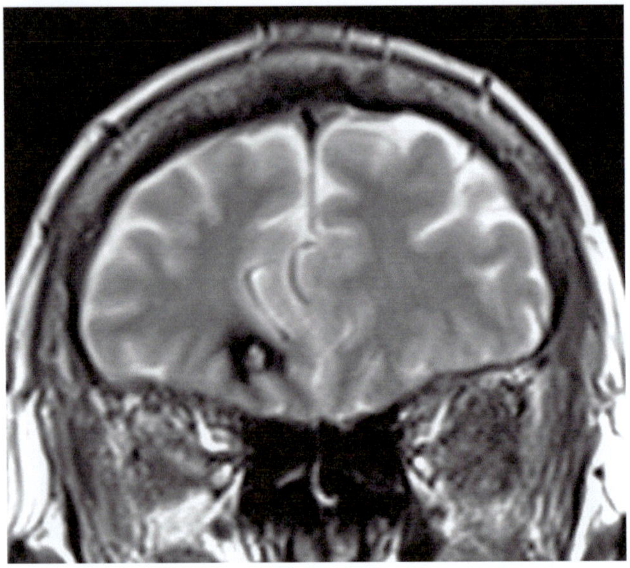

Fig. 46.7 MRI coronal T2 sequence at a frontal pole level. A right frontal lobe hyperintensity is surrounded by hypointensity with extension to the right gyrus rectus. The lesion demonstrates a combination of subacute and chronic hemorrhage and has no edema or mass effect. No other abnormality is present

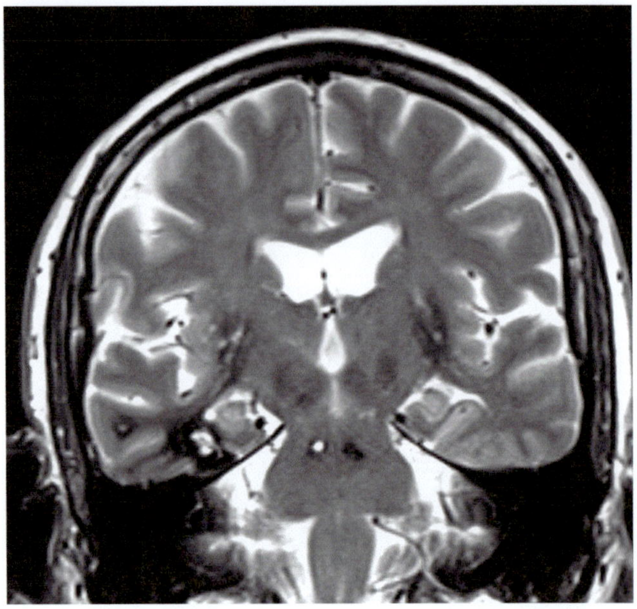

Fig. 46.9 MRI coronal T2 sequence at a hippocampal body level. A large hypointense abnormality with central hyperintensity is evident in the right fusiform gyrus and inferior temporal gyrus. The adjacent hippocampus is normal, as is the left hippocampus. The right middle temporal gyrus has an additional hypointensity with internal hyperintensity, which corresponds to the lateral cavernous malformation in the axial hippocampal head level images. Two foci of hypointense signal abnormality are in the central pons, indicating two more cavernous malformations. The right-sided pontine lesion has prominent central hyperintensity, indicating a subacute hemorrhage. The remaining punctate hypointensities are normal blood vessels

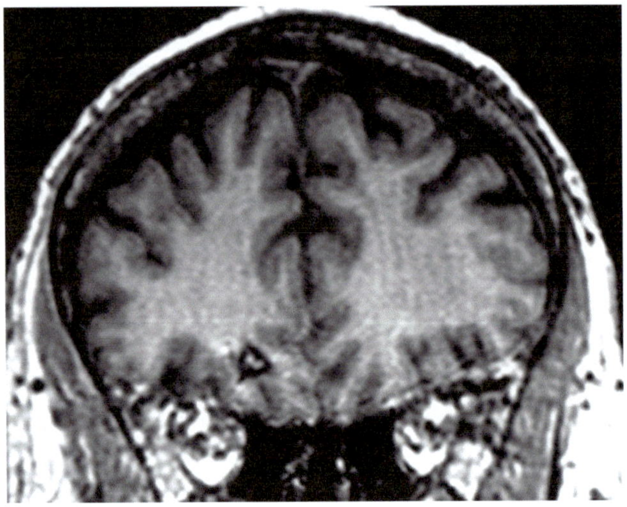

Fig. 46.8 MRI coronal T1 sequence at a frontal pole level similar to Fig. 46.7. The right frontal lobe has a triangular hypointense focus with a hyperintense signal within it. Compared to the GRE in Fig. 46.7, the surrounding hypointensity is less, and the internal hyperintensity is similar

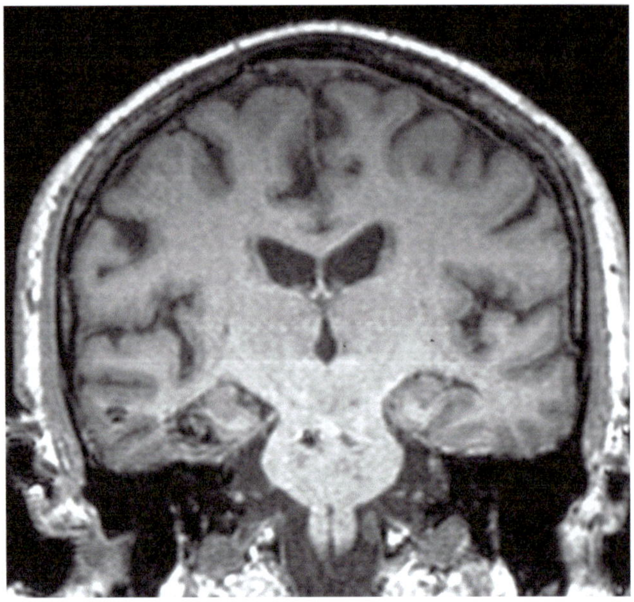

Fig. 46.10 MRI coronal T1 sequence at hippocampal body level similar to Fig. 46.9. The cavernous malformations are evident as mixed intensity foci in the right fusiform gyrus and the right middle temporal gyrus and two irregular foci of hypointensity in the central pons. The hemosiderin staining is much less prominent than with the T2 sequence. The hippocampi are normal

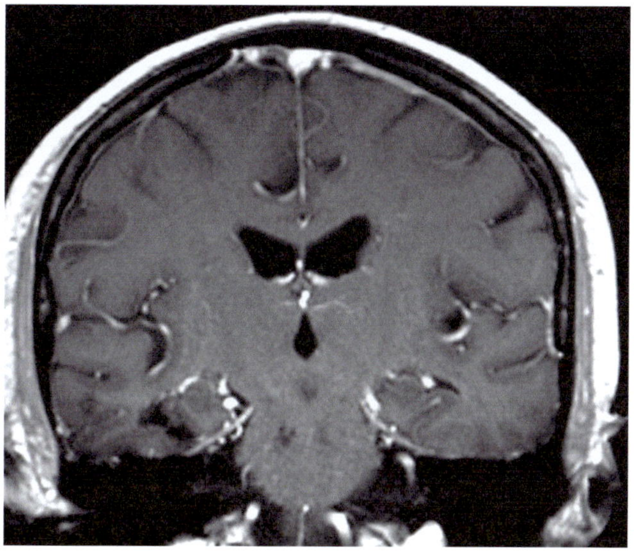

Fig. 46.11 MRI coronal T1 sequence after contrast administration and at the same hippocampal body level as Fig. 46.10. No developmental venous anomalies are evident. No abnormal enhancement is present. The two right temporal cavernous malformations are evident as hypointense foci

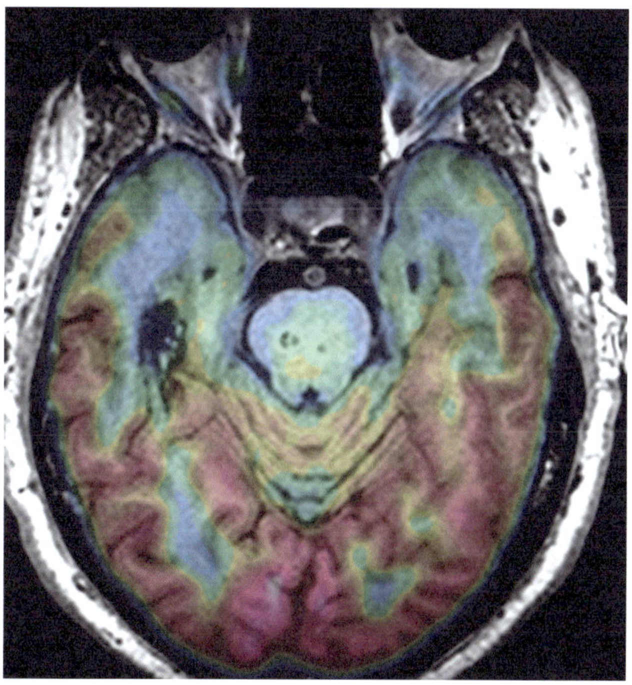

Fig. 46.12 PET-MRI co-registration with color-scale FDG tracer in an axial plane at a temporal pole level. Bilateral anterior temporal hypometabolism is evident. The right temporal white matter cavernous malformation is evident as MRI hypointensity. Because the level's angle differs from the MRI images in the preceding axial plane figures, the right middle temporal gyrus cavernous malformation is not included, but the two pontine cavernous malformations are visible

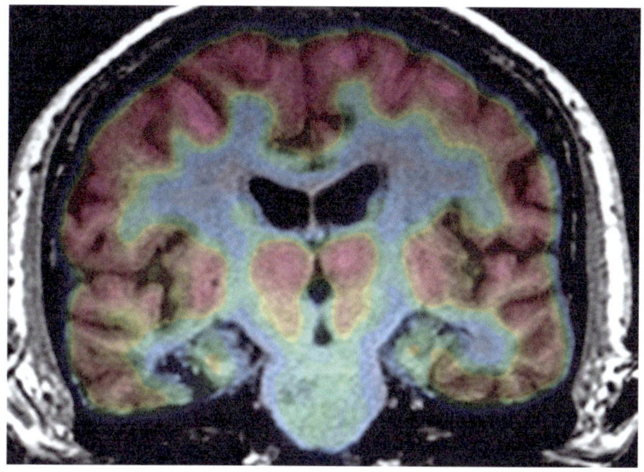

Fig. 46.13 PET-MRI co-registration with color-scale FDG tracer in a coronal plane at a hippocampal body level. Bilateral mesial temporal hypometabolism and right fusiform gyrus hypometabolism are evident. No other metabolism abnormality is present

Arteriovenous Malformation 47

Clinical History

The first recognized seizure occurred at age 22 years as a tonic-clonic convulsion. An evaluation at that time identified a left frontal lobe arteriovenous malformation (AVM).

The habitual seizures manifested as bilateral tonic-clonic convulsions that sometimes followed a stereotyped aura described as a heightened awareness of an imminent danger. The aura also occurred in isolation. Focal seizures with impaired awareness were rare and had a pattern of none occurring for years and several occurring within a day. When progressing to bilateral tonic-clonic movements, the seizures included asymmetric posturing of the arms, but witnesses' lateralization of the asymmetry was not known. Treatment included multiple anti-seizure medications with a seizure frequency of one tonic-clonic seizure every 1–3 months and no focal seizures with impaired awareness for several years.

The only epilepsy risk factor was the vascular malformation.

Neurological examination identified word finding and language fluency deficits. The deficit severity fluctuates and was most evident after a seizure. Neuropsychological testing identified borderline performance across multiple domains that suggested a decline from premorbid levels.

Interictal EEG depicted broad left-sided abnormal slowing that was maximal in the central-temporal region and epileptiform discharges over the left frontal and temporal regions. Video-EEG monitoring identified focal seizures manifested as left manual automatisms with clonic movements of the right arm and clonic turning of the head to the right. The ictal EEG's seizure onset was broadly across the left hemisphere with prominence in the left anterior frontal region before extending posteriorly.

MRI and CT identified a large, left frontal AVM with the superior frontal gyrus demonstrating the most prominent encephalomalacia. The temporal lobes were not affected. PET identified a large, left frontal, ametabolic region with a margin of hypometabolism.

The history and evaluation indicate focal seizures with ictal motor behavior that lateralizes the seizures to the left hemisphere, and the imaging identifies a large, left, superior frontal lesion. Propagation into the limbic system is a possible explanation for the aura and focal seizures with impairment that do not progress to tonic-clonic, but an aura of sensing imminent danger is not necessarily limbic. Furthermore, the observed quick progression to asymmetric clonic movements is more suggestive of a neocortical onset and is referrable to the AVM location. Because of the AVM's features, two or more discrete epileptogenic regions may be producing the differing seizure manifestations, and this further complicates the epileptogenic zone localization.

The size of the AVM precludes complete resection, and the evaluation did not produce a reliable localization of a resectable epileptogenic zone within it. After discussing this with the patient, palliative radiosurgery was chosen (see 82 in the Treatment Related Findings section)

J. M. Stern, N. Salamon, *Imaging of Epilepsy*, https://doi.org/10.1007/978-3-030-86672-3_47

Imaging

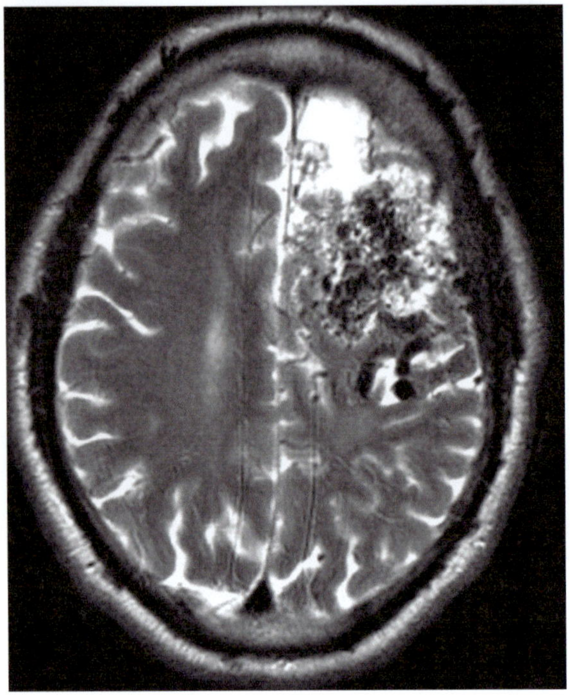

Fig. 47.1 MRI axial T2 sequence at a high lateral ventricle level. A large tangle of vessels is evident as flow voids in the left frontal lobe. Posterior to the nidus, a large vessel and draining veins are present. Anterior to the nidus, the left superior frontal gyrus includes encephalomalacia. The right hemisphere is normal

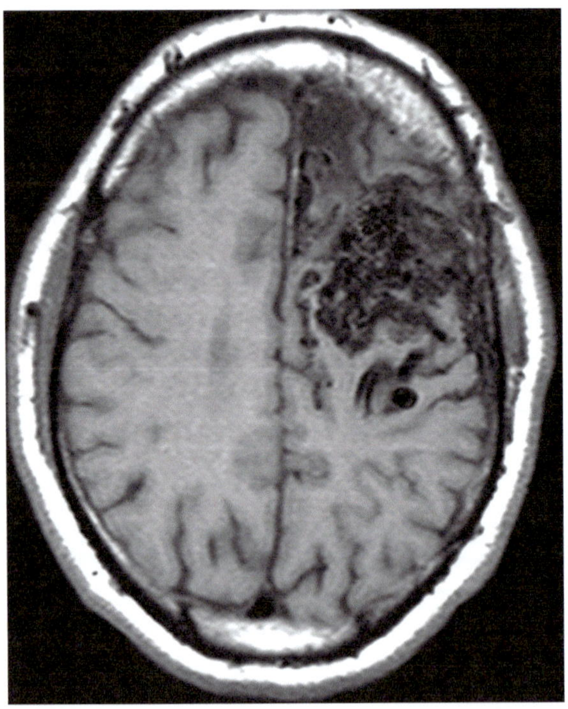

Fig. 47.2 MRI axial T1 sequence at the same high lateral ventricle level as Fig. 47.1. A large tangle of vessels is evident in the left frontal lobe adjacent to encephalomalacia of the superior frontal gyrus. The regions of hypointensity are the same as with the T2 sequence in Fig. 47.1, which indicates the high flow of an arteriovenous malformation

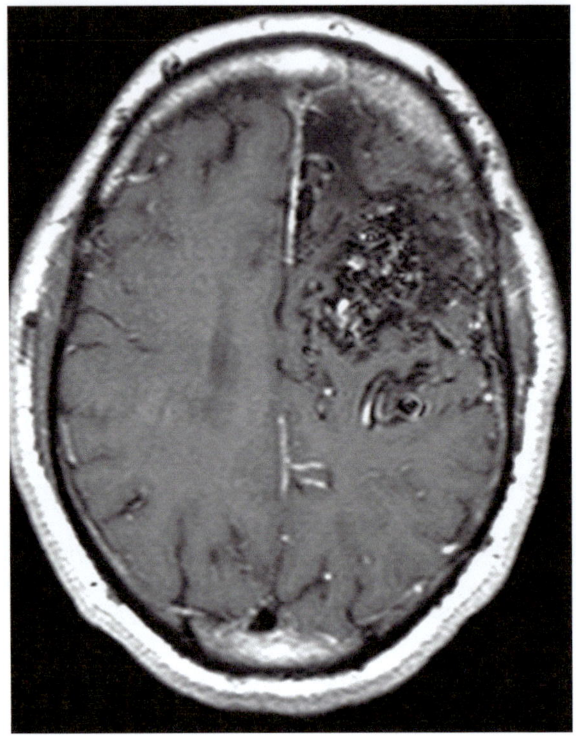

Fig. 47.3 MRI axial T1 sequence after contrast administration at the same high lateral ventricle level as Figs. 47.1 and 47.2. The majority of the vascular malformation does not demonstrate enhancement. Small areas of scattered enhancement are present internally and also in portions of the draining vein. The enhancement is likely due to flow turbulence because of its partial presence

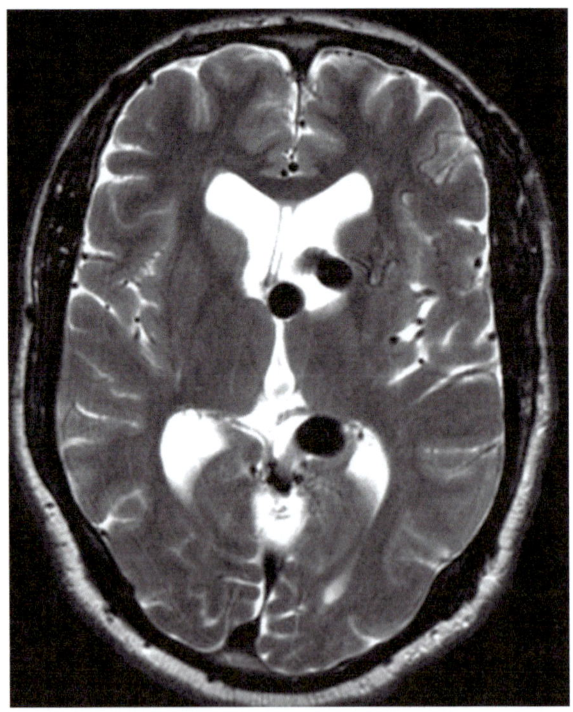

Fig. 47.4 MRI axial T2 sequence at a thalamus level. The enlarged vessels in the left lateral ventricle are components of the draining vein. The arterial branches visible in the left Sylvian fissure and the left anterior interhemispheric fissure are abnormally larger than their corresponding right-sided vessels

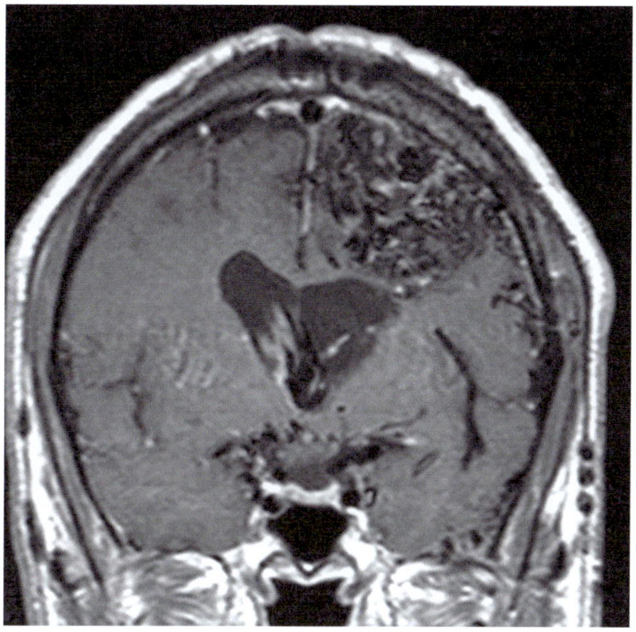

Fig. 47.5 MRI coronal T1 sequence after contrast administration at a temporal pole level. A large nidus is evident in the left frontal lobe with displacement of the horn of the left lateral ventricle. Scattered enhancement is evident within the nidus due to turbulent flow. The superior sagittal sinus is rounded, indicating increased flow

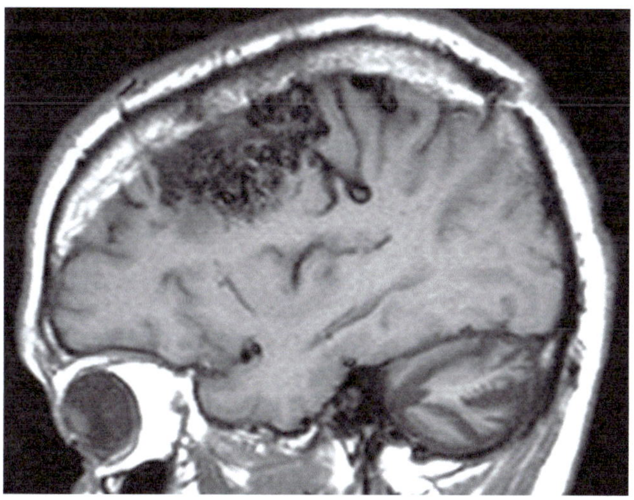

Fig. 47.6 MRI sagittal T1 sequence at a left insula level. The left frontal lobe nidus is evident anterior to the central sulcus. Inferior-posterior to the nidus, a dilated draining vein is evident as a circular hypointensity. Cerebellar atrophy also is present

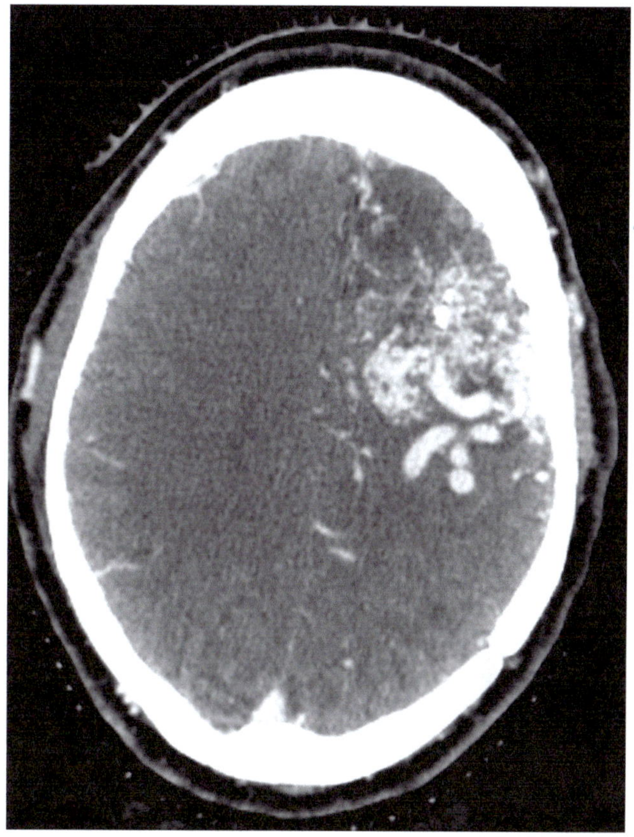

Fig. 47.7 CT in an axial plane after contrast administration at a centrum semi-ovale level similar to Fig. 47.1. A contrast-enhanced tangle of vessels is evident in the left frontal lobe with serpentine vessels corresponding to the draining vein. The low density anterior to the nidus is encephalomalacia of the superior frontal gyrus

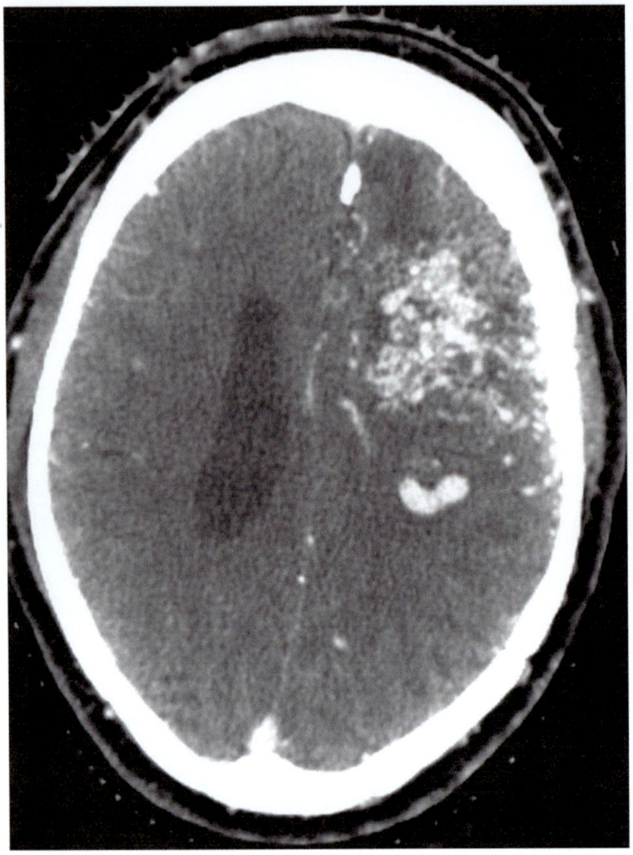

Fig. 47.8 CT in an axial plane after contrast administration at a lateral ventricle level. The left lateral ventricle is not visible because of its inferior displacement by the AVM. The AVM is visible as a scattered, enhancing, tangle of vessels in the left frontal lobe with a posterior draining vein

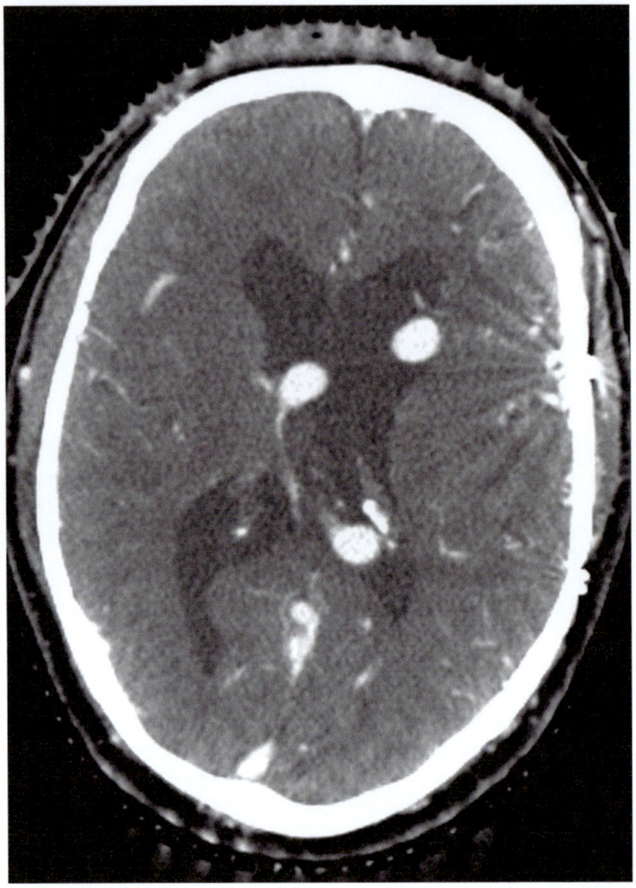

Fig. 47.9 CT in an axial plane after contrast administration at a lateral ventricle level slightly superior to Fig. 47.4. Dilated draining veins are evident in the lateral ventricles, and the lateral ventricles are abnormally enlarged. Streak artifact is present across the left frontal lobe due to the staples from a prior craniotomy

Ischemic Infarction

48

Clinical History

The first recognized seizure occurred at age 19 years as an episode of involuntary flexion of the right hip followed by flexion of the right arm and curling of the right foot's toes. An alteration in awareness or memory did not occur. An evaluation at that time included an extended EEG recording that identified left-sided interictal epileptiform abnormality.

The habitual seizures were similar at their onset to the first seizure with the same spreading motor abnormality, and the seizures caused a fall when they occurred while standing. However, the habitual seizures differed by quickly progressing to a sensory experience that did not have the marching progression of the motor abnormality. The sensory manifestation was a right hemibody sensory loss or paresthesia accompanied by an abnormal sensation in the throat that interfered with speech and sometimes produced choking. Understanding, awareness, and memory were never impaired during the seizures. The total seizure duration was less than 1 minute, and recovery was immediate and without fatigue, confusion, or focal deficits. Treatment included multiple anti-seizure medications with a seizure frequency of typically one or several seizures daily and a frequency range that spans up to 3 weeks of seizure freedom and up to 20 seizures in 1 day.

The epilepsy risk factor was a stroke. At age 16 years, problems with right-hand coordination and walking were evaluated with an MRI that identified a left caudate infarction. A cause for the stroke was not identified.

Neurological examination identified compensatory left-handedness because of stroke-related right-hand clumsiness. Right facial droop, right pronator drift, right-hand postural tremor, and right-sided hypertonia were present. Neuropsychological testing identified difficulties in verbal expression, impaired executive function, and reduced processing speed. Medical history was not relevant to epilepsy or cerebrovascular disease.

Interictal EEG depicted broadly distributed, left-sided epileptiform discharges that often occurred in runs. Video-EEG monitoring recorded focal seizures without impaired awareness manifested as eye fluttering with right arm clonus. The ictal EEG's seizure onset was broad, rhythmic slowing that was best formed over the left hemisphere and maximal over the left frontal-central region.

MRI identified a chronic infarction of the left basal ganglia with gliosis in the adjacent insula. PET identified hypometabolism of the left caudate head and adjacent regions. MEG identified dipoles in the left insula, left fusiform gyrus, and broadly across the left frontal lobe. Language functional MRI identified bilateral activation of Broca's and Wernicke's areas.

The history and evaluation indicate focal seizures with possibly frontal and insular features. The early, spreading motor features may be left frontal, and the subsequent hemibody and throat sensory features suggest the left insula. The imaging and scalp EEG findings provide a regional localization in the left anterior quadrant. This does not differentiate between the frontal neocortex and the insula, so localization was not sufficient to offer a resection. To further the localization, intracranial EEG was obtained using 12 depth electrodes with bilateral coverage of the entorhinal and orbitofrontal cortices and left-sided coverage of the amygdala, hippocampus, cingulate cortex, and insula. Interictal depth EEG recordings identified frequent epileptiform discharges across the left-sided electrodes, including both medial and lateral contacts. The ictal depth EEG seizure onset included the left inferior frontal and anterior insula regions.

The depth EEG recordings narrowed the localization but did not provide adequate evidence for a resectable epileptogenic region, so treatment with a responsive neurostimulator was offered. The neurostimulator's recording electrodes were placed according to intraoperative electrocorticography's identification of the greatest interictal epileptiform abnormality, which was in the left inferior frontal lobe and left anterior insula and also the locations of the depth EEG ictal onsets.

J. M. Stern, N. Salamon, *Imaging of Epilepsy*, https://doi.org/10.1007/978-3-030-86672-3_48

Seizures have continued for the year since the responsive neurostimulator placement. During this time, the seizure detector and stimulation settings have been adjusted to optimize the detection and seizure termination. Because of an insufficient response with stimulation at the two electrodes, the stimulation pathway is now between the two electrodes, which provides stimulation to a larger region.

Imaging

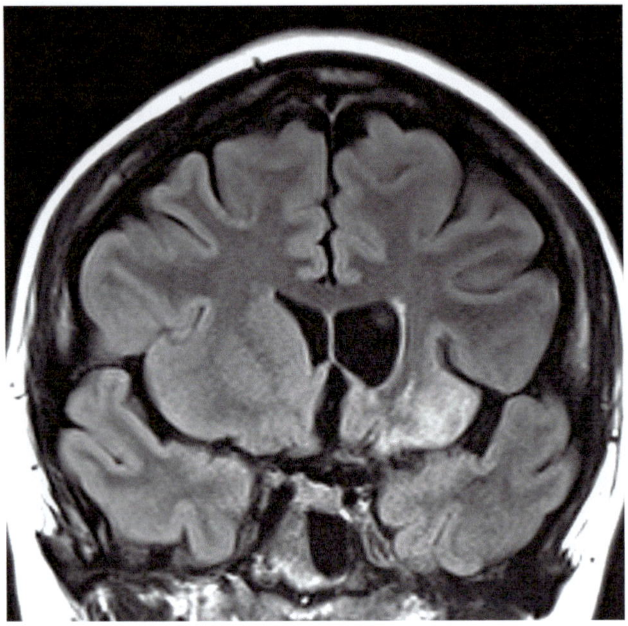

Fig. 48.1 MRI coronal FLAIR sequence at a temporal pole level. Hyperintensity extends from the left anterior insula to the basal forebrain, and a linear hyperintensity is present in the region of the left putamen. The left frontal horn of the lateral ventricle is enlarged with a high intensity lining that corresponds to an atrophic caudate nucleus. The temporal lobes and frontal lobes are normal

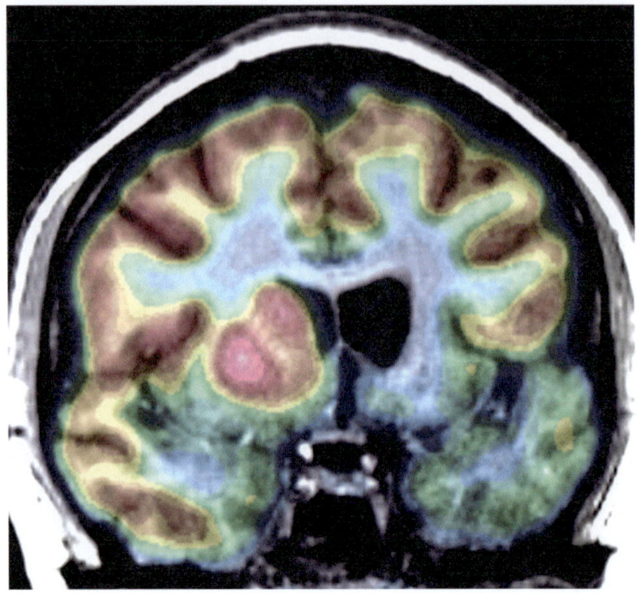

Fig. 48.2 PET-MRI co-registration with color-scale FDG tracer in a coronal plane at the same temporal pole level as Fig. 48.1. Hypometabolism is evident within the left anterior insula, left residual caudate and putamen, and also the left temporal pole. The right temporal lobe and bilateral frontal lobes are normal, but the left frontal lobe is subtly, asymmetrically decreased in metabolism, which may be due to the left basal ganglia abnormality and deafferentation

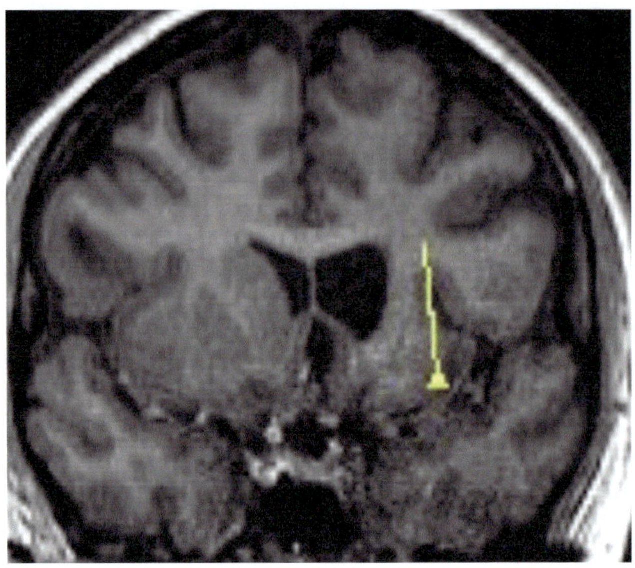

Fig. 48.3 MEG co-registered to MRI coronal T1 sequence at the same level temporal pole level as Figs. 48.1 and 48.2. A single epileptiform dipole has been localized to the left anterior insula

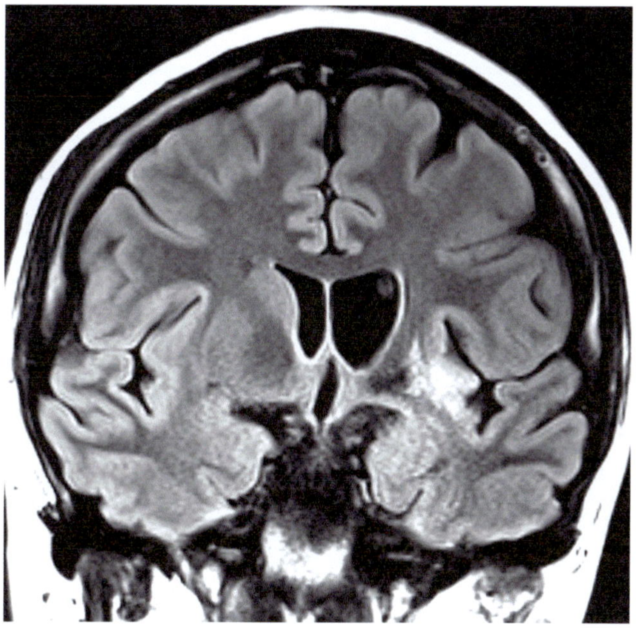

Fig. 48.4 MRI coronal FLAIR sequence at an amygdala level. Hyperintensity is evident in the left insula and left putamen, and hypointensity is evident in the left globus pallidus. With the ischemic injury to these structures, the left lateral ventricle has ex-vacuo enlargement. The amygdalae along with the remaining temporal lobes and also frontal lobes are symmetric and normal

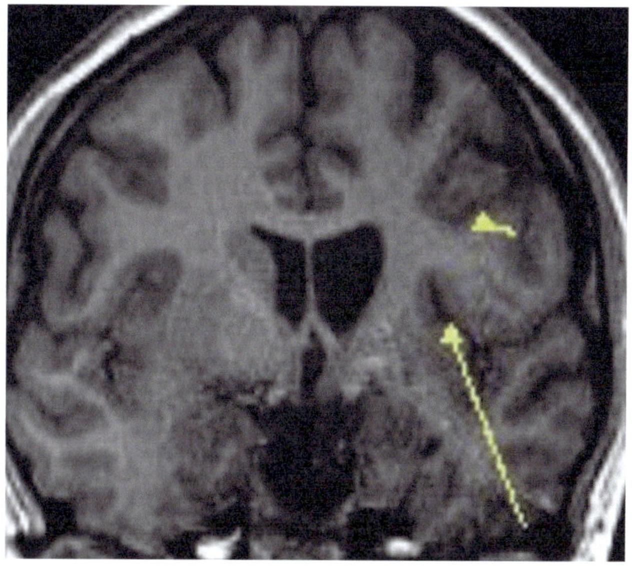

Fig. 48.6 MEG co-registered to MRI coronal T1 sequence at the same amygdala level as Figs. 48.4 and 48.5. Two epileptiform dipoles were localized with one in the left insula and the other in the left middle frontal gyrus

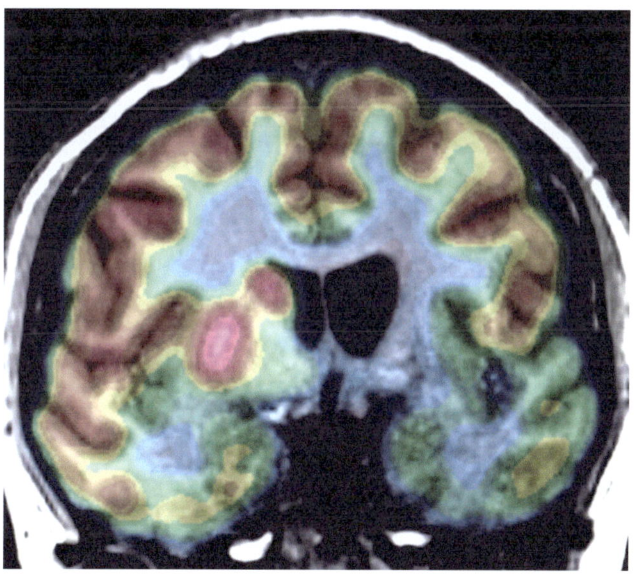

Fig. 48.5 PET-MRI co-registration with color-scale FDG tracer in a coronal plane at the same amygdala level as Fig. 48.4. The left insula, left basal ganglia, and most prominently left inferior lobe are hypometabolic. The remaining left temporal is hypometabolic but not as prominently as the inferior aspect. To a lesser extent, the entire left frontal lobe also is hypometabolic

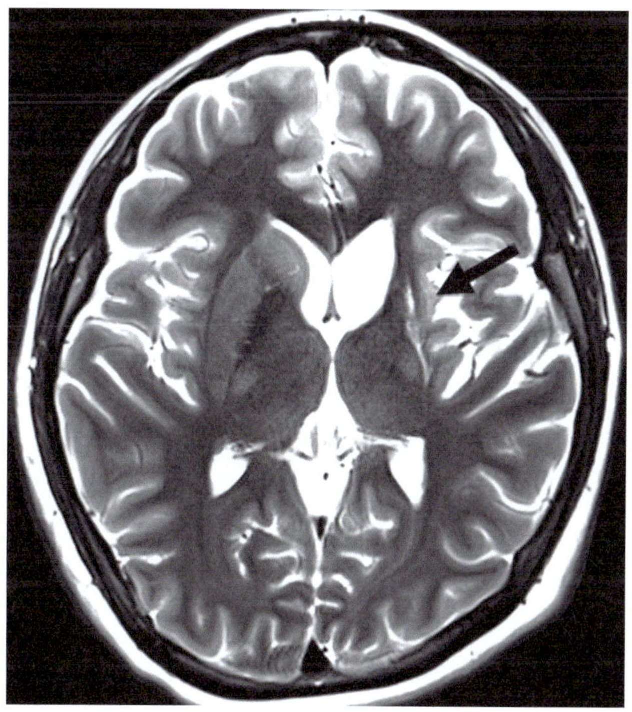

Fig. 48.7 MRI axial T2 sequence at a thalamus level. The left insular cortex is atrophic (arrow). The linear hyperintensity medial to the left insula is the encephalomalacia of the left putamen. The left caudate nucleus is not visible, which corresponds to the enlargement of the left lateral ventricle's frontal horn and the atrium. The infarction territory is constant with a deep middle cerebral artery perforator. Overall, the left hemisphere is subtly atrophic

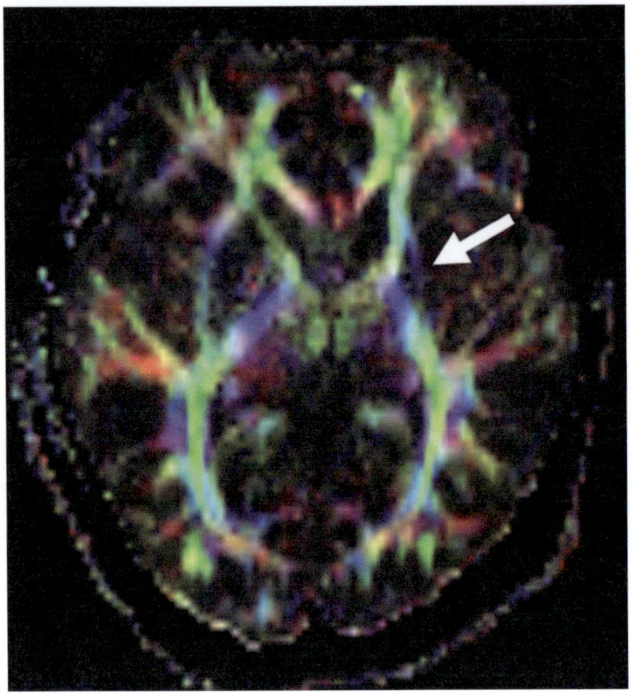

Fig. 48.8 MRI with axial diffusion tensor imaging at the same thalamus level as Fig. 48.7. The left external capsule is faintly visible (arrow) while clearly evident on the right. The optic radiations are also asymmetric with light green compared to the blue green, indicating loss of anisotropy. The atrophic left putamen is depicted by the asymmetry of the internal capsule

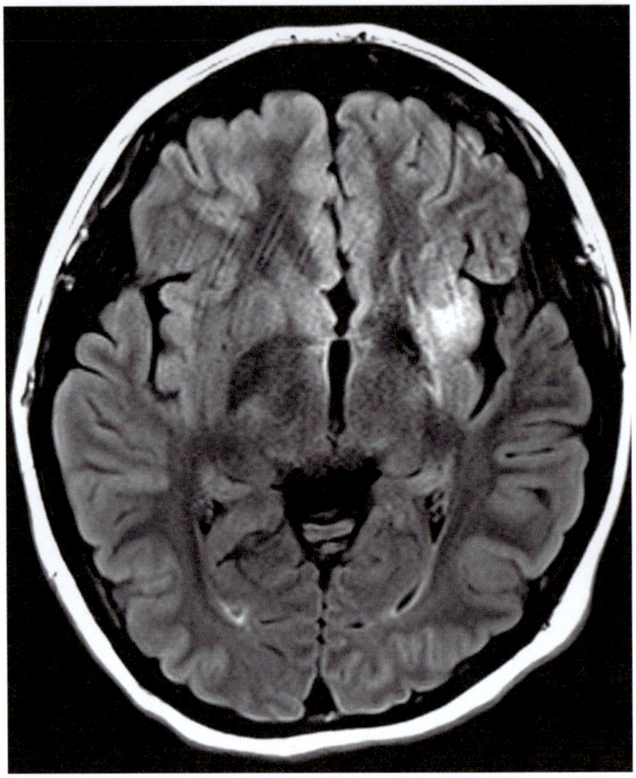

Fig. 48.10 MRI axial FLAIR sequence at the same posterior commissure level as Fig. 48.9. Hyperintensity is evident in the left insula and left putamen, but the atrophy of these structures is not as apparent as with the T2 sequence in Figs. 48.7 and 48.9. The right hemisphere is normal

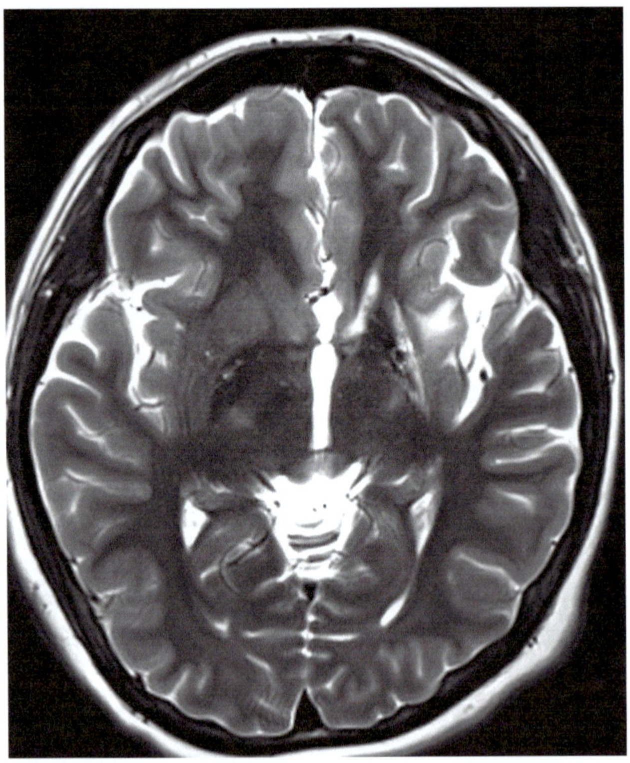

Fig. 48.9 MRI axial T2 sequence at a posterior commissure level, slightly inferior to the thalamus. Hyperintensity is evident in the left insula and left putamen, and the left putamen along with the remainder of the left basal ganglia are atrophic. The left hemisphere has a subtle, overall atrophy. The right hemisphere is normal

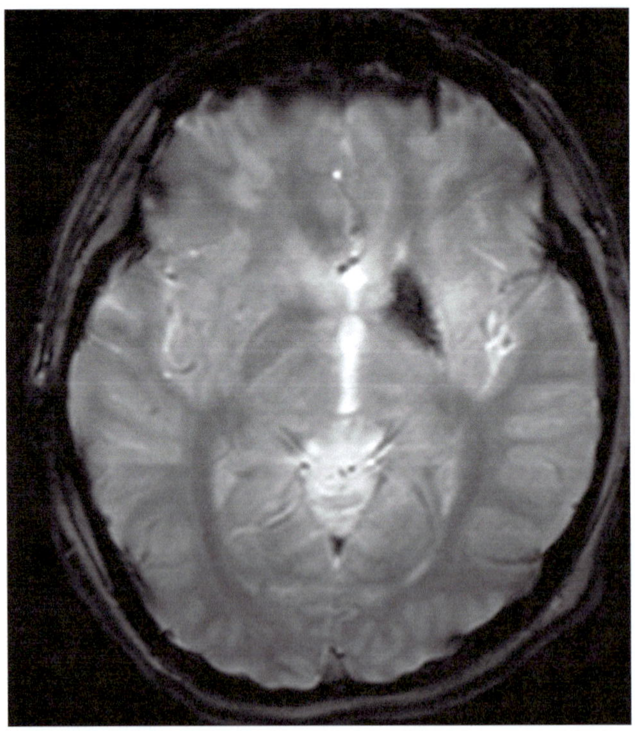

Fig. 48.11 MRI axial GRE sequence at the same posterior commissure level as Figs. 48.9 and 48.10. Abnormal hypointense signal, which is a sequelae (plural) of hemorrhagic infarction, extends across the left putamen and includes a portion of the left caudate nucleus. No other abnormal is present

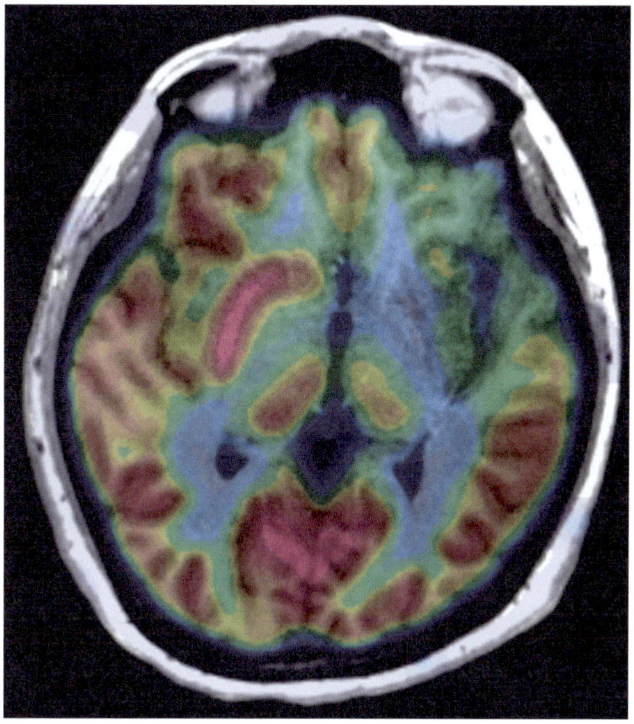

Fig. 48.12 PET-MRI co-registration with color-scale FDG tracer at a thalamus level. Hypometabolism is evident in the left orbitofrontal cortex, left insula, left basal ganglia, left temporal pole, and anterior portion of the left superior temporal gyrus. The left thalamus is slightly hypometabolic. Metabolism is normal in the medial frontal lobes, posterior temporal lobes, and occipital lobes

49 Porencephaly

Clinical History

The first recognized seizure occurred as an infant and in the context of bacterial meningitis. The features of these seizures were no longer known, but seizures during childhood were recalled, and these manifesteded as oral automatisms with left arm stiffening and leftward head turning.

The habitual seizures typically manifesteded as behavioral arrest, salivation, and staring with a glazed facial expression for a duration of typically 30–60 seconds. Infrequently, the seizures progressed to loss of postural tone or falling, and the drop seizures occurred with and without tonic-clonic movements. Treatment included multiple anti-seizure medications, and a three-medication combination has provided seizure freedom for the past year. Prior to this, the staring seizures occurred two to three times daily, and the drop seizures were infrequent with seizure-free periods for as long as several years.

The epilepsy risk factor was early childhood meningitis.

Neurological examination identified intellectual disability and left hemiparesis. Communication was achieved through pointing, and verbal interactions were limited to single words and occasional several word sentences. Overall, the communication was sufficient for expressing essential needs. Independence for activities of daily living was not present, and a wheelchair was used for safety and increased mobility.

Interictal EEG in adulthood depicted mild intermittent right temporal slowing and frequent epileptiform discharges across the right mid-temporal and posterior temporal regions. The epileptiform discharges occurred in isolation and in runs lasting up to 8 seconds. During childhood, video-EEG monitoring recorded focal seizures manifested as lip smacking, left arm stiffening, and head turning to the left. The ictal EEG's seizure onset depicted artifact from muscle and movement without an epileptiform abnormality.

MRI identified left peri-insular gliosis and a right porencephalic cyst within a large portion of the right cerebral hemisphere. PET identified right frontal and parietal photopenia that corresponded to the right hemispheric encephalomalacia.

The history and evaluation indicate medication-resistant epilepsy in the context of intellectual disability and bilateral cerebral injury. Although the imaging and interictal EEG identified a region of abnormality that may produce focal seizures, the diffuse cerebral dysfunction and non localizing ictal EEG was interpreted as indicating an inadequate likelihood of success from epilepsy surgery. Fortunately, pharmacotherapy later provided seizure freedom.

J. M. Stern, N. Salamon, *Imaging of Epilepsy*, https://doi.org/10.1007/978-3-030-86672-3_49

Imaging

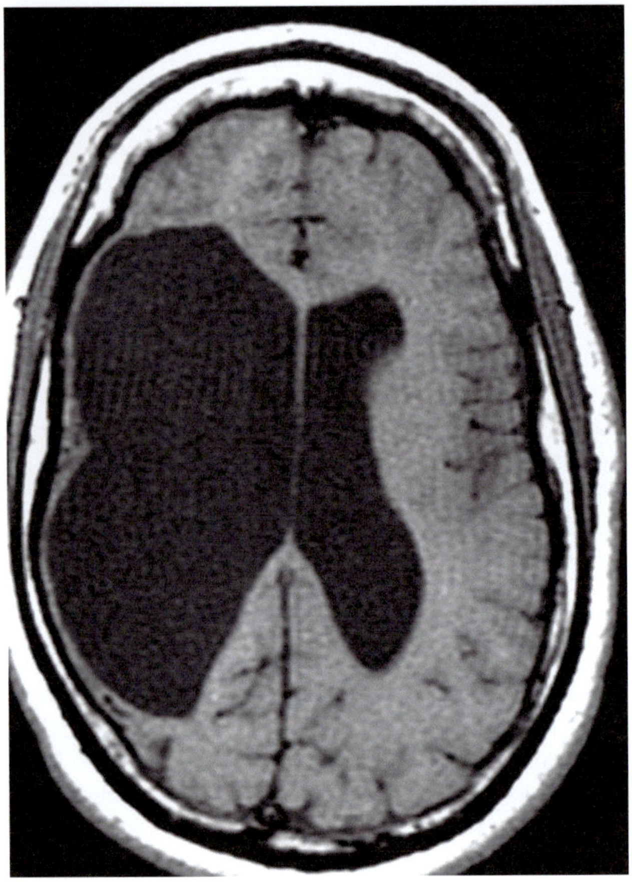

Fig. 49.1 MRI axial T1 sequence at a lateral ventricle level. The right lateral ventricle is markedly dilated with thinning of the lateral cortical surface. Unlike ex-vacuo enlargement of a lateral ventricle into space produced by parenchymal infarction, a porencephalic cyst does not have an ependymal margin, so the cyst comprises both the ventricle and infarction-producing cerebrospinal fluid (CSF) space. No midline shift is present

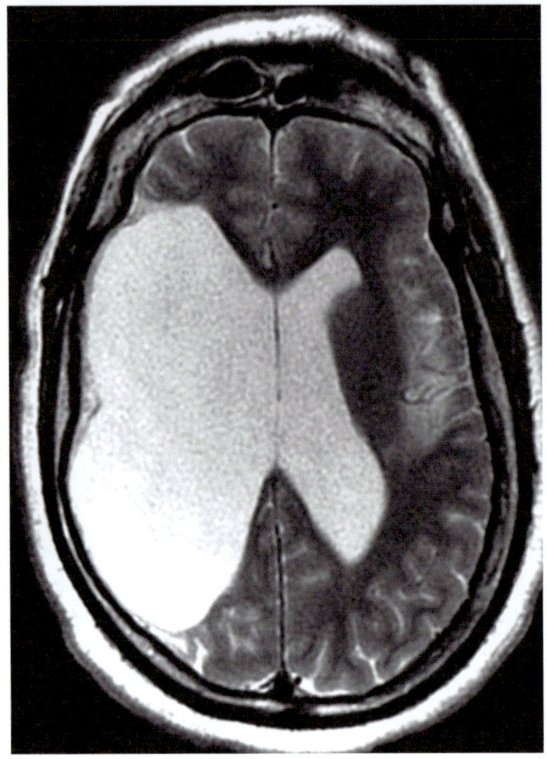

Fig. 49.2 MRI axial T2 sequence at the same level lateral ventricle level as Fig. 49.1. A right porencephalic cyst is evident with subtle hyperintensity at the anterior margin, along the frontal cortex, and at the posterior margin, along the parietal lobe. Similar hyperintensity is present in the left insula. The hyperintense regions are gliosis and probably related to the intrauterine vascular occlusion that produced the porencephalic cyst

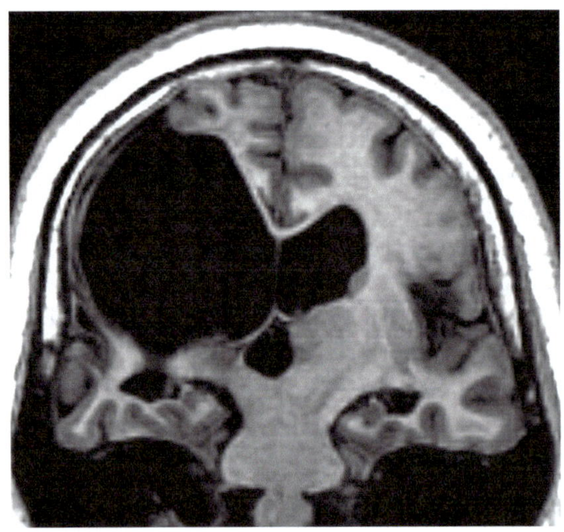

Fig. 49.3 MRI coronal T1 sequence at a hippocampal body level. The right lateral ventricle is markedly dilated and communicates with the territory of a right middle cerebral artery infarction. The third ventricle is asymmetrically dilated with deviation toward the right. The right superior frontal gyrus, right cerebral peduncle, and right temporal lobe are asymmetrically smaller than the left. The temporal lobe abnormality includes encephalomalacia in the right superior temporal gyrus, enlargement of the temporal horn of the right lateral ventricle, and atrophy of the right hippocampal body. The left insula and neighboring perisylvian region have subtle hypointensity indicating gliosis. The left temporal lobe is normal

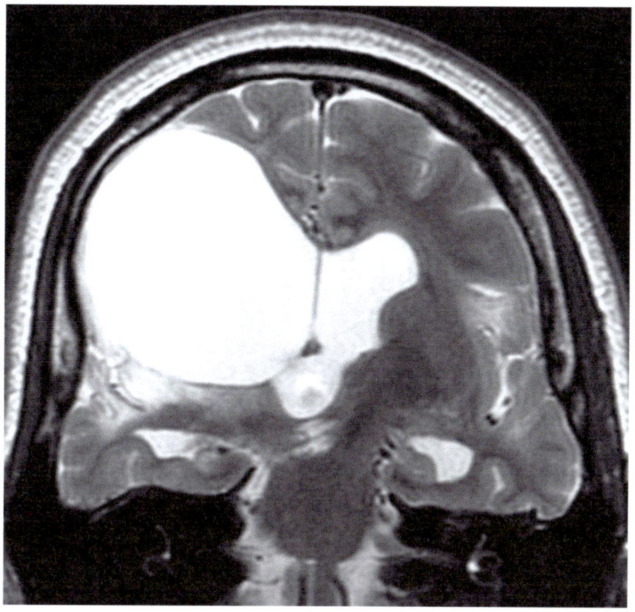

Fig. 49.4 MRI coronal T2 sequence at the same hippocampal body level as Fig. 49.3. Hyperintensity is evident inferior to the dilated ventricle and within the right superior temporal gyrus, which more clearly indicates gliosis than is evident with the T1 sequence. Hyperintensity is faintly visible in the right hippocampal body, which also more clearly indicates abnormality than the T1 sequence and suggests hippocampal sclerosis. Gliosis also is evident on the left, as is evident as hyperintensity within the left insula, frontal operculum, and superior temporal gyrus. The corpus callous is thinned bilaterally

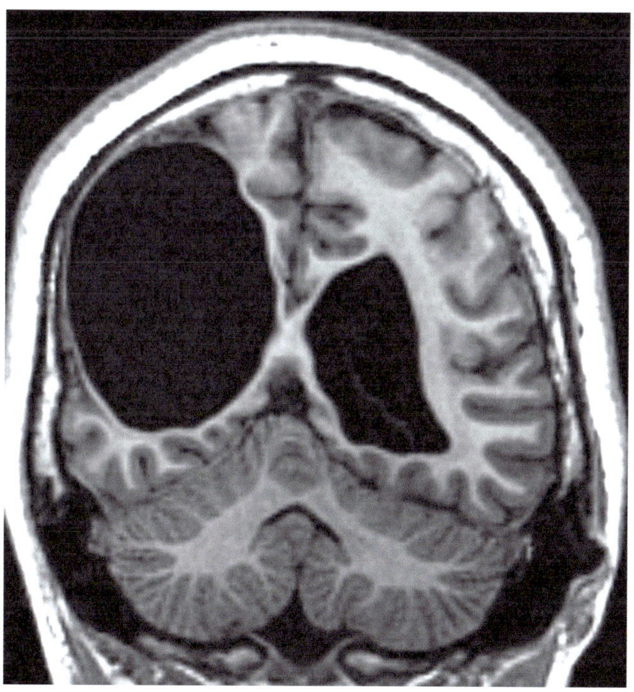

Fig. 49.5 MRI coronal T1 sequence at a splenium of the corpus callosum level. Hypointensity is evident along the margin of the right porencephalic cyst. The left cerebellum has a minor inferior deformity, but cerebellar diaschisis is not present. Because of the developmental age of the infarction, which is before cerebral to cerebellar connections are formed, cerebellar diaschisis is not expected

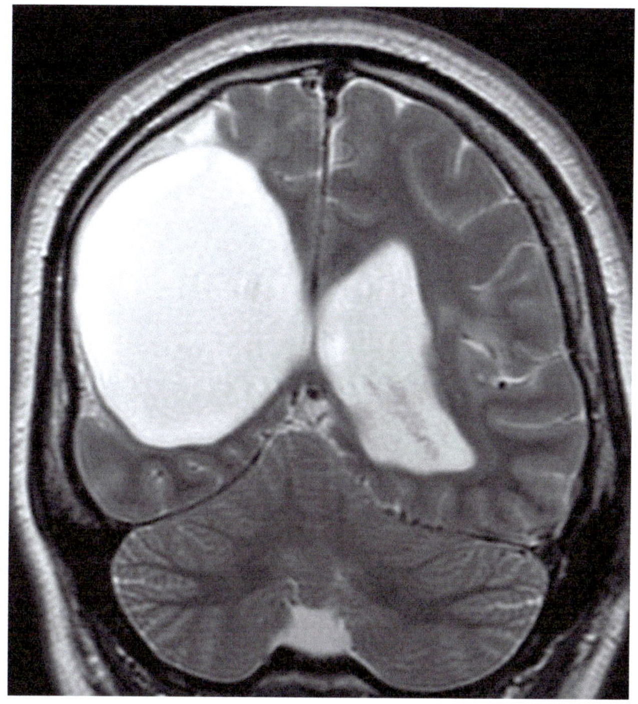

Fig. 49.6 MRI coronal T2 sequence at the same splenium of the corpus callosum level as Fig. 49.5. Hyperintensity is evident along the superior and lateral margins of the right porencephalic cyst. The left lateral ventricle has ex-vacuo enlargement, as is evident in the intact ventricular margin, and is due to left cerebral ischemia. The left cerebral ischemia also is evident as gliosis-related hyperintensity in the left posterior Sylvian region

Sturge-Weber Syndrome in an Infant

50

Clinical History

The first recognized seizure occurred at age 3 days as twitching of the right arm and leg. Soon after this, seizures with tonic stiffening, flexion of the torso, and abnormal eye movements also were identified. An evaluation at that time produced a diagnosis of Sturge-Weber syndrome.

Habitual seizures manifested as right hand and foot twitching that typically lasted 25 seconds and recurred about 15 times daily. Some seizures were prolonged with durations of several minutes and one lasted 20 minutes. After 2 months of successive pharmacotherapies, seizure freedom was achieved, and this persisted for 2.5 months. At age 4 months, status epilepticus occurred and was followed by several weeks of frequent and prolonged seizures that were similar to the seizures from the neonatal period.

The epilepsy risk factor was Sturge-Weber syndrome.

Neurological examination identified developmental delay with developmental regression as the seizure burden increased. Motor asymmetry is evident in poor control of the right hand and resultant left-handedness.

Medical history includes a normal gestation and delivery.

Interictal EEG depicted disorganized and attenuated left-sided rhythms with increased slowing in bilateral posterior quadrants and the absence of a posterior dominant rhythm. The left posterior quadrant had asymmetrically greater slowing and an absence of faster frequencies. Vertex sharp waves and sleep spindles were asymmetric and better formed on the right. Spikes and spike and slow-wave complexes were occasionally present over the left occipital pole and the left frontal parasagittal region. Video-EEG monitoring did not record the habitual behavioral seizures but identified electrographic seizures over the left frontal-central region with expansion anteriorly and posteriorly with ultimately including the left parietal and occipital regions.

MRI identified progressive left cerebral volume loss. PET identified a large region of left hemispheric hypometabolism and normal metabolism across the right hemisphere.

The history and evaluation indicated medication-resistant epilepsy related to Sturge-Weber syndrome with left hemispheric structural and epileptiform abnormalities. The high seizure burden and the developmental regression led to consideration of epilepsy surgery, and the existing motor deficits and broad seizure onset were an indication for an extensive resection.

A left functional hemispherectomy was performed at age 7 months. Histopathological examination identified meningeal angiomatosis consistent with Sturge-Weber syndrome, focal cortical dysplasia, and cerebral calcifications. No seizures have occurred for the 2 years since surgery, and three of the four anti seizure medications have been tapered to discontinuation. Neurological examination at age 2.5 years identified intact movements bilaterally with a preference for the left hand, independence for sitting up, and inability for ambulation

J. M. Stern, N. Salamon, *Imaging of Epilepsy*, https://doi.org/10.1007/978-3-030-86672-3_50

Imaging

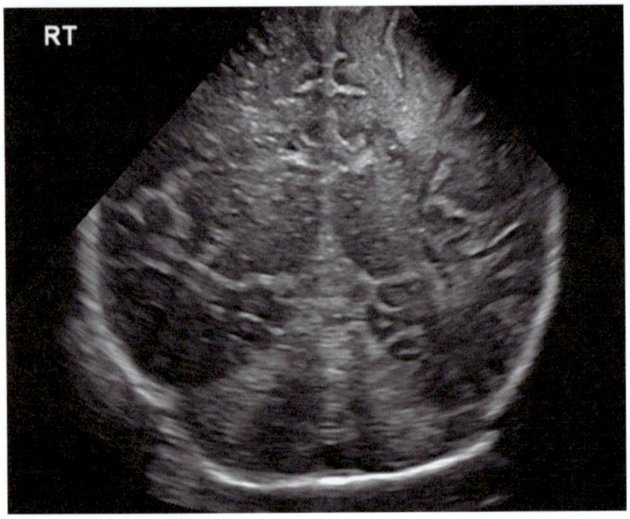

Fig. 50.1 Transcranial ultrasound in a coronal plane at a thalamus level. The image was obtained on postpartum day 1. Increased echogenicity is evident across the left hemisphere with enlargement of the left hemisphere's cortical sulci, as compared to the right. Hydrocephalus is not present

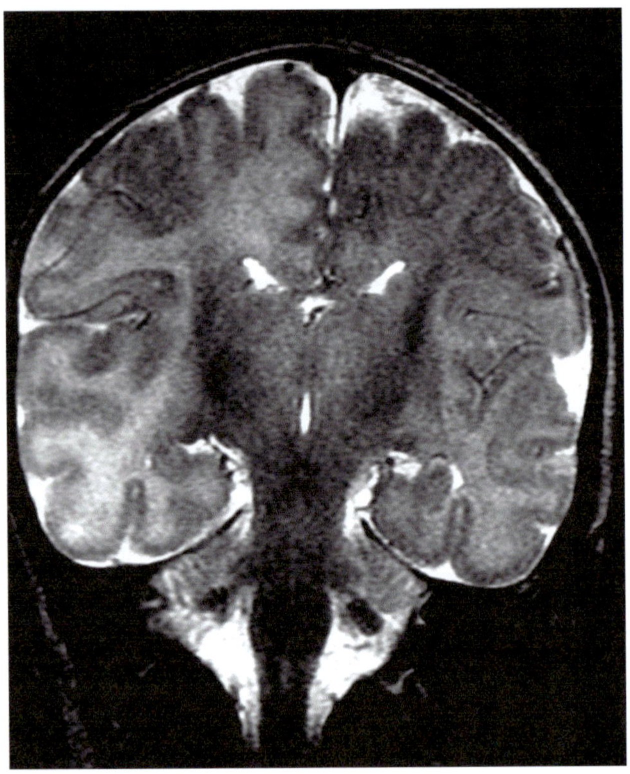

Fig. 50.2 MRI T2 coronal sequence at a thalamus level. The image was obtained on postpartum day 2 along with the images in Figs. 50.3, 50.4, 50.5, and 50.6. Hypointense signal is evident in the left frontal cortex and is a sign of hypermyelination. The left temporal lobe also is hypointense and hypermyelinated. The left temporal lobe hypointensity is not as abnormal as the left frontal lobe, but it is asymmetrically decreased when compared to the right temporal lobe. Overall, the left hemisphere is atrophic, and its corticospinal tract is hypointense with the abnormality decreasing in a cranial to caudal direction. The combination of hemispheric atrophy and hypermyelination suggests Sturge-Weber syndrome. The lateral ventricles are symmetric, as expected

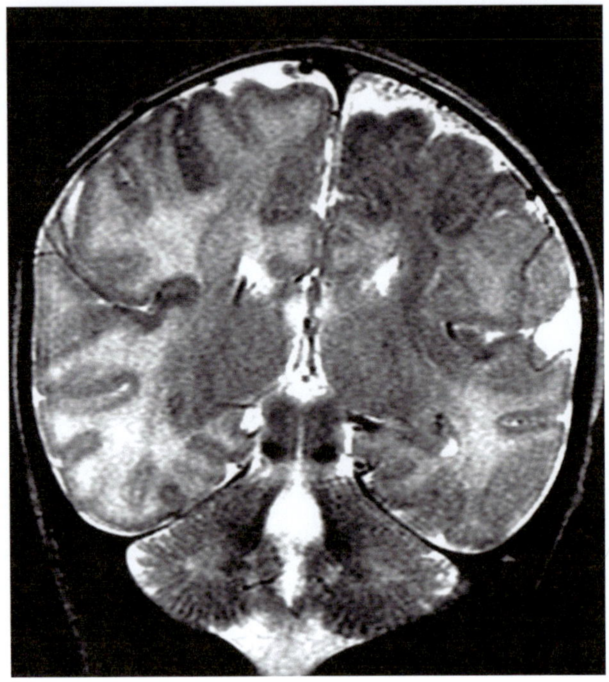

Fig. 50.3 MRI T2 coronal sequence at a colliculi level on postpartum day 2. The left hemisphere is atrophic and has decreased white matter signal indicating hypermyelination. Small vasculature is evident in the subarachnoid space across the superior surface, which suggests the venous collaterals with dilated leptomeningeal vessels of Sturge-Weber syndrome. The cerebellum is normal

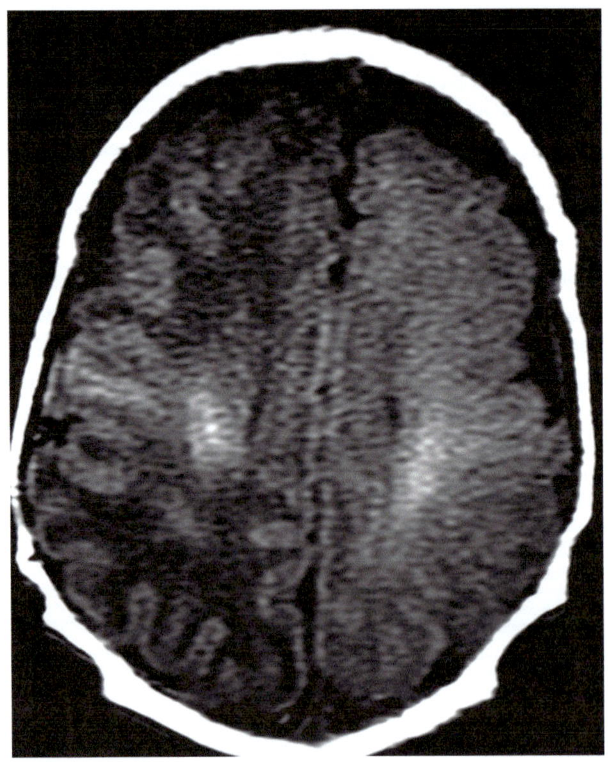

Fig. 50.4 MRI T1 axial sequence at a superior ventricle level on postpartum day 2. The left hemisphere is atrophic and has diffuse, hyperintense signal, suggesting hypermyelination. Higher T1 signal is evident bilaterally in the sensorimotor cortex, which is normal for developmental age. Normal myelination is present across the right hemisphere. The cortical ribbon is normal bilaterally

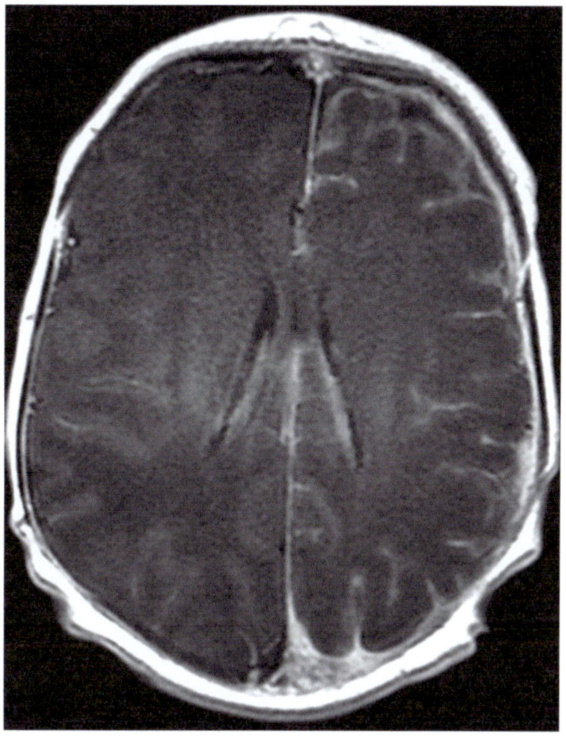

Fig. 50.5 MRI T1 axial sequence at a lateral ventricle level on postpartum day 2 after contrast administration. The left hemisphere is atrophic, and increased enhancement is evident along its pial surface and subarachnoid space and within the sulci. This abnormal enhancement indicates leptomeningeal vascular engorgement. The lateral ventricles are normal

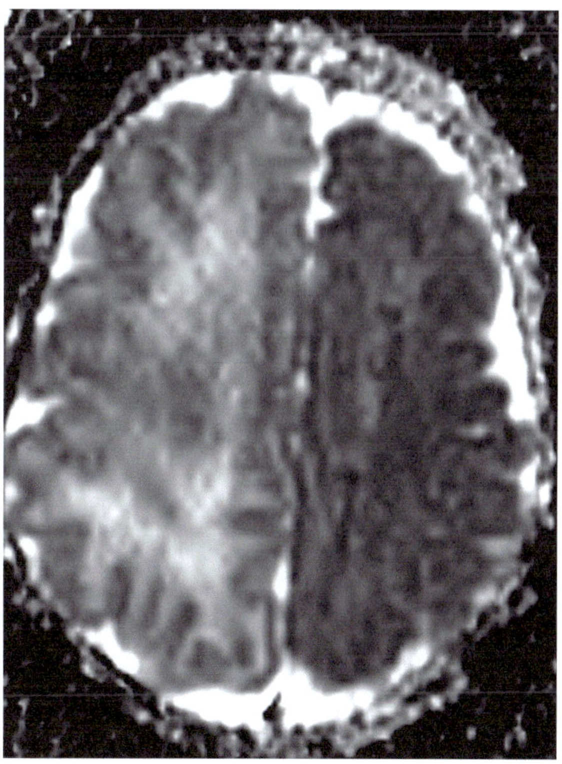

Fig. 50.6 MRI diffusion-weight imaging with an apparent diffusion coefficient map at a centrum semi-ovale level on postpartum day 2. The left hemisphere atrophic and the entire left hemisphere has an abnormally decreased apparent diffusion coefficient value indicating hypermyelination. The right hemisphere is normal

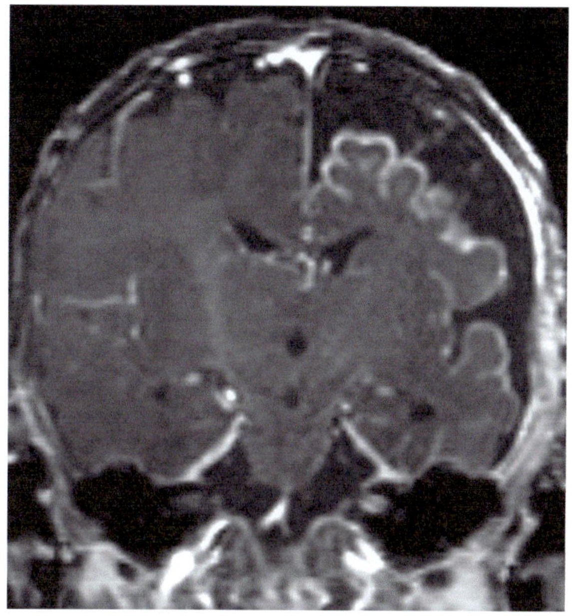

Fig. 50.7 MRI T1 coronal sequence at a thalamus level after contrast administration. The image was obtained at age 4 months along with the images in Figs. 50.8, 50.9, 50.10, 50.11, 50.12 and 50.13. Marked atrophy of the left frontal and temporal lobes is evident. The atrophy has progressed, and the asymmetry is greater than it was at age 2 days. The left lateral ventricle is now larger than the right. The left thalamus has less marked atrophy. Leptomeningeal and dural enhancement is present around the left hemisphere. The right hemisphere is normal

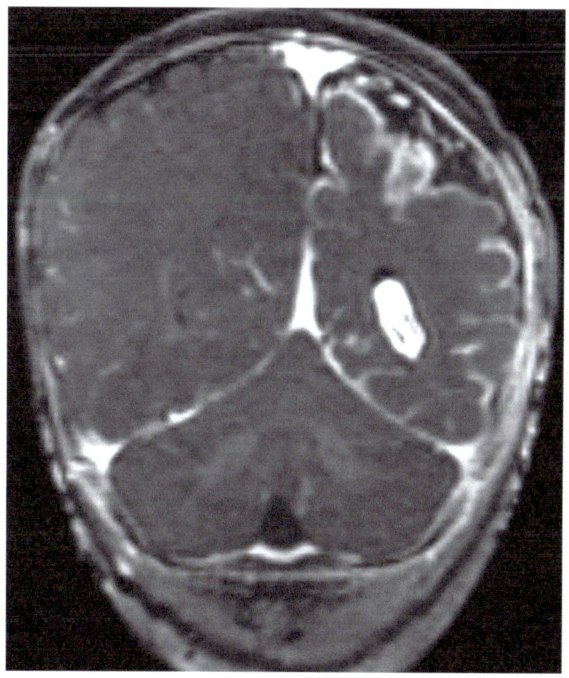

Fig. 50.8 MRI T1 coronal sequence at an atrium of the lateral ventricle level at age 4 months after contrast administration. The left hemisphere is atrophic, and left leptomeningeal enhancement is present. The left choroid plexus is enlarged, which is characteristic of Sturge-Weber because of the increased deep venous drainage. An increased venous presence also is evident in the subarachnoid space superior and lateral to the parietal lobe. The left dura is thickened and enhanced. The right hemisphere is normal

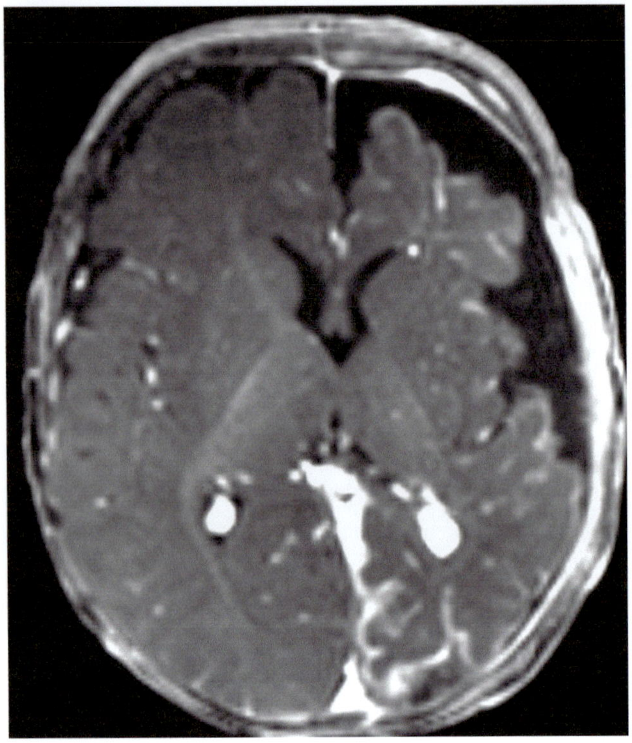

Fig. 50.9 MRI T1 axial sequence at a basal ganglia level at age 4 months after contrast administration. Marked atrophy of the left frontal and temporal lobes is evident along with leptomeningeal enhancement of the left hemisphere. Choroid plexus is abnormally larger on the left. Dural enhancement is present on the left

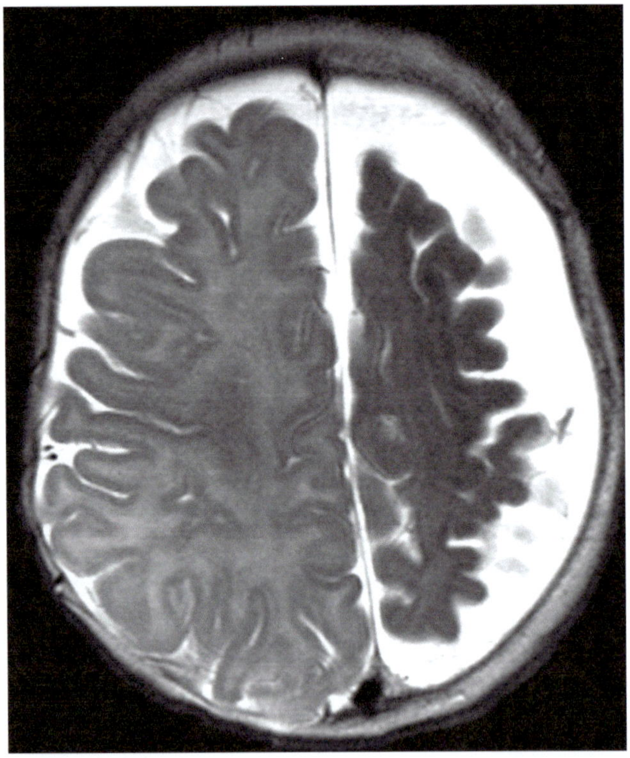

Fig. 50.10 MRI T2 axial sequence at a centrum semi-ovale level at age 4 months. Marked atrophy of the left hemisphere is evident along with decreased signal in the white matter, suggesting hypermyelination. The left skull is asymmetrically thickened. The right hemisphere and skull are normal

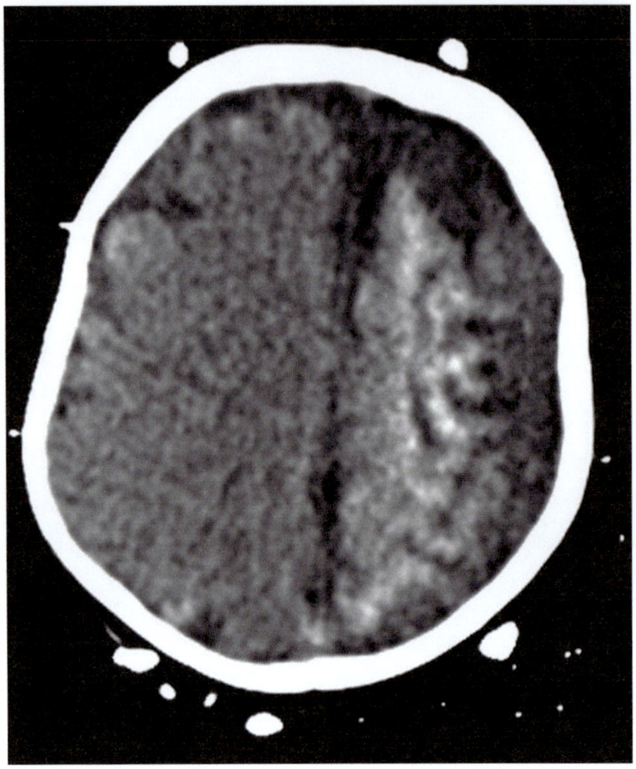

Fig. 50.11 CT in an axial plane at age 4 months and at the same centrum semi-ovale level as Fig. 50.10. Left hemispheric atrophy is evident with a thickened skull. The left cerebrum has increased radiodensity because of parenchymal calcification, and this increases the gyral contour visibility. The hyperdense spots around the head are EEG electrodes

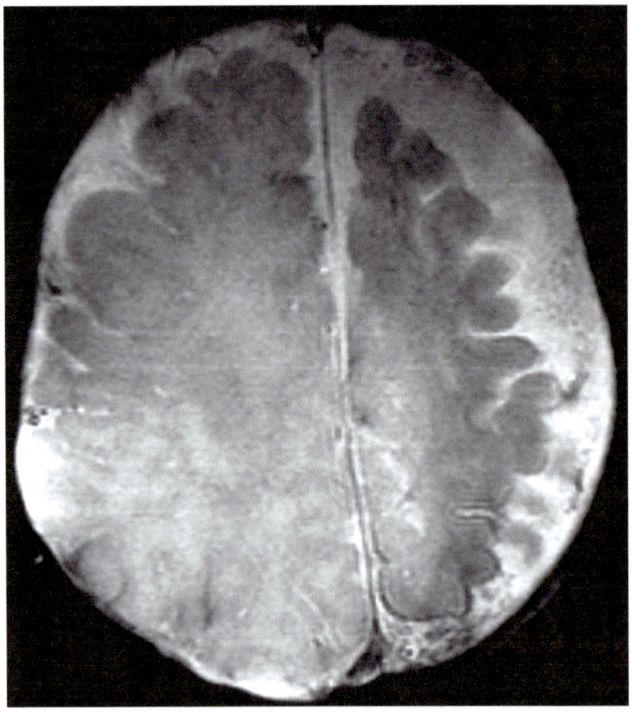

Fig. 50.12 MRI gradient echo axial sequence at a centrum semi-ovale level. A hypointense line indicating calcification follows the cortical surface and is most prominent across the parietal lobe but also evident along the frontal lobe. The subarachnoid space is dilated and includes vascular structures

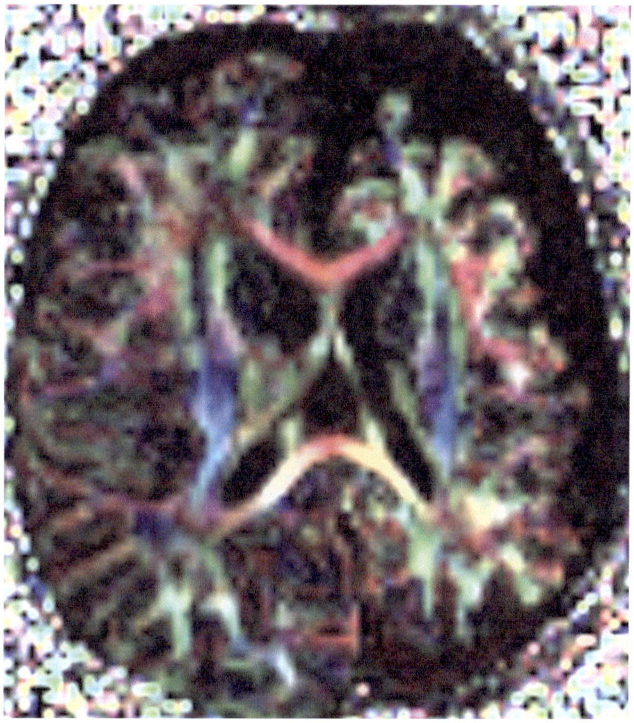

Fig. 50.13 MRI with axial diffusion tensor imaging color map at a lateral ventricle level. The left hemispheric atrophy is evident in the decreased fiber tract arborization. The genu of the corpus callosum has normal right-left orientation, as indicated by the red color. The splenium of the corpus callosum differs and is not red, indicating decreased fractional anisotropy and distortion of the fiber paths

51 Sturge-Weber Syndrome in a Child

Clinical History

The first recognized seizure occurred at age 8 months as left gaze deviation with continuous left face and arm twitching. Emergent care was obtained, and 2 weeks of inpatient care was needed to successfully treat focal motor status epilepticus.

Habitual seizures developed after 4 months of seizure freedom that followed the episode of status epilepticus. The habitual seizures initially manifested as left face, chin, and arm twitching with a postictal left-sided paresis. Treatment included multiple anti-seizure medications without seizure freedom but with a seizure frequency that varied over 15 months from several seizures daily to seizure freedom for months. The focal status epilepticus recurred at age 2 years as motor seizures producing simultaneous left arm twitching and left toes curling.

The epilepsy risk factor was Sturge-Weber syndrome.

Neurological examination at age 9 months identified developmental delay. At age 2 years, verbal language was highly limited, and communication was mostly through hand gestures. A port-wine stain was present immediately above the right eye.

Medical history included a normal gestation, delivery, and neonatal period. No ocular abnormality was evident in the ophthalmologic exam.

Interictal EEG depicted abnormal bilateral slowing with attenuation and asymmetrically greater slowing across the right hemisphere. Slowing was maximal in the right posterior quadrant, and the posterior dominant rhythm was present only on the left.

Video-EEG monitoring recorded focal seizures manifested as left-hand twitching that did not have an accompanying EEG abnormality, and no electrographic seizures were present.

MRI identified a venous malformation of the right temporal, parietal, and occipital lobes. PET identified hypometabolism that corresponded to the MRI abnormality.

The history and evaluation indicate medication-resistant focal motor seizures due to Sturge-Weber syndrome with seizures occurring individually and as epilepsia partialis continua. The EEG finding of asymmetric slowing without epileptiform correlates to the behavioral seizures and is typical of epilepsia partialis continua. The slowing corresponds to the broad cerebral dysfunction, and the seizures do not produce a sufficiently expansive synchronization to be visible with scalp electrode EEG.

Because of the epilepsia partialis continua, motor deficits, and developmental delay, a right hemispherotomy was performed at age 2 years. Histopathological examination identified leptomeningeal angiomatosis consistent with Sturge-Weber syndrome, focal cortical dysplasia, and focal dystrophic calcifications. No seizures have occurred for the 12 years since surgery, and anti-seizure medications were tapered with final discontinuation 4 years ago. Verbal language improved within months of surgery to include multiple words. Speaking and walking were regained by age 3.5 years. As a teenager, a left hemiparesis was present, and school performance was reading at grade level and math lagging by 2–3 grade levels.

J. M. Stern, N. Salamon, *Imaging of Epilepsy*, https://doi.org/10.1007/978-3-030-86672-3_51

Imaging

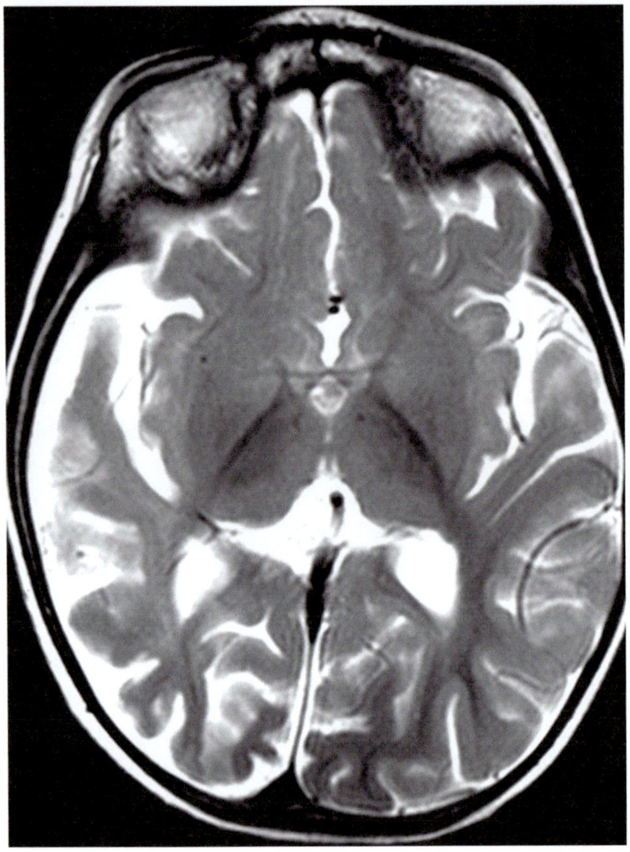

Fig. 51.1 MRI axial T2 sequence at a basal ganglia level. The right temporal and occipital lobes are atrophic with enlargement of the right Sylvian fissure. The inferior right frontal lobe has minor atrophy. Hypomyelination is evident in the right temporal occipital white matter. The basal ganglia, thalamus, and left hemisphere are normal

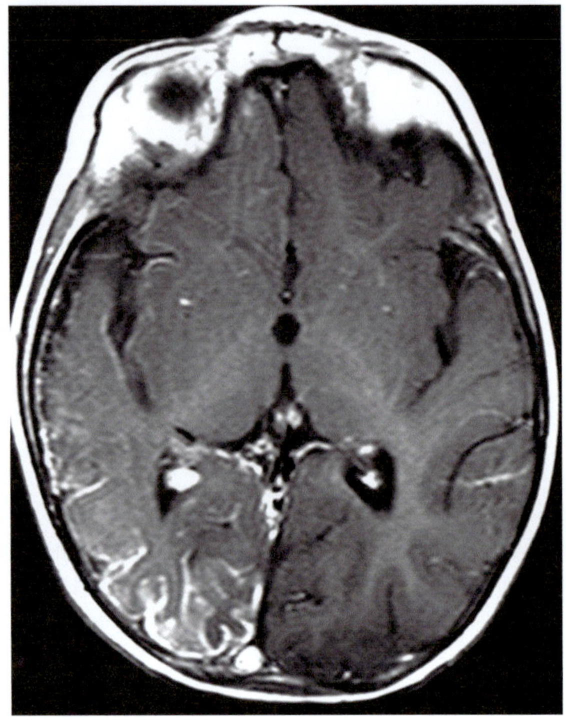

Fig. 51.2 MRI axial T1 sequence after contrast administration at the same basal ganglia level as Fig. 51.1. Leptomeningeal enhancement of right temporal occipital lobe is prominent. Subtle pial surface enhancement is evident across the right superior temporal gyrus, right inferior frontal lobe, and right insula. The right choroid plexus is enlarged, indicating abnormally increased deep venous drainage. The linear signal across left lateral temporal lobe is pulsation artifact

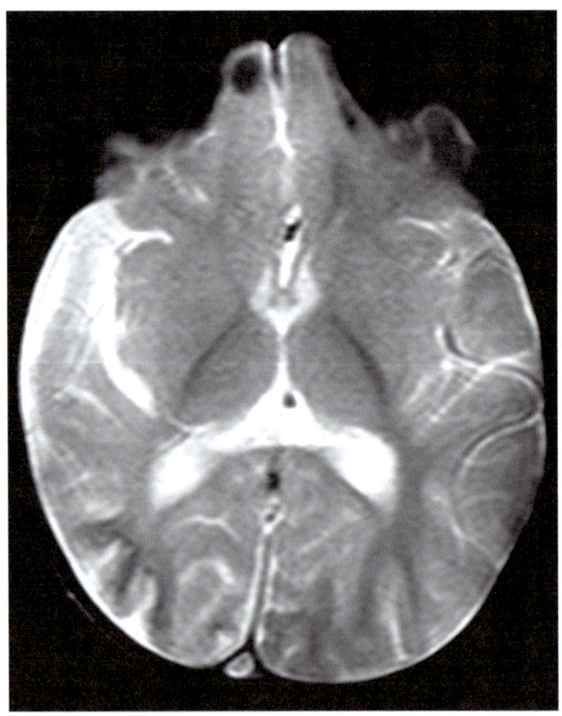

Fig. 51.3 MRI axial gradient echo sequence at the same basal ganglia level as Figs. 51.1 and 51.2. Susceptibility artifact that is evident across the right occipital lobe's cortical ribbon indicates calcification. The ovoid hypointensity in the right gyrus rectus is susceptibility artifact from the air sinus

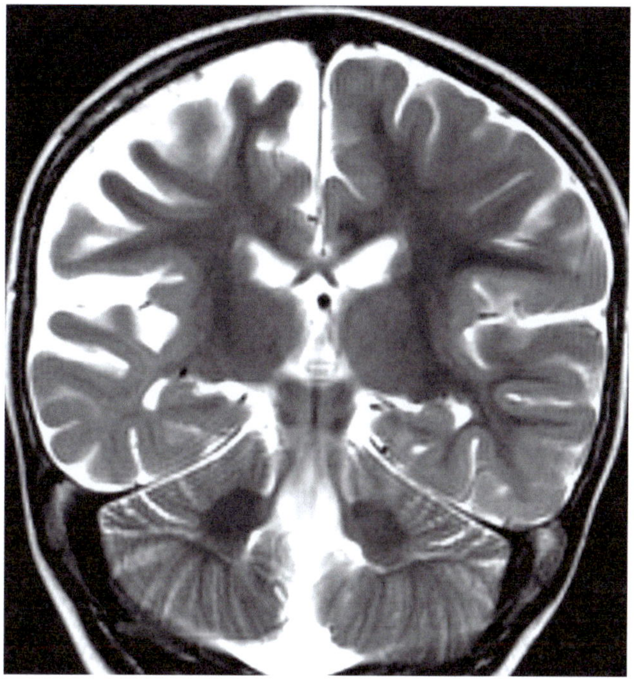

Fig. 51.4 MRI coronal T2 sequence at a colliculi level. The right hemisphere is atrophic with an enlarged right Sylvian fissure. Hypomyelination is evident within the right temporal lobe white matter. The thalamus, lateral ventricles, and cerebellum are symmetric and normal. The left hemisphere also is normal

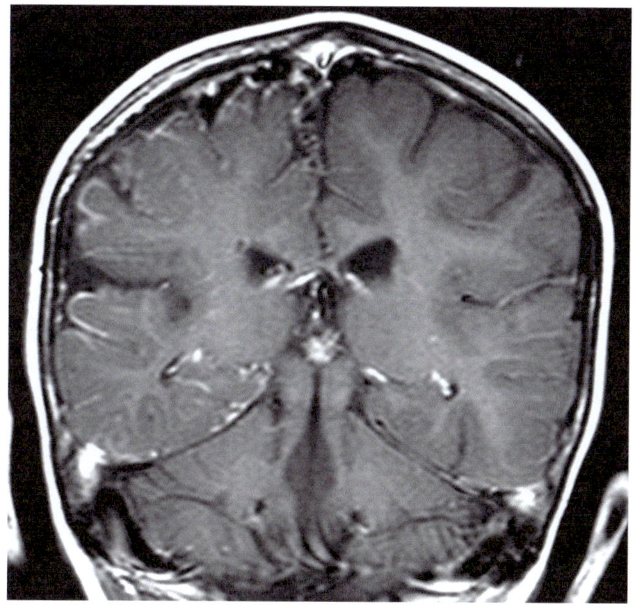

Fig. 51.5 MRI coronal T1 sequence after contrast administration at a colliculi level that is slightly posterior to Fig. 51.4. The right hemisphere's atrophy is evident but not as prominent as in Fig. 51.4. Leptomeningeal enhancement is present across the surface of the right hemisphere. The left hemisphere and cerebellum are normal

52 Sturge-Weber Syndrome in an Adult

Clinical History

The first recognized seizure occurred at age 5 years as an experience of a "funny feeling" with staring and behavioral arrest, and evaluation for this seizure produced the diagnosis of Sturge-Weber syndrome. In retrospect, the first seizures occurred before age 1 year as shaking episodes that were not recognized at that time as abnormal.

The habitual seizures manifested as the aura of a "funny feeling" and then depersonalization and sometimes singing a specific verse from a particular song. This was followed by tonic posturing of the left arm and then flexion of the right arm and bilateral tonic extension of the legs. A fall resulted if a seizure occurred while standing. The seizures impairing awareness were sometimes evident as a brief period of amnesia, but clear loss of consciousness was never present. Auras in isolation occurred infrequently, and an aura always precedes the seizures with amnesia or motor involvement. The seizure duration was 20 to 30 seconds, and postictal state was 1 minute with nausea and confusion. Treatment included multiple anti-seizure medications and vagus nerve stimulation with a seizure frequency of about three to four seizures on most days and occasional seizure-free days.

The epilepsy risk factors were Sturge-Weber syndrome and meningitis at age 2.5 years that produced several days of coma.

Neurological examination identified asymmetric limb sizes with a smaller left side, especially at the hand and foot. Mild left hemiparesis was present and produced an asymmetric gait. Developmental delay was evident in early childhood, and an individualized education program was used through high school graduation. A port-wine stain was present bilaterally across the three divisions of cranial nerve V. Medical history included monocular glaucoma with blindness since age 11 years.

Interictal EEG depicted an asymmetric posterior dominant rhythm due to a poorly formed rhythm on the right and a normal rhythm on the left. During sleep, vertex sharp waves were unilaterally present on the left. No epileptiform abnormality was present. Video-EEG monitoring recorded focal seizures manifested as auras in isolation that had no abnormal EEG correlate. The ictal EEG's onset for seizures with impaired memory was rhythmic slowing broadly across the left hemisphere.

MRI identified right hemispheric atrophy with gray matter calcifications and right hippocampal sclerosis. CT identified right hemispheric atrophy and extensive gyral calcifications across the right occipital and posterior temporal and posterior parietal lobes. PET identified marked hypometabolism of the right cerebral hemisphere with relative sparing of the anterior and inferior right frontal lobe and right thalamus. Mild left cerebellar hypometabolism also was present.

The history and evaluation indicate focal seizures that follow a limbic aura and include asymmetric posturing supportive of a right-sided seizure onset. The imaging and the ictal EEG supports this lateralization, but the extensive structural abnormality and broad electrographic seizure onset preclude localization. The limbic aura may be due to propagation even with the imaging evidence of hippocampal sclerosis. Surgical treatment was not offered because of the apparent need for a large, disabling resection to provide a reasonable likelihood of improved seizure control and the low likelihood of seizure freedom.

J. M. Stern, N. Salamon, *Imaging of Epilepsy*, https://doi.org/10.1007/978-3-030-86672-3_52

Imaging

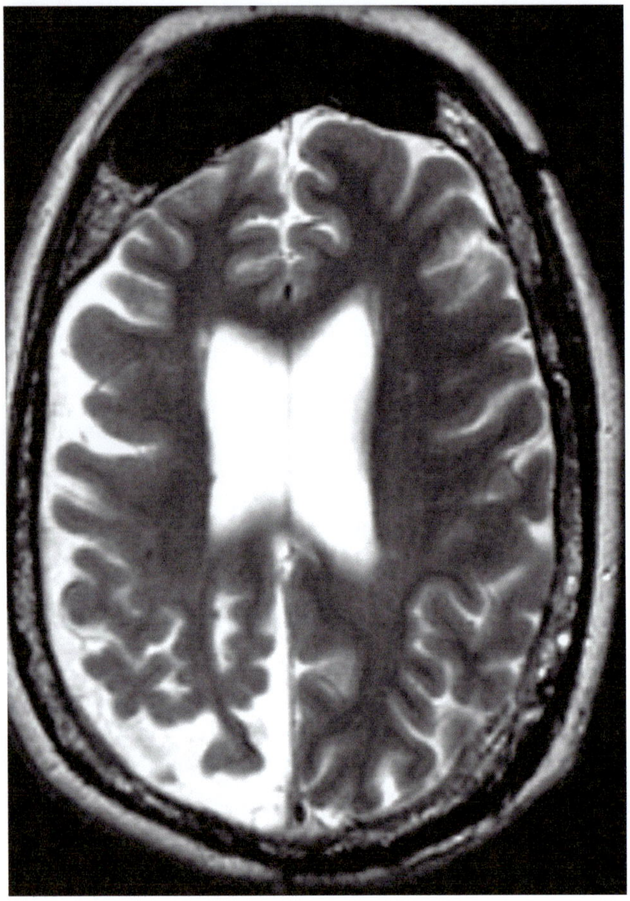

Fig. 52.1 MRI axial T2 sequence at a lateral ventricle level. The right hemisphere has marked atrophy that is especially prominent posteriorly. The cerebral tissue loss is associated with an enlargement of the right frontal sinus. The ventricles are symmetric and normal. The left hemisphere is normal

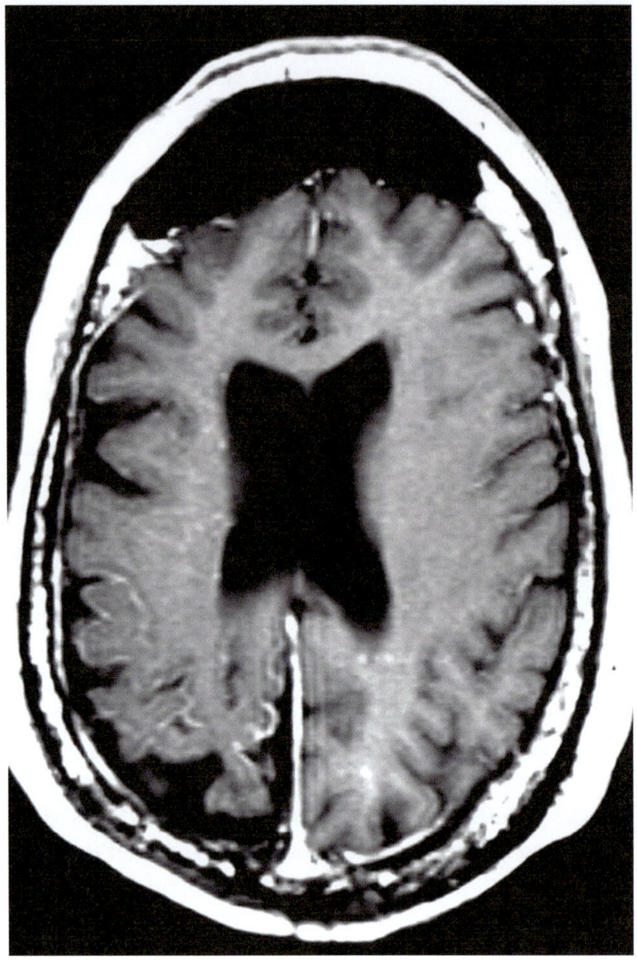

Fig. 52.2 MRI axial T1 sequence after contrast administration at the same lateral ventricle level as Fig. 52.1. Right hemisphere atrophy is evident with greater involvement of the parietal lobe. Leptomeningeal enhancement has greatest prominence across the right parietal lobe. No abnormal enhancement is present in the left hemisphere

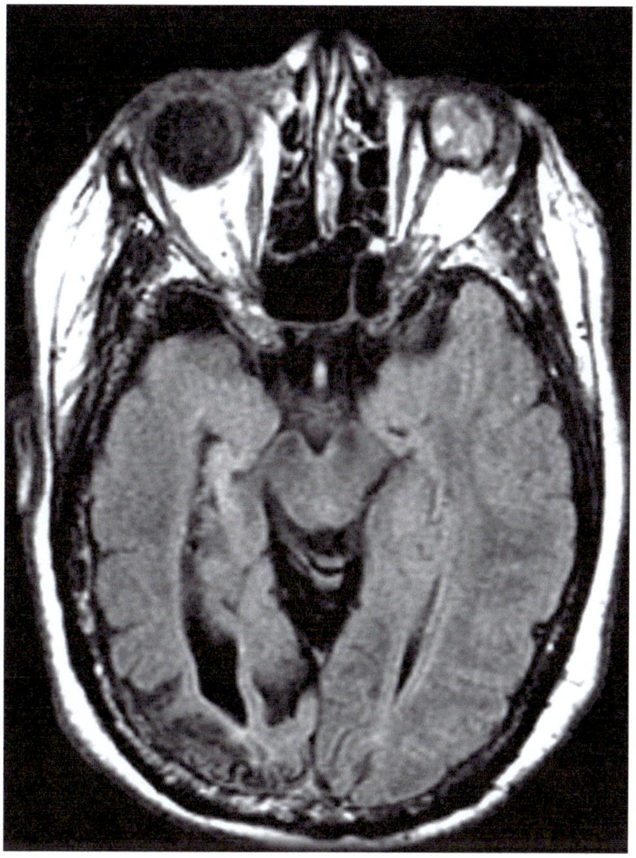

Fig. 52.3 MRI axial FLAIR sequence at a hippocampus level. The right temporal and occipital lobes are atrophic with dilation of the right lateral ventricle's temporal occipital horn. A hypointense signal indicating calcification is evident along the surface of the right occipital lobe. The left eye is smaller and malformed with abnormal heterogeneous signal intensity within the globe that suggests remote hemorrhage

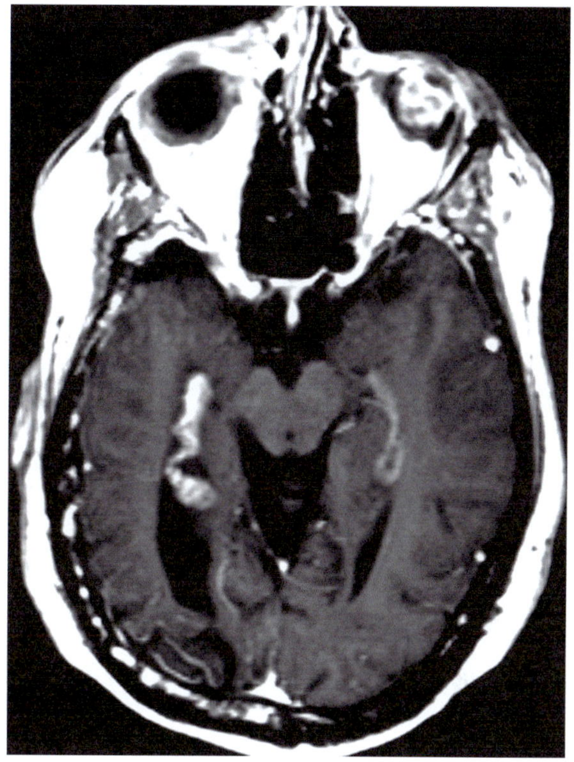

Fig. 52.4 MRI axial T1 sequence after contrast administration at the same hippocampus level as Fig. 52.3. The right temporal and occipital lobes are atrophic with dilatation of the right lateral ventricle's temporal horn. The right choroid plexus is abnormally enlarged. Leptomeningeal enhancement is evident across the right occipital lobe with pronounced enhancement in the diploic space of the right temporal occipital bone. Abnormal enhancement is evident within the left eye's vitreous fluid

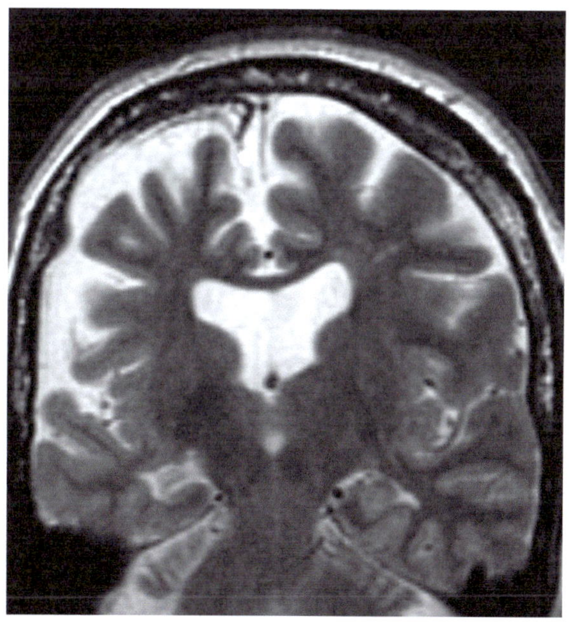

Fig. 52.5 MRI coronal T2 sequence at a hippocampal body level. The right hemisphere is atrophic with an enlarged vein in the right superior convexity. Myelination of the right hemisphere is decreased compared to the left, and the right hippocampus is asymmetrically smaller. The basal ganglia is normal bilaterally

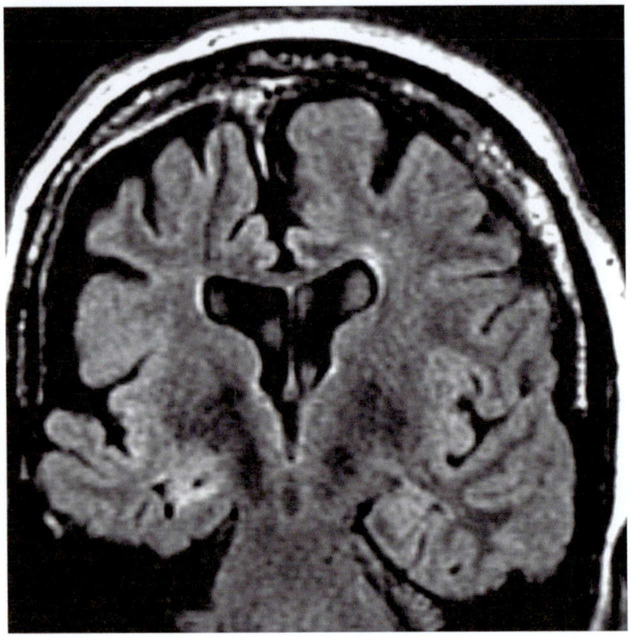

Fig. 52.6 MRI coronal FLAIR sequence at the same hippocampal body level as Fig. 52.5. The right hemisphere is atrophic. The hyperintensity of the atrophic right hippocampus suggests hippocampal sclerosis. The left hemisphere is normal

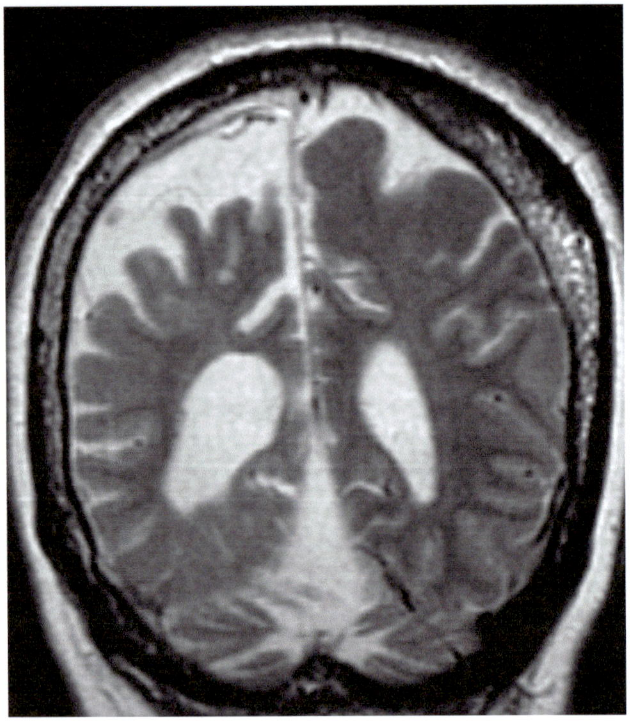

Fig. 52.7 MRI coronal T2 sequence at an occipital horn of the lateral ventricle level. The right parietal and occipital lobes are atrophic with enlargement of the right lateral ventricle. Hypomyelination is evident in the right occipital lobe. The left hemisphere is normal

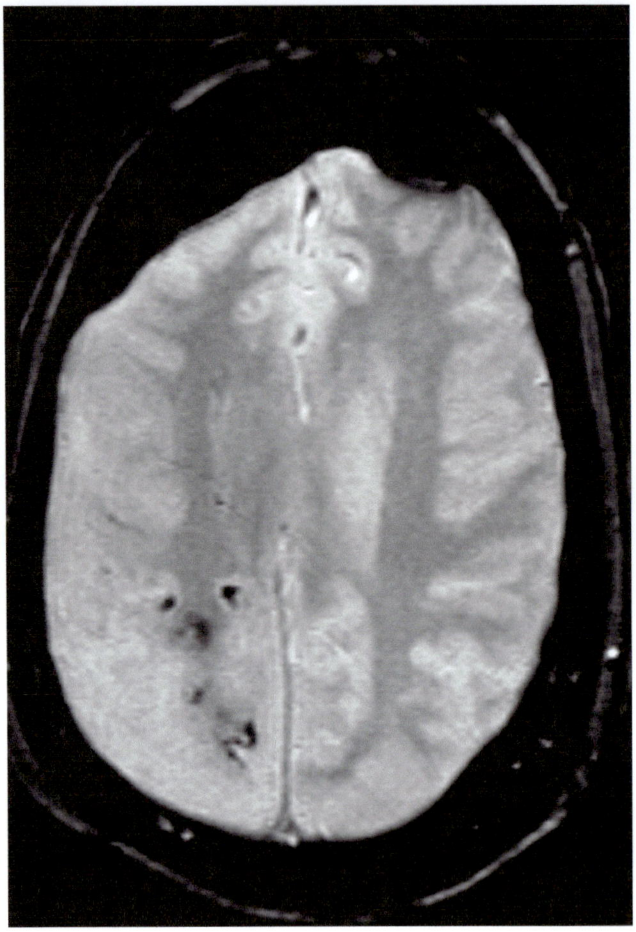

Fig. 52.8 MRI axial gradient echo sequence at a high lateral ventricle level. Multiple punctate hypointensities are present across the right parietal lobe. These are susceptibility artifact and indicate cortical calcification

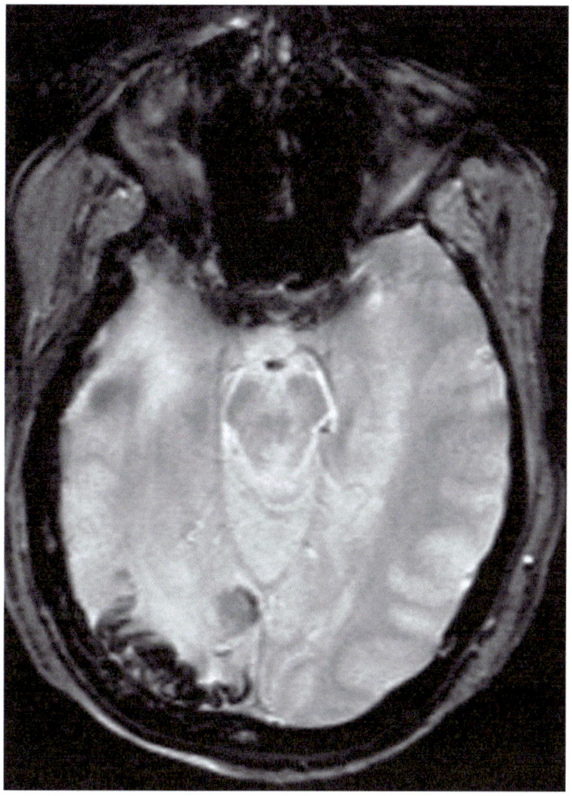

Fig. 52.9 MRI axial gradient echo sequence at a midbrain level. Serpentine susceptibility artifact is present across the right posterior cortical surface and indicates gyriform calcification

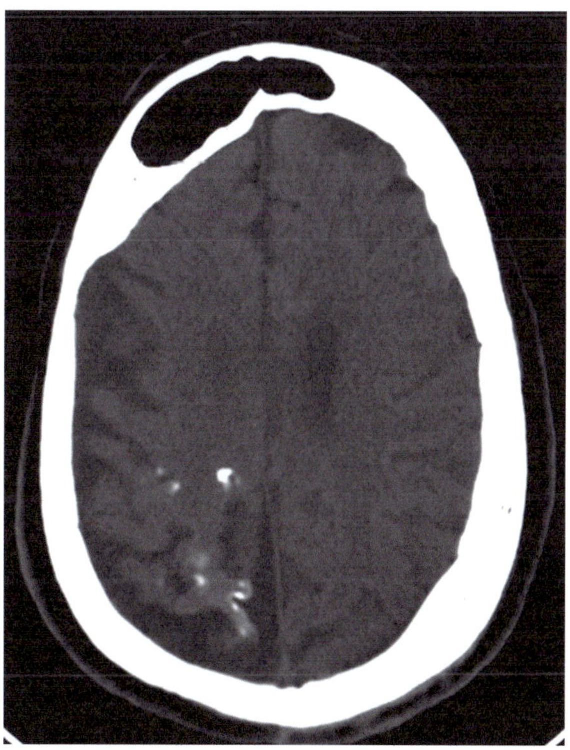

Fig. 52.10 CT in an axial plane at the same high ventricle level as Fig. 52.8. Hyperdensities indicating calcification correspond to the gradient echo susceptibility artifact

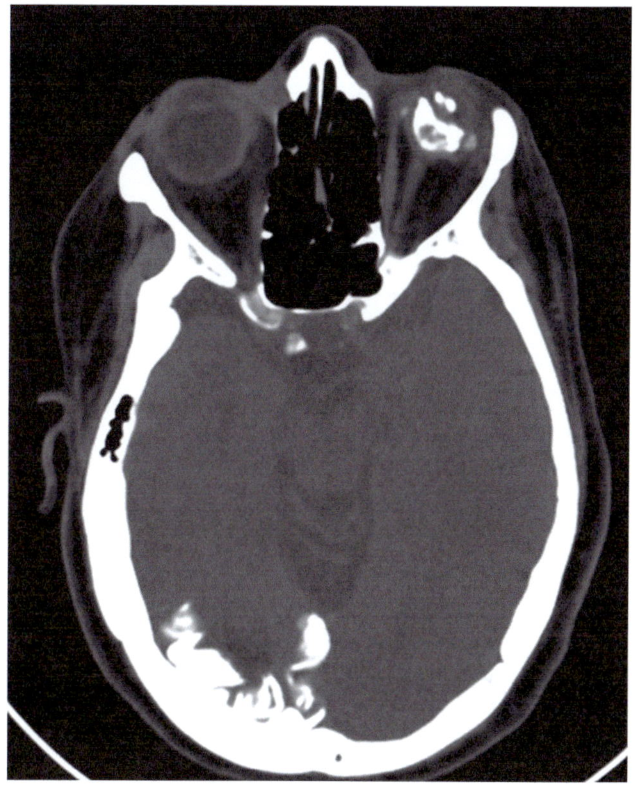

Fig. 52.11 CT in an axial plane at a midbrain level similar to Fig. 52.9. Gyriform hyperdensity with serpentine appearance is evident in the right posterior cortical surface and corresponds to the gradient echo susceptibility artifact. Abnormal calcification also is present in the left globe

Part VI

Tumors

Brain tumor
Brain cancer
Astrocytoma
Oligodendroglioma
Dysembryoplastic neuroepithelial tumor
Ganglioglioma
Hamartoma
Meningioma

Astrocytomas on an unenhanced CT appear as either a hypodense or isodense mass lesion and rarely contain calcification. With MRI, their common appearance is as a lesion of abnormal signal with minor, if any, mass effect. The surrounding tissue may demonstrate an associated focal cortical dysplasia (Type IIIb). Pilocytic astrocytomas are distinct because of a commonly occurring cystic component with an enhancing mural nodule. Calcification may be present in up to 25% of instances, and internal hemorrhage has been reported. Pleomorphic xanthoastrocytomas (PXA) are classically a circumscribed, nodular mass involving cortex, and they usually enhance along with adjacent leptomeninges.

Oligodendrogliomas are hyperintense with T2 weighted imaging and often include calcification that is most evident with susceptibility weighted MRI or CT imaging. They may or may not enhance with contrast. Minimal to moderate patchy, multifocal enhancement with a dot-like or lacy pattern is evident in up to 50% of occurrences.

Dysembryoplastic neuroepithelial tumors (DNET) appear with CT scans as hypoattenuating masses with sporadic calcifications across the cortical-subcortical region. With MRI, their appearance is more distinct and are well-demarcated, wedge shaped, multinodular, "bubbly" or pseudocystic intracortical tumors that are hypointense with T1 weighted and hyperintense with T2 weighted images. They have minimal or no mass effect and do not produce vasogenic edema. Scalloping of the adjacent inner table of the skull may also be present. Their multicystic form is helpful in differentiating them from gangliogliomas. Contrast enhancement is present for about 30% of occurrences.

Gangliogliomas and gangliocytomas have similar imaging characteristics and are differentiated histologically. Both occur as 2 to 3 cm lesions with the most common location at the periphery of a cerebral hemispheres. They usually have little associated mass effect and peripheral vasogenic edema, but superficial gangliogliomas and gangliocytomas may expand cortex and remodel bone. Their MR signal is variable and inhomogeneous due to the presence of a combination of solid, cystic and calcified components. Calcifications can be conspicuous as areas of hypointensity on T2* gradient echo weighted images and are even more evident with unenhanced CT. Contrast enhancement is variable and may be none, nodular, or as a ring. Extremely rarely, they produce focal leptomeningeal involvement.

Hypothalamic hamartomas are congenital malformations arising from the tuber cinereum, a structure between the mammillary bodies and pituitary stalk. They are most evident with a sagittal midline level and have either a pedunculated or sessile attachment to the hypothalamus. With T1 and T2 weighted imaging, the signal is typically isointense to gray matter, but T2 signal sometimes is hyperintense. Contrast enhancement does not occur, and repeated imaging does not depict an interval change in size. When growth occurs, the abnormality is more likely to be a glioma.

Meningiomas are dural based masses with gray matter isointense signal with T1 and T2W sequences. The underlying cerebral cortex may be displaced and demonstrates normal signal abnormality or edema when a cortical vein is compressed. Invasive meningiomas appear as larger masses and may have cortical surface contrast enhancement. Meningiomas are related to seizures only when they are supratentorial, and seizures are more likely when peri-tumoral edema is evident and the location is not along the skull base.

Key References

Castillo M, Davis PC, Takei Y, Hoffman JC. Intracranial ganglioglioma: MR, CT, and clinical findings in 18 patients. Am J Roentgenology. 1990;154:607–12.

Englot DJ, Magill ST, Han SJ, et al. Seizures in supratentorial meningioma: a systematic review and meta-analysis. J Neurosurg. 2016;124:1552–61.

Fernandez C, Girard N, Paredes AP, et al. The usefulness of MR Imaging in the diagnosis of dysembryoplastic neuroepithelial tumor in children: a study of 14 cases. AJNR Am J Neuroradiol. 24:829–34.

Freeman JL, Coleman LT, Wellard RM, et al. MR imaging and spectroscopic study of epileptogenic hypothalamic hamartomas: Analysis of 72 cases. AJNR 2004;25:450–62.

She D, Liu J, Xing Z, et al. MR imaging features of anaplastic pleomorphic xanthoastrocytoma mimicking high-grade astrocytoma. AJNR Am J Neuroradiol 2018;39:1446-52.

Smith M. Imaging of Oligodendroglioma. Br J Radiol 2016;89:20150857.

Astrocytoma

53

Clinical History

The first recognized seizure occurred at age 5 years as nocturnal tonic-clonic without lateralizing features. An evaluation at that time identified a left frontal mass.

Subsequent nocturnal tonic-clonic seizures were behaviorally similar and had observed durations of about 1 minute. An additional habitual seizure manifestation was identified after the epilepsy diagnosis and occurred in both wakefulness and sleep. This seizure manifested as a sudden change to facial expression with widening of the eyes suggesting being startled or frightened. When occurring during wakefulness, behavioral arrest accompanied the brief facial expression, and the seizure resolved with an immediate return to baseline interaction; however, autism and language disability impacted the baseline interaction. Treatment included multiple anti-seizure medications with a nocturnal tonic-clonic seizure frequency of about one seizure every 1 to 2 weeks with up to two seizures weekly and none for up to 4 weeks. The frequency of the brief seizures with facial expression change was estimated to be about six weekly with up to several in 1 day.

The epilepsy risk factors were a left frontal tumor and developmental disability.

Neurological examination identified language delay and autism. Medical history included a normal gestation and delivery.

Interictal EEG depicted generalized slowing that was maximal over the left hemisphere with absence of the left-sided mu rhythm. Interictal epileptiform discharges were in the left central region and were rare with occurrences only during sleep. Video-EEG monitoring recorded the habitual tonic-clonic seizures as an arousal from sleep with forward staring and sometimes manual automatisms for about 30 seconds that was followed falling toward the right, sometimes right-sided jerks, and then progression to bilateral tonic-clonic movements. Ictal EEG's seizure onset was left frontal-temporal slowing that evolved into 1 to 2 Hz generalized spike discharges and then generalized fast activity. The total seizure durations were about 2 minutes. The episodes of widening of the eyes and facial expression change also were recorded, and the corresponding EEG depicted a seizure onset of brief rhythmic theta activity across the left temporal region.

MRI identified a homogeneous, enhancing lesion in the inferior left frontal lobe without surrounding edema. Surveillance of the tumor identified growth without a change to internal features or the development of edema. PET identified hypometabolism within the lesion.

The history and evaluation indicate focal and bilateral tonic-clonic seizures. The focal seizures were evident in the stereotyped episodes of a frightened facial expression, which suggests a limbic involvement and is consistent with the ictal rhythm across the temporal lobe. Limbic features were also evident in the behavioral arrest, staring, and manual automatisms at the onset of the bilateral tonic-clonic seizures, and these features are consistent with the cingulate gyrus location of the frontal lobe tumor. The secondary bilateral synchrony that is evident in the generalized EEG abnormalities is also consistent with a medial frontal abnormality.

After radiologic monitoring of the frontal lobe lesion identified an increase in size and multiple anti-seizure medications failed to produce seizure freedom, a left frontal resection was performed. Histopathological examination identified a pilocytic astrocytoma. No focal seizures or bilateral tonic-clonic seizures have occurred for the 4 years since surgery.

J. M. Stern, N. Salamon, *Imaging of Epilepsy*, https://doi.org/10.1007/978-3-030-86672-3_53

Imaging

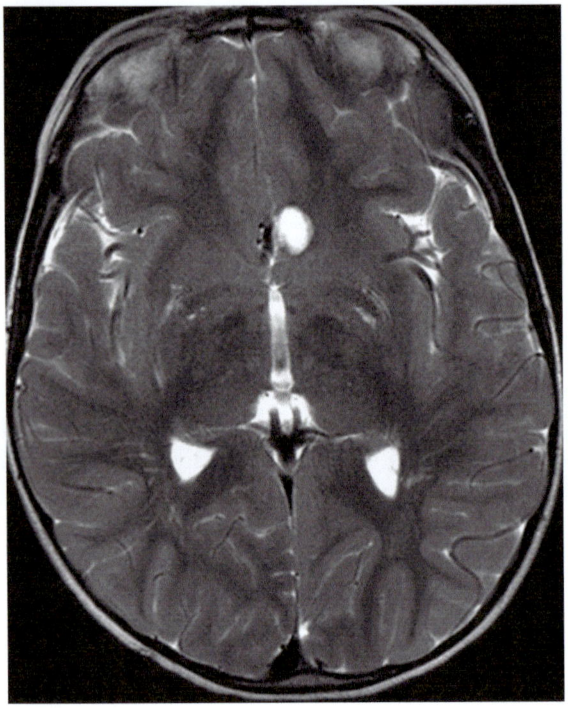

Fig. 53.1 MRI axial T2 sequence at an anterior commissure level. A well-defined hyperintense mass is evident in the left subcallosal cingulate gyrus, near the superficial gray matter surface and adjacent to the anterior cerebral artery. The mass has no surrounding edema. No other abnormality is present

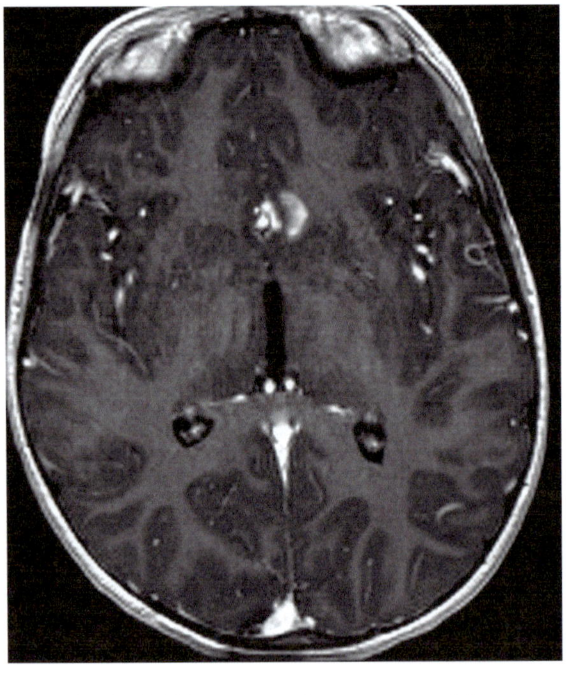

Fig. 53.2 MRI axial T1 sequence after contrast administration at the same anterior commissure level as Fig. 53.1. The left cingulate gyrus mass has homogeneous enhancement that does not extend to include the gray matter that is medially adjacent. The gray matter separates the mass from the normal, vascular hyperintensity within the interhemispheric fissure, partly from the anterior cerebral artery

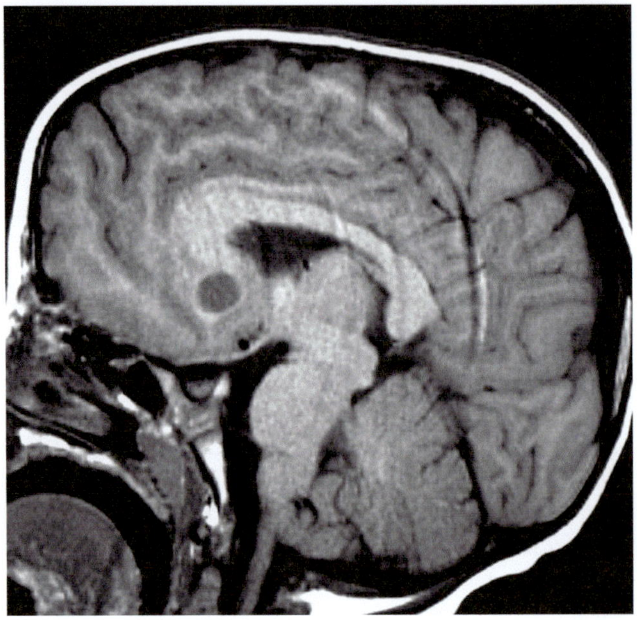

Fig. 53.3 MRI sagittal T1 sequence at a midline corpus callosum level. A well-defined round focus of hypointensity is evident in the left subcallosal cingulate gyrus. There is no mass effect or edema. No other abnormality is present

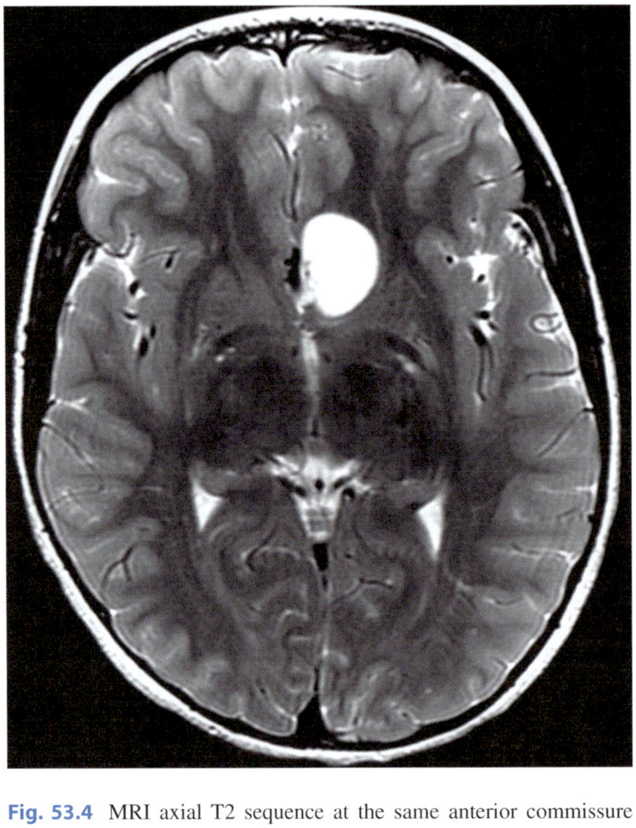

Fig. 53.4 MRI axial T2 sequence at the same anterior commissure level as Figs. 53.1 and 53.2. This image and the images in Figs. 53.5, 53.6, 53.7, 53.8, 53.9, and 53.10 were obtained four years after Figs. 53.1, 53.2, and 53.3. Over the interval period, the left cingulate gyrus mass had a marked increase in size, and it now produces mass effect on the left basal ganglia. However, its internal, homogeneous signal has not changed, and no edema is present

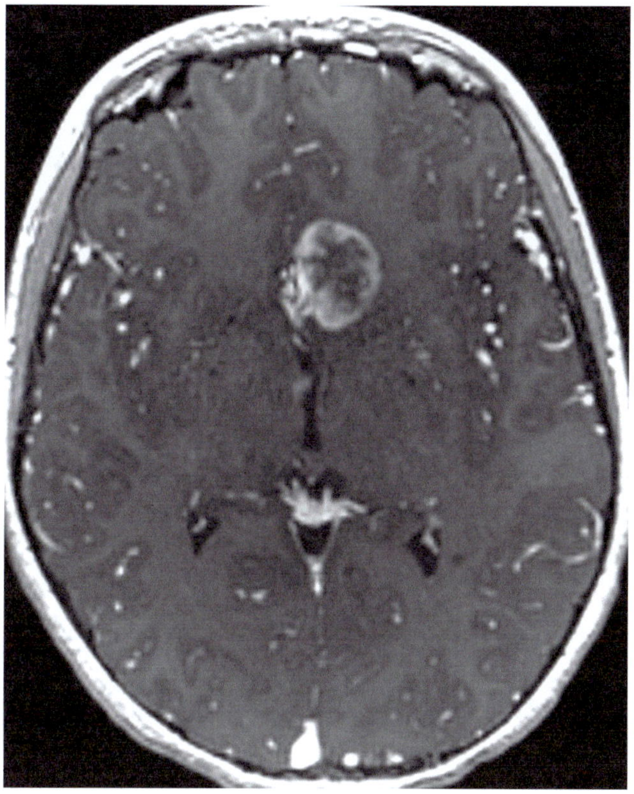

Fig. 53.5 MRI axial T1 sequence after contrast administration at the same anterior commissure level as Fig. 53.4 and earlier Figs. 53.1 and 53.2. The left cingulate gyrus mass demonstrates heterogenous enhancement with the peripheral portion enhancing more than central portion. Normal vascular enhancement is evident medial to the mass and is separate from the mass. Unlike Fig. 53.2, the enhancement now extends to include the cortical surface of the left subcallosal cingulate cortex. However, it does not include the leptomeninges

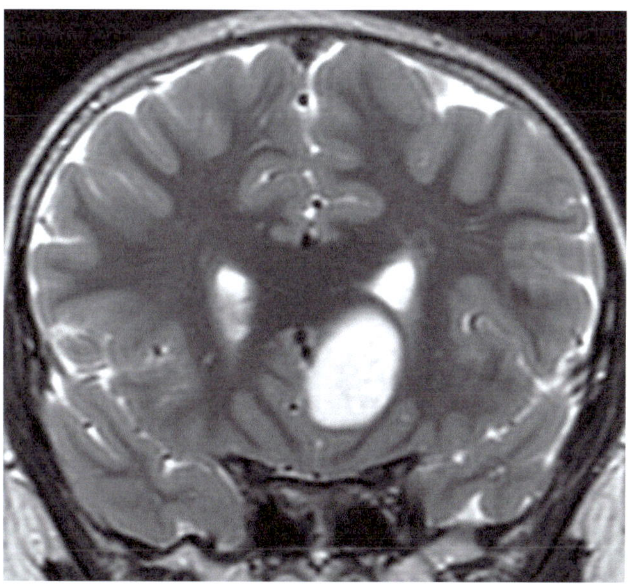

Fig. 53.6 MRI coronal T2 sequence at a genu of the corpus callosum level. A well-circumscribed, oval-shaped hyperintense mass is evident in the left subcallosal cingulate gyrus and abuts the gyrus' cortical surface. The anterior cerebral artery is displaced, and the mass effect also produces a deformation of the frontal horn of the lateral ventricle with displacement of the corpus callosum. No edema is present

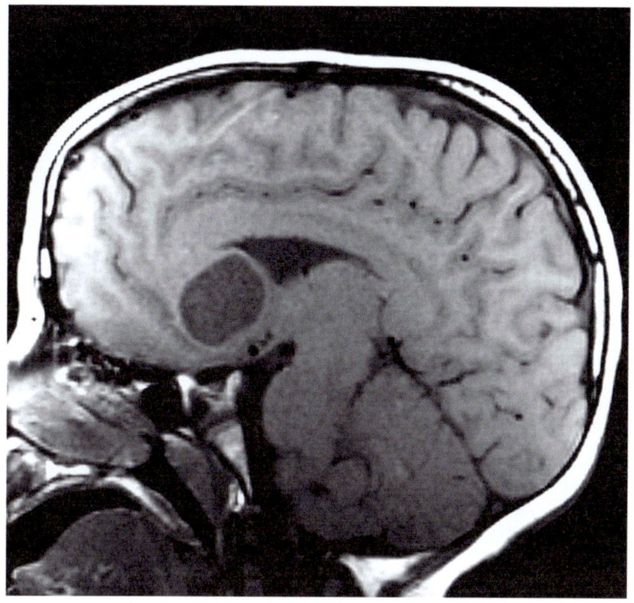

Fig. 53.7 MRI sagittal T1 sequence at the same midline corpus callosum level as Fig. 53.3. A well-circumscribed, oval, hypointense mass is evident in the left subcallosal cingulate gyrus with associated deformation of the rostrum of the corpus callosum. No edema or other abnormality is present

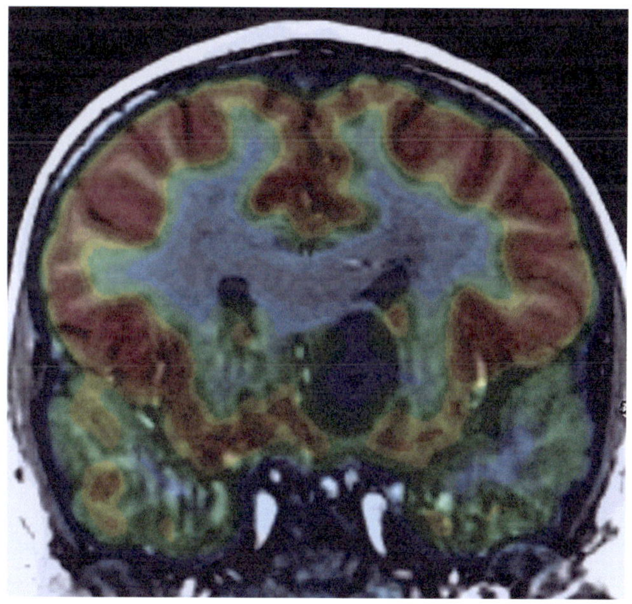

Fig. 53.8 PET-MRI co-registration with color-scale FDG tracer in a coronal plane at a genu of the corpus callosum level similar to Fig. 53.6. The left cingulate gyrus mass has marked hypometabolism. Beyond the mass's margins, less pronounced hypometabolism is evident. The left orbitofrontal region and temporal pole are asymmetrically hypometabolic. The right temporal pole and bilateral frontal convexities are normal

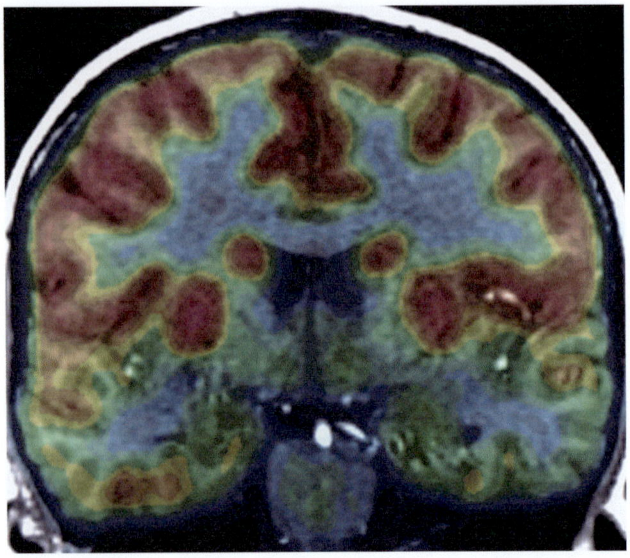

Fig. 53.9 PET-MRI co-registration with color-scale FDG tracer in a coronal plane at a hippocampal head level. The left temporal lobe is asymmetrically hypometabolic, along the lateral and inferior aspects in particular. The hippocampi are bilaterally symmetric. The frontal lobes are normal

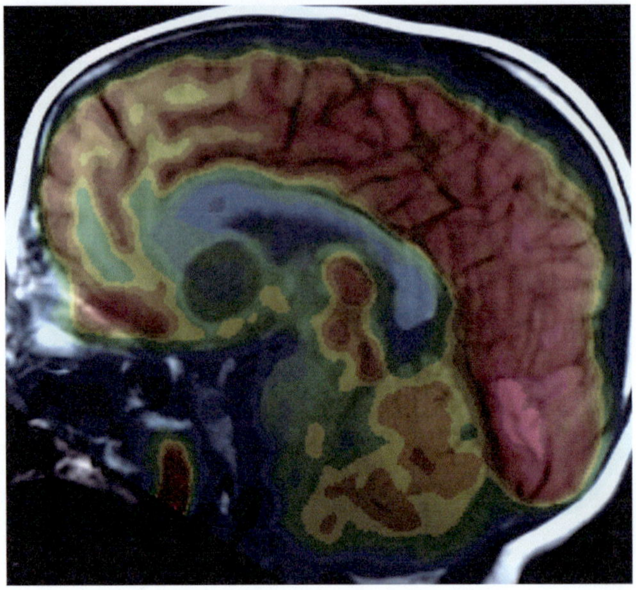

Fig. 53.10 PET-MRI co-registration with color-scale FDG tracer in a sagittal plane at the same midline corpus callosum level as Figs. 53.3 and 53.7. A well-circumscribed, hypometabolic mass is evident in the subcallosal anterior cingulate gyrus. No other abnormality is present

Oligodendroglioma

54

Clinical History

The first recognized seizure occurred during infancy with seizures described as bilateral rhythmic shaking. Epilepsy treatment began at about the age of 1 year, and the details of the evaluation at that time were no longer known. Tonic-clonic seizures continued to occur for about 2 years, and seizure freedom then was present through childhood. Treatment was discontinued at about age 3 years.

The epilepsy recurrence was at age 16 years as nocturnal tonic-clonic status epilepticus. Treatment was resumed, and the next seizure was a nocturnal tonic-clonic seizure at age 17 years. Seizure freedom continued until the development of the habitual seizures at age 21 years. These manifested as a feeling of warmth and dizziness followed by behavioral arrest, looking to the left, loss of awareness, and sometimes stepping movements. The seizure duration was 30 to 90 seconds, and resolution included postictal fatigue. Rarely, the focal seizures progressed to bilateral tonic-clonic seizures. Treatment included multiple anti-seizure medications with a focal seizure frequency of one seizure every 2 to 4 days. The most recent tonic-clonic seizure was several years ago. Prior to this, the tonic-clonic seizure frequency was one every few months.

The epilepsy risk factor was a parietal lobe lesion that was identified in adulthood.

Neurological examination was normal. Neuropsychological testing identified reading difficulty, mild left parietal dysfunction, normal memory function, and an IQ in the superior range.

Interictal EEG depicted epileptiform discharges that were maximum in the left central region. Video-EEG monitoring recorded focal seizures manifested as leftward head turning, right-hand dystonic posturing, and left-hand automatisms, followed by laterally directed hyperkinetic movements of the head and arms for 30 seconds to 2 minutes. Minimal postictal confusion was present. Ictal EEG's seizure onset was clear for only one of the recorded seizures, and it depicted parasagittal slowing as the ictal rhythm.

MRI identified a 6-mm left superior parietal lobule lesion that was hypointense with both T1 and T2 sequences. PET identified a hypometabolic region that corresponded to the MRI finding. Ictal SPECT identified hyperperfusion of the high left frontal and parietal regions.

The history and evaluation indicate focal seizures that follow a nonspecific aura. The right-hand dystonic posturing suggests a left-sided lateralization, which is not contradicted by the leftward turning that may be due to right-sided ictal neglect. The hyperkinetic movements and quick recovery of mentation suggest a neocortical epilepsy, and this is consistent with the lesion identified by MRI and the neuropsychological testing results. The ictal EEG was localizing for only one seizure, so an ictal SPECT was obtained, and this provided additional support for the localization.

A left superior parietal lobe resection was performed at age 44 years.

Histopathological examination identified an oligodendroglioma with large concretions of calcium, decreased brain tissue cellularity, and infiltrative glia with a preponderance of oligodendroglia. No seizures or auras occurred for 10 years since surgery, and subsequent MRIs have no evidence of residual or recurrent tumor. Anti-seizure medications are being gradually tapered with the plan of discontinuation.

J. M. Stern, N. Salamon, *Imaging of Epilepsy*, https://doi.org/10.1007/978-3-030-86672-3_54

Imaging

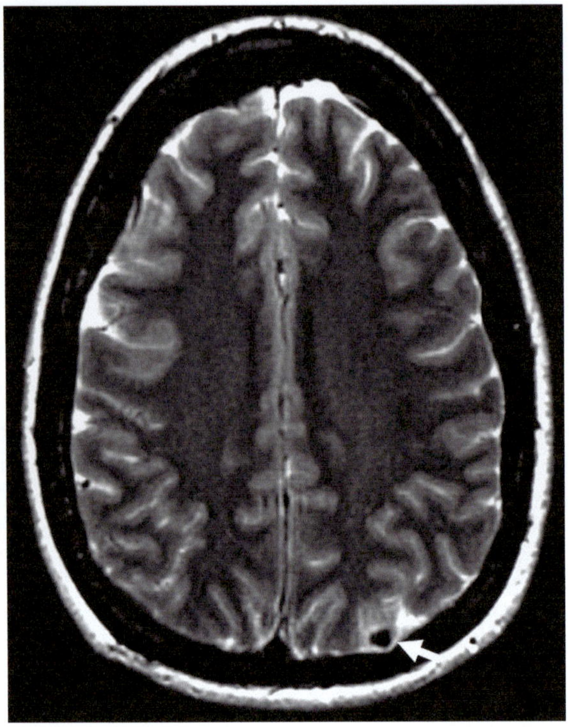

Fig. 54.1 MRI axial T2 sequence at a centrum semi-ovale level. Hypointense signal (arrow) is evident in the superficial surface of the left superior parietal lobule and has surrounding hyperintensity across the gray-white junction. No edema is present

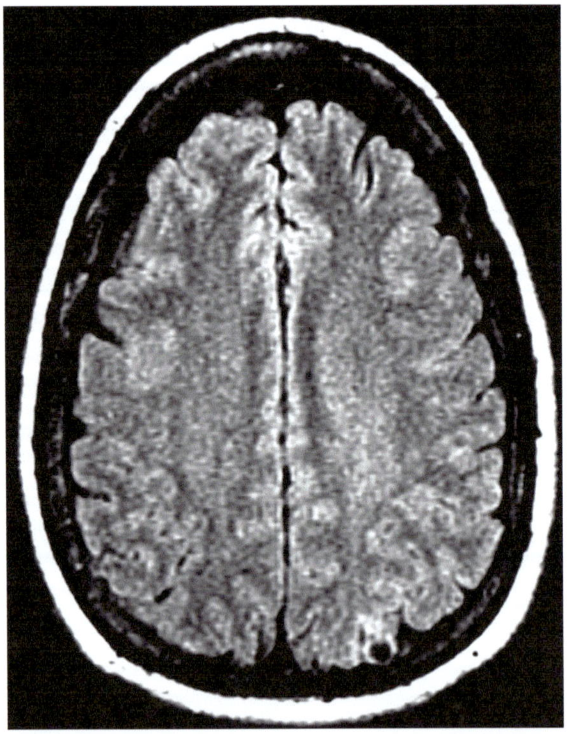

Fig. 54.2 MRI axial FLAIR sequence at the same centrum semi-ovale level as Fig. 54.1. A hypointense focus is present at the surface of the left superior parietal lobule with an associated hyperintense focus immediately anterior to it. No edema is present

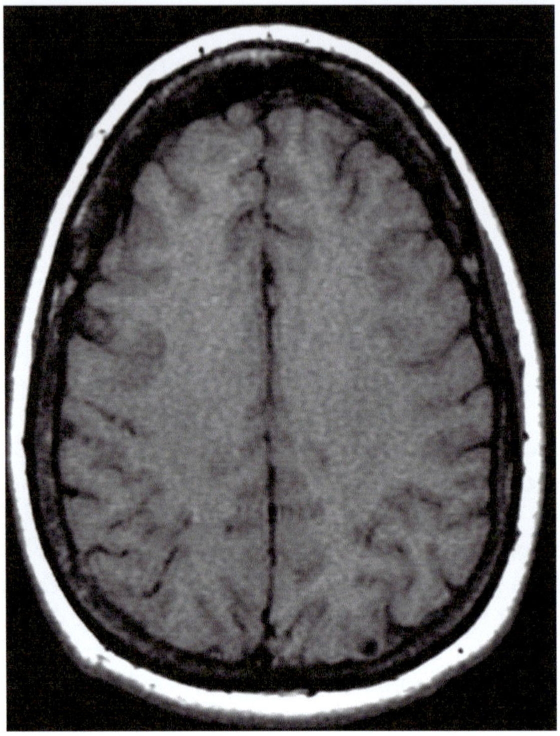

Fig. 54.3 MRI axial T1 sequence at the same centrum semi-ovale level as Figs. 54.1 and 54.2. A hypointense signal is evident at the surface of the left superior parietal lobule without signal abnormality immediately anterior to it, as is visible with the FLAIR sequence

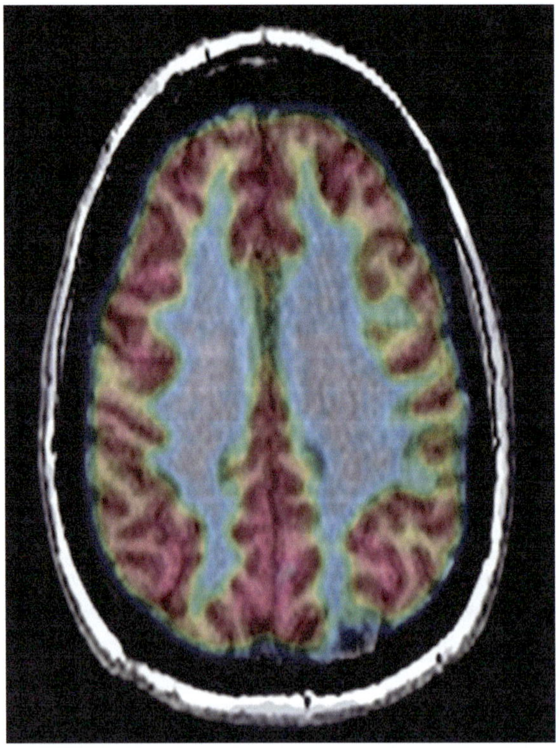

Fig. 54.4 PET-MRI co-registration with color-scale FDG tracer in an axial plane at the same level centrum semi-ovale level as the three preceding Figs. A region of hypometabolism surrounds the left superior parietal lobule lesion, which is evident as smaller region of hypointensity from the co-registered T1 sequence MRI that is within the hypometabolic abnormality

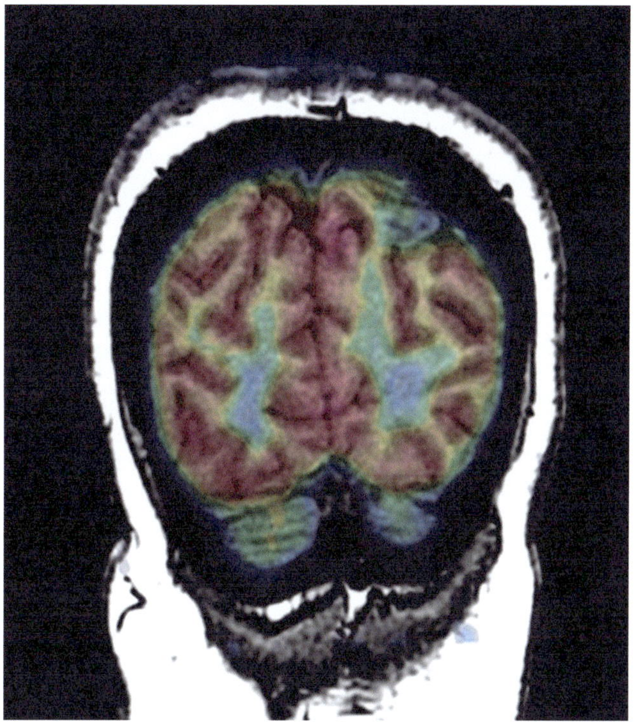

Fig. 54.5 PET-MRI co-registration with color-scale FDG tracer in a coronal plane at a posterior parietal level. The region of hypometabolism within the left superior parietal lobule extends farther from the MRI lesion and includes the intraparietal sulcus. No other abnormality is present

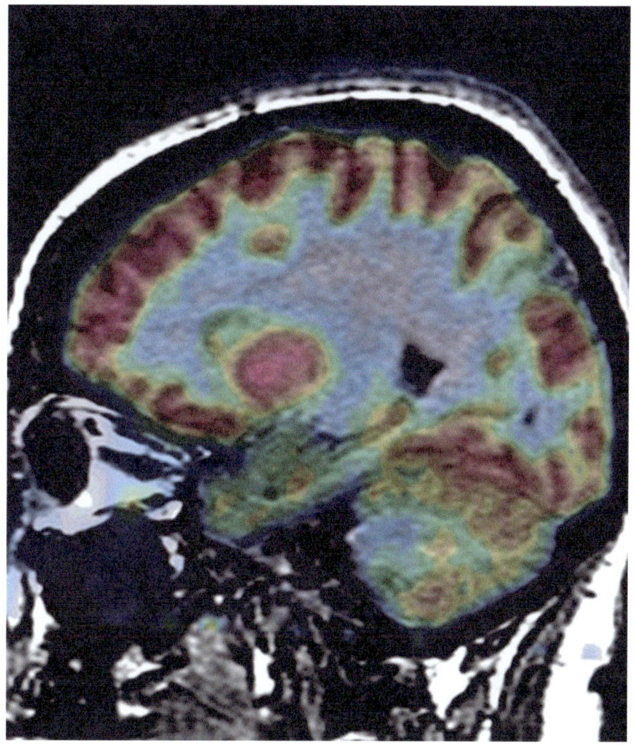

Fig. 54.6 PET-MRI co-registration with color-scale FDG tracer in a sagittal plane at a left hippocampal level. Focal hypometabolism is evident in the left superior parietal lobule and surrounds the triangular, hypointense lesion. No other abnormality is present

55 Dysembryoplastic Neuroepithelial Tumor

Clinical History

The first recognized seizure occurred at age 11 years as an episode of drooling and word repetition. An emergent evaluation at that time identified a left temporal-parietal mass. During the inpatient evaluation because of the mass, a second seizure occurred, had the same initial features, and progressed to bilateral tonic-clonic.

The habitual seizures manifested as an auditory hallucination aura of tones and then either speech arrest with retained awareness for 15 to 75 seconds or speech arrest that progressed to rightward head turning and then a bilateral tonic-clonic seizure. Treatment included multiple anti-seizure medications with a focal seizure frequency that varied from several daily to one every 5 days and a bilateral tonic-clonic seizure frequency that increased over years from none for years to three during 1 month.

The epilepsy risk factor was the temporal-parietal lesion.

Neurological examination identified minor pronunciation difficulty. Neuropsychological testing identified minor deficits in auditory comprehension.

Interictal EEG depicted epileptiform discharges over the left central region. Video-EEG monitoring recorded focal seizures manifested as speech arrest that corresponded to an ictal rhythm of delta activity maximal in the left central region that progressed once to include most of the left hemisphere. One motor seizure was recorded, and this manifested as vocalization with rightward head turning and then bilateral clonic activity. Ictal EEG's seizure onset was generalized rhythmic delta activity.

MRI identified a lesion in the left superior temporal lobe and supramarginal gyrus that has a heterogeneous internal structure and an enhancing ring. PET identified hypometabolism within the lesion. Functional MRI identified bilateral language regions.

The history and evaluation indicate focal seizures with auditory and language features, which suggests a localization in the region of the language dominant hemisphere's posterior temporal lobe. The initial seizures also included salivation, which suggests limbic and possibly insular involvement at that time. Establishing the lateralization was complicated by the fMRI evidence of bilateral language function, and this is likely related to the lesion, as its location may have impacted the lateralization of language during development.

A left temporal-parietal resection with an awake intraoperative language mapping was performed. Histopathological examination identified a low-grade glial neoplasm consistent with a dysembryoplastic neuroepithelial tumor. No postoperative language deficit was present. One seizure occurred at about 6 weeks after surgery, and no additional seizures have occurred over the subsequent 1.5 years.

J. M. Stern, N. Salamon, *Imaging of Epilepsy*, https://doi.org/10.1007/978-3-030-86672-3_55

Imaging

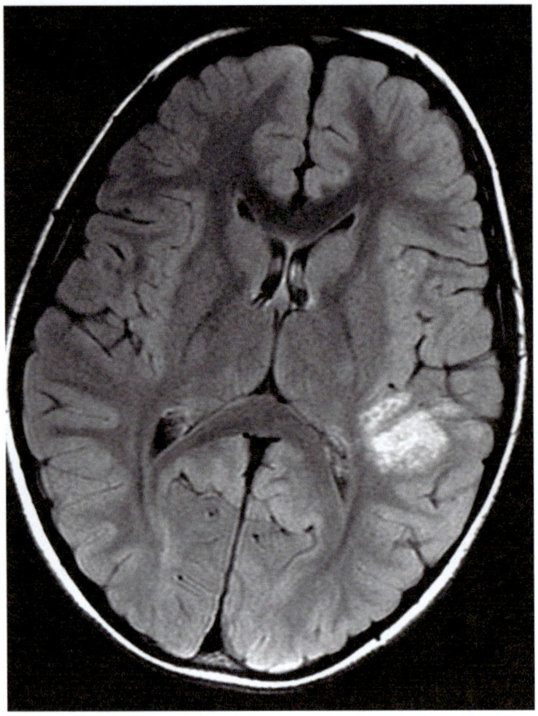

Fig. 55.1 MRI axial FLAIR sequence at a basal ganglia level. A hyperintense lesion is evident in the left Heschl's gyrus, posterior superior temporal gyrus, and supramarginal gyrus. It is not involving the adjacent insula, but it is abutting the optic radiations. The lesion has no surrounding edema or mass effect

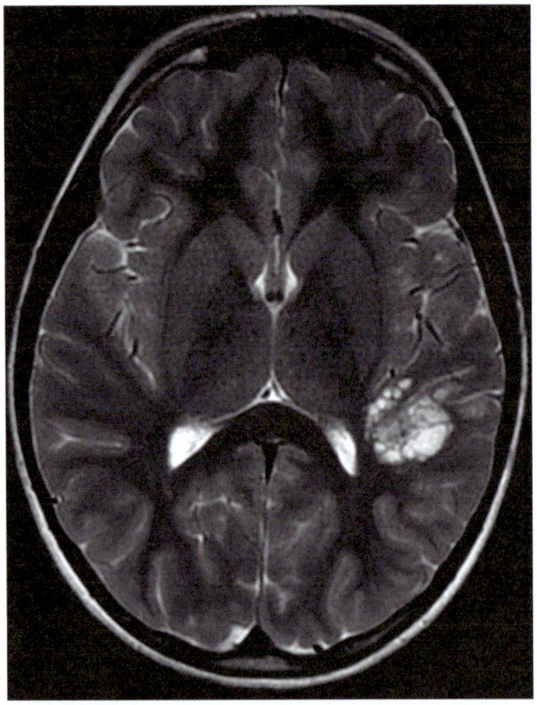

Fig. 55.2 MRI axial T2 sequence at a basal ganglia level slightly inferior to Fig. 55.1. A well-defined, multi-septated, hyperintense lesion is evident in the left Heschl's gyrus and posterior superior temporal gyrus with a heterogenous internal signal. The lesion abuts the insula without involving it. There is no edema or mass effect

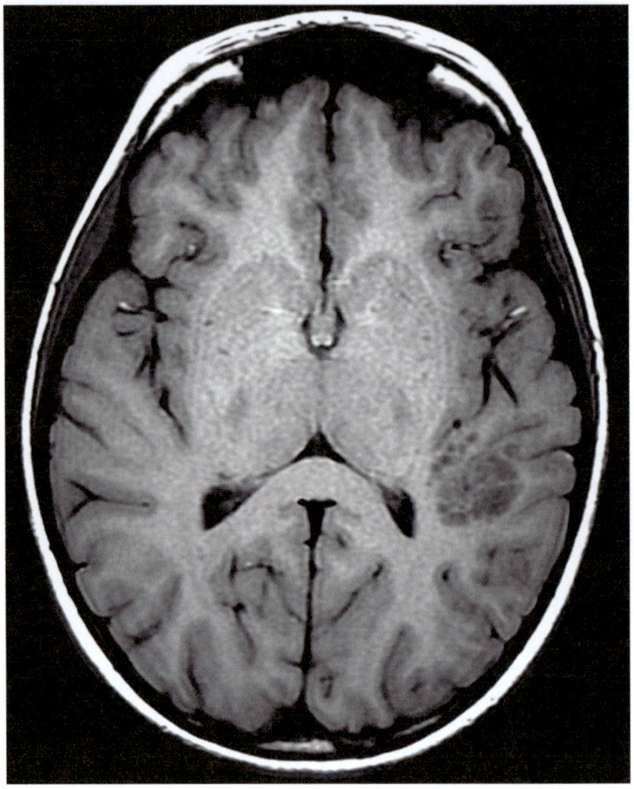

Fig. 55.3 MRI axial T1 sequence at the same basal ganglia level as Fig. 55.2. A hypointense, multi-septated lesion is evident in the left Heschl's gyrus and supramarginal gyrus with an internal signal that has minor heterogeneity. No edema is present

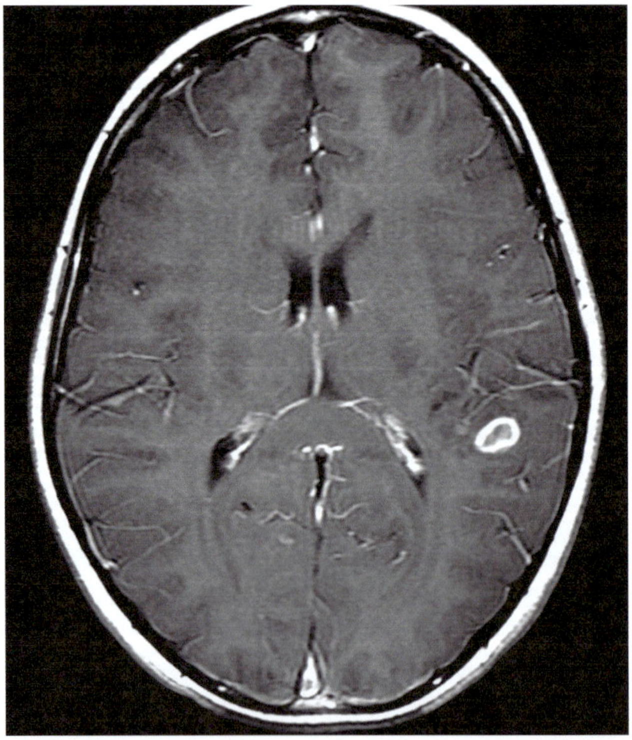

Fig. 55.4 MRI axial T1 sequence after contrast administration at a basal ganglia slightly superior to Figs. 55.2 and 55.3. A ring enhancing lesion is evident in the left supramarginal gyrus. Heschl's gyrus is not involved at this level. No edema is present

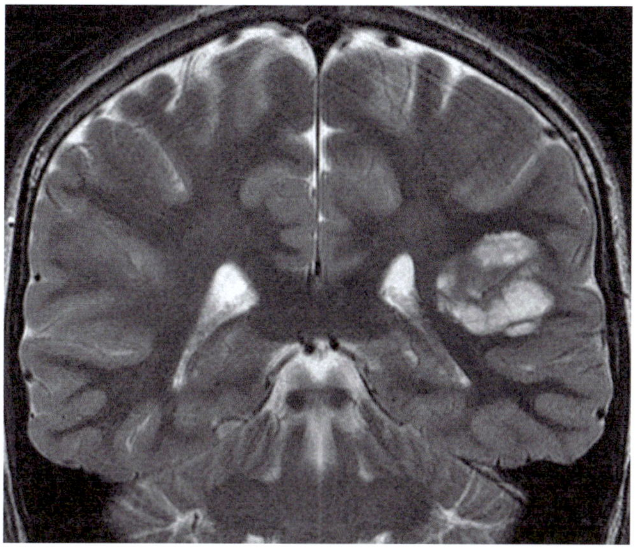

Fig. 55.5 MRI coronal T2 sequence at a splenium of the corpus callosum level. A multi-septated heterogeneous hyperintense lesion is evident in the posterior portion of the left superior temporal gyrus and supramarginal gyrus. No edema is present

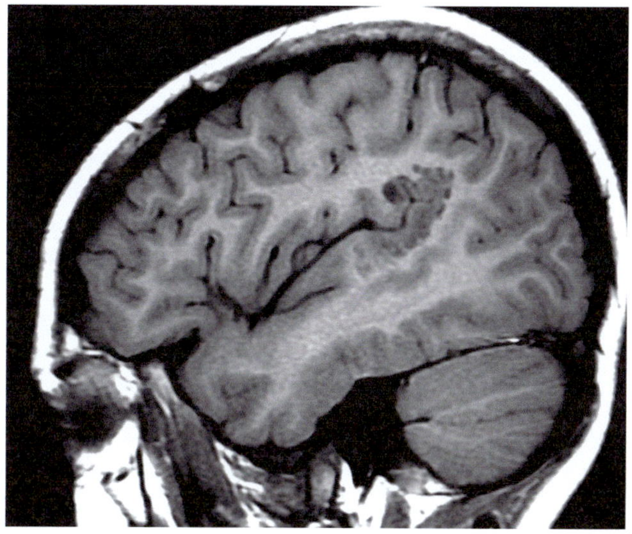

Fig. 55.7 MRI sagittal T1 sequence at a left Sylvian fissure level. A multi-septated, hypointense lesion is evident across the posterior aspect of the Sylvian fissure and involves the u-fibers adjacent to the gray matter. The lesion includes the posterior superior temporal gyrus and the supramarginal gyrus

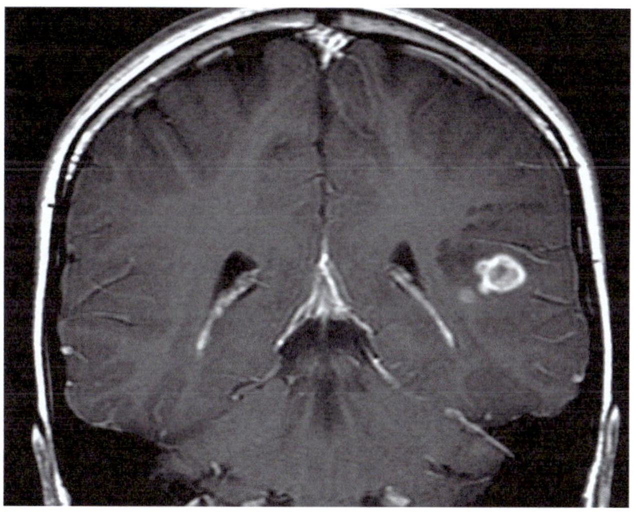

Fig. 55.6 MRI coronal T1 sequence after contrast administration at an atrium of the lateral ventricles level, slightly posterior to Fig. 55.5. A ring enhancing lesion is evident in the left supramarginal gyrus. Hyperintense protrusions medially include an additional ring enhancing abnormalities that indicate septation of the lesion

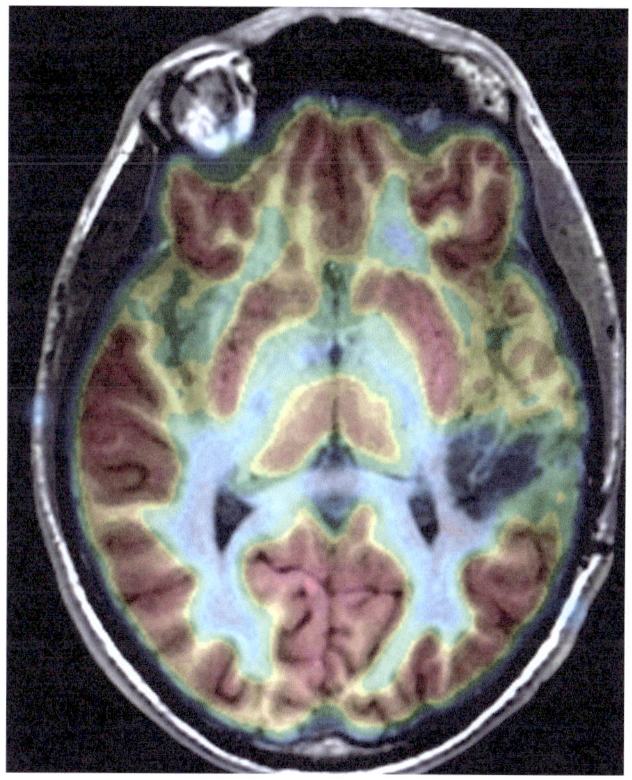

Fig. 55.8 PET-MRI co-registration with color-scale FDG tracer in an axial plane at a basal ganglia level similar to Fig. 55.2. The left superior temporal gyrus is hypometabolic with a more pronounced hypometabolism in its posterior aspect. The thalamus is asymmetric with subtle left-sided hypometabolism. The other cortex and the basal ganglia are normal

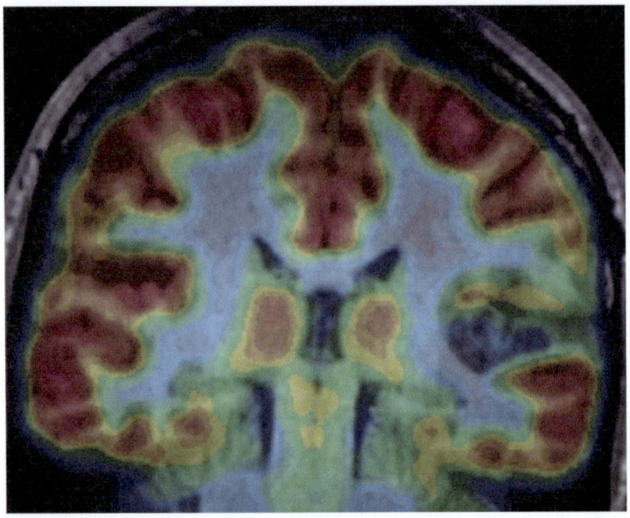

Fig. 55.9 PET-MRI co-registration with color-scale FDG tracer in a coronal plane at a pulvinar level anterior to Fig. 55.5. Hypometabolism is evident in the left parietal operculum and superior temporal gyrus with a visible lesion visible in the left superior temporal gyrus. The left thalamus and the left inferior and mesial temporal lobe also are hypometabolic

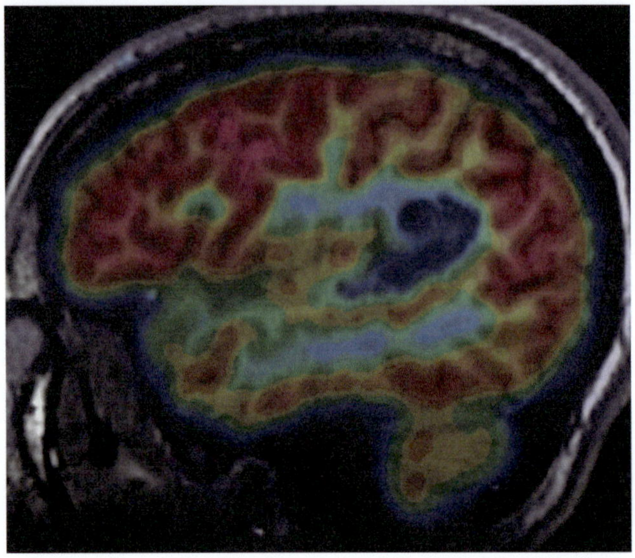

Fig. 55.10 PET-MRI co-registration with color-scale FDG tracer in a sagittal plane at a left Sylvian fissure level similar to Fig. 55.7. The left superior temporal gyrus and supramarginal gyrus are hypometabolic with a region of greater hypometabolism corresponding to the lesion

56 Ganglioglioma of the Mesial Temporal Lobe

Clinical History

The first recognized seizure occurred while in school at age 7 years as suddenly feeling unwell, experiencing a strange taste, and reverting to the foreign language spoken at home. This was followed by staring with facial pallor and then post-ictal sleepiness. In retrospect, the parents realized that the seizures first occurred several years earlier, but they had not recognized them as abnormal. The evaluation at age 7 years identified a right temporal tumor. An intracarotid amobarbital test identified left hemisphere dominance for language, and a tumor resection was performed within weeks of the diagnostic testing. Histopathological examination identified a ganglioglioma with microcalcification. No seizures or auras occurred for several years, and anti-seizure treatment was discontinued.

At about age 10 years, a new habitual seizure first occurred. Initially, the seizures were subtle and brief episodes of anxiety. By age 15 years, they became more intense and prolonged, and medical attention was sought. By then, the manifestation was a combination of anxiety and shivering, left-hand tremor, and brief "blackouts." The anxiety, shivering, and tremor had a duration of minutes, and the "blackouts" were evident in retrospect as amnesia for periods lasting seconds. Treatment included multiple anti-seizure medications with a seizure frequency of several times weekly.

The epilepsy risk factor was a right temporal lobe lesion.

Neurological examination was normal. Scholastic performance was very high.

Interictal EEG after the recurrence of epilepsy with the new habitual seizures depicted frequent epileptiform discharges over the right temporal region. Video-EEG monitoring recorded focal seizures manifested as shivering without an impairment of awareness. The ictal EEG was unchanged from the baseline, interictal EEG.

Postoperative MRI was unchanged at ages 7, 10, and 15 years. Each identified a right anterior temporal lobe resection cavity that extended to the amygdala, no abnormal enhancement, and signal abnormality of the right temporal pole indicating likely focal cortical dysplasia.

Treatment was resumed with the recognition of the seizures and diagnostic testing at age 15 years. Since resuming treatment, seizure freedom has been present for 8 years with monotherapy.

The history and evaluation indicate focal seizures with limbic features at the time of presentation. A tumor resection guided by the tumor's margins was provided upon presentation, and this provided seizure control for several years. The seizures after the seizure recurrence differed in manifestation but also had limbic features, and the interictal EEG supported the prior diagnosis of right mesial temporal lobe epilepsy. However, the ictal EEG did not confirm the diagnosis, as the seizures did not impair awareness so the scalp EEG's sensitivity to the seizures was insufficient to provide the confirmation. Nevertheless, a change to anti-seizure medications led to full seizure control, and the follow-up MRI had no evidence of tumor recurrence, so surgical treatment was not indicated.

J. M. Stern, N. Salamon, *Imaging of Epilepsy*, https://doi.org/10.1007/978-3-030-86672-3_56

Imaging

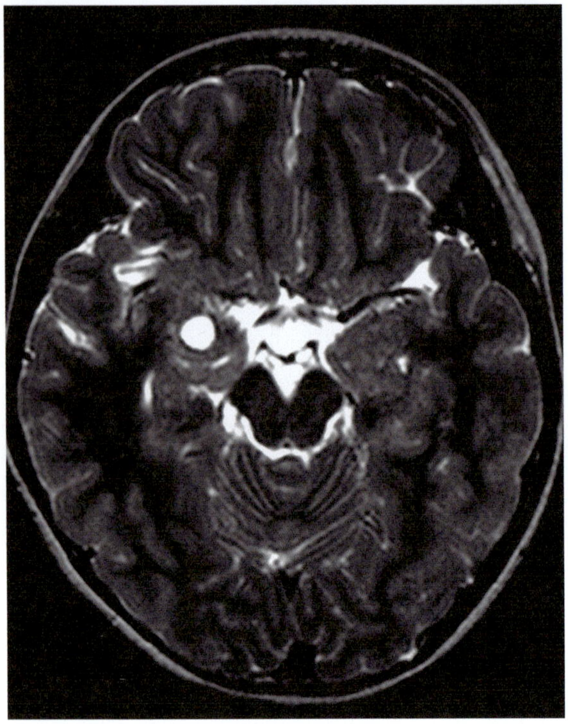

Fig. 56.1 MRI axial T2 sequence at a midbrain level. A round focus of hyperintensity is evident in the right amygdala with distortion of the amygdalar anatomy but no surrounding edema. The right hippocampal head and bilateral lateral temporal lobes are normal

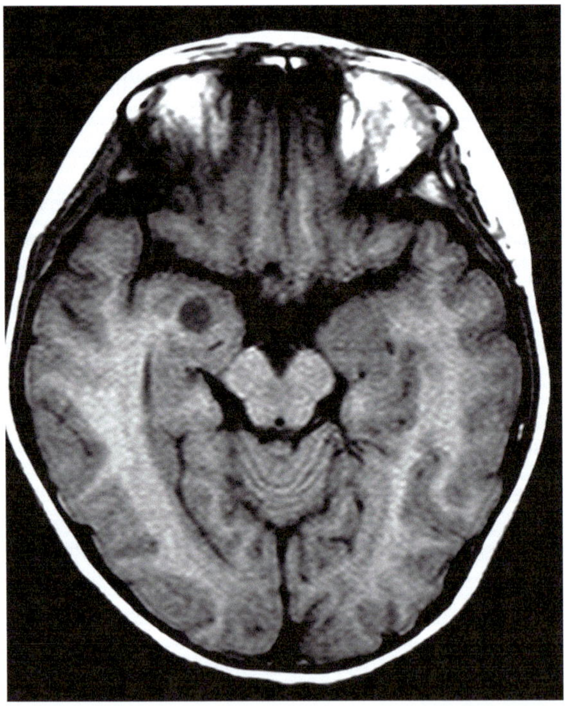

Fig. 56.2 MRI axial T1 sequence at a similar midbrain level as Fig. 56.1. A round hypointense lesion is in the right amygdala. No edema is present. The remainder of the right temporal lobe is normal

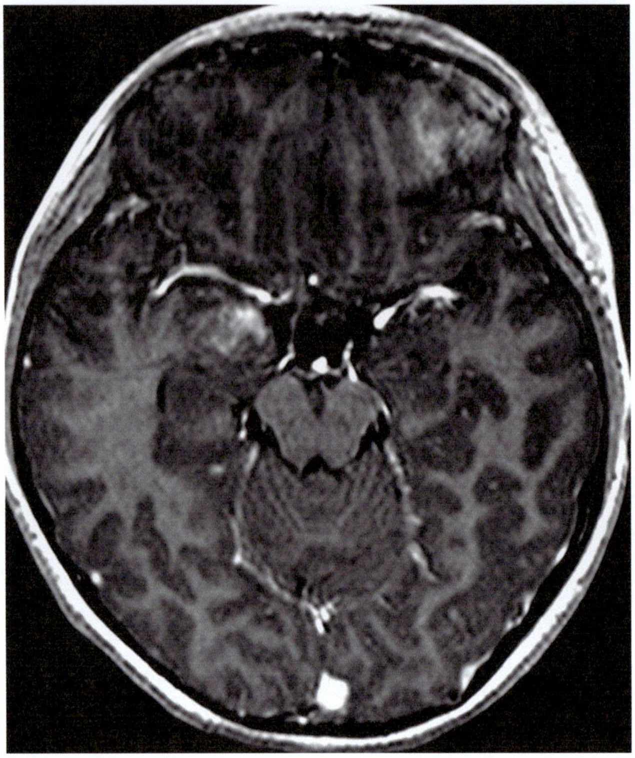

Fig. 56.3 MRI axial T1 sequence after contrast administration at the same midbrain level as Fig. 56.1. The round right amygdalar lesion has heterogeneous enhancement. No other abnormal enhancement is present

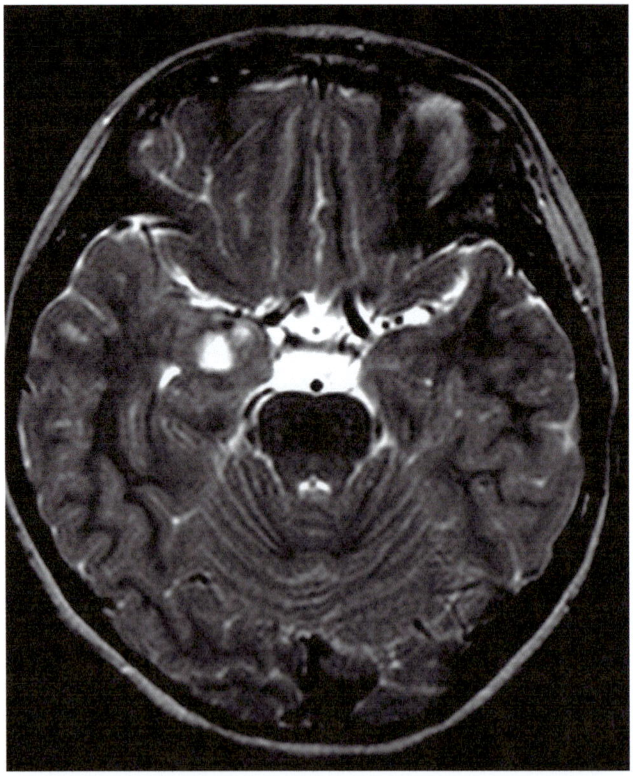

Fig. 56.4 MRI axial T2 sequence at a pons level. Mixed intensity signal is evident in the round lesion within the right amygdala with evidence of a solid component in the anterior portion. The posterior-lateral portion has homogeneously hyperintense signal, which suggests fluid, but the T1 sequence in Fig. 56.5 indicates a mixed composition

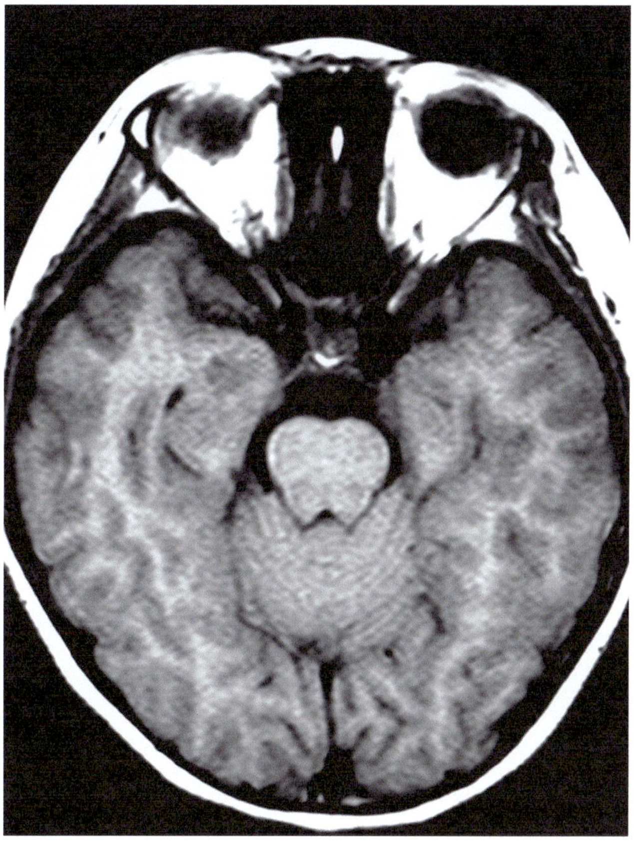

Fig. 56.5 MRI axial T1 sequence at a pons level similar to Fig. 56.4. Subtle hypointense signal is evident within the right amygdala. The lack of clear hypointensity suggests a mixed composition instead of fluid. The amygdala's external contour is anatomically normal

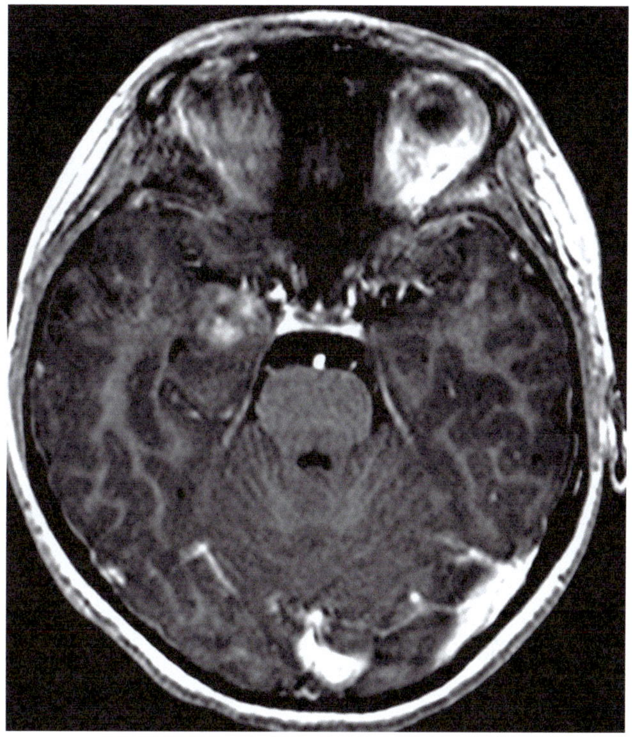

Fig. 56.6 MRI axial T1 sequence after contrast administration at the same pons level as Fig. 56.5. Heterogeneous enhancement is evident in the right amygdala with extension of enhancement to the amygdala's anterior surface. This distribution of the enhancement indicates that the lesion is larger than it appears with the T1 sequence before contrast administration or with the T2 sequence

Ganglioglioma of the Lateral Temporal Lobe

57

Clinical History

The first recognized seizure occurred at age 13 years as a loss of consciousness with a generalized convulsion. An evaluation at that time identified a right temporal lobe lesion.

The habitual seizures never followed an aura and manifested as clenching of the left hand with head turning to the left, followed by left hemibody shaking and loss of consciousness. The seizure duration was seconds with postictal fatigue and word finding difficulty for several additional seconds. Seizures usually occurred at the time of sleep onset. Treatment included multiple anti-seizure medications with a seizure frequency that was initially one to two weekly and increased to one daily after a few months.

The epilepsy risk factor was a right temporal lobe lesion.

Neurological examination was normal. Neuropsychological testing identified borderline cognitive performance with disproportionately greater deficits in visuospatial functioning. Verbal and nonverbal memory was intact.

Interictal EEG depicted epileptiform discharges during sleep broadly distributed across the right frontal-temporal region. Video-EEG monitoring recorded focal seizures manifested as impaired awareness that sometimes progressed to left-sided clonus. Ictal EEG's seizure onset was broad and spanned the right temporal lobe.

MRI identified a multilobulated, enhancing, cortically based lesion in the right superior temporal lobe. PET identified hypometabolism within the right superior temporal gyrus. Functional MRI depicted left-sided language dominance with bilateral activation in Wernicke's area.

The history and evaluation indicate focal seizures lateralized to the right hemisphere that occurred without auras and have quick postictal recovery. These features and the broad EEG abnormality that extends to the right frontal lobe are consistent with the superior temporal lobe lesion on MRI. The cognitive testing further supported a right hemispheric abnormality but also demonstrated normal mesial temporal lobe function. Based on the functional and structural findings, the epileptogenic zone was localized to the region of the lesion without inclusion of the mesial temporal lobe.

A right temporal lobe resection with sparing of the mesial structures was performed. Histopathological examination identified a ganglioglioma described as a glial tumor with dysplastic, binucleate ganglioid cells. No seizures or auras have occurred for the 2.5 years since surgery. Anti-seizure medications were tapered to discontinuation 2 years after surgery.

J. M. Stern, N. Salamon, *Imaging of Epilepsy*, https://doi.org/10.1007/978-3-030-86672-3_57

Imaging

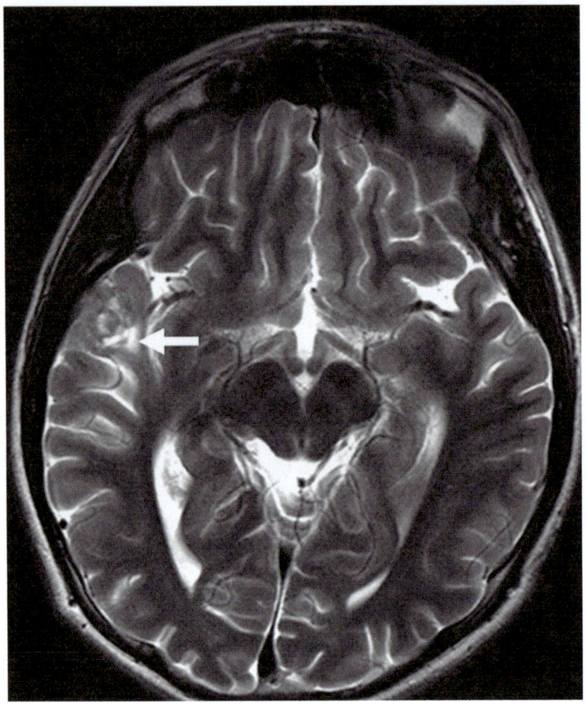

Fig. 57.1 MRI axial T2 sequence at a midbrain level. A heterogeneous signal lesion is evident in the right anterior superior temporal gyrus' gray matter with hyperintense signal extending medially into the white matter (arrow). The lesion has no surrounding edema and does not produce mass effect

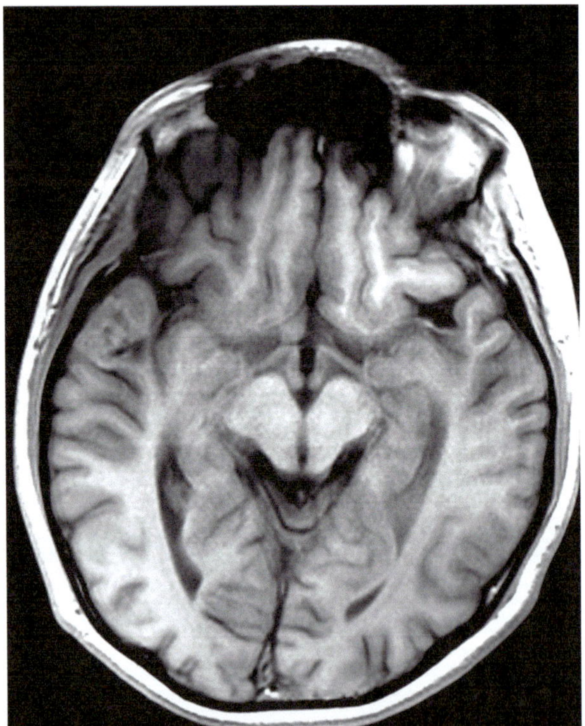

Fig. 57.2 MRI axial T1 sequence at the same midbrain level as Fig. 57.1. A heterogeneous signal intensity lesion is within the right anterior superior temporal gyrus. A hypointense signal is within the adjacent white matter and corresponds to Fig. 57.1's T2 hyperintense signal abnormality

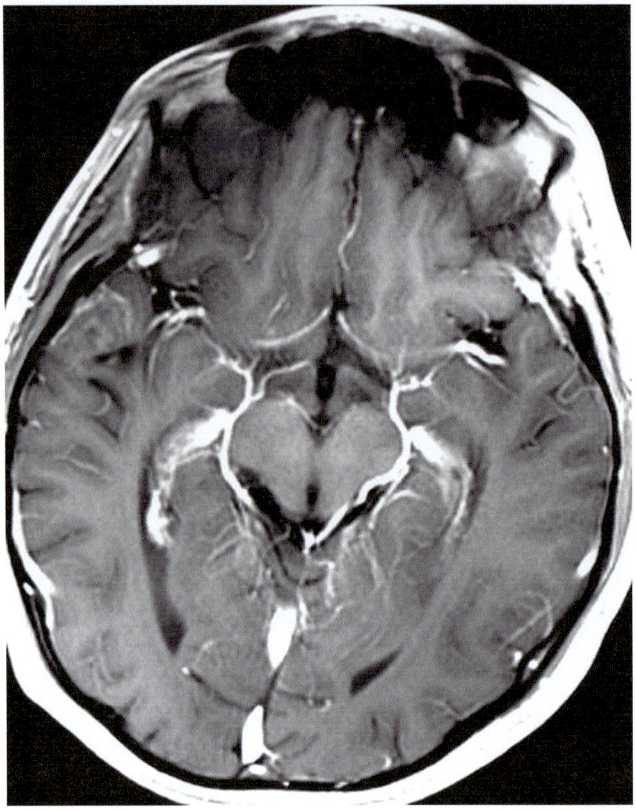

Fig. 57.3 MRI axial T1 sequence after contrast administration at the same midbrain level as Figs. 57.1 and 57.2. Abnormal enhancement is evident along the periphery of the right superior temporal gyrus' lesion. This pial surface hyperintensity suggests a vascular-based enhancement overlying the mass. No enhancement is within the lesion, and there is no other abnormal enhancement

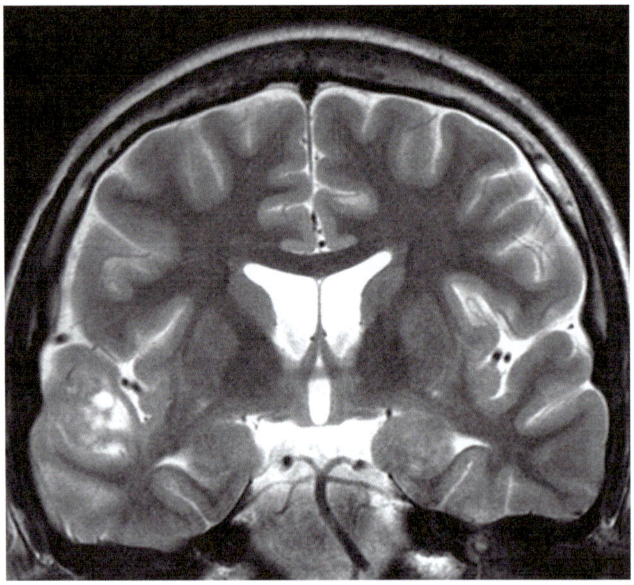

Fig. 57.4 MRI coronal T2 sequence at an amygdala level. An expansile heterogeneous lesion is evident in the right superior temporal gyrus. The lesion's lateral aspect has solid components, and medial aspect has a cystic component with hyperintense T2 signal. The remainder of the right temporal lobe is normal

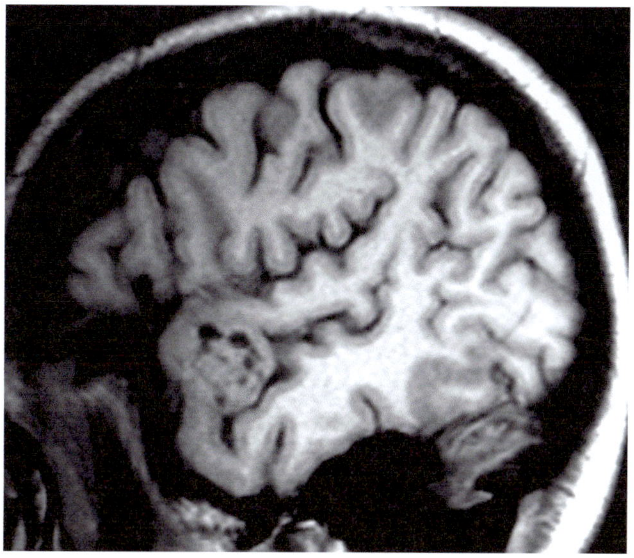

Fig. 57.5 MRI sagittal T1 sequence at a right Sylvian fissure level. An expansile heterogeneous lesion is evident in the right superior temporal gyrus with multiple, internal cystic components that are isointense to cerebrospinal fluid (CSF)

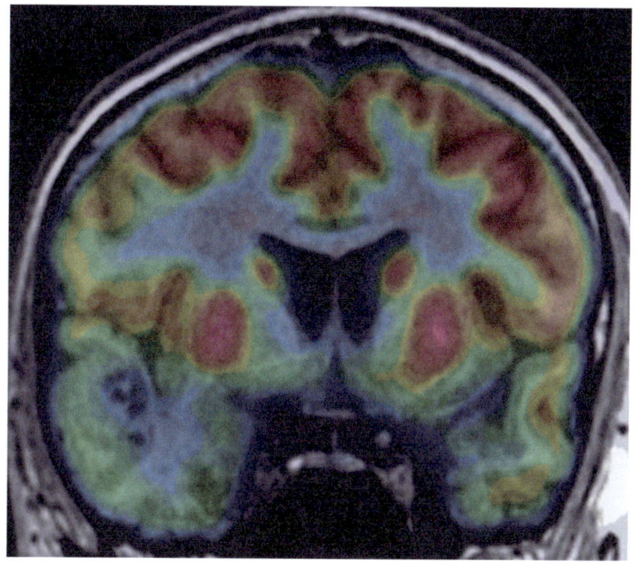

Fig. 57.7 PET-MRI co-registration with color-scale FDG tracer in a coronal plane at amygdala level similar to Fig. 57.4. A hypometabolic lesion is evident in the right superior temporal gyrus with an internal region of greater hypometabolism. The right temporal lobe is abnormal due to asymmetrically greater hypometabolism, compared to the left temporal lobe. This includes the right temporal lobe's lateral and inferior aspects. The minor metabolic asymmetry to the lateral frontal lobes and caudates is normal

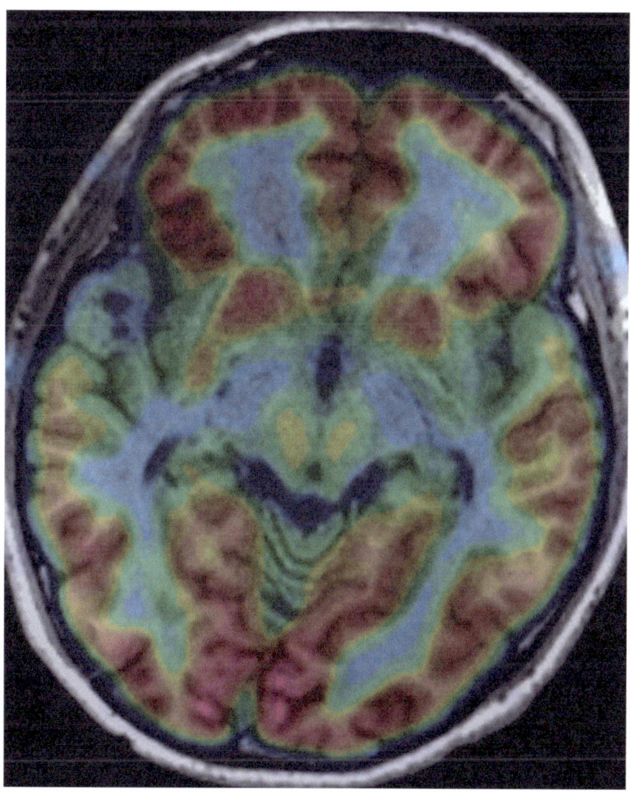

Fig. 57.6 PET-MRI co-registration with color-scale FDG tracer in an axial plane at a similar midbrain level as Figs. 57.1 and 57.2. The anterior portion of the right superior temporal gyrus is hypometabolic with greater hypometabolism within the lesion. The right temporal lobe beyond the lesion is normal. The left temporal lobe and bilateral insulae also are normal

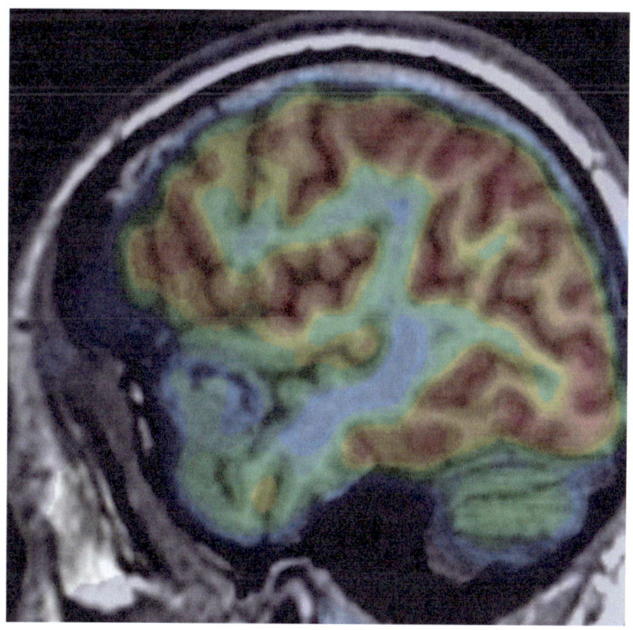

Fig. 57.8 PET-MRI co-registration with color-scale FDG tracer in a sagittal plane at a right Sylvian fissure level. A hypometabolic lesion is evident in the anterior superior temporal gyrus with mixed metabolic signal within the lesion

Hamartoma

58

Clinical History

The first recognized seizure occurred at age 7 years as a 2-minute episode of loss of consciousness with tonic-clonic activity of all limbs. An evaluation at that time included EEG and MRI that are recalled by the parents as normal.

A second tonic-clonic seizure occurred 2 months after the first, and treatment was then begun. The evaluation that followed the second seizure included a more detailed MRI, and this depicted a hypothalamic hamartoma. Upon discussing the finding with the parents, a history of spontaneous "giggles" was obtained. These episodes occurred since infancy with durations of 10 to 15 seconds followed by fatigue or sleep. Not recognizing the abnormality, the giggles were interpreted by the parents as a sign of fatigue or sleepiness. Prior to treatment, the giggle episode frequency was about two times daily. Treatment included multiple anti-seizure medications without significant change to the giggle episodes, but no tonic-clonic seizures occurred after beginning anti-seizure medications.

The epilepsy risk factor was a hypothalamic hamartoma.

Neurological examination was normal. School performance has produced high grades. Medical history was normal.

Interictal EEG depicted occasional right central-parietal epileptiform discharges that were activated by sleep. Video-EEG monitoring recorded focal seizures during wakefulness manifested as giggling without motor abnormality. For these seizures, ictal EEG's seizure onset was a gradual emergence of bifrontal slowing for 20 to 25 seconds. Focal seizures during sleep produced arousal with a facial expression of fear or bewilderment followed by leftward gaze, oral automatisms, and leftward jerks of the head. For the nocturnal seizures, ictal EEG's seizure onset was generalized, polymorphic slowing with gradually resolution.

MRI identified a non-enhancing mass in the posterior hypothalamus. PET identified no abnormality.

The history and evaluation indicate gelastic epilepsy, as evident in the seizures of mechanical laughter without amusement and the identification of a hypothalamic hamartoma. The seizures' lateralizing behavioral features do not preclude the hypothalamic epileptogenic lesion as the features may instead indicate a right-sided propagation pathway and not necessarily the seizure onset zone. The broad, nonfocal EEG findings are consistent with the deep location of the seizure onset zone and provide further support for an epileptogenic hamartoma.

A stereotactic interstitial laser ablation of the hamartoma was performed. No seizures have occurred for 2 years since surgery, and anti-seizure medications have been reduced to monotherapy.

J. M. Stern, N. Salamon, *Imaging of Epilepsy*, https://doi.org/10.1007/978-3-030-86672-3_58

Imaging

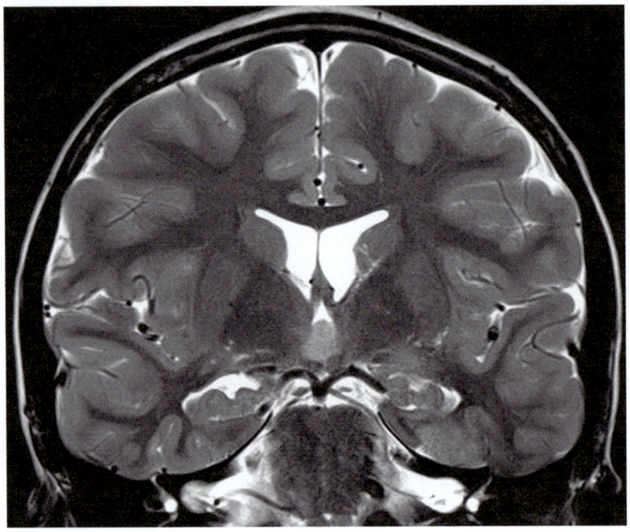

Fig. 58.1 MRI coronal T2 sequence at a hippocampal head level. A mass within the third ventricle has homogeneous signal intensity that is isointense to the gray matter. Mass effect is evident with compression of the right mammillary body present. The linear hyperintensity within the left caudate relates to a remote, minor infarction. The hippocampi and ventricles are bilaterally normal

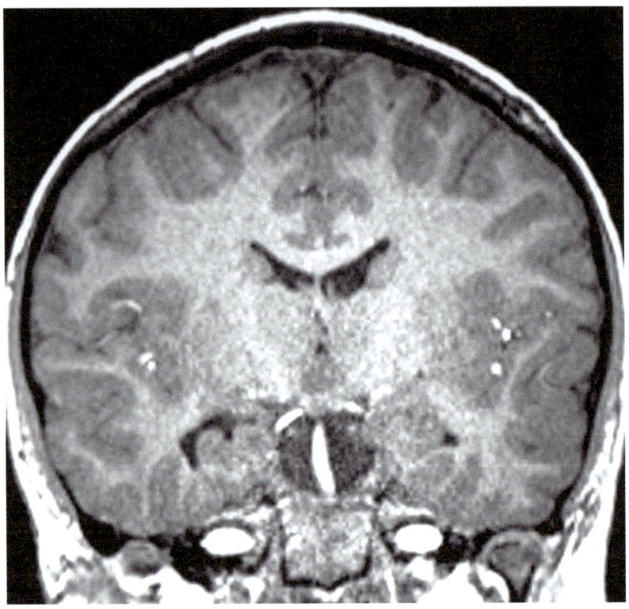

Fig. 58.2 MRI coronal T1 sequence at a similar hippocampal head level as Fig. 58.1. The mass within the third ventricle is isointense to gray matter and less apparent than with a T2 sequence. The cortical ribbon and gray white junction are normal. Slightly tilting of the imaging level gives the appearance of hippocampal asymmetry, but no abnormality is present

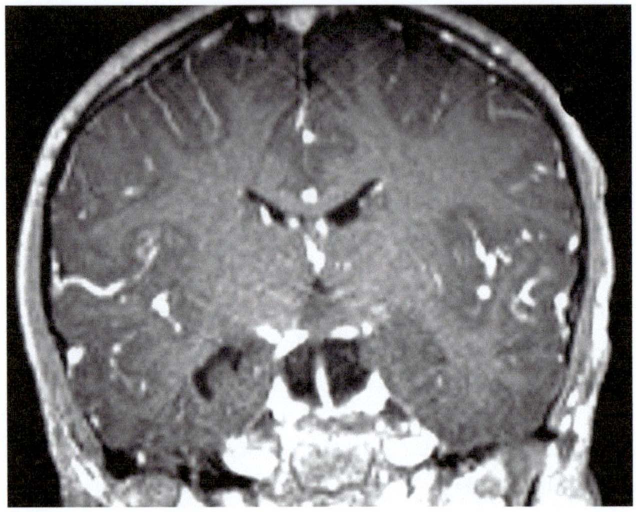

Fig. 58.3 MRI coronal T1 sequence after contrast administration at the same hippocampal head level as Fig. 58.2. The mass within the third ventricle does not enhance. No abnormal enhancement is present elsewhere

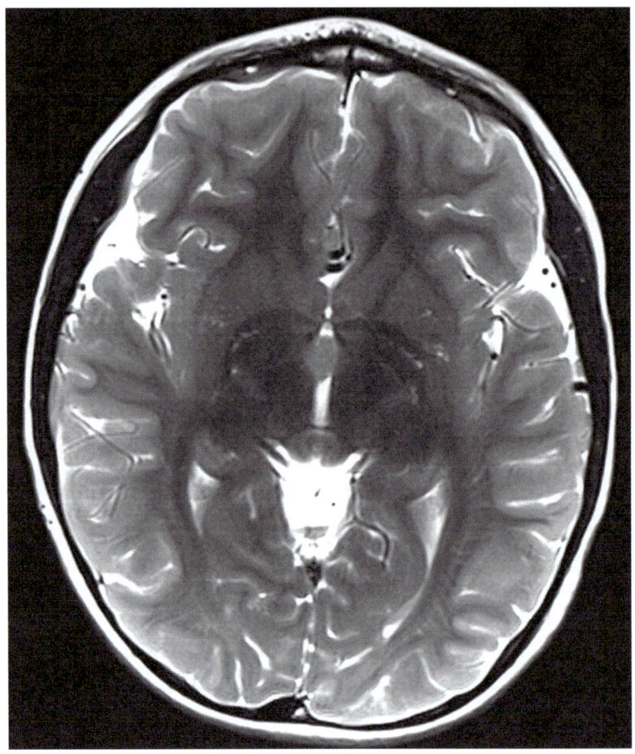

Fig. 58.4 MRI axial T2 sequence at a basal ganglia level. An oblong mass is evident in the anterior portion of the third ventricle and is isointense to gray matter. No edema is present around the mass

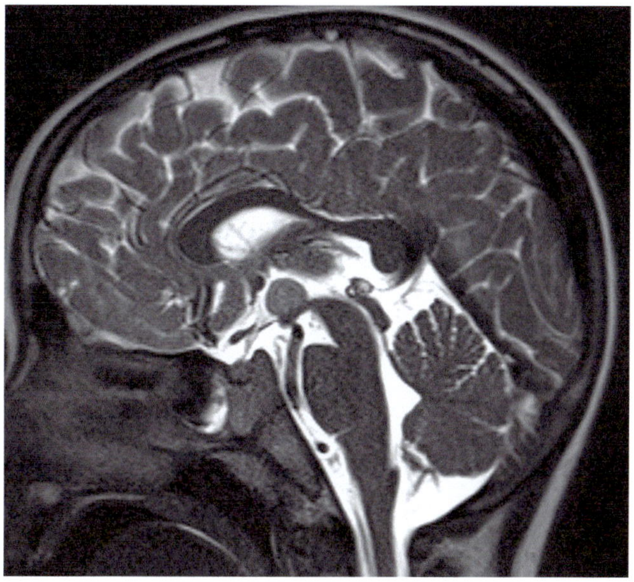

Fig. 58.5 MRI sagittal T2 sequence at a midline of the corpus callosum level. A round mass is evident superior to the mammillary body and projecting into the third ventricle without obstruction of the ventricular system. No other abnormality is present

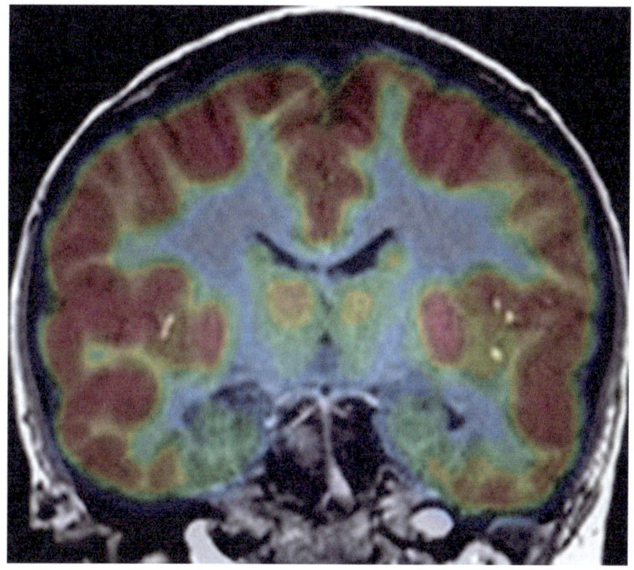

Fig. 58.7 PET-MRI co-registration with color-scale FDG tracer in a coronal plane at the same hippocampal head level as Figs. 58.2 and 58.3. The mass within the third ventricle has a metabolic signal similar to white matter. The hippocampi and bilateral frontal and temporal cortex are normal and symmetric

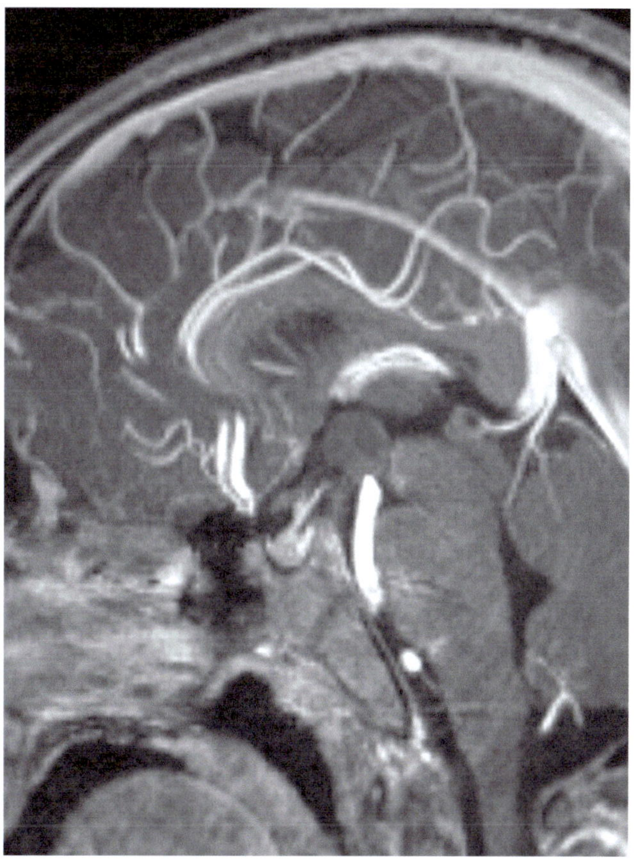

Fig. 58.6 MRI sagittal T1 sequence after contrast administration at the same midline of the corpus callosum level as Fig. 58.5. The round mass superior to the mammillary body does not enhance. No abnormal enhancement is present elsewhere

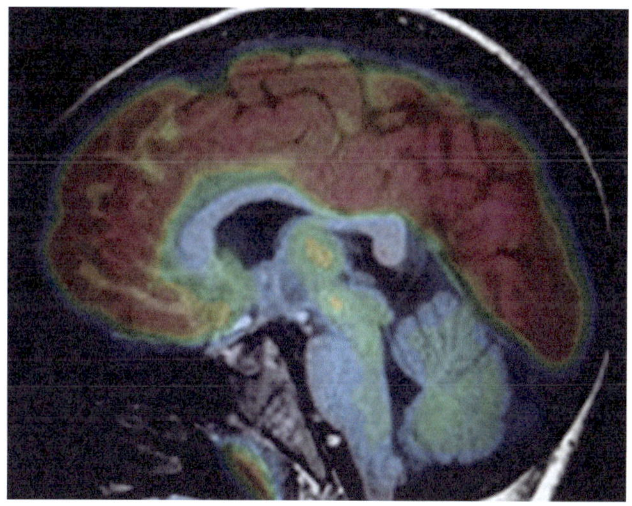

Fig. 58.8 PET-MRI co-registration with color-scale FDG tracer in a sagittal plane at a midline of the corpus callosum level similar to Figs. 58.5 and 58.6. A round mass is superior to the mammillary body and has a low metabolic signal that is lower than the corpus callosum

Meningioma

59

Clinical History

The first recognized seizure occurred at age 28 years as a subtle feeling of fear that lasted seconds. The manifestation progressed over months to episodes with greater intensity and duration. After presentation at this later time, anxiety disorder was diagnosed, and a benzodiazepine treatment began that produced a minor benefit. After the benzodiazepine was discontinued, episodes of urinary incontinence developed. During a urologic evaluation for the incontinence, an episode with impairmed awareness was witnessed, and the urologist provided the diagnosis of seizures.

The habitual seizures manifested as a sense of fear with an epigastric rising sensation that is followed by a gasp, confusion, rightward head turning, and urinary incontinence. Rarely, a seizure produced a fall, but none of the seizures have progressed to convulsive motor features. The typical duration was about 10 seconds, and the postictal state was anxiety without confusion. The period of impairment was not perceived, but recollection of each seizure was possible because of the aura. Treatment included multiple anti-seizure medications with a seizure frequency of one to three daily with up to five seizures in one day. However, no seizures have occurred over the 9 months after a change to anti-seizure medications was provided during the epilepsy surgery evaluation.

The epilepsy risk factor was a right petroclival meningioma that was diagnosed at age 32 years and was first symptomatic at age 28 years with diplopia right facial numberless, and the seizures. Radiation treatment at age 33 years led to resolution of the diplopia and numbness, and the seizures. Radiation treatment at age 33 years led to resolution of the diplopia and numbness but no change to the seizures.

Neurological examination was normal.

Interictal EEG depicted frequent epileptiform discharges over the right anterior temporal region. Video-EEG monitoring recorded focal seizures manifested as a facial expression change suggesting discomfort followed by oral automatisms and sometimes manual automatisms. Ictal EEG's seizure onset for five seizures was focal rhythmic slowing across the right anterior temporal region. Two behaviorally identical seizures had a seizure onset across the left anterior temporal region, and these followed seizures with a right-sided ictal onset pattern by less than 2 hours. Additional episodes were auras of anxiety without progression to impaired awareness, and their EEG correlates varied from no change to subtle right anterior temporal rhythmic slowing.

MRI at the time of the epilepsy evaluation at age 41 years identified a large right petroclival, extra-axial lesion with mass effect on the right mesial temporal lobe. PET identified hypometabolism of the right parahippocampal gyrus.

The history and evaluation indicate focal seizures with a limbic aura but brief duration and quick recovery. As such, the seizures have features of both limbic and neocortical epileptogenic zones. The EEG suggests a right temporal lobe epilepsy. The occurrence of two left-sided seizures may be related to the brief time after right temporal lobe seizures and the clustering phenomenon. The imaging provides an anatomic diagnosis with evidence of a meningioma compressing the parahippocampal gyrus with apparent production of an anterior-mesial temporal lobe seizure. Surgical treatment has been deferred and will ultimately depend on continued seizure control and the effects of the meningioma.

J. M. Stern, N. Salamon, *Imaging of Epilepsy*, https://doi.org/10.1007/978-3-030-86672-3_59

Imaging

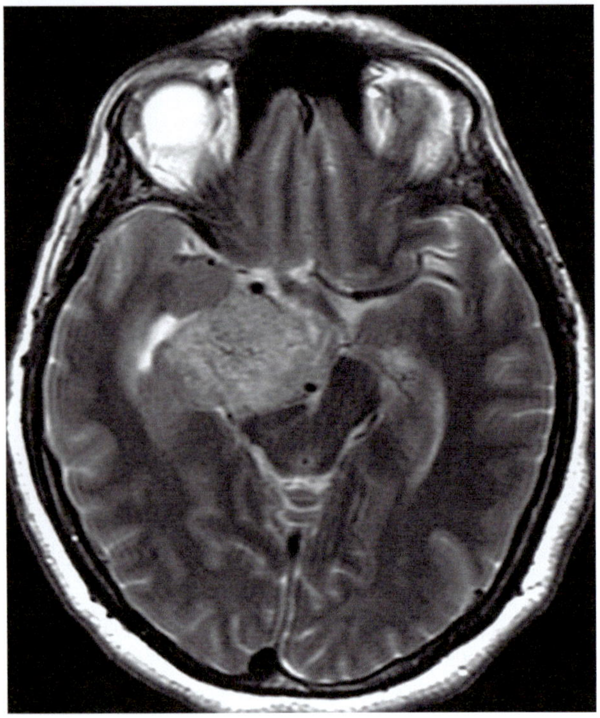

Fig. 59.1 MRI axial T2 sequence at a hippocampal head level. A hyperintense extra-axial mass is medial to right hippocampus and anterior to midbrain. It is displacing the basilar artery posterior-medially and abutting the right internal carotid artery terminus anteriorly. No edema is evident in the mesial temporal lobe or midbrain. The mass is hypointense internally, which suggests hypervascularity. The right hippocampus is displaced laterally but has normal signal and volume

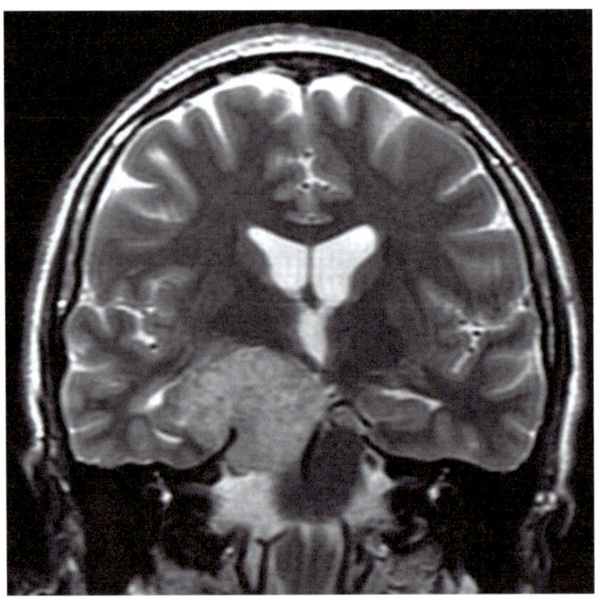

Fig. 59.2 MRI coronal T2 sequence at a hippocampal head level. An extra-axial mass is evident at the edge of the right tentorium with displacement of the basal forebrain and compression of the mammillary body superiorly. The right hippocampal head is compressed by the mass and vertically oriented but has normal signal. The basilar artery is displaced laterally. The third ventricle is deformed but is not obstructing cerebrospinal fluid (CSF) flow, as hydrocephalus is not present. The left hippocampus is normal

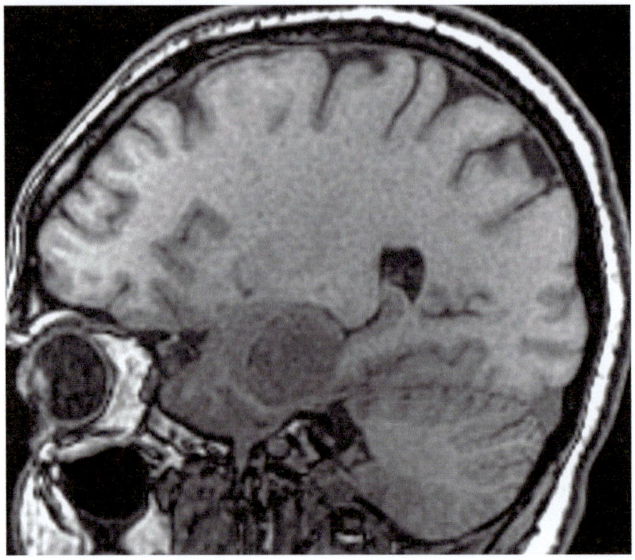

Fig. 59.3 MRI sagittal T1 sequence at a right hippocampus level. A well-defined, extra-axial, homogeneously hypointense mass is evident adjacent to the temporal horn of the right lateral ventricle with displacement of the right hippocampus and parahippocampal gyrus. No internal hemorrhage is evident within the mass

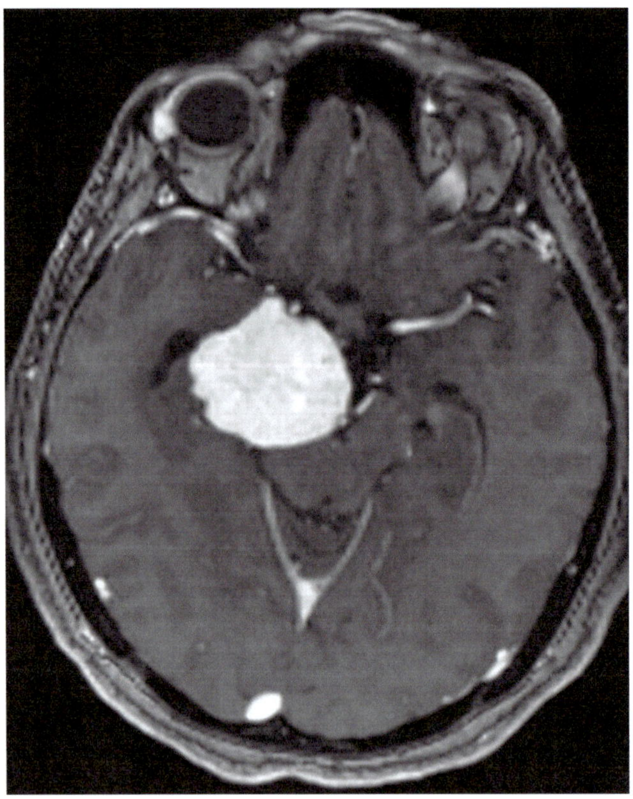

Fig. 59.4 MRI axial T1 sequence after contrast administration at the level as Fig. 59.1. Homogeneous, abnormal enhancement is evident within the extra-axial mass that is medial to the right hippocampus. No other abnormal enhancement is present. The normal enhancement of the vessels highlights the mass touching the right internal carotid artery terminus anteriorly and the basilar artery posterior-laterally

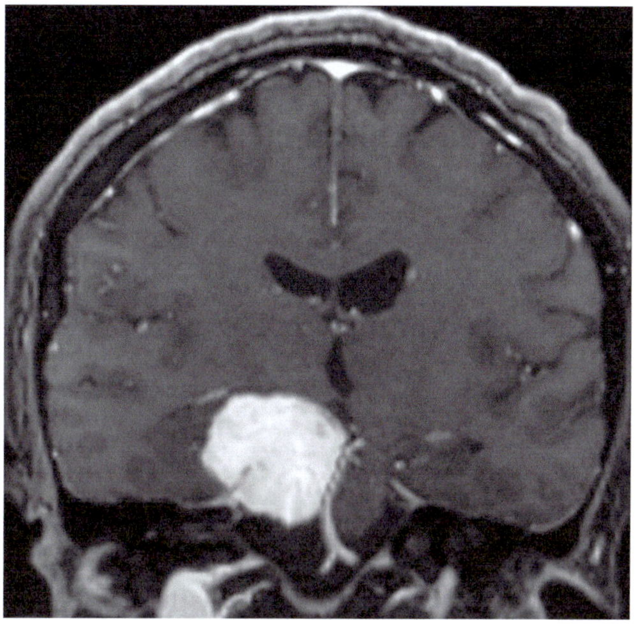

Fig. 59.5 MRI coronal T1 sequence after contrast administration at the same hippocampal head level as Fig. 59.2. A homogeneously enhancing mass is evident in the right mesial temporal region along the right tentorium. The enhancement includes a small tail along the tentorium's dura lateral to the mass, which suggests a meningioma. No edema or other abnormal enhancement is present. The basilar artery is displaced but patent

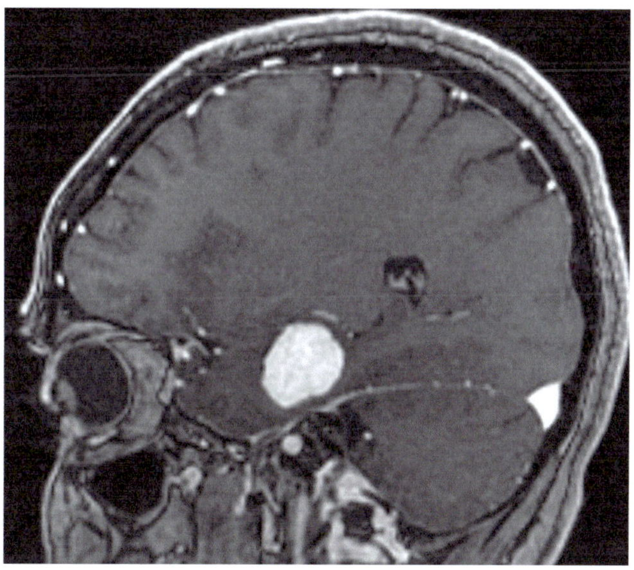

Fig. 59.6 MRI sagittal T1 sequence after contrast administration at a right hippocampus level. A homogeneously enhancing mass is evident along the temporal horn of the right lateral ventricle. No surrounding edema or other abnormal enhancement is present

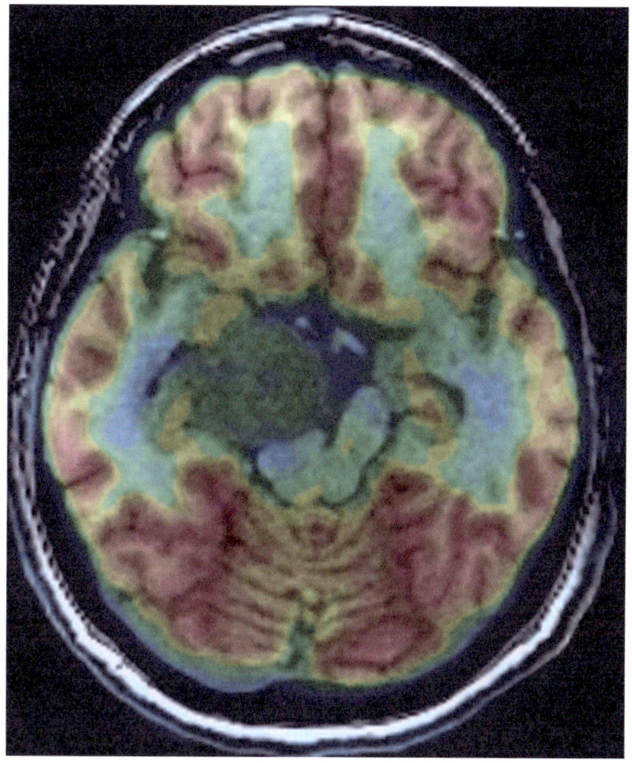

Fig. 59.7 PET-MRI co-registration with color-scale FDG tracer in an axial plane at a level slightly superior to Figs. 59.1 and 59.4. The right medial temporal region extra-axial mass does not demonstrate hypometabolism. The adjacent mesial and lateral temporal lobe is symmetric to the left mesial and lateral temporal lobe

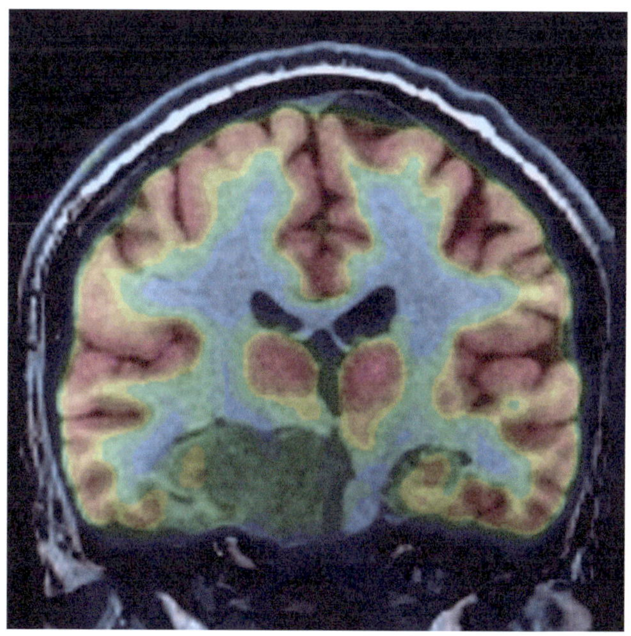

Fig. 59.8 PET-MRI co-registration with color-scale FDG tracer in a coronal plane at a level similar to Figs. 59.2 and 59.5. The extra-axial mass in the right medial temporal region is hypometabolic. The adjacent right hippocampus and right lateral temporal lobe are metabolically normal and symmetric to the left-sided structures, but the right parahippocampal gyrus is hypometabolic compared to left parahippocampal gyrus. The thalamus is symmetric and normal

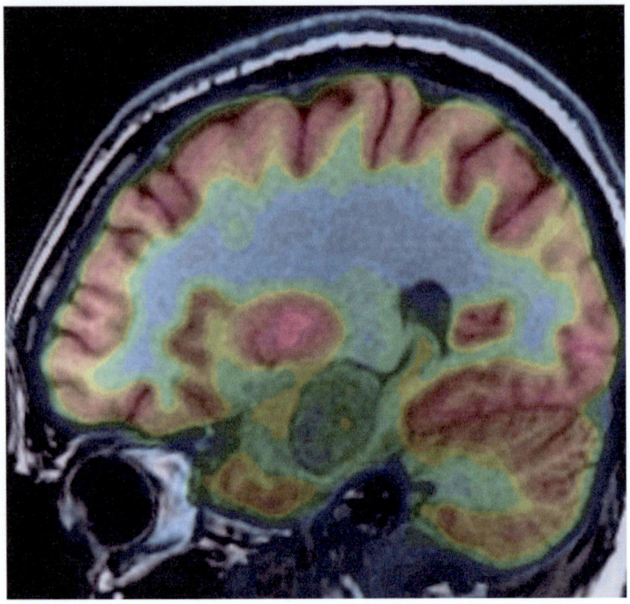

Fig. 59.9 PET-MRI co-registration with color-scale FDG tracer in a sagittal plane at the same right hippocampus level as Figs. 59.3 and 59.6. The extra-axial mass adjacent to the temporal horn of the right lateral ventricle is hypometabolic, as is the right parahippocampal gyrus inferior to the mass. The temporal pole is normal

Part VII

Tuberous Sclerosis

Tuberous sclerosis
Tuber
Subependymal nodular heterotopia
Subependymal giant cell astrocytoma

In children and adults with tuberous sclerosis complex (TSC), tubers at the cortex or the subcortical region are usually hypointense with T1-weighted and hyperintense with T2-weighted MRI, but the signal features differ during infancy. Before age 3 months, tubers are hyperintense with T1-weighted MRI and closer to isointense with T2-weighting, especially before white matter myelination. At about age 6 months, tubers are isointense with both the T1-weighted and T2-weighted imaging. After age 8 months, the child and adult pattern is present. Regardless of age, contrast enhancement may be present, and the apparent diffusion coefficient (ADC) of surrounding tissue may be increased. Occasionally, cysts are present within tubers. With CT, tubers are hypodense, sometimes include calcification, and rarely enhance. FDG PET depicts the tubers as hypometabolic. Epileptogenic tubers often have similar appearance, but they may have lower tracer update and a larger area of surrounding hypometabolism. Cerebellar tubers are present for about half of patients with TSC. The cerebellar tubers may expand and have internal changes, and sometimes they develop abnormal vessels that can cause hemorrhage.

Subependymal nodules have variable signal and often have hyperintense T1-weighted and isointense T2-weighted signal that differs from normal gray matter signal. Calcification is common with about 90% having this feature by adulthood. Although, subependymal nodules can be evident by age 6 months, calcification is not present in early childhood. Enhancement is variable and is not a useful feature in distinguishing subependymal nodules from subependymal giant cell astrocytomas (SEGAs). However, SEGAs tend to have intense enhancement. Ultimately, only serial imaging and evidence of growth can reliably identify the lesion as a SEGA. SEGAs have a peak occurrence between ages 8 and 18 years and tend to be large if present for years because of their growth.

Additional white matter abnormality occurs in TSC and has a variable appearance. Often the abnormality is nodular, ill-defined, or cystic. Band-like lesions with a radial migration appearance is relatively specific for TSC.

Key References

Chan DL, Calder T, Lawson JA, Mowat D, Kennedy SE. The natural history of subependymal giant cell astrocytomas in tuberous sclerosis complex: a review. Rev Neurosci. 2018;29:295–301.

Krishnan A, Kaza RK, Vummidi D. Cross-sectional imaging review of tuberous sclerosis. Radiol Clin North Am. 2016;54:423–40.

Russo C, Nastro A, Cicala D, De Liso M, Covelli EM, Cinalli G. Neuroimaging in tuberous sclerosis complex. Childs Nerv Syst. 2020;36:2497–509.

Sun K, Cui J, Wang B, et al. Magnetic resonance imaging of tuberous sclerosis complex with or without epilepsy at 7 T. Neuroradiology. 2018;60:785–94.

Tubers of Tuberous Sclerosis

60

Clinical History

The first recognized seizures occurred at age 4 months as infantile spasms. A head CT at that time identified tubers and provided the diagnosis of tuberous sclerosis. After an anti-seizure medication failed to produce seizure freedom, ACTH was started and produced 5 months of seizure freedom.

The habitual seizures began at about age 1 year and manifested as lapses in awareness that sometimes included head drops and then brief tonic posturing with facial flushing. The duration was about 10 seconds and was followed by sleepiness. Treatment included multiple anti-seizure medications and the ketogenic diet with a seizure frequency of 10 to 12 and up to 30 daily.

The epilepsy risk factor was tuberous sclerosis.

Neurological examination identified developmental delay and autism spectrum disorder. Medical history included a cardiac rhabdomyoma and a renal angiomyolipoma.

Interictal EEG during early childhood depicted moderate, generalized slowing without a posterior dominant rhythm and with occasional runs of greater slowing that was lateralized with a shifting asymmetry. Epileptiform discharges were frequent and independent over the left and right posterior temporal regions. Occasionally, bursts of paroxysmal fast activity, electrodecrements, and 2-Hz generalized epileptiform discharges also were present. Video-EEG monitoring recorded seizures manifested as brief neck flexion (head drops) and episodes of staring. Ictal EEG's seizure onset during the head drops was generalized sharp and slow-wave discharges with a maximal field over the posterior temporal regions. Each was followed by an electrodecrement with superimposed fast activity. Ictal EEG onset for the staring episodes was a right posterior temporal sharp wave followed by an electrodecrement with right-sided fast activity and then a posterior temporal theta frequency rhythm.

At age 3 years, MRI identified multiple tubers, as evident as focal abnormalities in the subcortical white matter, and small subependymal nodules. Also at age 3 years, PET identified multiple regions of hypometabolism that corresponded to the tubers evident with MRI.

The history and evaluation indicate a generalized epilepsy due to multiple tubers of tuberous sclerosis and a resulting, distributed, functional abnormality. The developmental delay, generalized EEG abnormalities, and seizures during infancy and childhood correspond to the generalized cerebral dysfunction. The presence of asymmetric or focal features reflects focality within the distributed abnormality, but the findings are not sufficient to indicate a reasonable likelihood of epilepsy surgery producing seizure freedom and development improvement. Additional anti-seizure medications and vagus nerve stimulation were recommended.

J. M. Stern, N. Salamon, *Imaging of Epilepsy*, https://doi.org/10.1007/978-3-030-86672-3_60

Imaging

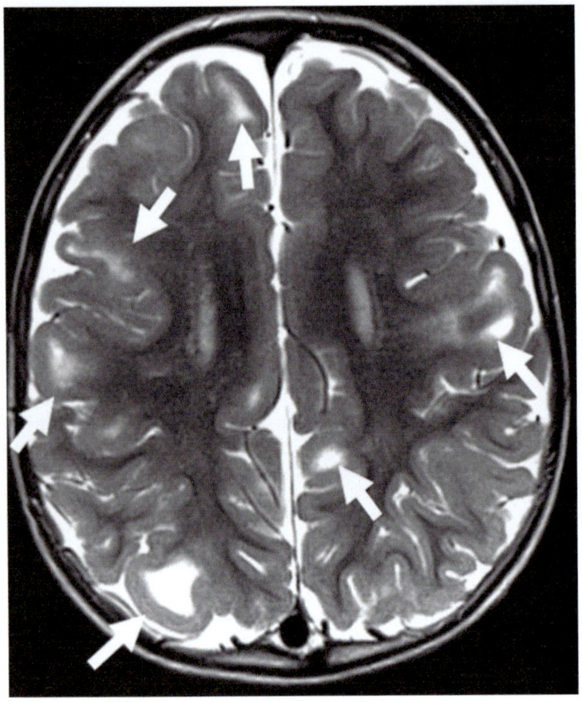

Fig. 60.1 MRI axial T2 sequence at a super-ventricular level. Multiple foci of hyperintense abnormality are evident in the subcortical white matter with six of the foci indicated by arrows. The locations and signal characteristics are typical for cortical tubers. No edema or other abnormality is present. The cortical ribbon is normal

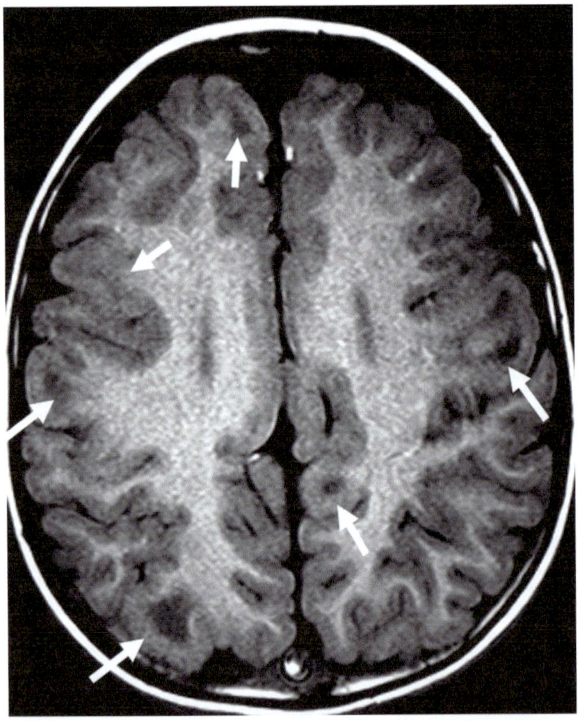

Fig. 60.2 MRI axial T1 sequence at the same super-ventricular level as Fig. 60.1. Multiple foci of hypointense abnormality are evident in the subcortical white matter with arrows indicating the same lesions as in Fig. 60.1 for a comparison to the T1 sequence. No other abnormality is present

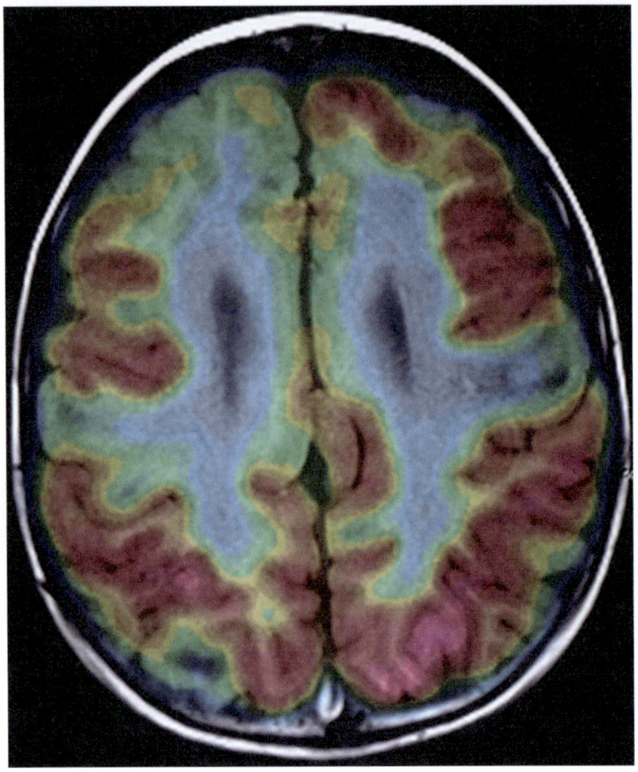

Fig. 60.3 PET-MRI co-registration with color-scale FDG tracer in an axial plane at the same super-ventricular level as Figs. 60.1 and 60.2. Multiple foci of hypometabolism correspond to the tubers in Figs. 60.1 and 60.2. The right frontal lobe hypometabolic abnormality is much larger than the corresponding tuber

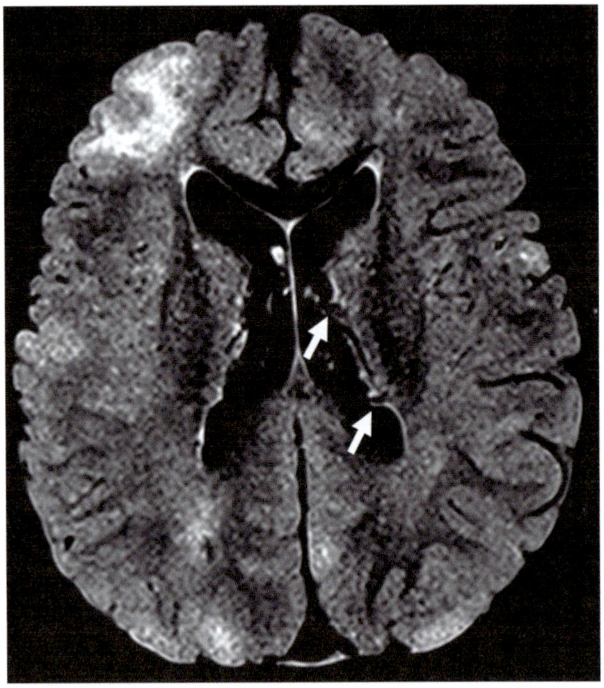

Fig. 60.4 MRI axial FLAIR sequence at a lateral ventricle level. Multiple foci of hyperintense abnormality are evident in the right frontal and bilateral lateral frontal and parietal regions. The anterior and posterior cingulate gyrus on the left has subtle hyperintense abnormality. Small subependymal nodules are present bilaterally with the more prominent nodules indicated by arrows

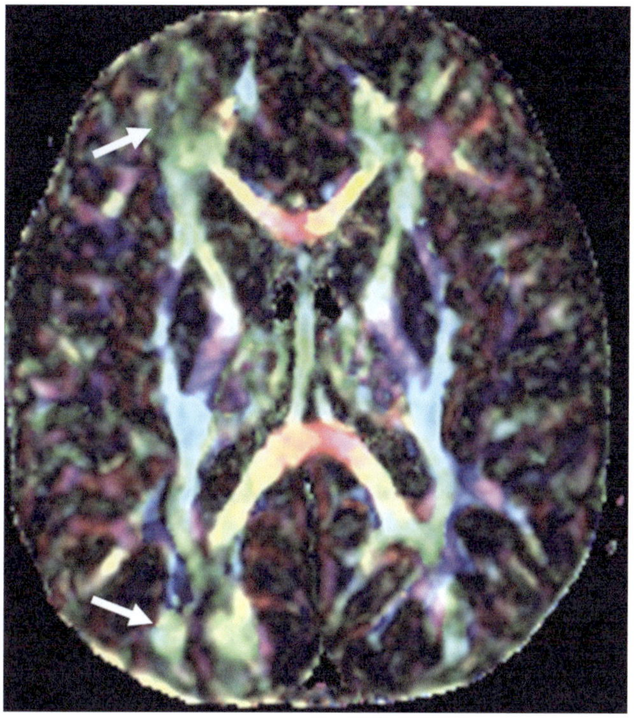

Fig. 60.5 MRI with axial diffusion tensor imaging at the same lateral ventricle level as Fig. 60.4. The asymmetries within the color map (arrows) indicate locations of tubers in the right frontal and right parietal areas

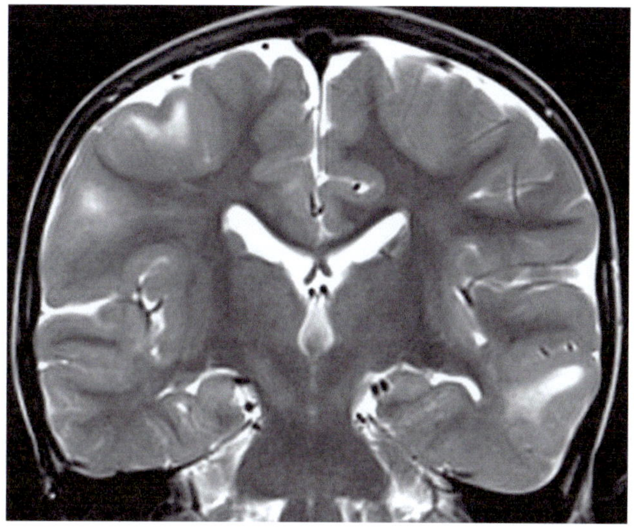

Fig. 60.7 MRI coronal T2 sequence at a hippocampal body level. Multiple foci of hyperintensity are evident in the right frontal and left temporal subcortical white matter with two prominent regions of abnormality within the right frontal lobe and one in the left temporal lobe. The cortical ribbon, subependymal margins, and hippocampi are normal

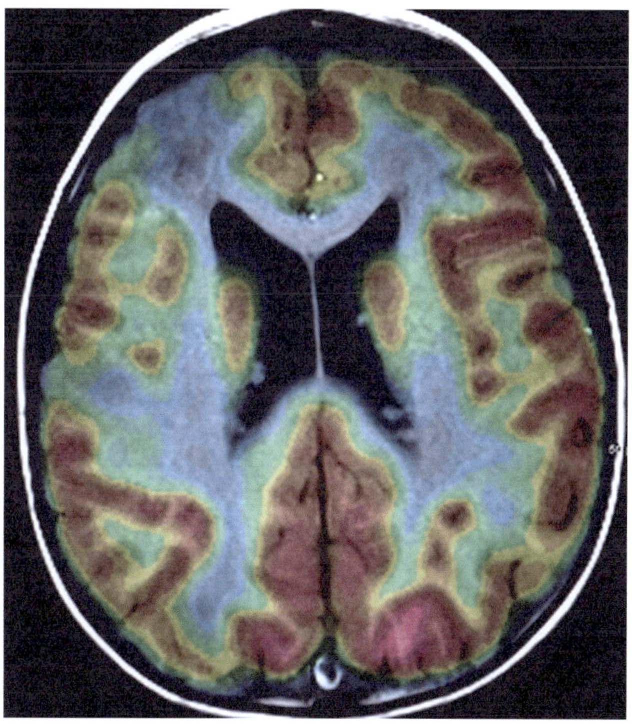

Fig. 60.6 PET-MRI co-registration with color-scale FDG tracer in an axial plane at a similar level as Figs. 60.4 and 60.5. Regions of hypometabolism are evident surrounding the tubers with the regions varying in size and metabolic signal. The subependymal nodules are evident bilaterally along the walls of the lateral ventricles as low metabolic signal protrusions into the ventricles

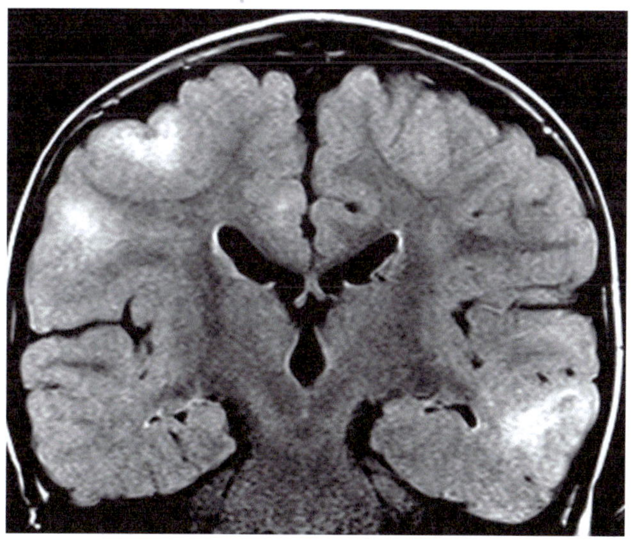

Fig. 60.8 MRI coronal FLAIR sequence at the same hippocampal body level as Fig. 60.7. The three prominent tubers are evident as hyperintensities in the right frontal lobe and left temporal lobe. A more subtle right cingulate gyrus tuber is evident and more clearly visible than with the T2 sequence. The cortical ribbon and gray-white junction are normal

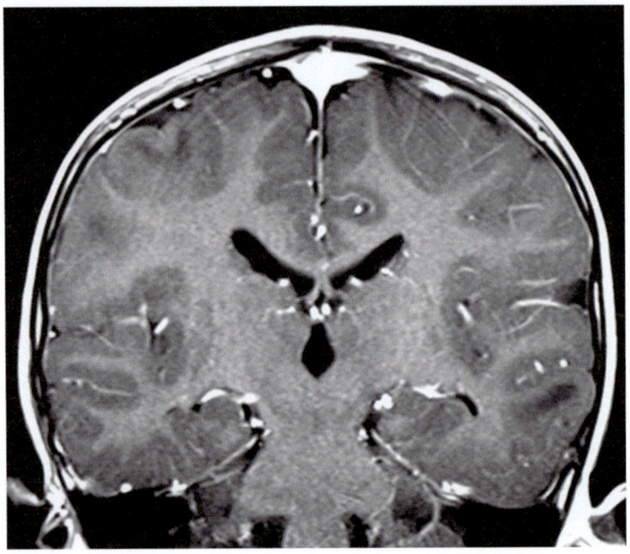

Fig. 60.9 MRI coronal T1 sequence after contrast administration at the same hippocampal body level as Figs. 60.7 and 60.8. The two right frontal lobe tubers and one left temporal lobe tuber correspond to regions hypointense signal that are less prominent than the signal abnormality with FLAIR and T2 sequences. The right cingulate gyrus tuber is isointense and not clearly present. No abnormal contrast enhancement is present

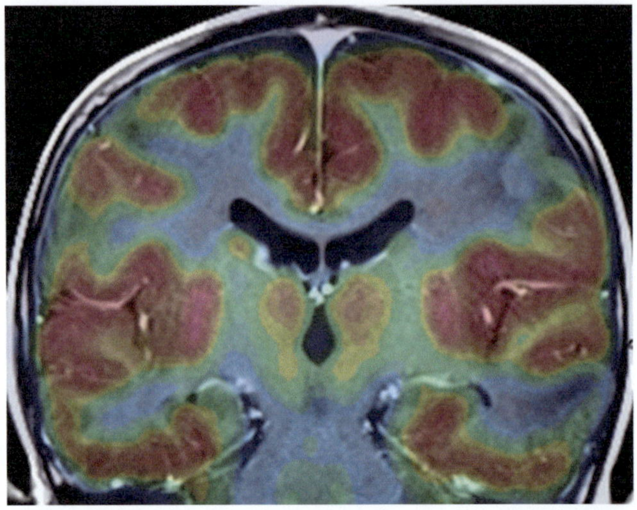

Fig. 60.10 PET-MRI co-registration with color-scale FDG tracer in a coronal plane at the same level as Figs. 60.7, 60.8, and 60.9 but with a slightly different angle. Multiple foci of hypometabolism are evident, and each corresponds to tubers in the preceding figures. In addition, a region of hypometabolism in the left frontal lobe indicates an additional tuber that was not clearly visible with MRI. The subependymal region, mesial temporal lobes, and hippocampi are normal

Subependymal Nodules of Tuberous Sclerosis

61

Clinical History

The first recognized seizures occurred at age 5 months as infantile spasms that occurred 30 times daily and had a left-sided predominance that included clenching of the left hand. An evaluation at that time identified tuberous sclerosis with brain, kidney, and heart involvement.

After treatment with multiple anti-seizure medications and ACTH, seizure freedom was briefly achieved, but this was followed by the emergence of focal seizures at about age 1 year. The focal seizures manifested in the left hand as extension of the first and second digits followed by flexion of the fourth and fifth digits and then progression proximally over 20 seconds to include extension of the left arm, left facial movements, and left leg extension. These seizures occurred about 5 times daily until age 3 years. From then until about age 11 years, seizures were typically manifested as staring episodes that lasted about 15 seconds and sometimes included a smile. These seizures occurred at least daily, but the actual frequency could not be estimated because of the subtle manifestation. During this time, several generalized tonic-clonic seizures also occurred.

The habitual seizures since age 11 years manifested as a left-hand tremor that sometimes progressed to left arm twitching and facial grimacing without an impairment of awareness. The motor component had similar distribution to the seizures in early childhood, but the movements differed. The frequency was several weekly until everolimus was added to the treatment regimen. Since then, the habitual seizures manifested as a sensation that the left hand is shaking without any actual movement of the hand. The seizure duration was 20 seconds, and there was no change to external awareness or ictal or postictal weakness of the hand. For this seizure, the frequency was typically one or two daily with seizure-free periods as long as 3 days.

The epilepsy risk factor was tuberous sclerosis.

Neurological examination identified mild dysmetria of the right upper extremity. Neuropsychological testing identified an IQ in the normal range and learning disabilities requiring educational accommodations. Medical history included ash leaf spots, angiofibromas, hypertension, and bilateral polycystic kidney disease with moderate renal insufficiency. A cardiac rhabdomyoma was present and resolved by about age 3 years.

Interictal EEG depicted intermittent, abnormal generalized slowing and greater slowing that occurred rarely and with a higher amplitude and a right posterior hemisphere predominance. Occasional epileptiform discharges occurred in the right central region with a field that extended to the left central region. Interictal MEG depicted similarly localized epileptiform abnormalities. Video-EEG monitoring recorded focal seizures manifested as a sensation of left arm shaking followed by voluntary extension of the arm due to the sensory experience. Interaction and awareness remained intact. Ictal EEG was unchanged from the baseline interictal recording.

MRI identified cortical tubers and nonobstructive subependymal nodules, and these findings were unchanged across multiple MRIs until age 12 years. At age 12 years, transformation of a subependymal nodule into a subependymal giant cell astrocytoma (SEGA) was evident, and this led to starting everolimus. The subsequent MRIs identified a SEGA volume decrease. PET identified multifocal hypometabolism, including regions corresponding to tubers, subependymal nodules, and the subependymal giant cell astrocytoma. CT identified tuber and subependymal nodule calcifications.

The history and evaluation include two epilepsy manifestations of tuberous sclerosis with spasms during infancy and focal seizures in childhood. Both indicate a right cerebral abnormality, but the focal seizures are more localizing and suggest an epileptogenic zone in the right central region. Both the EEG and the MRI depict a distributed abnormality consistent with the history of infantile spasms. Specifically, the MRI identified multiple potentially epileptic tubers, and both the EEG and the MEG depicted diffuse dysfunction with superimposed focal abnormality in the right posterior region. However, the EEG's right posterior cerebral focal abnormality is most consistent with the likely seizure

J. M. Stern, N. Salamon, *Imaging of Epilepsy*, https://doi.org/10.1007/978-3-030-86672-3_61

localization. After beginning treatment for the SEGA with everolimus, the seizure changed to become purely sensory and thereby less disabling. Ongoing epilepsy care continues with anti-seizure medications.

Imaging

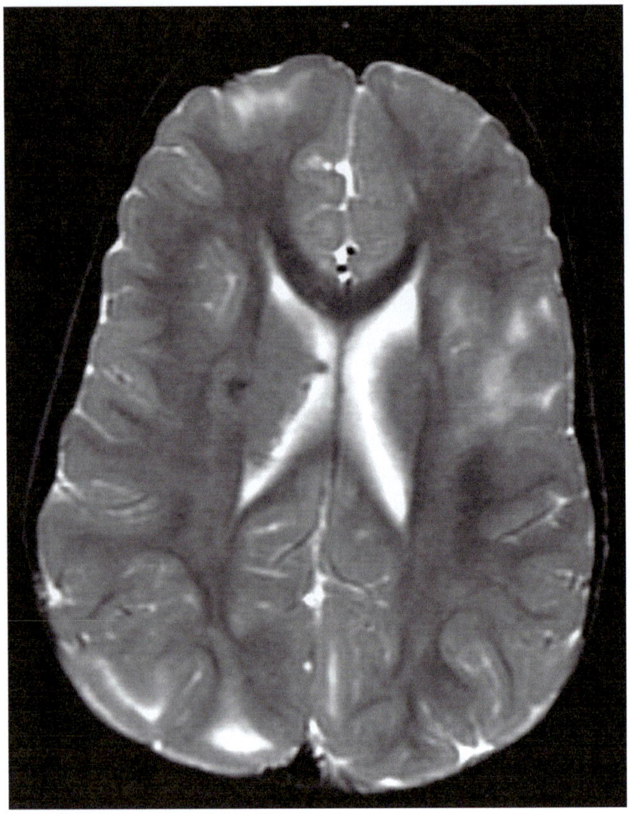

Fig. 61.1 MRI axial T2 sequence at a lateral ventricle level. Along the margin of right lateral ventricle, a prominent, round hypointense focus protrudes into the ventricle and is consistent with a subependymal nodule. A smaller hypointense focus is immediately posterior to the prominent nodule without protrusion into the ventricle, and it possibly another subependymal nodule. Tubers are evident as multiple foci of hyperintense signal in the subcortical white matter of bilateral frontal and right parietal lobes and one hypointense calcified focus in the right corona radiata

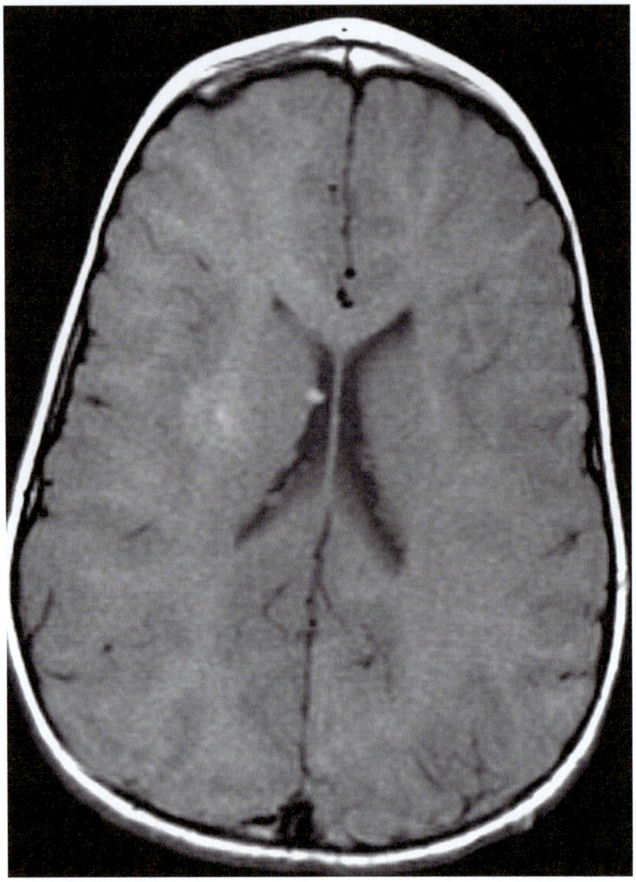

Fig. 61.2 MRI axial T1 sequence at the same lateral ventricle level. A punctate hyperintensity is evident along right lateral ventricle's margin and corresponds to the prominent subependymal nodule in Fig. 61.1. A smaller subependymal nodule is faintly visible posterior to the hyperintense abnormality. Other than the hyperintense focus in the right corona radiata, the subcortical tubers evident in Fig. 61.1 are highly subtle

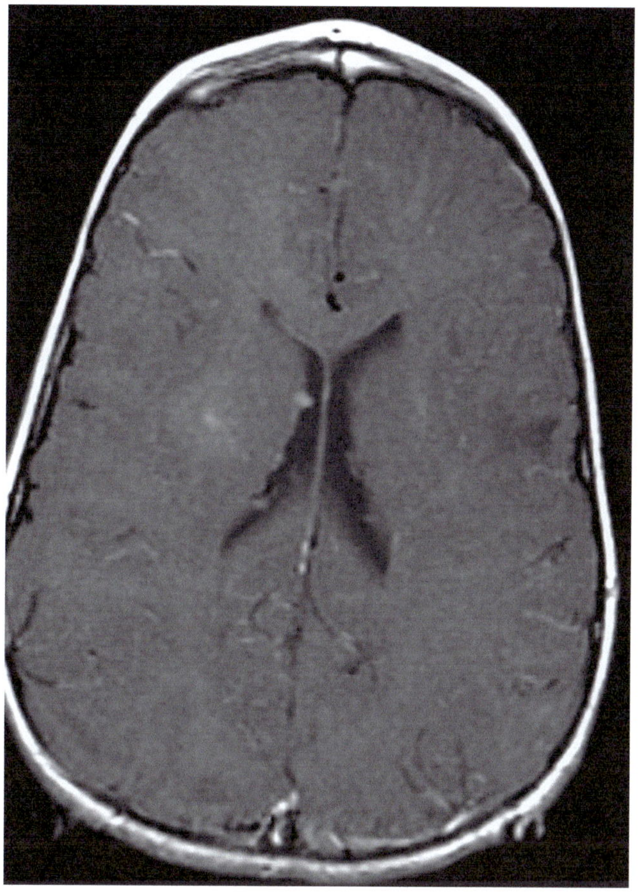

Fig. 61.3 MRI axial T1 sequence after contrast administration at the same lateral ventricle level as Figs. 61.1 and 61.2. The hyperintense subependymal nodule that protrudes into the right lateral ventricle is unchanged and so is not enhanced. The smaller subependymal nodule posterior to the prominent protruding has minor enhancement. No other abnormal enhancement is present

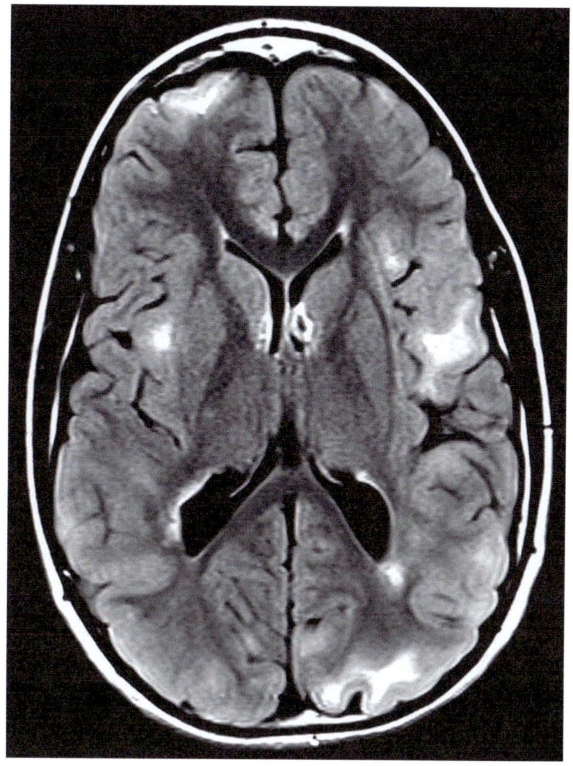

Fig. 61.4 MRI axial FLAIR sequence at a thalamus level. Subependymal nodules are present near the foramen of Monro in the posterior frontal horns of both lateral ventricles. The left subependymal nodule protrudes into the ventricle and the right does not. The hypointense central portion within the left subependymal nodule is due to internal calcification. Tubers are evident as hyperintensities in the right and left insula, right frontal pole, left operculum, and left occipital pole

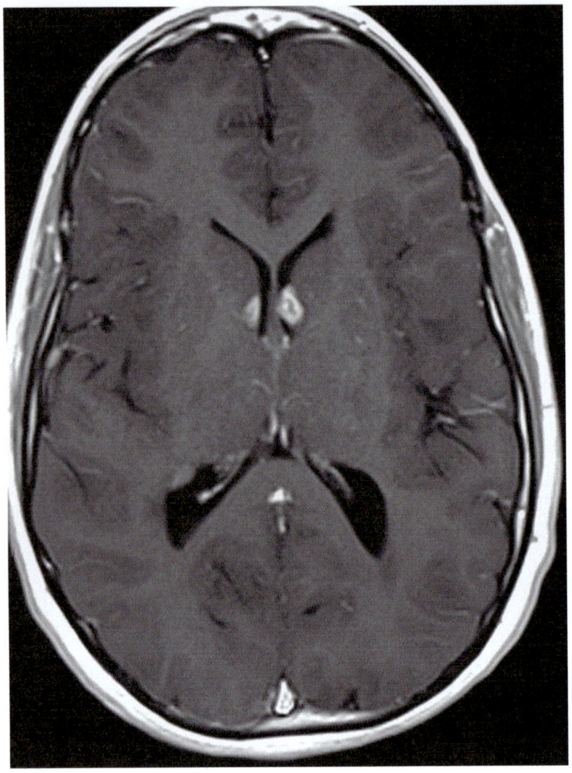

Fig. 61.5 MRI axial T1 sequence after contrast administration at the same thalamus level as Fig. 61.4. Enhancement of the bilateral frontal horn subependymal nodules is evident. Hypointensity is present in both nodules and indicates calcification in both. The multiple subcortical tubers are not evident

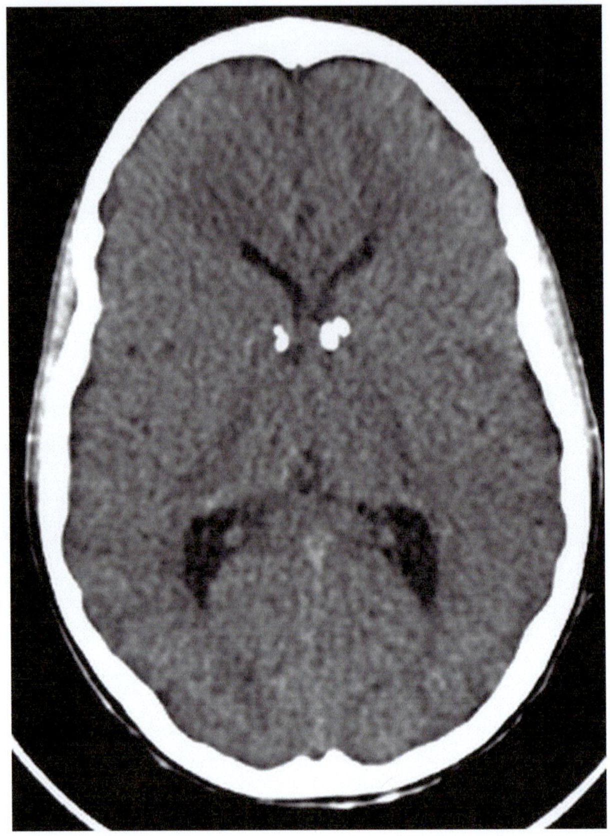

Fig. 61.7 CT axial plane at a low lateral ventricle that is similar to Fig. 61.4. Prominent calcification is evident in each of the bilateral subependymal nodules that are in the frontal horns of bilateral lateral ventricles near the foramen of Monro. No other calcification or abnormality is evident

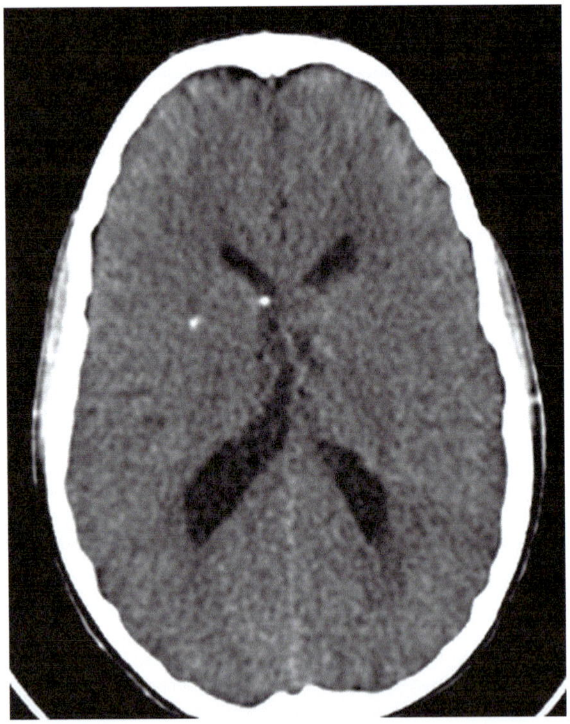

Fig. 61.6 CT axial plane at a lateral ventricle level that is between Figs. 61.1 and 61.4. The right lateral ventricle subependymal nodule is hyperdense, including calcification. An additional calcification is within the right corona radiata and is due to a calcified tuber

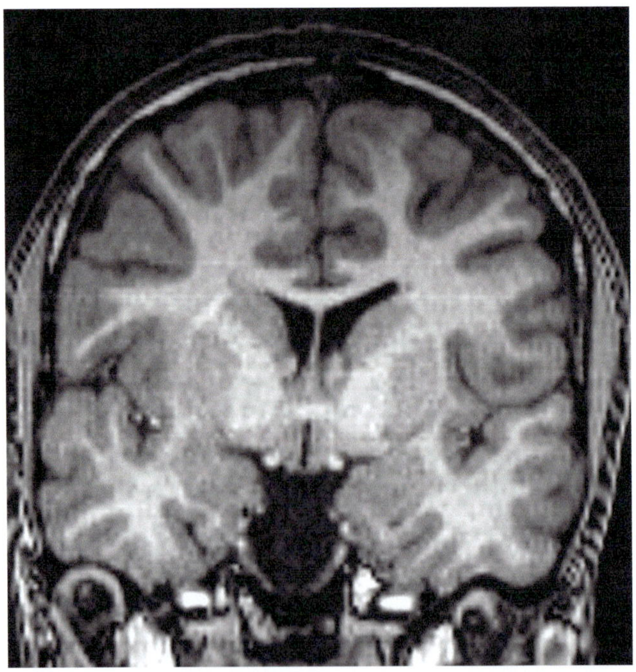

Fig. 61.8 MRI coronal T1 sequence at an amygdala level. Subependymal nodules are evident in the inferior aspect of bilateral frontal horns of the lateral ventricles with protrusion into the ventricles. The nodules are isointense to gray matter. No other abnormality is evident

Subependymal Giant Cell Astrocytoma of Tuberous Sclerosis

62

Clinical History

See Subependymal Nodules of Tuberous Sclerosis.

Imaging

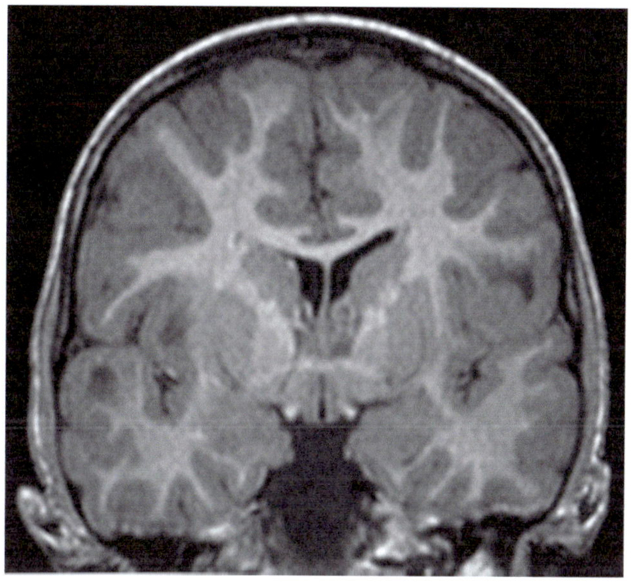

Fig. 62.1 MRI coronal T1 sequence at an amygdala level. Subependymal nodules are evident in the inferior aspects of bilateral frontal horns of the lateral ventricles. Hypointensity is present at the center of each nodule, suggesting internal calcification. Subcortical tubers are present in the right superior temporal gyrus, the right insula, and the left frontal operculum. A subependymal giant cell astrocytoma (SEGA) is not evident

J. M. Stern, N. Salamon, *Imaging of Epilepsy*, https://doi.org/10.1007/978-3-030-86672-3_62

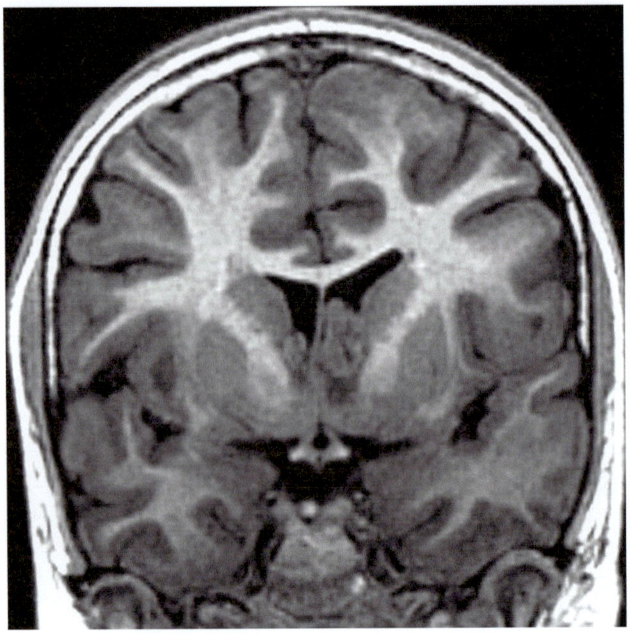

Fig. 62.2 MRI coronal T1 sequence at the same amygdala level. The image was obtained 7 years after Fig. 62.1. The left frontal horn subependymal lesion has an interval increase in size, indicating transformation into a SEGA. The growth has resulted in a slight increase in ventricle volume bilaterally. The right frontal horn subependymal nodule and the subcortical tubers are unchanged

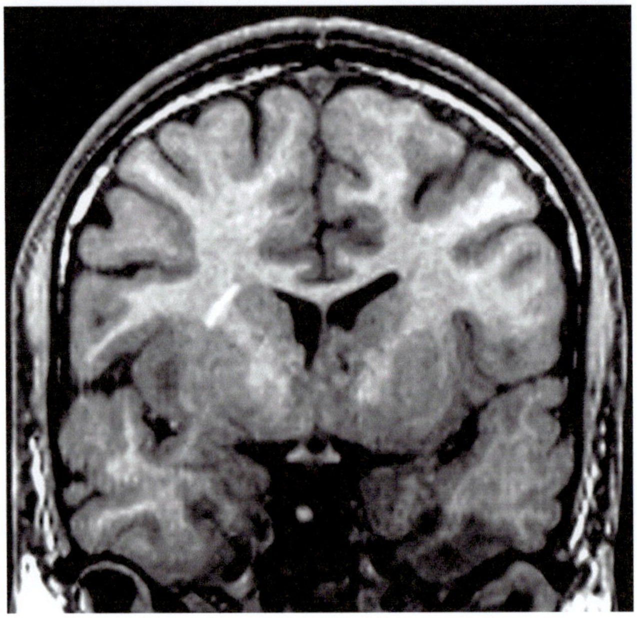

Fig. 62.4 MRI coronal T1 sequence at a level that is slightly anterior to Figs. 62.1, 62.2, and 62.3. The image was obtained 3 years after Figs. 62.2 and 62.3. An interval volume decrease is evident for the bilateral subependymal nodules and the left SEGA in particular. The ventricular volume is unchanged

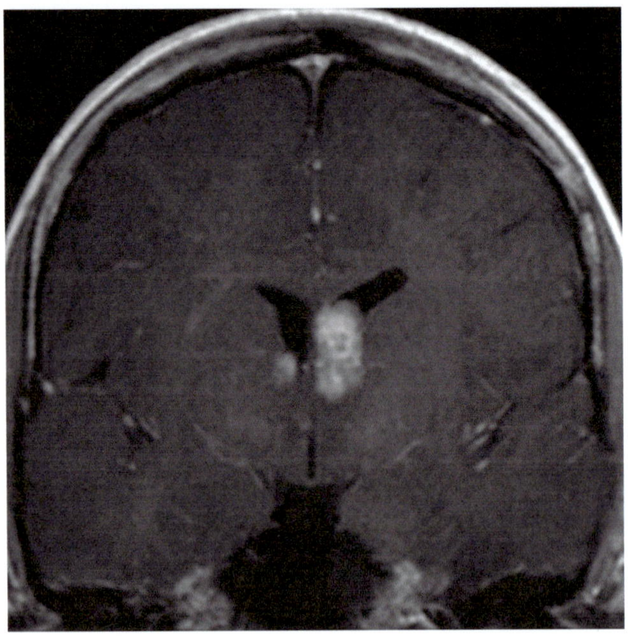

Fig. 62.3 MRI coronal T1 sequence after contrast administration at the same level and imaging session as Fig. 62.2. Enhancement is evident within the bilateral frontal horn intraventricular nodules and the left-sided SEGA. No other abnormal enhancement is present

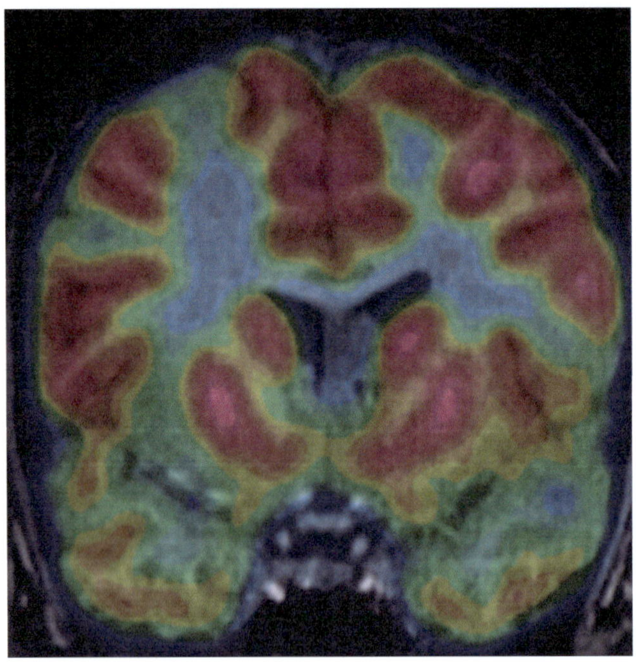

Fig. 62.5 PET-MRI co-registration with color-scale FDG tracer in a coronal plane that is similar to Fig. 62.4. The bilateral subependymal modules and the left-sided SEGA are hypometabolic. Hypometabolism also is evident in the multiple tubers, including in bilateral superior temporal gyri, left middle temporal gyrus, left inferior frontal gyrus, and right superior frontal gyrus

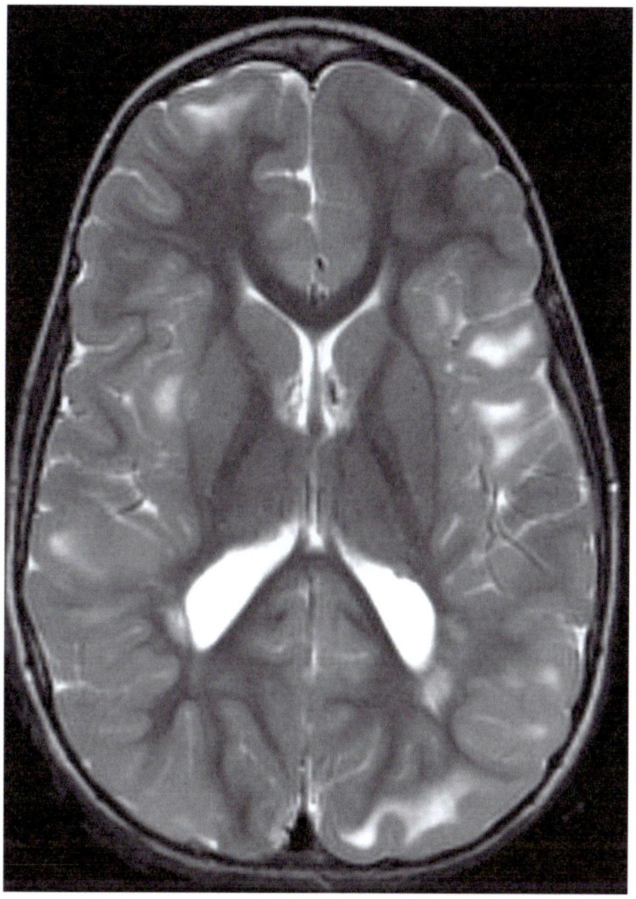

Fig. 62.6 MRI axial T2 sequence at a thalamus level. The image was obtained at the time of Fig. 62.1. Subependymal nodules are evident in bilateral frontal horns of the lateral ventricles. Each has a central hypointensity suggesting calcification. No hydrocephalus is present. Multiple subcortical tubers are evident, including in right frontal pole, right insula, left operculum, and left occipital pole

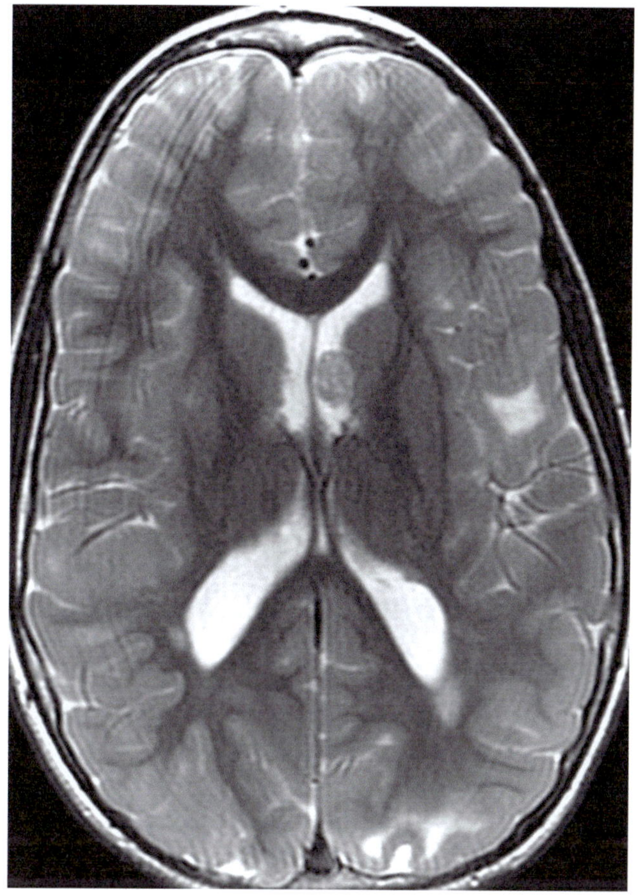

Fig. 62.7 MRI axial T2 sequence at a thalamus level that is similar to Fig. 62.6. The image was obtained 7 years after Fig. 62.6 and at the time of Fig. 62.2. An interval increase in size of the left frontal horn subependymal nodule indicates a SEGA. An interval increase in ventricular volume also is present. There is no other change

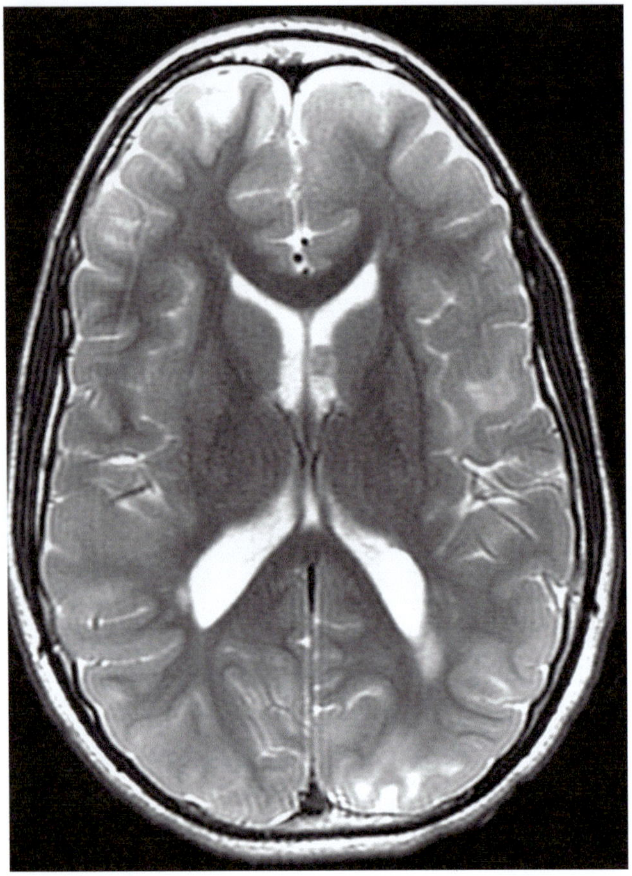

Fig. 62.8 MRI axial T2 sequence at same thalamus level as Fig. 62.7. The image was obtained 3 years after Fig. 62.7 and at the time of Fig. 62.4. The left frontal horn SEGA has decreased in volume. The ventricular volumes and the subcortical tubers are unchanged

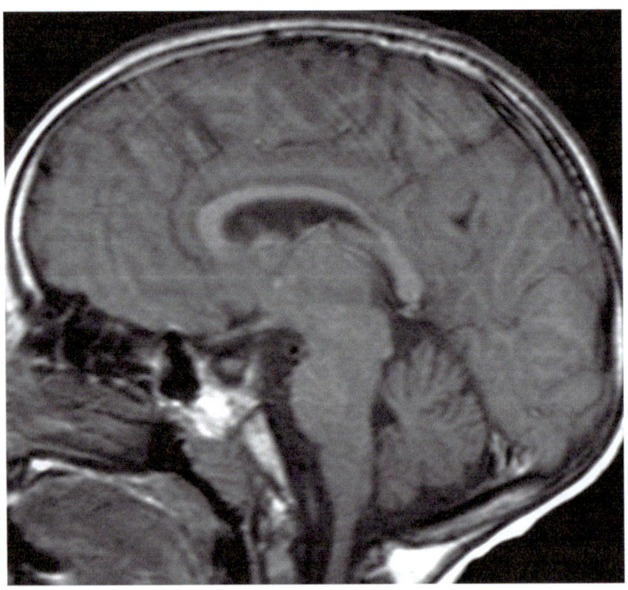

Fig. 62.9 MRI sagittal T1 sequence at a corpus callosum midline level. The image was obtained at the same time as Figs. 62.1 and 62.6. The subependymal nodules are evident adjacent to the foramen of Monro in the frontal horn of the lateral ventricle. The lateral ventricle has normal volume

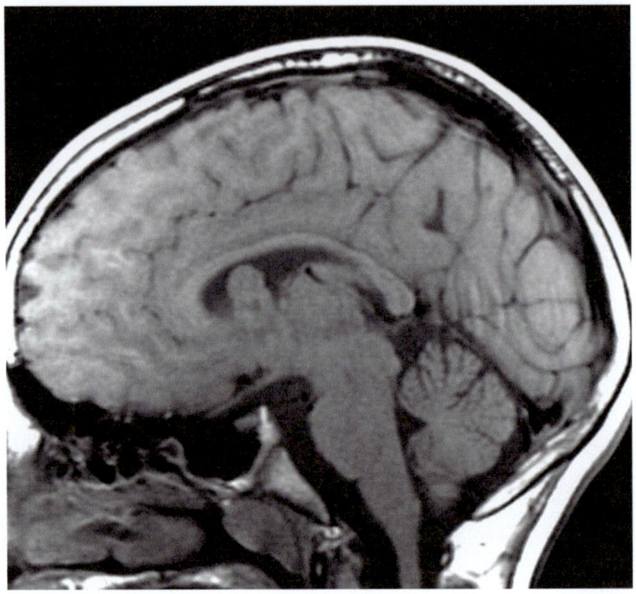

Fig. 62.10 MRI sagittal T1 sequence at the same corpus callosum midline level as Fig. 62.9. The image was obtained 7 years after 62.9 and at the same time as Figs. 62.2 and 62.7. The subependymal lesion near the foramen of Monro has increased in volume and has prominent protrusion into the lateral ventricle, indicating SEGA. The ventricular volume has not changed at this level

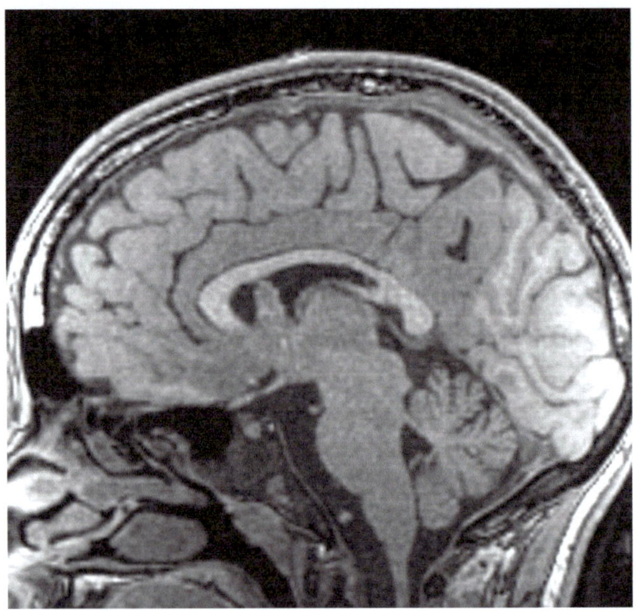

Fig. 62.11 MRI sagittal T1 sequence at the same corpus callosum midline level as Figs. 62.9 and 62.10. The image was obtained 3 years after Fig. 62.10 and at the same time as Figs. 62.4 and 62.8. The SEGA near the foramen of Monro has decreased in volume. There is no change to the ventricular volume

Part VIII

Non-epileptogenic Findings

Hippocampal atrophy
Hippocampal inversion
Hippocampal malrotation
Developmental venous anomaly
Venous angioma
Arachnoid cyst
Epidermoid cyst
Cerebellar atrophy
Splenium signal abnormality
Status epilepticus

Hippocampal atrophy is evident in several features that may be considered together to identify the loss of hippocampal volume. Most often, hippocampal atrophy is evident in the ex vacuo widening of the temporal horn of the lateral ventricle. Other changes include a widening of the choroid fissure, loss of hippocampal height as compared to its width, and a greater volume of cerebrospinal fluid (CSF) around the hippocampus. When these changes occur without an abnormality within the hippocampus, such as loss or blurring of internal architecture or the presence of hyperintensity, the finding is atrophy without evidence of sclerosis.

Incomplete hippocampal inversion (IHI), which has also been called hippocampal malrotation, appears as a round, vertical, and medially rotated hippocampus. By itself, IHI has been reported as more common in epilepsy than when epilepsy is not the diagnosis and it has a prevalence of 30 to 50% in temporal lobe epilepsy. However, it also occurs in people without any neurologic diagnosis. The association with epilepsy is complicated by its association with sulcal structural abnormalities that are most often in the limbic system and with malformations of cortical development that are not limited to one region. The left hippocampus is more likely to have this finding.

Developmental venous anomalies (DVA) are an intrauterine complication of an arrest of venous development. This results in retention of primitive medullary veins, and they are visible pathologically and radiologically as radially arranged (caput medusae) vessels. Rarely, DVAs may be associated with potentially epileptogenic abnormalities, such as a partially thrombosed DVA with associated gliosis, cavernous malformation, or cortical dysplasia; however, DVAs that are not associated with such other findings should be considered unrelated to epilepsy.

Arachnoid cysts have the signal intensity of CSF on T1- and T2-weighted images and do not show restriction on diffusion-weighted images. Epidermoid cysts also have the signal intensity of similar to the CSF signal on T1- and T2-weighted images, but they demonstrate restricted diffusion and no enhancement. Furthermore, they may have mildly heterogeneous signal intensity with FLAIR sequences. Both cysts are congenital, incidental findings and do not reflect the localization of epileptogenic abnormality.

Cerebellar atrophy has been reported as associated with chronic epilepsy for almost a century and has been considered either to be a due to cumulative seizure-mediated cell loss or an adverse effect of phenytoin or other pharmacotherapies. More recent studies have redirected the etiology from phenytoin to epilepsy duration. The atrophy typically is symmetric and involves both the cerebellar midline and hemispheres, the atrophy does not relate to the seizure lateralization.

Splenium signal abnormality is evident as a cytotoxic abnormality with restricted diffusion and high T2/FLAIR signal in the central portion of the splenium of the corpus callosum. Abnormal contrast enhancement does not accompany the abnormality. The finding is well defined clinically and consistently reversible. In most instances, the clinical history alone includes recent status epilepticus or a cluster of seizures and an increase in anti-seizure medication.

Status epilepticus appears with MRI as T2 and diffusion-weighted imaging (DWI) hyperintense gray matter within the region engaged in the seizure production, including the possibility of broad hemispheric neocortex and the hippocampus or mesial temporal lobe. When the seizure involves the temporal, parietal, or occipital lobes, the ipsilateral pulvinar of the thalamus can also demonstrate DWI, T2, and FLAIR signal abnormality. Vascular dilatation may be associated with the seizure, which can be evident in hyperperfusion visible as increased hemispheric cerebral blood volume. The diffusion-weighted and perfusion-weighted changes typically are resolved by 2–7 days after resolution of the seizure.

Key References

Cury C, Toro T, Cohen F, et al. Incomplete hippocampal inversion: a comprehensive MRI study of over 2000 subjects. Front Neuroanat. 2015;9:160.

Dussaule C, Masnou P, Nasser G, et al. Can developmental venous anomalies cause seizures? J Neurol. 2017;264:2495–505.

Osborn AG, Preece MT. Intracranial cysts: adiologic-pathologic correlation and imaging approach. Radiology. 2006;239:650–64.

Sandok EK, O'Brien TJ, Jack CR, So EL. Significance of cerebellar atrophy in intractable temporal lobe Epilepsy: a quantitative MRI study. Epilepsia. 2000;41:1315–20.

Starkey J, Kobayashi N, Numaguchi Y, et al. Cytotoxic lesions of the corpus callosum that show restricted diffusion: mechanisms, causes, and manifestations. RadioGraphics. 2017;37:562–76.

Szabo K, Poepel A, Pohlman-Eden B, et al. Diffusion-weighted and perfusion MRI demonstrates parenchymal changes in complex partial status epilepticus. Brain. 2005;128:1369–76.

63 Hippocampal Atrophy

Clinical History

The first recognized seizure occurred at age 35 years and was bilateral tonic-clonic without focal features. In retrospect, several episodes of confusion likely occurred without motor activity before the first recognized seizure. An evaluation after the recognized seizure included an MRI that was consistent with the previously identified diagnosis of multiple sclerosis.

The habitual seizures did not follow an aura or warning. They manifested as a collapse with loss of awareness and generalized stiffening. The duration was several minutes and postictal confusion, and lethargy then typically lasted 30 minutes. No consistent focal features were present during the seizures. Distinct from the motor seizures, seizures manifested as only confusion also occur. These did not include stereotyped or unusual movements or behaviors, and they were noted when disorientation developed during a conversation. The confusion lasted up to 30 minutes. Treatment has included multiple anti-seizure medications with a motor seizure frequency of once every few months and a non-motor, confusion seizure once every week.

The epilepsy risk factors were multiple sclerosis, which was diagnosed at age 30; Hashimoto's encephalopathy, which was diagnosed several years after the multiple sclerosis diagnosis; and possibly a concussion as a teenager.

Neurological examination was significant for memory impairment requiring residence in an assisted living facility. Neuropsychological testing identified impaired cognitive function with partial orientation and dysphasia. Medical history included immunosuppression.

Interictal EEG depicted mild generalized slowing with intermittent moderate generalized slowing. Asymmetric slowing across the left temporal region also was present. Epileptiform discharges were present independently across bilateral anterior temporal regions with a greater number on the right. Video-EEG monitoring recorded focal seizures manifested as impaired awareness and subtle oral automatisms and other seizures that were bilateral tonic-clonic. Most of the ictal EEG's seizure onsets were across the left anterior temporal region, and some were across the right anterior temporal region.

MRI identified generalized atrophy and periventricular, subcortical, and brainstem signal abnormalities consistent with a high burden of multiple sclerosis. Bilateral hippocampal atrophy without signal abnormality was present. PET identified no focal areas of hypometabolism.

The history and evaluation indicate focal epilepsy with both focal and bilateral tonic-clonic seizures. The seizures do not have features to indicate a region of onset, but the occurrence of seizures with impairment and oral automatisms suggest involvement of limbic regions. However, the MRI abnormalities indicate the reasonable possibility of propagation into the limbic regions and the mesial temporal lobes are not necessarily the epileptogenic regions.

J. M. Stern, N. Salamon, *Imaging of Epilepsy*, https://doi.org/10.1007/978-3-030-86672-3_63

Imaging

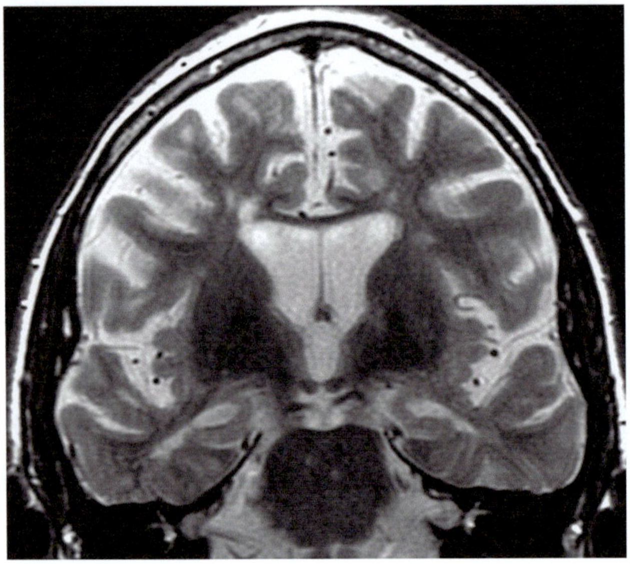

Fig. 63.1 MRI coronal T2 sequence at a hippocampal head level. The hippocampal head shape is abnormally flattening along the superior surface bilaterally, indicating atrophy. Diffuse cerebral atrophy is present, as evident the enlarged lateral and third ventricles, prominent cortical sulci, decreased white matter volume, and thin corpus callosum. Multiple periventricular foci of hyperintensity are also present. The basal ganglia are normal

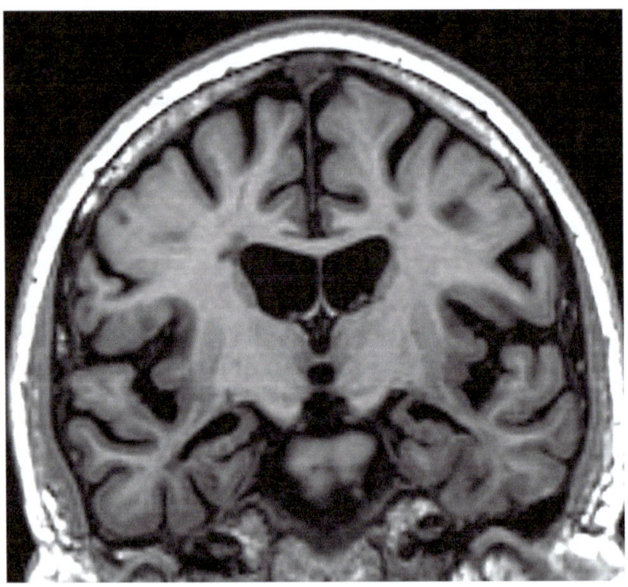

Fig. 63.2 MRI coronal T1 sequence at the same hippocampal head level as Fig. 63.1. The bilateral hippocampal atrophy is consistent with the bilateral temporal lobe atrophy. Additional atrophy is evident with the prominent cortical sulci and Sylvian fissures. Periventricular and subcortical hypointensities indicate chronic changes

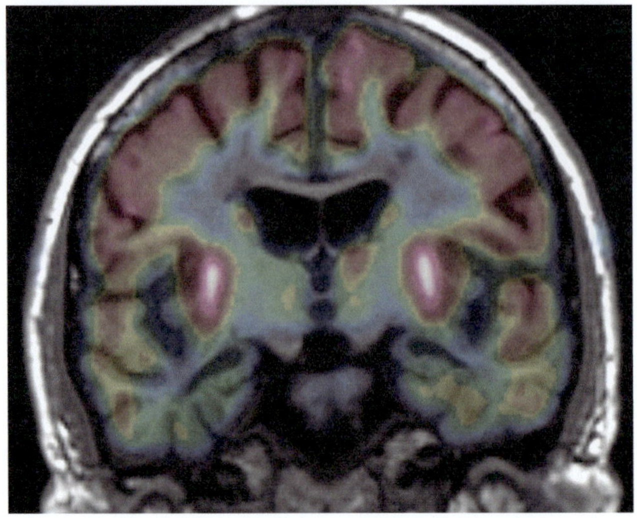

Fig. 63.3 PET-MRI co-registration with color-scale FDG tracer in a coronal plane at the same hippocampal head level as Figs. 63.1 and 63.2. Hypometabolism of the bilateral inferior and mesial temporal lobes is evident with relative sparing of the bilateral superior temporal gyri. The thalamus metabolic signal is asymmetric, but this is possibly due to the angle of the level. No other gray matter metabolic abnormality is present

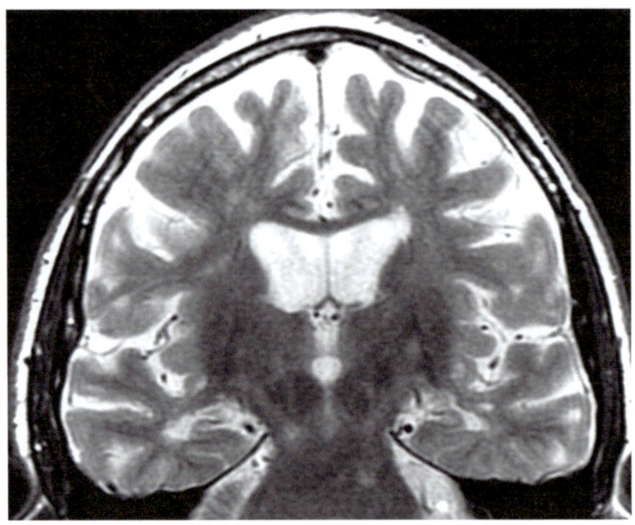

Fig. 63.4 MRI coronal T2 sequence at a hippocampal body level. The hippocampal bodies are bilaterally atrophic. The hippocampal internal signal intensity is normal bilaterally with subtly preserved internal architecture, which is not typical of hippocampal sclerosis. The internal architecture is clearer than in Fig. 63.1. The cortical sulci and ventricles are enlarged, suggesting global volume loss

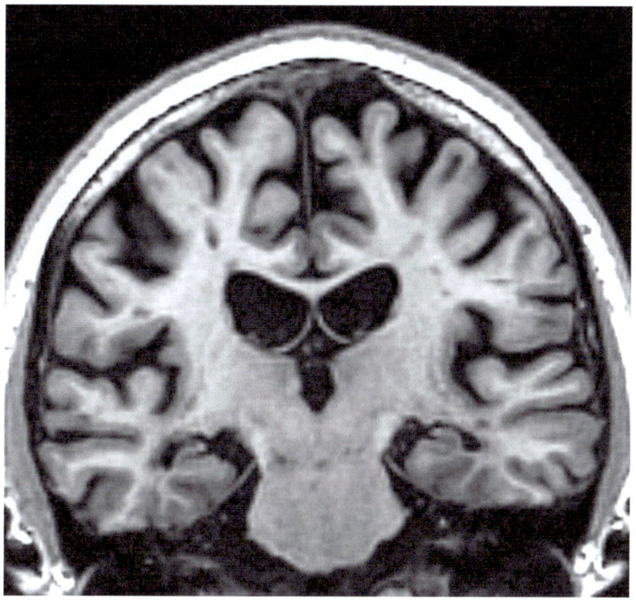

Fig. 63.5 MRI coronal T1 sequence at a similar hippocampal body level as Fig. 63.4. The hippocampi are bilaterally atrophic. The internal architecture is not as clear as Fig. 63.4. Global cerebral atrophy is evident. The pons and cerebral peduncles are normal

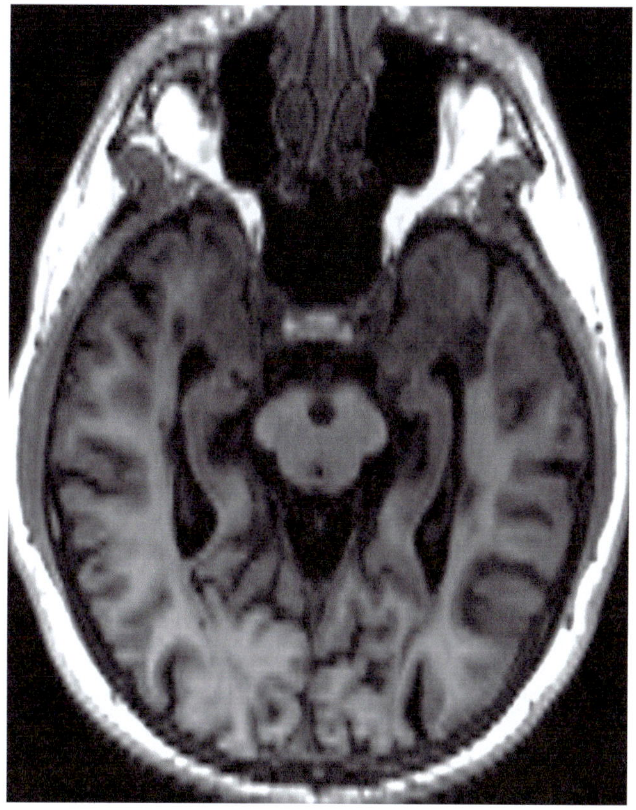

Fig. 63.7 MRI axial T1 sequence at a hippocampus level. Bilateral hippocampal and amygdalar atrophy are evident. Multiple foci of hypointensity are present in the temporal lobes' white matter, indicating chronic changes. The midbrain is normal

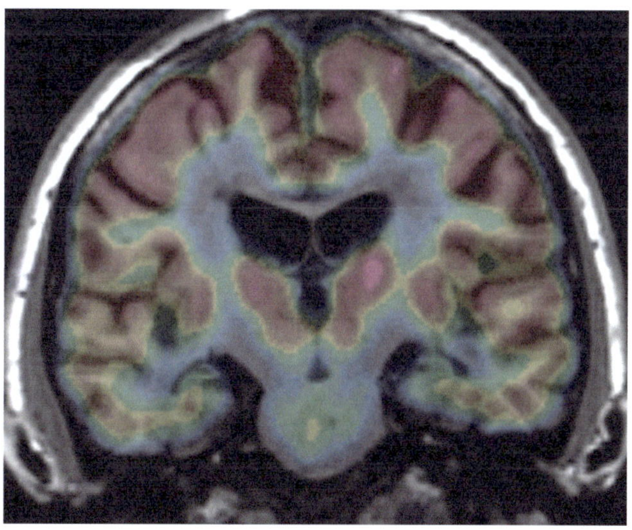

Fig. 63.6 PET-MRI co-registration with color-scale FDG tracer in a coronal plane at the same hippocampal body level as Fig. 63.5. Bilateral mesial temporal hypometabolism is evident with abnormal hypometabolism of the remaining temporal lobes bilaterally that is less prominent. The superior temporal gyri are relatively less hypometabolic but also are abnormal

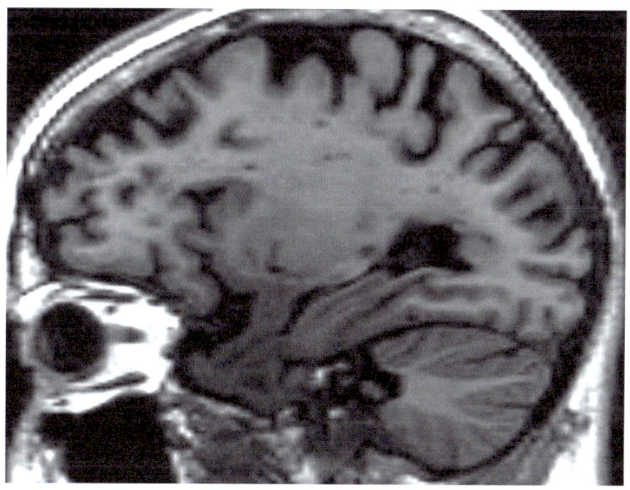

Fig. 63.8 MRI sagittal T1 sequence at a left hippocampus level. The hippocampal body volume is abnormally reduced with an associated, prominent anterior temporal lobe cerebrospinal fluid (CSF) space. Multifocal, abnormal hypointensities are in the cerebral white matter, and the cortical sulci are abnormally prominent

64 Incomplete Hippocampal Inversion

Clinical History

The first recognized seizure occurred at age 35 years as an episode of staring without awareness that progressed to bilateral stiffening and then shaking.

The habitual seizures occurred as two manifestations. One was similar to the first seizure and had durations of 3 to 5 minutes followed by postictal confusion and somnolence for hours. The other manifestation was a sense of warmth or clamminess that was followed by staring, atonia, and then bilateral stiffening with the same ictal and postictal period duration as the other seizure manifestation. Treatment has included multiple anti-seizure medications with a seizure frequency for the first manifestation of one to six seizures on most days of the week with occasional periods of up to 2 weeks of seizure freedom. The second manifestation occurred a few times weekly.

The epilepsy risk factors were traumatic loss of consciousness as a teenager when hit by a moving vehicle and also neurosurgery as an adult for decompression of an Arnold-Chiari malformation.

Neurological examination was normal. Medical history included anxiety and fibromyalgia.

Interictal EEG depicted excessive beta activity superimposed on a normal background. No epileptiform discharges were present. Video-EEG monitoring recorded seizures that followed the habitual aura and were manifested as sudden focal or generalized tonic posturing or atonia accompanied by unresponsiveness and then progressing to bilateral shaking. Ictal EEG's seizure seizure depiction was normal background activity.

MRI identified a vertical left hippocampus and bilateral hippocampi without atrophy or signal abnormality.

The history and evaluation indicate non-epileptic seizures, as was supported by a detailed review of video recordings of the ictal behaviors and the normal interictal and ictal EEG. The hippocampal finding is a normal variant. A subsequent psychological evaluation led to a diagnosis of conversion disorder with dissociative seizures, also called functional seizures and psychogenic non-epileptic seizures.

J. M. Stern, N. Salamon, *Imaging of Epilepsy*, https://doi.org/10.1007/978-3-030-86672-3_64

Imaging

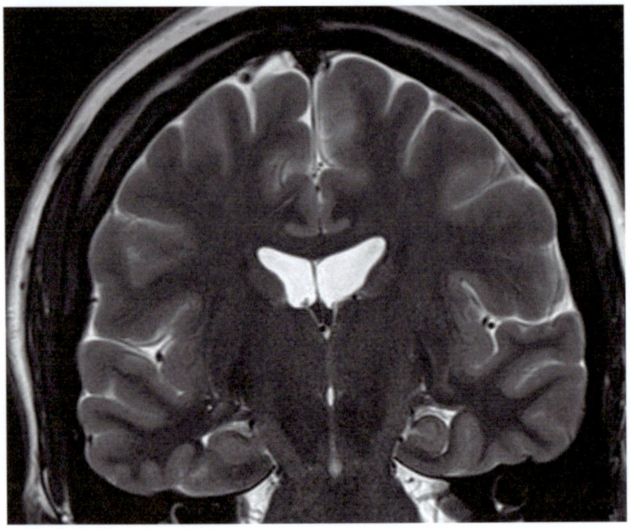

Fig. 64.1 MRI coronal T2 sequence at a hippocampal body level. The left collateral sulcus is oriented vertically and toward the temporal stem with an associated round shape to the left hippocampus. The left hippocampus' internal architecture and signal is normal and similar to the right hippocampus' architecture and signal. In contrast, the right hippocampus has a less round and more typical shape of a hippocampus. Its neighboring collateral sulcus is also typical by being oriented more obliquely toward the hippocampus

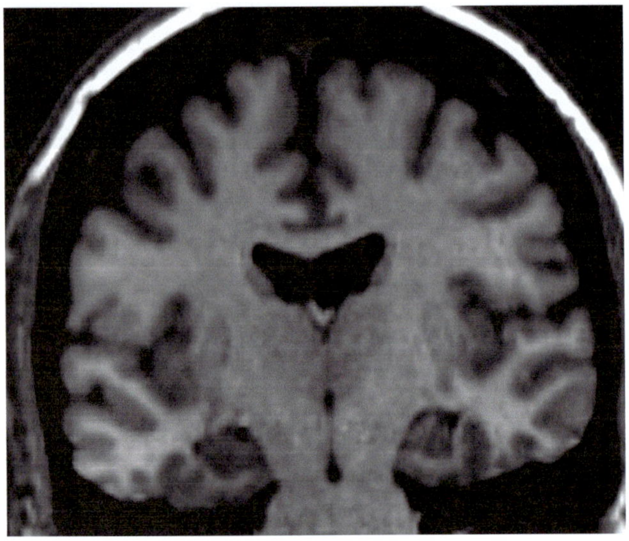

Fig. 64.2 MRI coronal T1 sequence at the same hippocampal body level as Figs. 64.1 and 64.2. Although the hippocampi differ in shape, their internal structure is symmetric and normal. No abnormality of the cortical ribbon is present

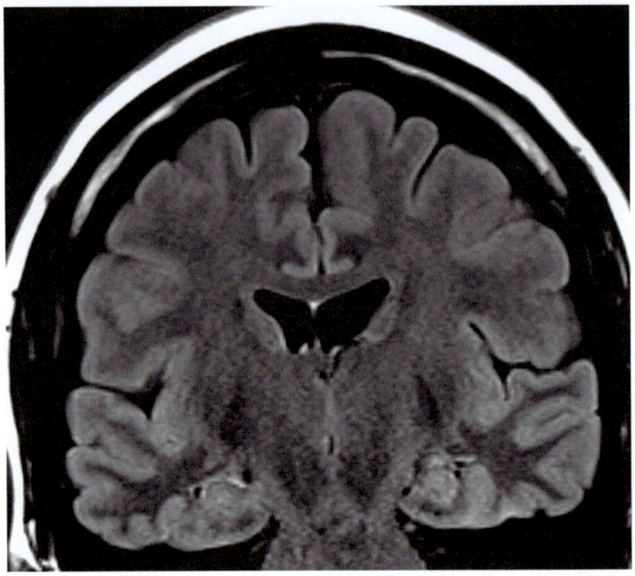

Fig. 64.3 MRI coronal FLAIR sequence at the same hippocampal body level as Fig. 64.1. The asymmetric shape of the hippocampi is apparent with rounded form on the left. The internal signal is normal and bilaterally symmetric. The left collateral sulcus is prominent, but its cortical ribbon is normal within the sulcus and in the remaining brain

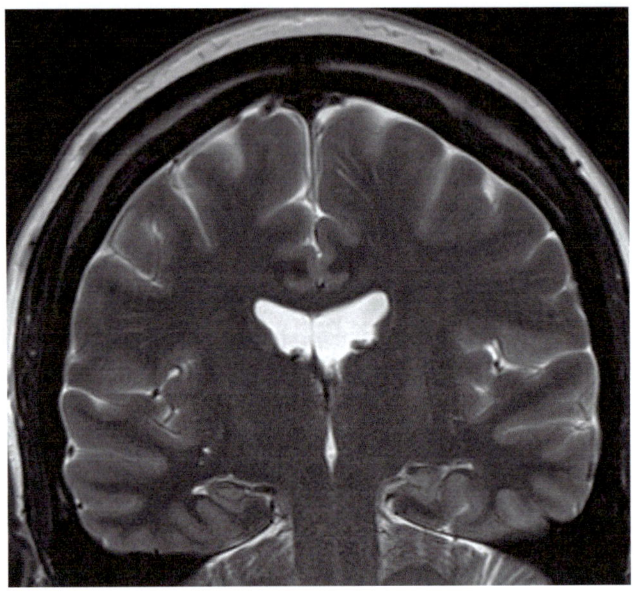

Fig. 64.4 MRI coronal T2 sequence of the hippocampal body at a level that is slightly posterior to Figs. 64.1, 64.2, and 64.3. The asymmetric collateral sulci are evident with the left collateral sulcus having a vertical orientation and the right collateral sulcus having a more laterally oblique orientation. The left hippocampus continues to have a rounded shape at this level

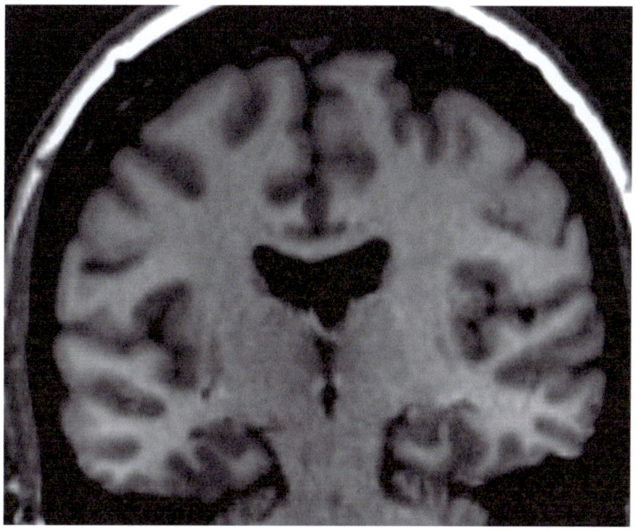

Fig. 64.5 MRI coronal T1 sequence at the same hippocampal body level as Fig. 64.4. The vertically oriented left collateral sulcus is evident along with the rounded shape of the left hippocampus, although the findings are not as clear as with the T2 sequence. The thalamic asymmetry is normal

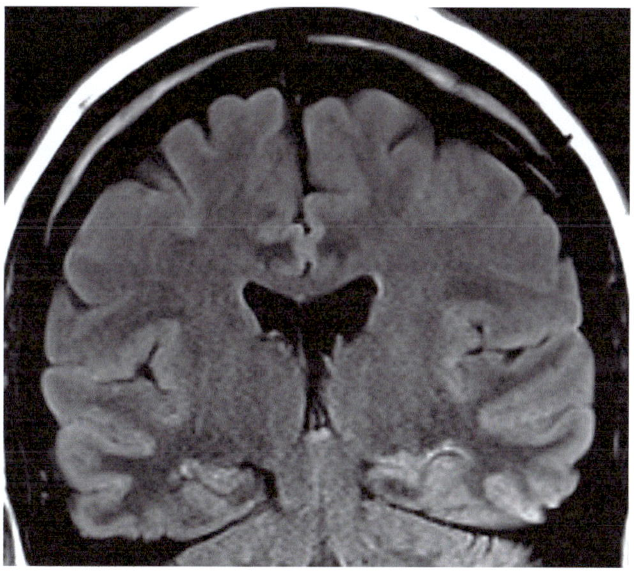

Fig. 64.6 MRI coronal FLAIR sequence at a similar hippocampal body levels as Figs. 64.4 and 64.5. The left collateral sulcus is vertically oriented and similar to Fig. 64.4, but the rounded shape of the left hippocampus is not as evident due to the difference in the level and the imaging sequence. The temporal lobe cortical ribbon is normal bilaterally and appears brighter on the left because of field inhomogeneity

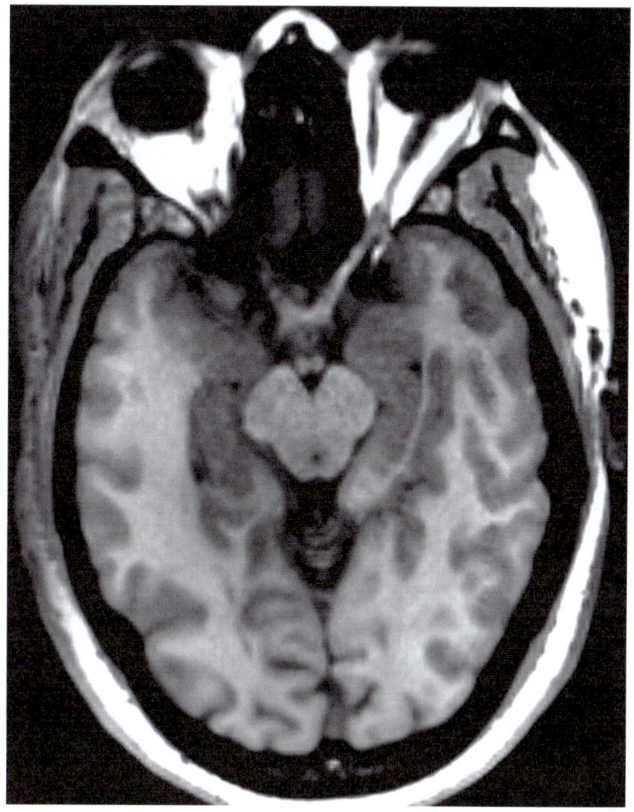

Fig. 64.7 MRI axial T1 sequence at a hippocampus level. The orientations of the mesial temporal lobes are asymmetric because of the collateral sulci. The left collateral sulcus is prominent and associated with the left hippocampus tilted mesially along both its anterior and posterior portions. The midbrain is normal

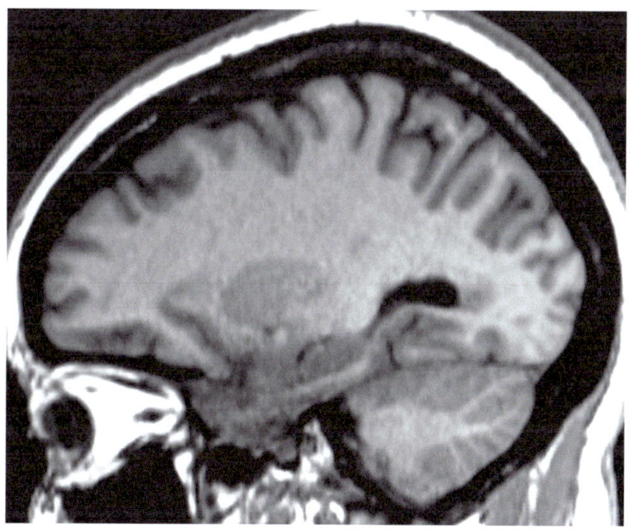

Fig. 64.8 MRI sagittal T1 sequence at a left hippocampus level. The posterior portion of the hippocampus is not in this level, and a vertically oriented deep portion of the collateral sulcus is evident along the inferior margin of the trigone of the lateral ventricles

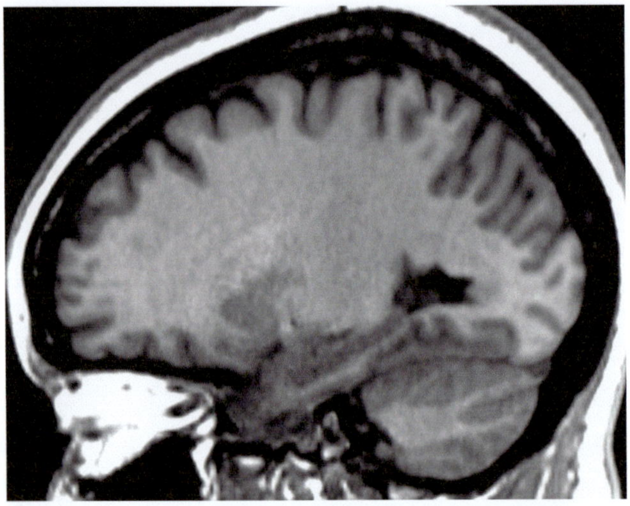

Fig. 64.9 MRI sagittal T1 sequence at a right hippocampus level. A normal hippocampus is evident with the entirety of the hippocampal body visible within the level. The collateral sulcus is visible inferior to the posterior hippocampus and has an orientation parallel to the hippocampus

65 Developmental Venous Anomaly

Clinical History

The first recognized seizure occurred at age 13 years as a nocturnal convulsion. An evaluation at that time included an EEG that depicted interictal epileptiform discharges across the anterior left temporal lobe and a brain MRI that identified a developmental venous anomaly in the left inferior frontal lobe. After a second nocturnal convulsion occurred several months later, treatment began.

The habitual seizures first occurred at age 20 years and after approximately 7 years of seizure freedom that followed starting anti-seizure medication. These seizures were during wakefulness and manifested as behavioral arrests and lapses in awareness without an aura or motor features. The seizure durations were about 1 minute. Treatment included multiple anti-seizure medications with a seizure frequency of two seizures during wakefulness weekly and one nocturnal tonic-clonic seizure yearly.

An epilepsy risk factor was not present.

Neurological examination was normal. Neuropsychological testing identified reduced confrontational naming and poor visuospatial skills.

Interictal EEG depicted left anterior and mid-temporal epileptiform discharges.

Video-EEG monitoring recorded focal seizures manifested as impairment of awareness with stereotyped right hand posturing with left arm flexion that lasted several seconds. Ictal EEG seizure onset was across the anterior left temporal lobe with expansion to include the entire left temporal region.

MRI identified a left orbitofrontal lobe developmental venous anomaly. PET identified left temporal hypometabolism. MEG identified a cluster of epileptiform dipoles across the anterior left temporal lobe, left insula, and left frontal operculum. Functional MRI identified left hemispheric dominance for language.

The history and evaluation indicate focal seizures with a likely left inferior frontal or anterior temporal neocortical temporal localization. The brief, motor asymmetric of the arms suggests left-sided lateralization, and the lack of an aura and brief seizure duration without postictal confusion suggest a neocortical origin. A neocortical origin is further supported by the neuropsychological testing identifying naming impairment with normal memory function. A left temporal lobe localization is most likely, as supported by the interictal and ictal EEG, interictal MEG, and PET; however, adjacent regions are also potential localizations because of the insular and opercular MEG dipoles and the possibility of an occult focal cortical dysplasia in the region of the orbitofrontal DVA. Stereotactic depth electrode video-EEG monitoring was recommended for narrowing the localization within these considerations prior to surgical treatment, and this invasive testing was deferred by the patient with a preference to continue treatment with anti-seizure medications.

J. M. Stern, N. Salamon, *Imaging of Epilepsy*, https://doi.org/10.1007/978-3-030-86672-3_65

Imaging

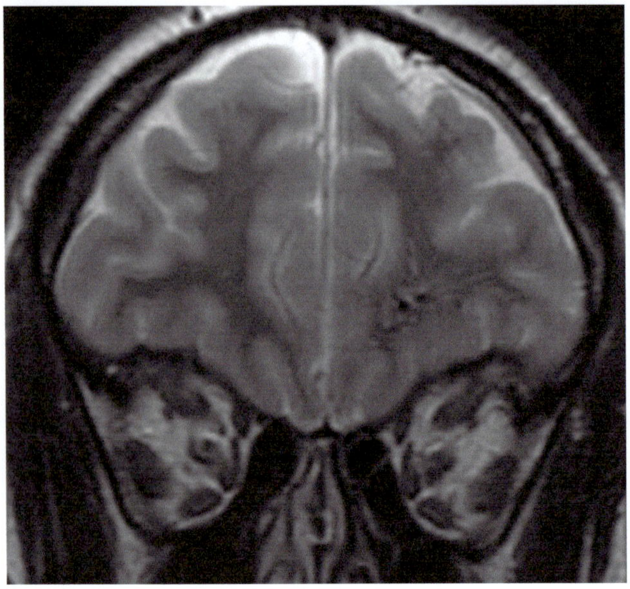

Fig. 65.1 MRI coronal T2 sequence at a frontal pole level. The two foci of hypointense signal within the left orbitofrontal white matter are due to flow voids from a developmental venous anomaly. Neither edema nor mass effects are adjacent to the foci. No other abnormality is present

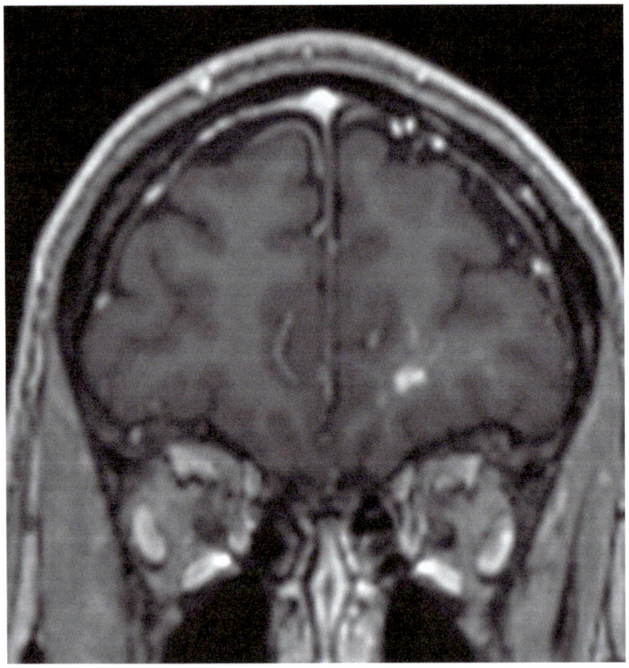

Fig. 65.2 MRI coronal T1 sequence after contrast administration at the same frontal pole level as Fig. 65.1. Contrast enhancement indicating a developmental venous anomaly is present in the same left orbitofrontal white matter location as the hypointensity in Fig. 65.1. Similar to the hypointensity in Fig. 65.1, the enhancement includes two components with one that is central and the other peripheral, which suggests one is a draining vein and the other is an element of a caput medusae. The linear enhancement that is radial from the enhancing couplet are normal veins in the cerebral white matter

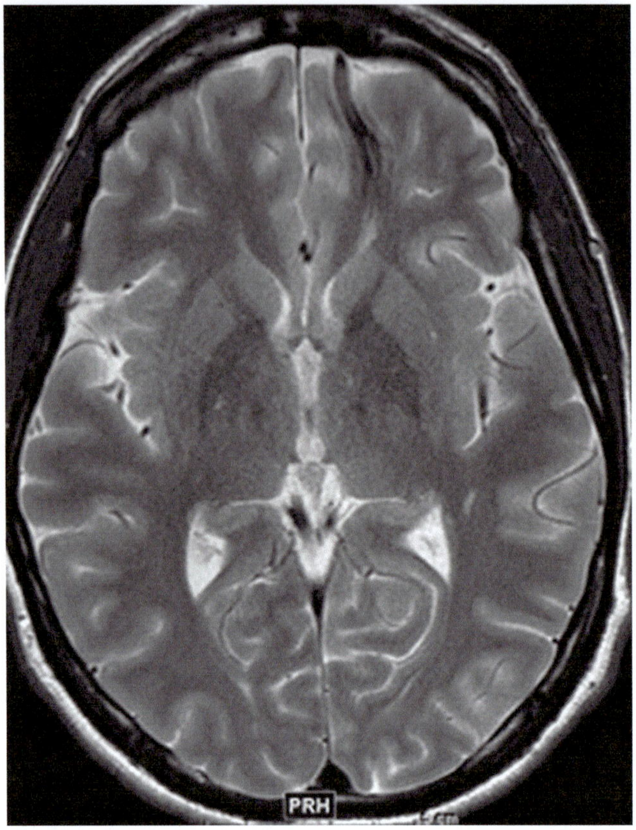

Fig. 65.3 MRI axial T2 sequence at a thalamus level. The developmental venous anomaly is visible as a draining vein with linear hypointense signal in the left orbitofrontal region that extends from superficial cortex toward through the deep white matter toward the ventral horn of the lateral ventricle. The abnormality does not produce edema or mass effect. The linear signal within the draining vein is pulsation artifact

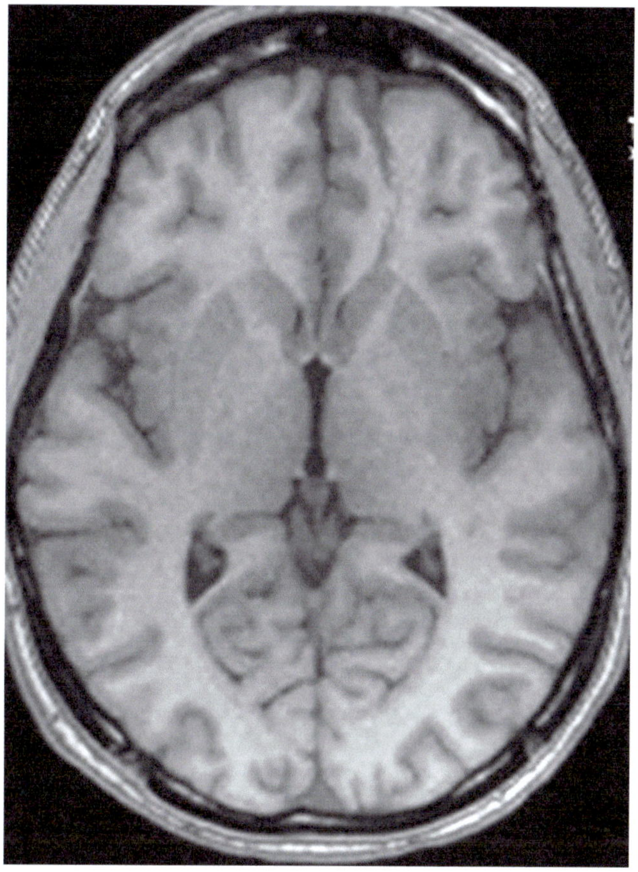

Fig. 65.4 MRI axial T1 sequence at the same thalamus level as Fig. 65.3. Similar to Fig. 65.3, the developmental venous anomaly is visible as linear hypointense signal due to a flow void within the left orbitofrontal region with draining from the frontal horn of the left lateral ventricle to the cortical surface. However, the abnormality is not as obvious with the T1 sequence in this figure as with the T2 sequence in Fig. 65.3

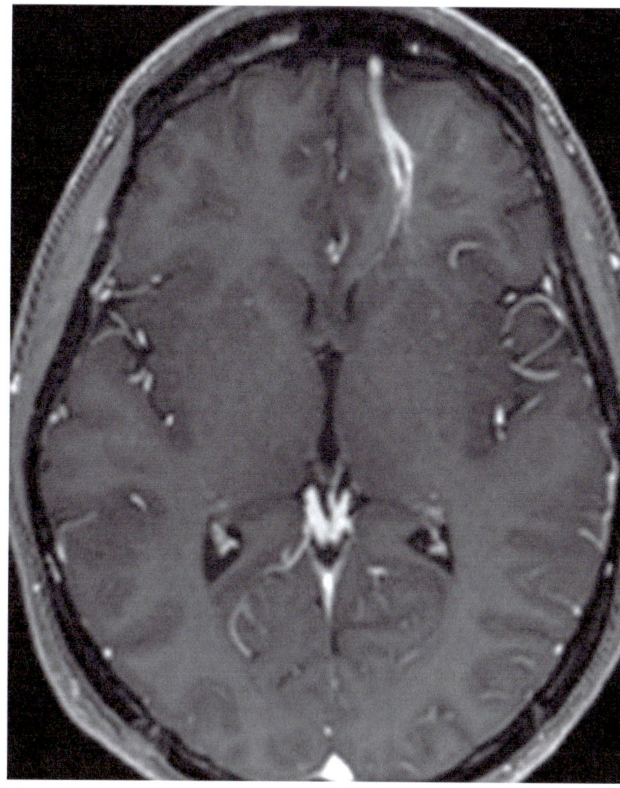

Fig. 65.5 MRI axial T1 sequence after contrast administration at the same thalamus level as Figs. 65.3 and 65.4. Linear contrast enhancement in the left orbitofrontal region extends from the frontal horn of the left lateral ventricle to the cortical surface with a branching in the mid-portion as the vein divides. Faint enhancement surrounds the tubular structure in left frontal white matter due to increased vascularity. The other enhancing venous structures in the figure are normal

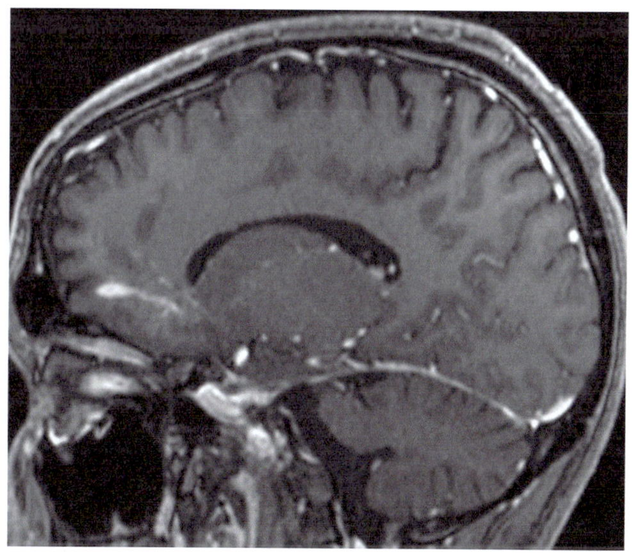

Fig. 65.6 MRI sagittal T1 sequence after contrast administration at a left thalamus level. Linear contrast enhancement in the orbitofrontal region extends between the frontal horn of the lateral ventricle surface to the cortical surface with minor enhancement that surrounds the linear enhancement due to increased vascularity. The remainder of enhancement in the figure is normal

Arachnoid Cyst

66

Clinical History

The first recognized seizure occurred at age 2 years as a nocturnal convulsion. An evaluation at that time that included head CT and EEG that were normal, and treatment was deferred. Two similar seizures occurred 1 year later, and treatment was deferred after an additional EEG was normal. At age 5 years, multiple nocturnal convulsions were observed with stereotyped occurrences about 20 minutes after sleep onset on 20 out of 30 consecutive nights, and treatment was initiated.

The habitual seizures manifested as bilateral stiffening with fist posturing and jaw tightening followed by generalized shaking with a total duration of about 30 to 60 seconds. Urinary incontinence or bilateral kicking sometimes occurred. Postictal fatigue was present without focal deficits. Treatment included multiple anti-seizure medications with a seizure frequency of five seizures monthly.

The epilepsy risk factors were mild autism and mild developmental delay.

Neurological examination identified mild autism and dysarthria. Neuropsychological testing identified a need for educational accommodations. Medical history included a chromosomal duplication.

Interictal EEGs were most often normal. One EEG identified left central epileptiform discharges, and another identified left frontal-temporal slowing. Video-EEG monitoring recorded nocturnal seizures manifested as right-upward gaze deviation and bilateral tonic-clonic movements. Ictal EEG seizure onset was bifrontal slowing followed by attenuation and then generalized rhythmic delta activity.

MRIs obtained over an 8-year period identified a right frontal arachnoid cyst and no other findings. PET was normal.

The history and evaluation indicate tonic-clonic seizures without clear evidence of either a focal or a generalized onset, as the history and video-EEG monitoring have not provided certainty in this differentiation. The interictal EEG suggests a left frontal abnormality, but the findings were subtle and rare. The MRI identification of an arachnoid cyst is apparently unrelated to the epilepsy, and a question remains whether the epilepsy is generalized or due to a left frontal structural abnormality that is not visible with MRI.

J. M. Stern, N. Salamon, *Imaging of Epilepsy*, https://doi.org/10.1007/978-3-030-86672-3_66

Imaging

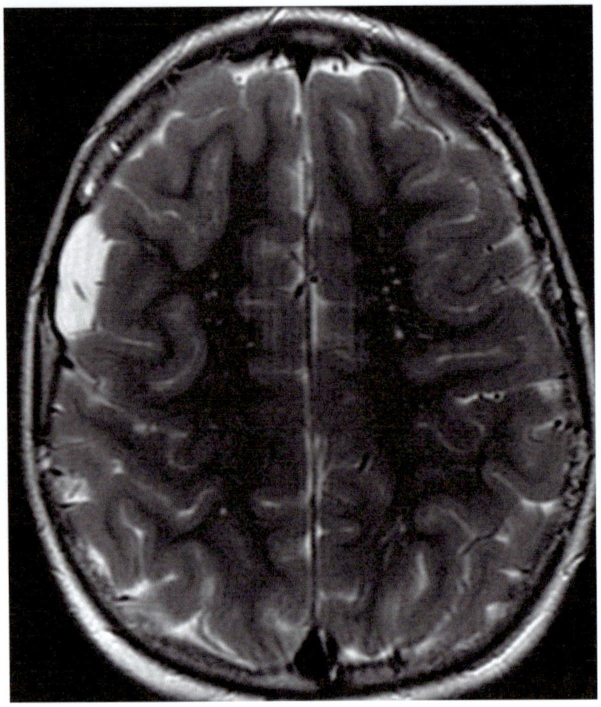

Fig. 66.1 MRI axial T2 sequence at a centrum semi-ovale level. An abnormal hyperintensity is present in the extra-axial space lateral to the right frontal lobe with associated displacement of the lateral aspect of the right middle frontal gyrus and bony erosion of the adjacent skull. The minor linear hypointensity within the abnormality probably represents a septum. The cerebrum is normal

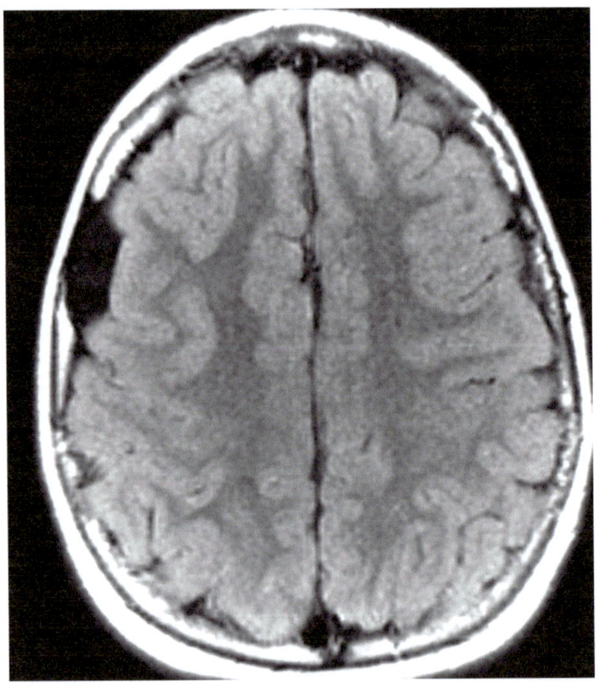

Fig. 66.2 MRI axial FLAIR sequence at the same centrum semi-ovale level as Fig. 66.1. A homogeneously hypointense oblong abnormality is within the extra-axial space lateral to the right frontal lobe. The adjacent right frontal lobe's signal intensity and cortical ribbon are normal along with the remainder of the visible cerebrum. The frontal bone is abnormally thinned

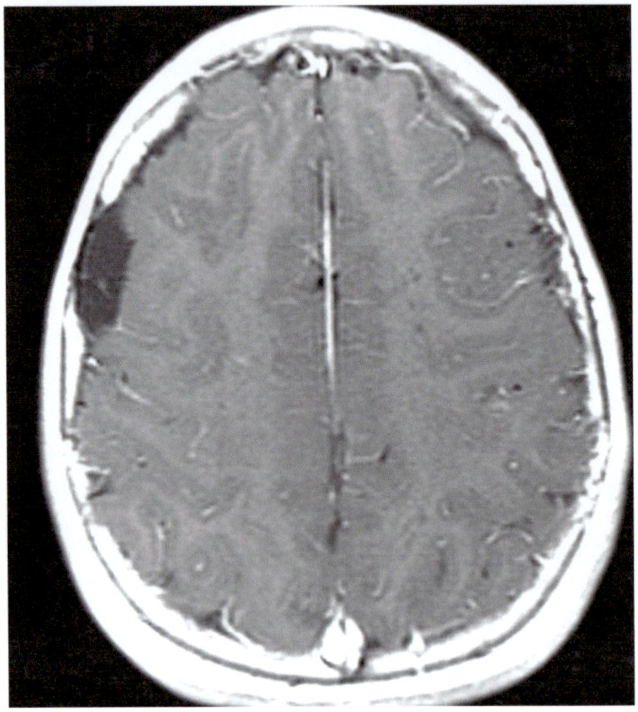

Fig. 66.3 MRI axial T1 sequence after contrast administration at the same centrum semi-ovale level as the preceding figures. A hypointense signal abnormality is lateral to the right frontal lobe. No abnormal enhancement is evident. The small linear feature within the abnormality is probably due to septation

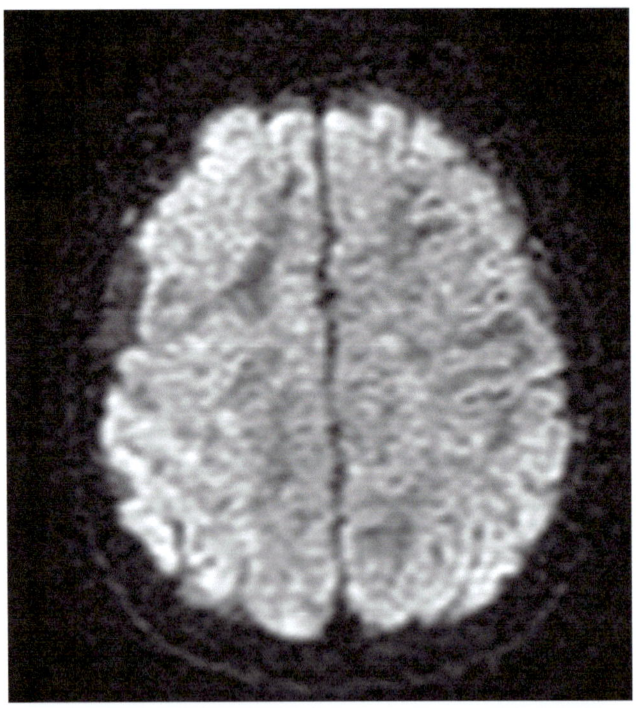

Fig. 66.4 MRI axial diffusion-weighted sequence at the same centrum semi-ovale level as the preceding figures. No restricted diffusion is present. The abnormality's signal intensity corresponds to cerebrospinal fluid (CSF)

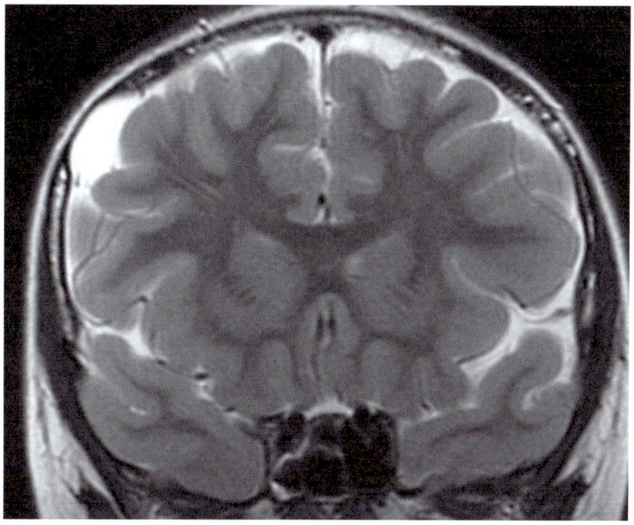

Fig. 66.5 MRI coronal T2 sequence at a genu of the corpus callosum level. A prominent CSF space is adjacent to the lateral aspect of right middle frontal gyrus. Lateral to the CSF space, the skull is thinned with bony erosion. The right middle frontal gyrus and remaining cerebrum are normal

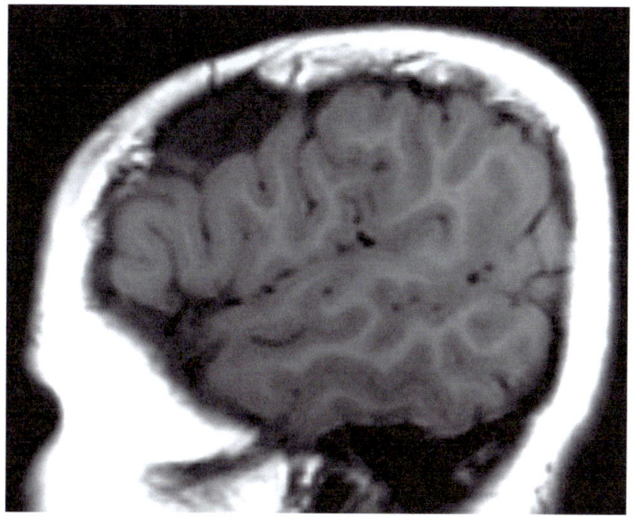

Fig. 66.7 MRI sagittal T1 sequence at a right Sylvian fissure level. An oblong hypointensity with signal consistent with CSF is adjacent to the right inferior frontal gyrus. The inferior frontal gyrus' cortical ribbon and the remaining cerebrum are normal. The skull adjacent to the hypointensity is abnormally thinned

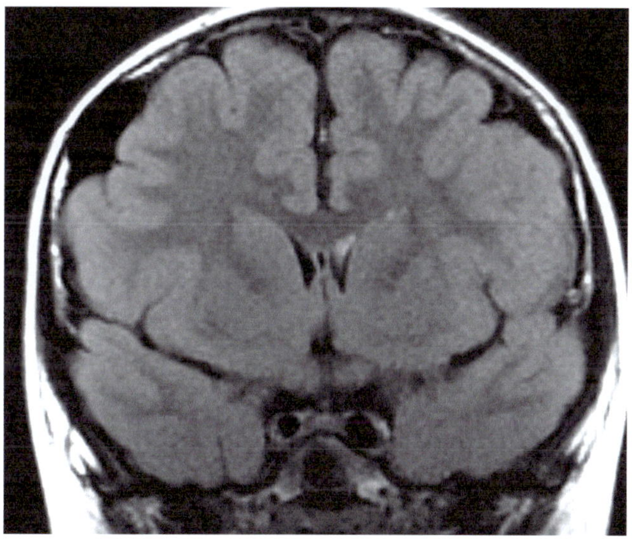

Fig. 66.6 MRI coronal FLAIR sequence at a level slightly posterior to Fig. 66.5. A hypointense abnormality with signal intensity corresponding to CSF is between the right middle frontal gyrus and a bony erosion of the skull. No other abnormality is present

Epidermoid Cyst

67

Clinical History

The first recognized seizures occurred at age 5 years as episodes of sudden bilateral arm abduction with a frequency of two to five daily. An evaluation at that time included an EEG that depicted generalized epileptiform abnormality.

The habitual seizures manifested as gaze deviation upward with or without rhythmic shaking of the arms. The duration was described as brief. Treatment has included multiple anti-seizure medications with a seizure frequency that decreased over the years from the onset to several annually.

The epilepsy risk factor was a diffuse cerebral dysfunction without a specific diagnosis. Based on non-neurologic abnormalities, mitochondrial disease was the presumed diagnosis, but testing has been negative.

Neurological examination identified a developmental age of between 1 and 2 years with almost no verbal ability. Hyperreflexia was present throughout and bilateral lower extremities have contractures. Bowel and bladder control were not present. Medical and neurologic history was normal until age 2 years when neurologic disability and rhabdomyolysis developed.

Interictal EEG that was obtained during the evaluation of the developmental delay was normal. One year later and after the occurrence of seizures, interictal EEG depicted mild to moderate abnormal generalized slowing, occasional to frequent right frontal-central and left occipital epileptiform discharges, and frequent, 3- to 4-second bursts of diffuse paroxysmal fast activity with a left-sided predominance. Video-EEG monitoring recorded focal seizures manifested as gaze deviation or staring for 1 to 2 seconds. Ictal EEG's seizure onset was 1- to 2-second bursts of high amplitude and sharply contoured, polymorphic slowing.

MRI identified a non-enhancing lesion in the left mesial temporal lobe and no other abnormality. PET was normal.

The history and evaluation indicate a generalized epilepsy that is likely due to a metabolic disorder. Laboratory testing including genetic analyses and muscle biopsy were not diagnostic. Imaging also was not diagnostic but depicted an epidermoid cyst that is not related to the clinical condition.

J. M. Stern, N. Salamon, *Imaging of Epilepsy*, https://doi.org/10.1007/978-3-030-86672-3_67

Imaging

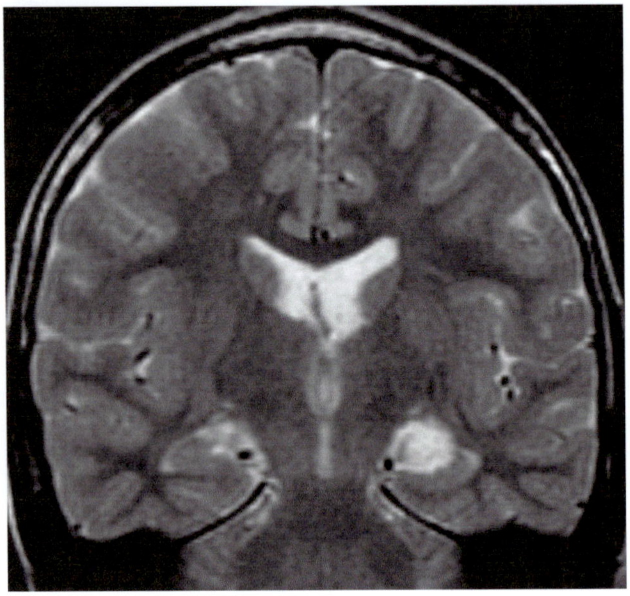

Fig. 67.1 MRI coronal T2 sequence at a hippocampal body level. A round, hyperintense lesion is evident in the left choroidal fissure and compressing the body of the left hippocampus. The lesion is isointense and is similar to cerebrospinal fluid (CSF) signal. The deformed hippocampal body has normal signal intensity. No other abnormality is present

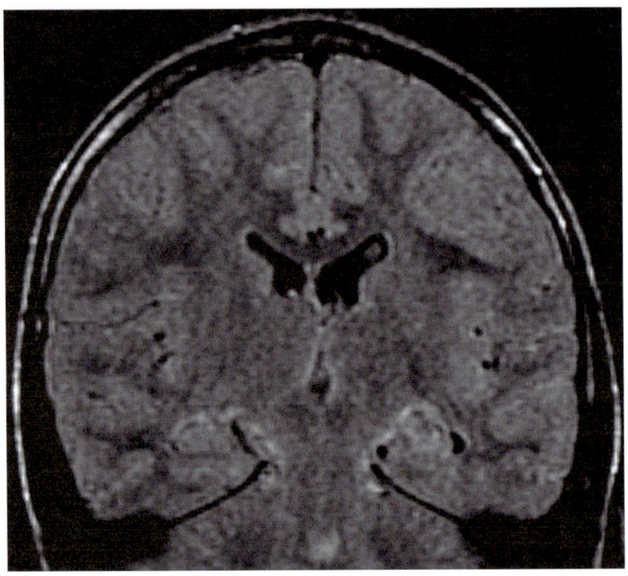

Fig. 67.2 MRI coronal FLAIR sequence at the same level hippocampal body level as Fig. 67.1. A lesion is evident in the left choroidal fissure and has signal that is isointense and is similar to cerebral tissue. Unlike the T2 sequence in Fig. 67.1, the lesion's signal differs from CSF. The left hippocampus is deformed and has normal signal intensity. No other abnormality is present

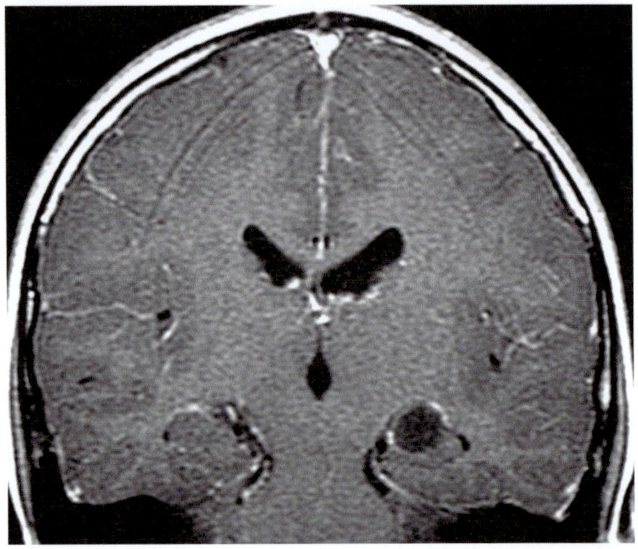

Fig. 67.3 MRI coronal T1 sequence after contrast administration at the same hippocampal body level as Figs. 67.1 and 67.2. A hypointense lesion is evident in the left choroidal fissure. The enhancement along the superior-lateral and medial margins of the cyst is normal choroid plexus enhancement. The internal content of the lesion does not enhance. The left hippocampus is deformed and otherwise normal

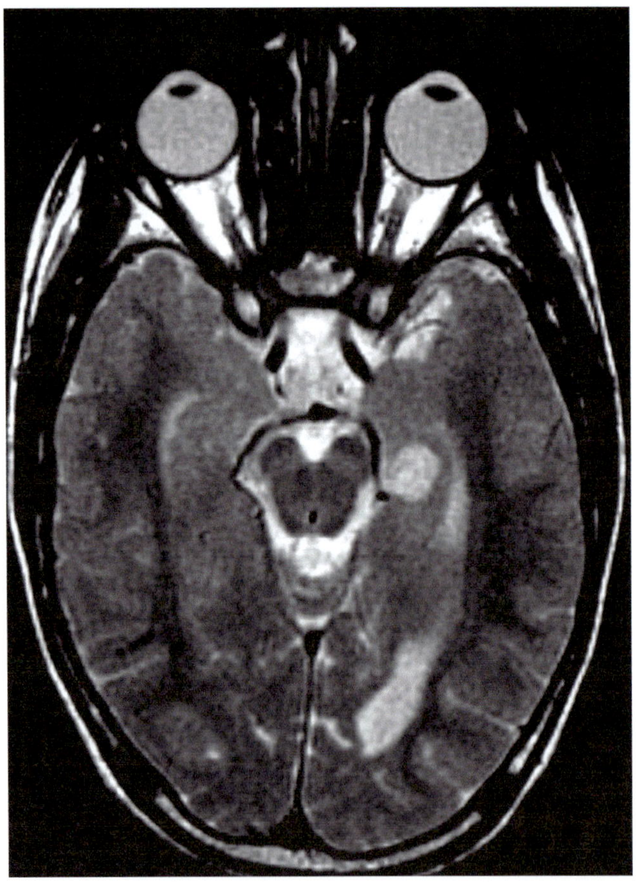

Fig. 67.4 MRI axial T2 sequence at a hippocampal body level. In the left mesial temporal lobe, a round hyperintense lesion with signal intensity similar to CSF protrudes into the anterior hippocampal body. The adjacent hippocampus has normal signal. The remainder of brain is normal

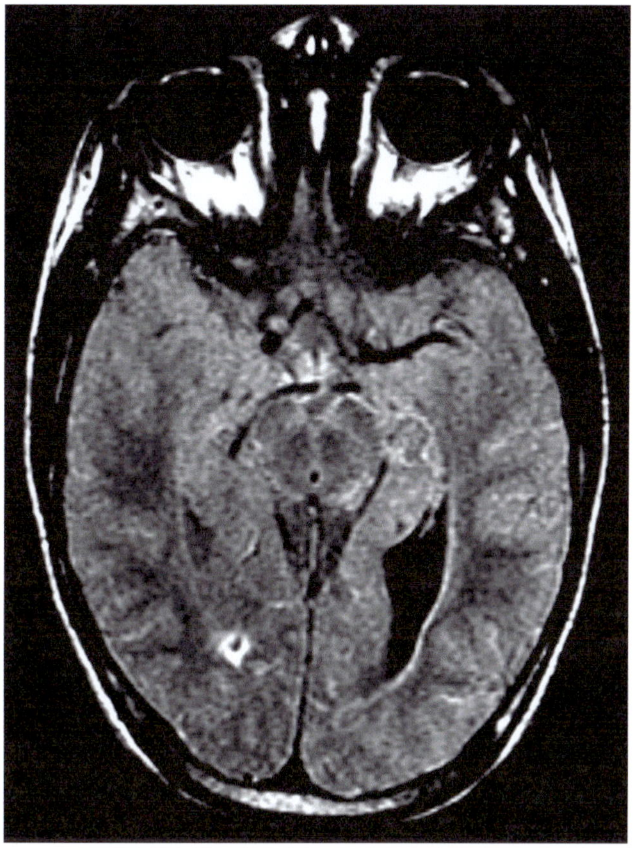

Fig. 67.5 MRI axial FLAIR sequence at the same hippocampal body level as Fig. 67.4. A round lesion is present in the left mesial temporal lobe, but it is subtle because its signal is isointense with the adjacent anterior body of the hippocampus, and it does not deform the hippocampus in this plane. A comparison to Fig. 67.4 helps identify the lesion's margins

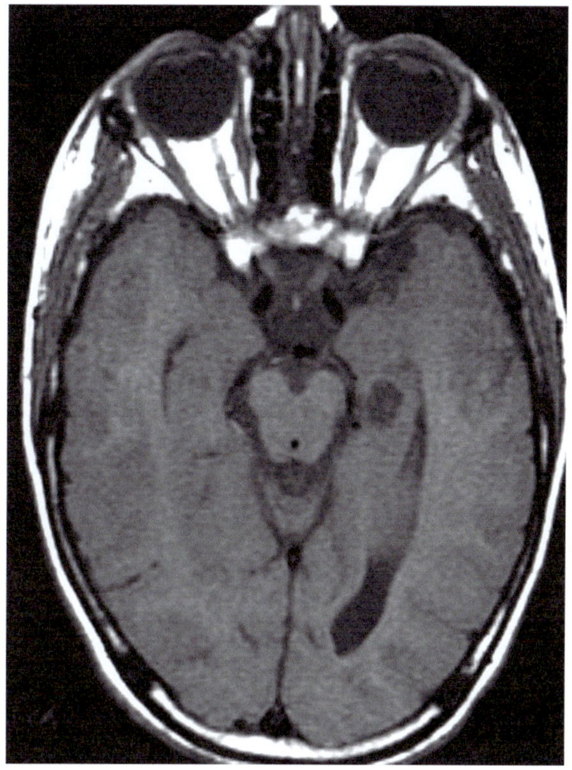

Fig. 67.6 MRI axial T1 sequence at the same hippocampal body level as Figs. 67.4 and 67.5. A round hypointense lesion is evident within the anterior body of the left hippocampus with signal intensity similar to CSF. The surrounding hippocampus is normal and without deformity

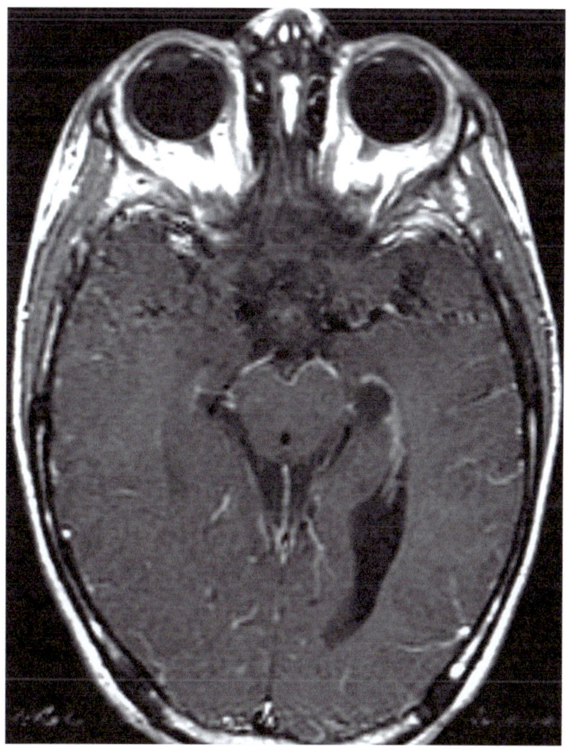

Fig. 67.7 MRI axial T1 sequence after contrast administration at the same hippocampal body level as Figs. 67.4, 67.5, and 67.6. A round lesion within the left hippocampal body has normal enhancement along its periphery due to the adjacent choroid plexus. No abnormal enhancement is present in the cyst or elsewhere in the image

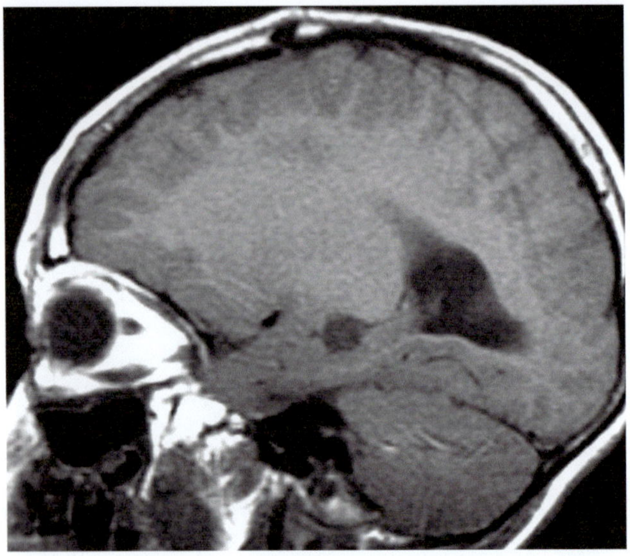

Fig. 67.8 MRI sagittal T1 sequence at a left hippocampus level. A round hypointense lesion is evident in the choroidal fissure and is compressing the hippocampal body. Compared to CSF signal, the lesion's signal intensity is similar but not as hypointense. Other than the deformity, the hippocampal body is normal

68 Cerebellar Atrophy

Clinical History

The first recognized seizure occurred at age 25 years as witnessed collapsing followed by a tonic-clonic convulsion. The details of the initial evaluation were no longer recalled.

The habitual seizures first occurred soon after the first seizure and around the time that treatment was begun. The seizures manifested as an aura of a sensation in the throat that produced gagging, and sometimes the aura also included deja vu. The auras never occurred in isolation and more recently ceased to consistently occur. With and without the aura, seizures produced impaired awareness with staring, patting the chest with the left hand, and kicking the left leg for 2 to 3 minutes. Occasionally, repetitive swallowing accompanied the left-hand automatism. Typically, the right body remained motionless throughout the seizure, and very rarely, urinary incontinence occurred. For several minutes after each seizure, fatigue and difficulty in speaking was present, but comprehension was intact. Treatment included multiple anti-seizure medications with a seizure frequency of 2 to 5 weekly. In total, 7 anti-seizure medications were tried, and phenytoin was a component of the treatment for 27 years. When phenytoin was discontinued, two additional tonic-clonic seizures occurred. No tonic-clonic seizures occurred during treatment with phenytoin.

An epilepsy risk factor was not present.

Neurological examination was normal.

Interictal EEG depicted left anterior temporal abnormal slowing, intermittent left anterior temporal epileptiform discharges, and rare right anterior temporal epileptiform discharges. Video-EEG monitoring recorded focal seizures manifested as a loss of awareness with repetitive oral and pharyngeal automatisms followed by left leg repetitive kicking. Ictal EEG's seizure onset was broad across the left hemisphere with suggestion of a left temporal maximum.

MRI identified bilateral hippocampal atrophy and signal abnormality with greater evidence of hippocampal sclerosis on the left. Cerebellar atrophy also was present.

PET was normal. An intracarotid amobarbital test identified episodic memory function bilaterally.

The history and evaluation indicate focal seizures with limbic auras and behavioral manifestations, including the experience of the throat sensation, deja vu, automatisms, and rare progression to bilateral tonic-clonic seizures. The bilateral interictal abnormality does not preclude a unilateral epileptogenic zone, and the left-sided automatisms with possibly right-sided posturing or neglect suggest a left-sided epilepsy. The MRI depicts bilateral hippocampal sclerosis that is asymmetrically greater on the left, but the intracarotid amobarbital test indicated a risk of a memory deficit from a left anterior temporal lobe resection. Based on the testing, the patient declined additional testing in consideration of a surgical treatment. The cerebellar atrophy may relate to the duration of the epilepsy, poor seizure control, and treatment with phenytoin.

J. M. Stern, N. Salamon, *Imaging of Epilepsy*, https://doi.org/10.1007/978-3-030-86672-3_68

Imaging

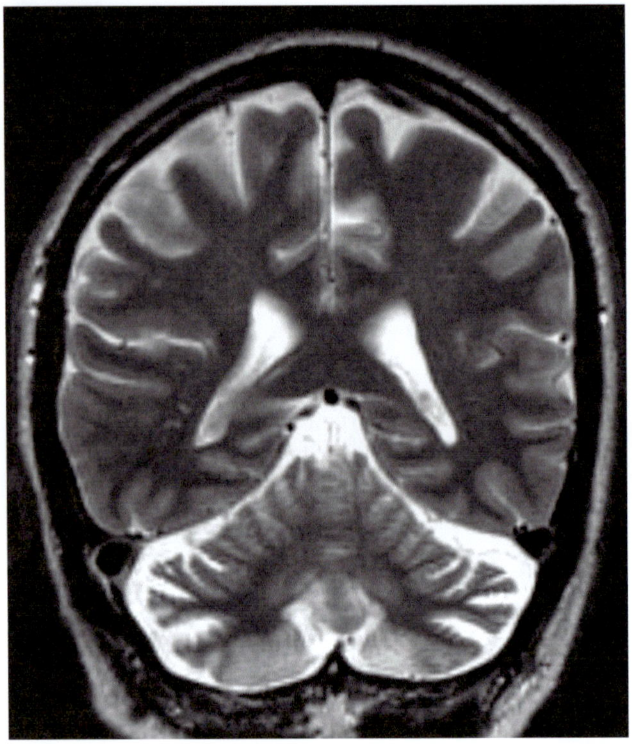

Fig. 68.1 MRI coronal T2 sequence at a splenium of the corpus callosum level. The cerebrospinal fluid (CSF) space is abnormally increased in the posterior fossa due to global volume loss of the cerebellar hemispheres bilaterally. No signal abnormality is evident within the cerebellum or the cerebrum. The cerebrum has normal volume and surrounding CSF space. The ventricles also are normal

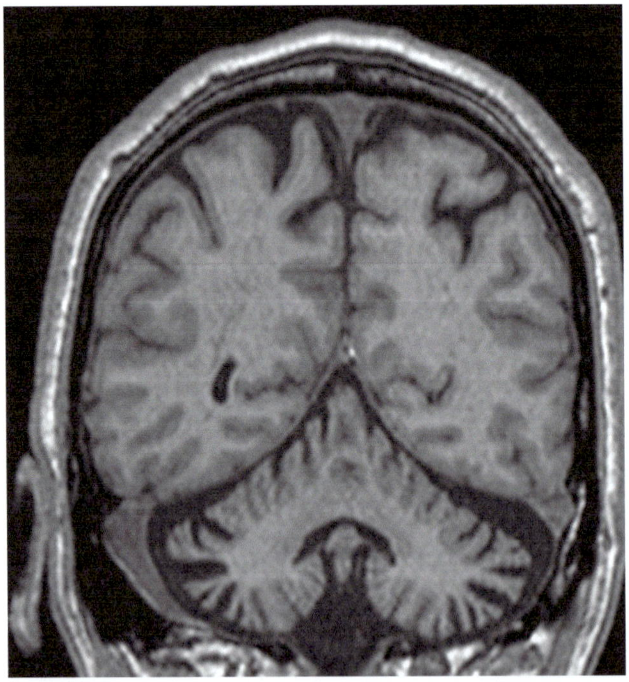

Fig. 68.2 MRI coronal T1 sequence at an occipital horn of the lateral ventricles level. Prominent CSF space is evident around the cerebellum with global volume loss of the cerebellar hemispheres. The cerebral volume is normal. The prominent left intraparietal sulcus is normal

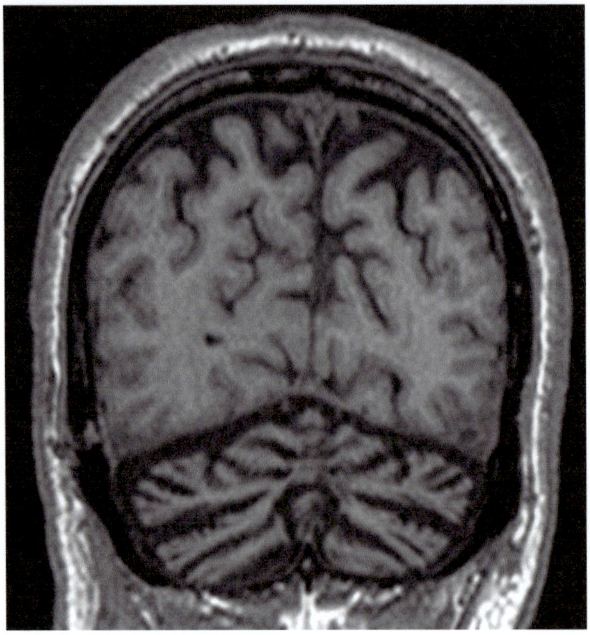

Fig. 68.3 MRI coronal T1 sequence at a level posterior to Fig. 68.2's occipital lobe level. Prominent CSF space is evident in the posterior fossa due to marked cerebellar volume loss with a particularly enlarged horizontal tissue within the cerebellar hemispheres. The cerebellar vermis is also atrophic but not as prominently as the hemispheres. The cerebrum is normal

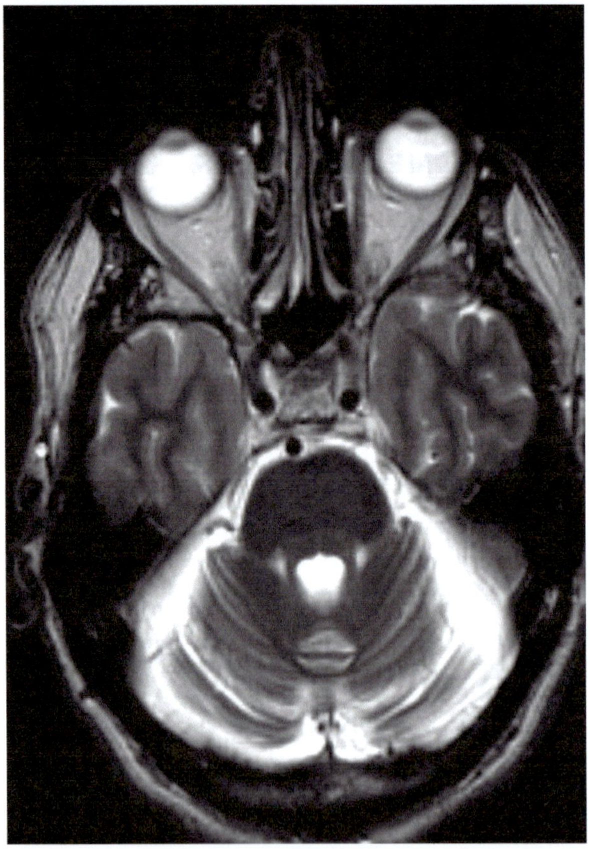

Fig. 68.4 MRI axial T2 sequence at a mid-pons level. Prominent CSF space is evident in the posterior fossa, especially around the cerebellum. Cerebellar vermis is slightly atrophic. The pons is normal in shape and size, and no abnormal signal is within the pons or cerebellum. The temporal lobes are normal

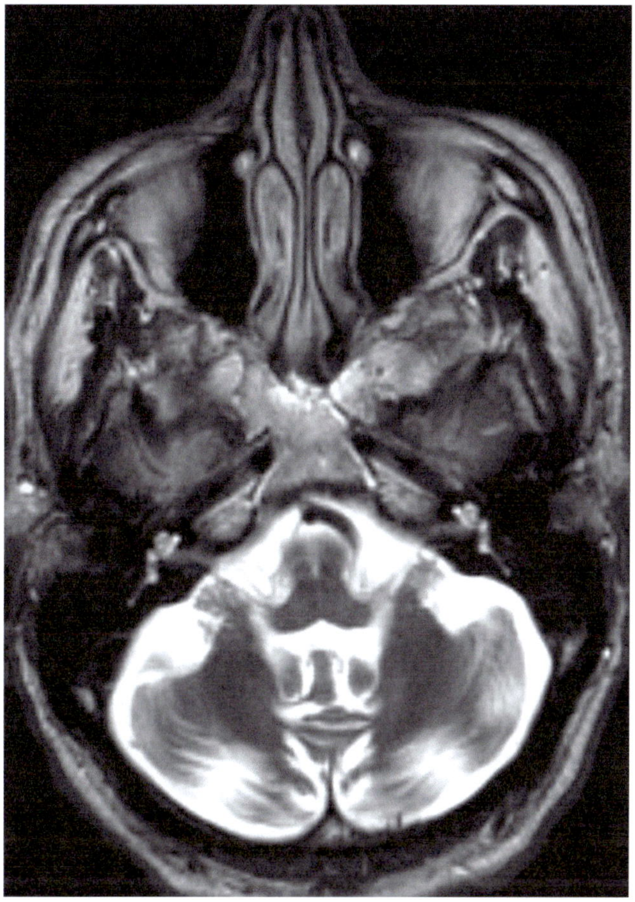

Fig. 68.5 MRI axial T2 sequence at a medulla level. Prominent CSF space surrounds the cerebellar hemispheres and vermis. The medulla and cerebellar white matter are normal

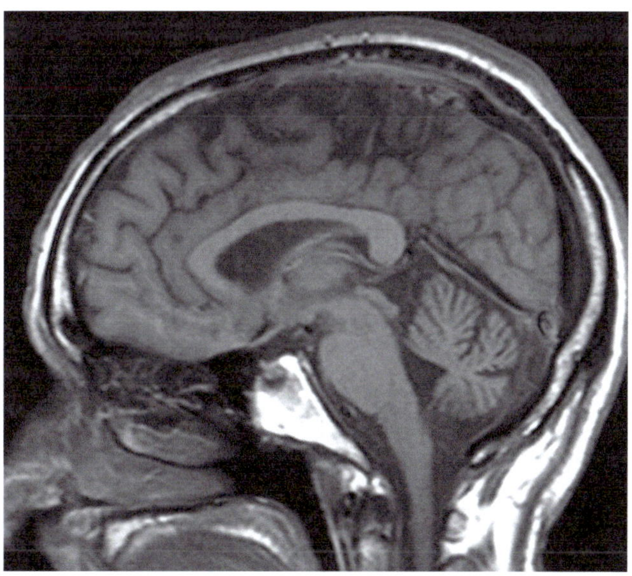

Fig. 68.6 MRI sagittal T1 sequence at a midline level. Prominent CSF surrounds the cerebellar vermis. The brainstem, cerebrum, and the ventricles are normal in size. The cerebellar and cerebral parenchyma are normal

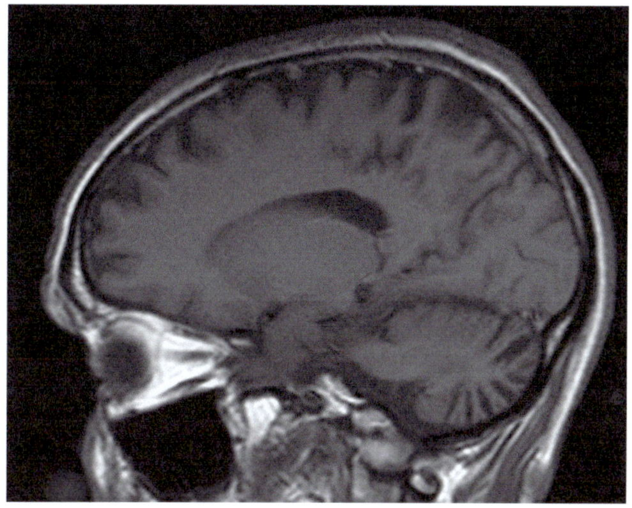

Fig. 68.7 MRI sagittal T1 sequence at a middle cerebellar peduncle level. A prominent CSF space is adjacent to the posterior inferior aspect of the cerebellum. The superior cerebellar atrophy is not as evident in this image. No other abnormality is present

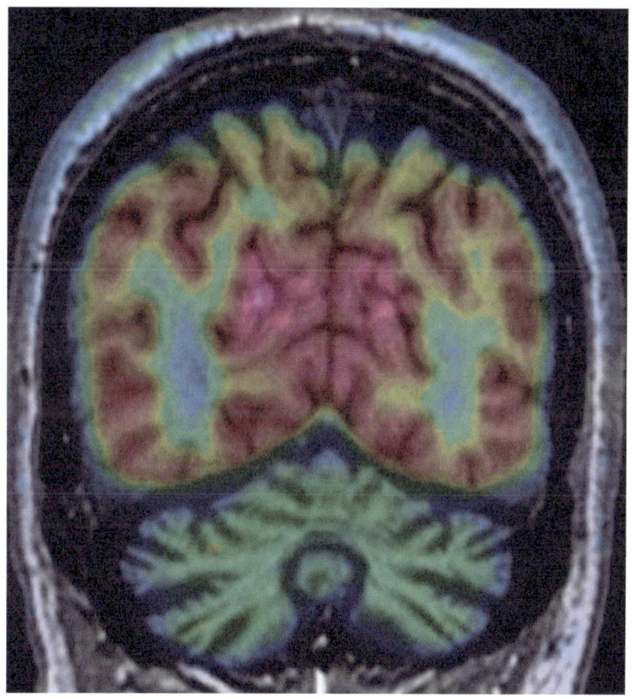

Fig. 68.8 PET-MRI co-registration with color-scale FDG tracer in a coronal plane at an occipital lobe level. The cerebellum has global hypometabolism. Normal cerebellar metabolism is similar to cerebral metabolism

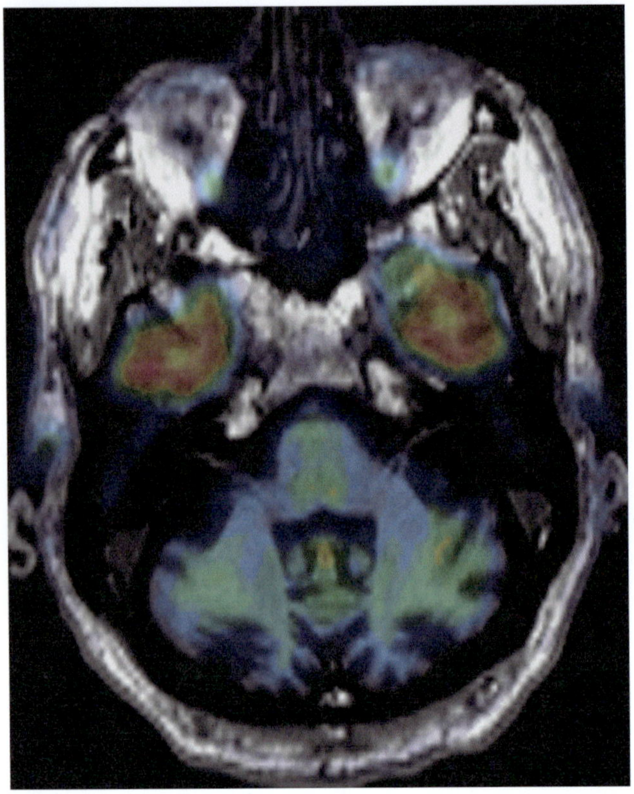

Fig. 68.9 PET-MRI co-registration with color-scale FDG tracer in an axial plane at a ponto-medullary junction level. Global hypometabolism of cerebellum includes the visible hemispheres and the vermis. The temporal lobe and brain metabolism are normal

69 Splenium Signal Abnormality

Clinical History

The first recognized seizure occurred at age 14 years as episodes described as inattention or confusion. The evaluation at that time was not recalled.

The habitual seizures manifested as tunnel vision accompanied by a sensation in the chest and have a duration of 30 seconds. Occasionally, the seizures progressed to include rightward twisting, and progression is less often to a tonic-clonic seizure. Treatment included multiple anti-seizure medications with a frequency of three to four seizures monthly. Tonic-clonic seizures occurred about once annually.

An epilepsy risk factor was not present.

Neurological examination was normal. Neuropsychological testing identified superior general intellectual function with deficits in attention, working memory, and executive functioning.

Interictal EEG depicted rare epileptiform discharges with a maximum in the left middle frontal lobe. Video-EEG monitoring recorded focal seizures manifested as right arm clonic movements followed by right arm dystonic posturing and rightward versive movements. Some seizures progressed further to include bilateral tonic-clonic movements. Ictal EEG's seizure onset was not clear, but a poorly formed rhythm across the left temporal lobe was present later during the seizures.

MRI obtained upon completion of video-EEG monitoring identified left precentral gyrus polymicrogyria and signal abnormality in the left hippocampal tail and the splenium of the corpus callosum. Specifically, the MRI was 2 days after a 5-day period during which seven seizures occurred. An MRI obtained 1.5 years later demonstrated resolution of the corpus callosum signal abnormality. PET was normal.

The history and evaluation indicate focal seizures with early motor signs, interictal EEG, and imaging findings indicating a left frontal lobe epileptogenic region. The neuropsychological testing also supports a frontal lobe abnormality. The ictal EEG rhythm across the left temporal lobe does not necessarily alter the localization as the finding occurred late in the seizure and may be related to propagation in the context of the hippocampal tail abnormality that indicates dual pathology. The abnormality within the splenium of the corpus callosum was present within a few days of a seizure cluster, which is typical of this finding. The MRI finding was not present years later.

J. M. Stern, N. Salamon, *Imaging of Epilepsy*, https://doi.org/10.1007/978-3-030-86672-3_69

Imaging

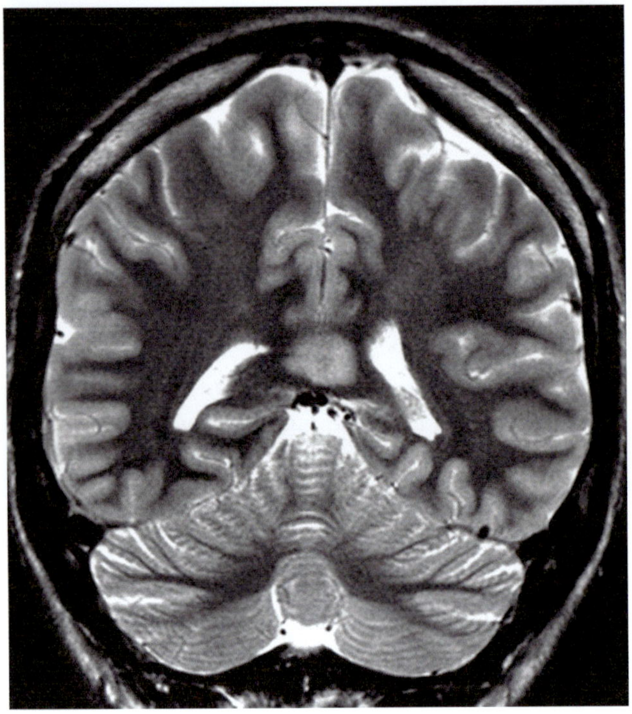

Fig. 69.1 MRI coronal T2 sequence at a splenium of the corpus callosum level. A well-defined hyperintensity in the center of splenium of the corpus callosum is consistent with focal edema. No other abnormalities are present

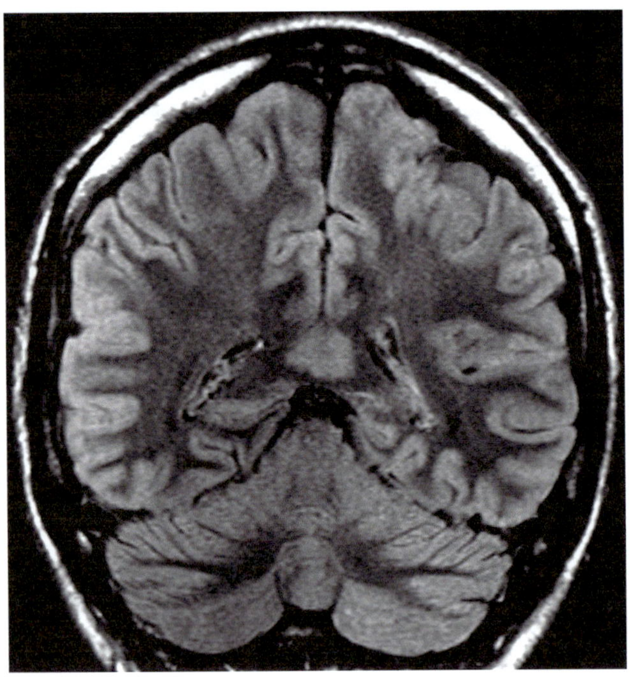

Fig. 69.2 MRI coronal FLAIR sequence at the same splenium of the corpus callosum level as Fig. 69.1. The hyperintense abnormality that is present in the center of splenium of the corpus callosum does not produce a deformation of the corpus callosum

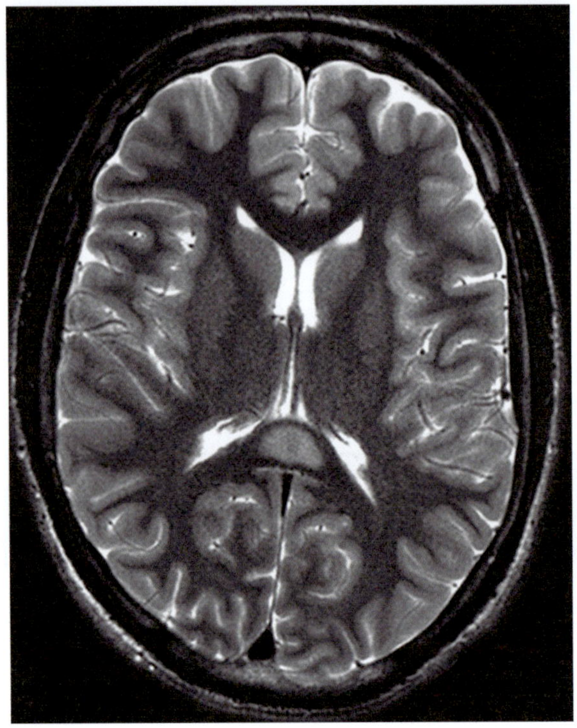

Fig. 69.3 MRI axial T2 sequence at a basal ganglia level. A well-defined homogenous hyperintense abnormality is in the center of splenium of the corpus callosum without deforming the corpus callosum's contour. The genu of the corpus callosum is normal. No other abnormality is present

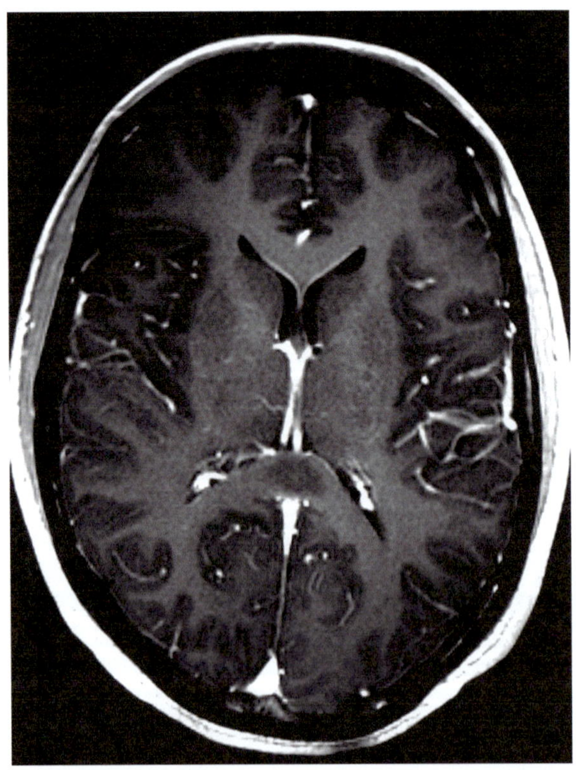

Fig. 69.4 MRI axial T1 sequence after contrast administration at the same basal ganglia level as Fig. 69.3. The well-defined hypointensity in the splenium of the corpus callosum does not enhance internally, and no enhancement surrounds the abnormality. The finding is consistent with focal edema

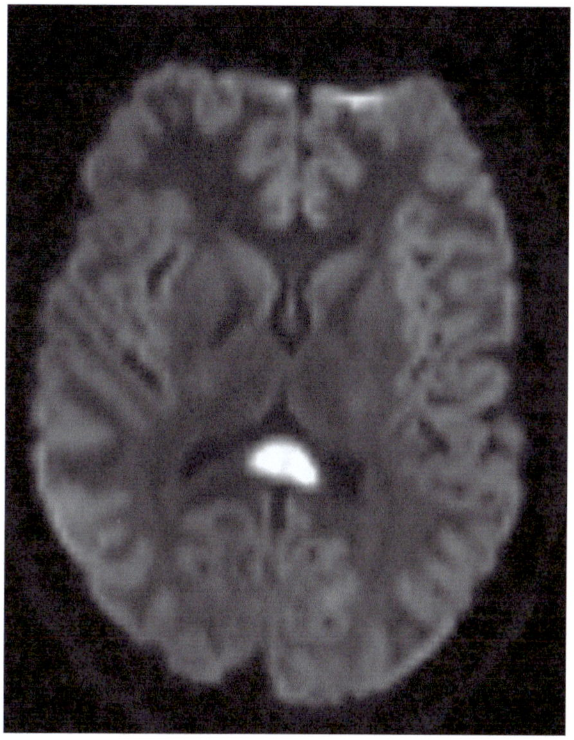

Fig. 69.5 MRI axial diffusion-weighted sequence at the same basal ganglia level as Figs. 69.3 and 69.4. Restricted diffusion is evident in the splenium of the corpus callosum and corresponds to other sequences' abnormalities. No other abnormality is present

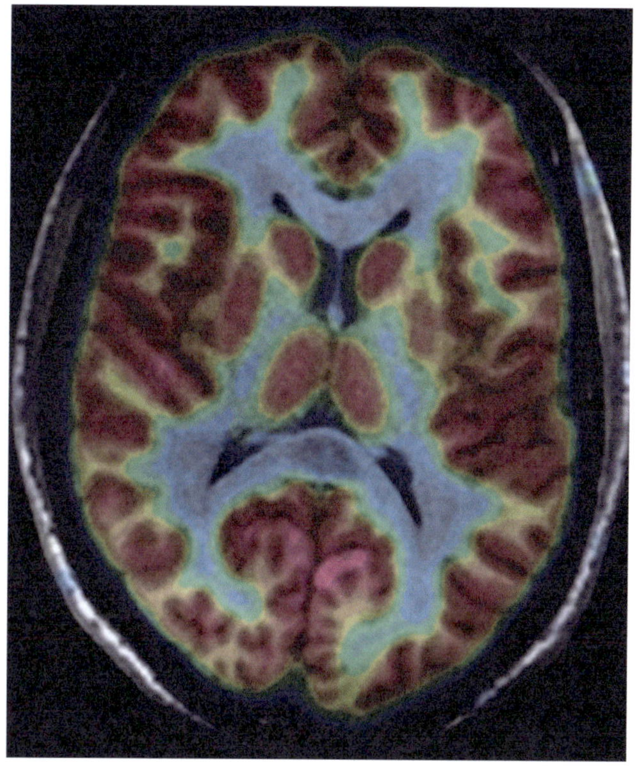

Fig. 69.7 PET-MRI co-registration with color-scale FDG tracer in an axial plane at the same basal ganglia level as Figs. 69.3 to 69.6. The splenium of the corpus callosum abnormality is isometabolic and similar in signal to the surrounding fiber tracts. It appears darker because of the hypointense signal of the co-registered MRI T1 sequence

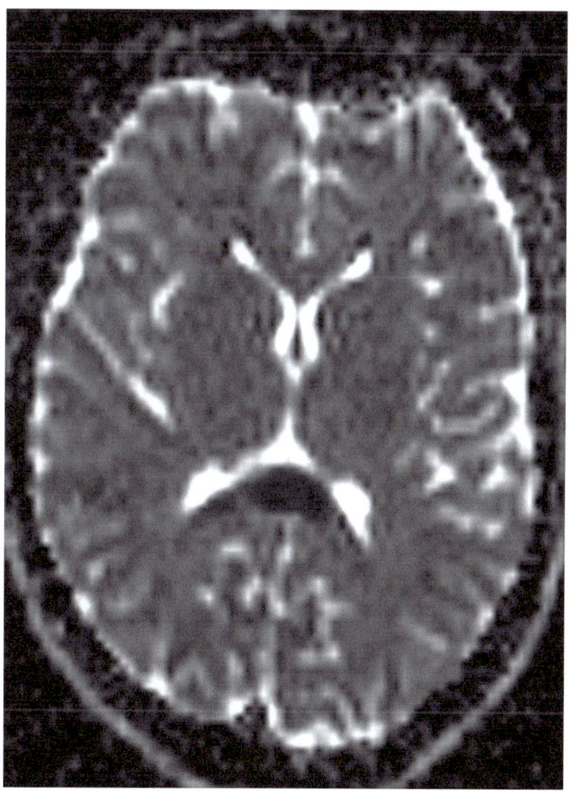

Fig. 69.6 MRI axial apparent diffusion coefficient map at the same basal ganglia level as Figs. 69.3 to 69.5. Hypointensity in the splenium of the corpus callosum suggests restricted diffusion within this abnormality that is consistent with intramyelinic edema

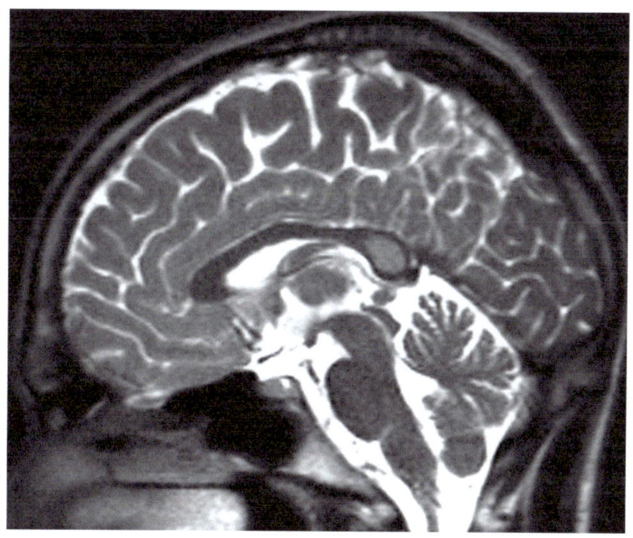

Fig. 69.8 MRI sagittal T2 sequence at a midline level. A hyperintensity with clear margins is in the center of the splenium of the corpus callosum without associated deformity. The remaining corpus callosum and brain are normal

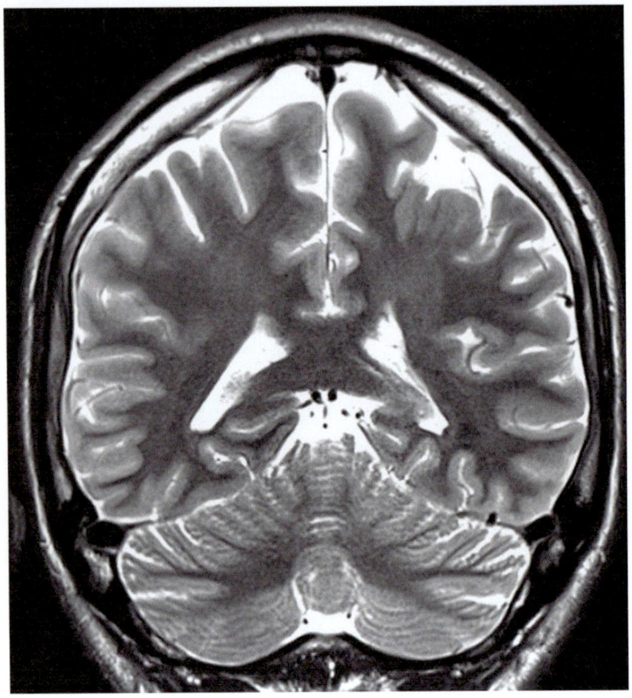

Fig. 69.9 MRI coronal T2 sequence at the same splenium of the corpus callosum level as Fig. 69.1 and obtained 3 years later. The splenium signal abnormality has completely resolved. No abnormality is present

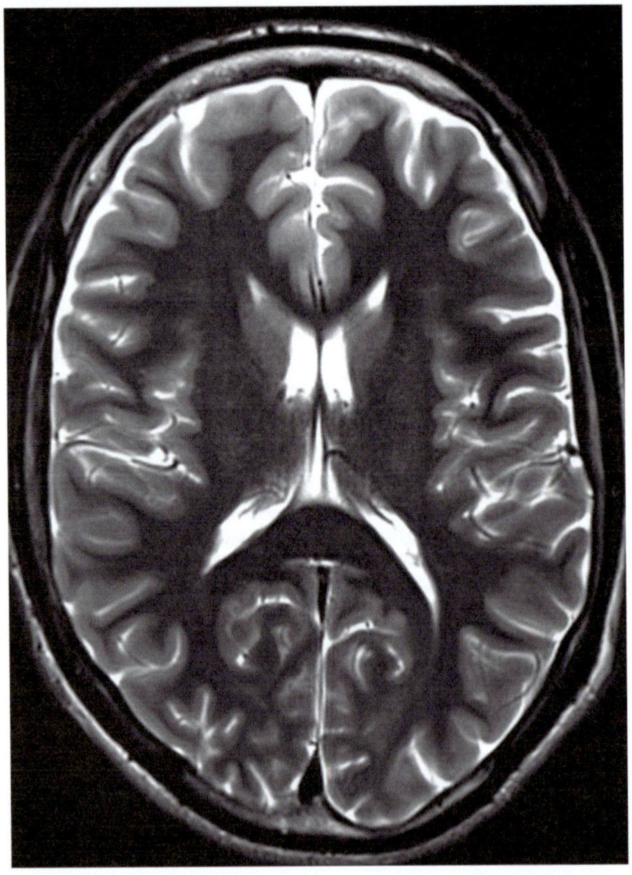

Fig. 69.10 MRI axial T2 sequence at the same basal ganglia level as the prior figures and obtained 3 years later. The splenium signal abnormality has completely resolved. No abnormality is present

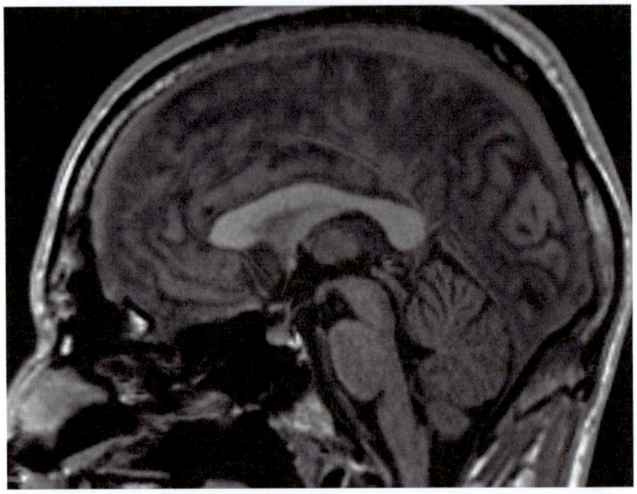

Fig. 69.11 MRI sagittal T1 sequence at the same midline level as Fig. 69.8 and obtained 3 years later. The corpus callosum is normal and without evidence of the prior splenium abnormality

Status Epilepticus Due to Epilepsy

70

Clinical History

The first recognized seizure occurred at age 12 years as a generalized tonic-clonic convulsion while swimming. The seizure was believed to have been triggered by shimmering light through the water, and it caused a near drowning. Generalized epilepsy was diagnosed after an evaluation that was not recalled, and an anti-seizure medication was started. Two additional tonic-clonic seizures occurred over the subsequent 9 years with one occurring during an attempted discontinuation of treatment and another after a change of anti-seizure medication.

At age 21 years, frequent left-hand myoclonus developed over days during a viral illness. Neither generalized nor focal myoclonus had previously occurred. Treatment with a benzodiazepine was initially successful, but the myoclonus worsened on the following day with extension to include the left face and an experience of left-hand weakness. An EEG on this day was normal, and additional benzodiazepine treatment was given. Two days later, seizures worsened and manifested as a left gaze preference with left hemibody contractions. Between seizures, somnolence was evident, and care was escalated to include intubation and treatment for status epilepticus with anesthetic medications.

The epilepsy risk factor was a family history with a sibling who had one tonic-clonic seizure in adolescence, was not treated, and remained seizure-free for years.

Neurological examination immediately prior to intubation identified unresponsiveness to verbal stimuli, left gaze preference with nystagmus to the left, and left hemibody weakness. Routine laboratory tests demonstrated minor abnormalities in serum chemistry and white blood cell count resulting from status epilepticus standard cerebrospinal fluid (CSF) analyses were normal.

Interictal EEG at the time of intubation depicted mild generalized slowing, right frontal rhythmic delta activity, and 1-Hz epileptiform discharges across the right hemisphere. Video-EEG monitoring recorded bilateral tonic-clonic seizures without asymmetry. Ictal EEG seizure onset prior to intubation was a 2-Hz delta rhythm. After anesthesia, the EEG depicted a burst-suppression pattern. Treatment, which included attempts at medication tapering, lasted 3 weeks and was followed by awakening with full recovery. Three months later, a follow-up interictal EEG depicted 3-Hz epileptiform discharges occurring in runs of up to 1 second with maximal amplitude over the right central region.

MRI was first obtained during the treatment for status epilepticus and while under anesthesia. It identified cerebral edema and right frontal lobe and thalamus signal abnormality. MRI soon after the resolution of status epilepticus identified a decrease in the signal abnormality and resolution of the edema.

The history and evaluation indicate focal status epilepticus in the context of generalized epilepsy diagnosis the focal motor seizure manifestation, focal EEG abnormality prior to intubation, and MRI signal abnormality were concordant in identifying right frontal lobe seizures. In retrospect, the prior tonic-clonic seizures apparently were focal-onset with quick propagation, and the interictal EEG after recovery from status epilepticus supports the right frontal epilepsy localization with its asymmetric epileptiform abnormality.

J. M. Stern, N. Salamon, *Imaging of Epilepsy*, https://doi.org/10.1007/978-3-030-86672-3_70

Imaging

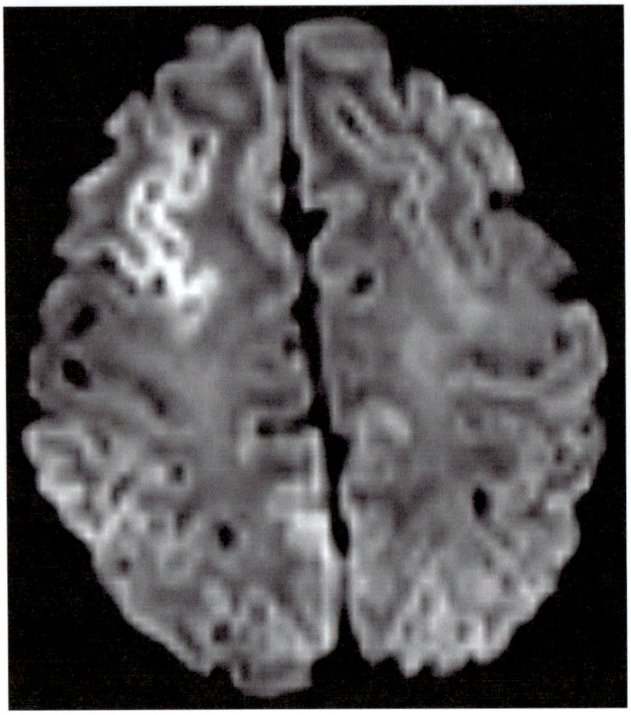

Fig. 70.1 MRI axial diffusion-weighted sequence at a high convexity level. Restricted diffusion is evident along the lateral margin of the right superior frontal gyrus and the medial margin of the right middle frontal gyrus. No other abnormality is present. The minor hyperintensities elsewhere in the image are due to signal inhomogeneity

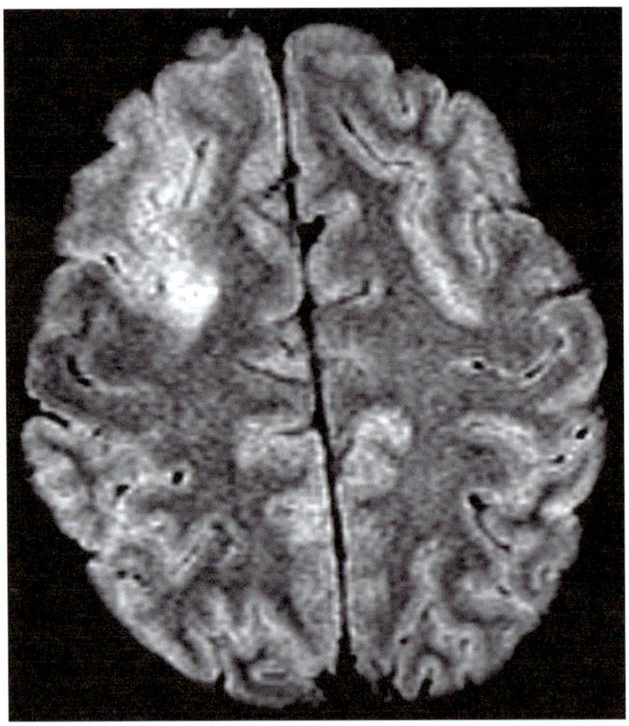

Fig. 70.2 MRI axial FLAIR sequence at the same high convexity level as Fig. 70.1. Abnormal hyperintense signal corresponds to gray matter edema along the lateral aspect of the right superior frontal gyrus and the medial middle frontal gyrus. The associated white matter and the remaining brain are normal

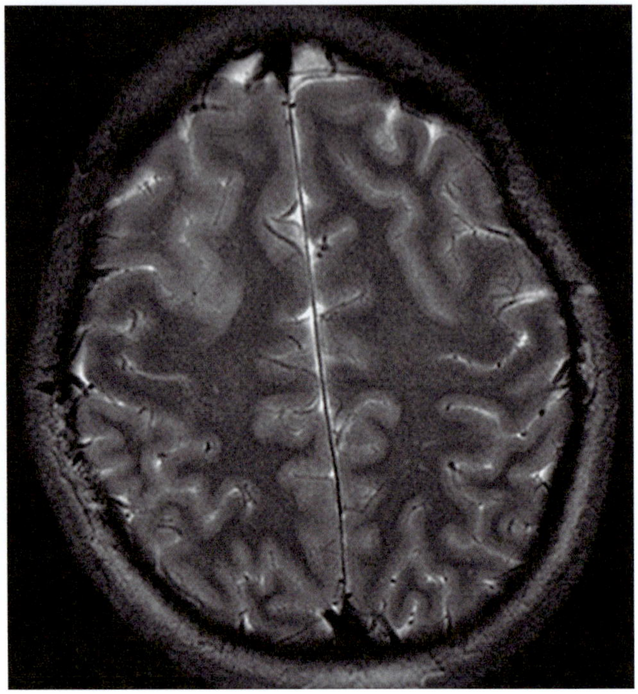

Fig. 70.3 MRI axial T2 sequence at a high convexity level similar to Figs. 70.1 and 70.2. Hyperintense signal abnormality corresponding to edema is present in the right frontal lobe gray matter with the same distribution as Fig. 70.2, but the finding is more subtle than with a FLAIR sequence

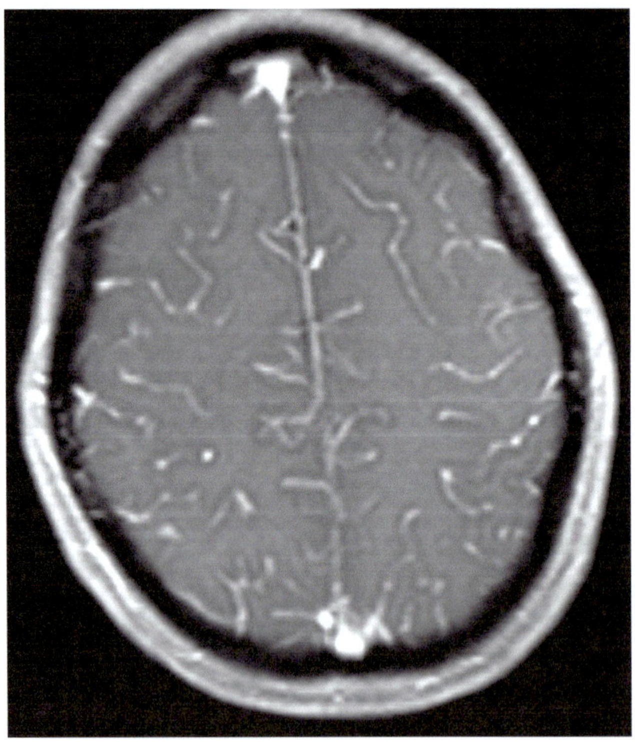

Fig. 70.4 MRI axial T1 sequence after contrast administration at the same high convexity level as Fig. 70.3. Enhancement is evident within the sulci bilaterally and throughout the level due to minor global edema producing effacement of the sulci with resultant engorgement of vessels within the sulci. The right frontal lobe focal edema is much less apparent than with the FLAIR and T2 sequences. The venous sinuses have normal enhancement

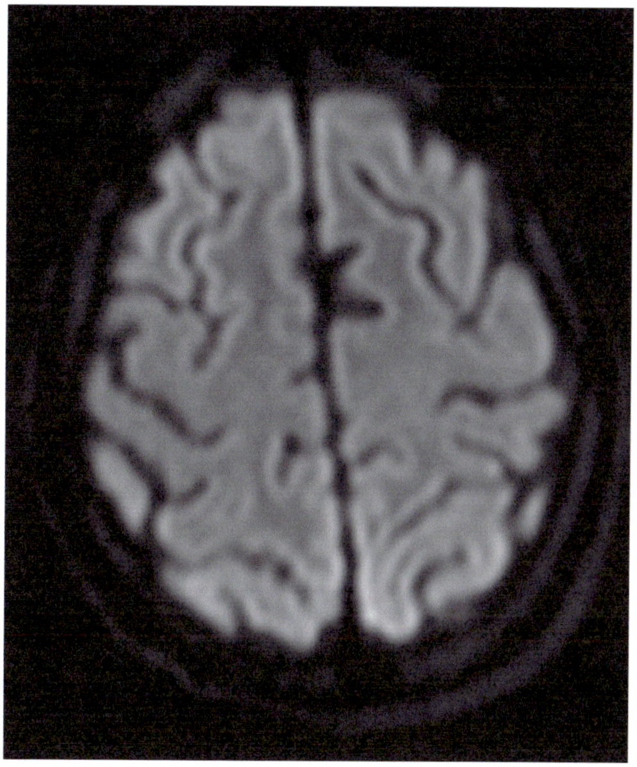

Fig. 70.5 MRI axial diffusion-weighted sequence at a high convexity level similar to Fig. 70.1 and obtained 3 weeks later. The signal abnormality of the right frontal lobe has resolved over the interval of weeks

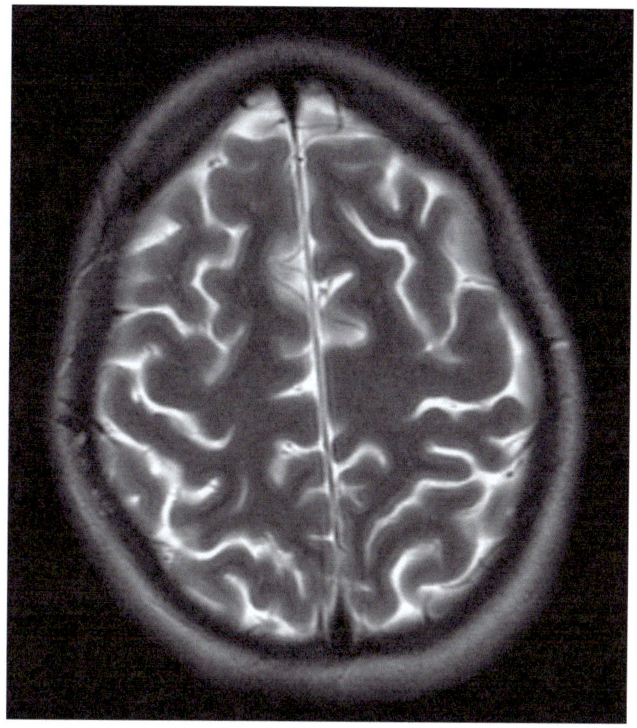

Fig. 70.7 MRI axial T2 sequence at a high convexity level similar to Fig. 70.3 and obtained 3 weeks later. No abnormality is evident. The subtle hyperintense abnormality has resolved. Because of the global edema resolution, the cortical sulci are larger than in Fig. 70.3

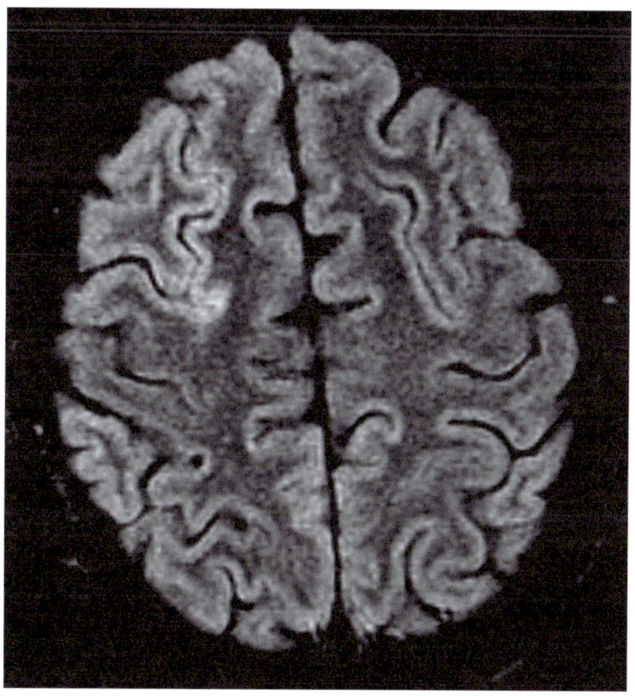

Fig. 70.6 MRI axial FLAIR sequence at the same high convexity level as Fig. 70.2 and obtained 3 weeks later. Subtle residual hyperintense signal abnormality is evident in the right superior frontal gyrus' most posterior aspect, which is at the depth of the right precentral sulcus. The abnormality does not include the precentral gyrus. The edema has otherwise resolved

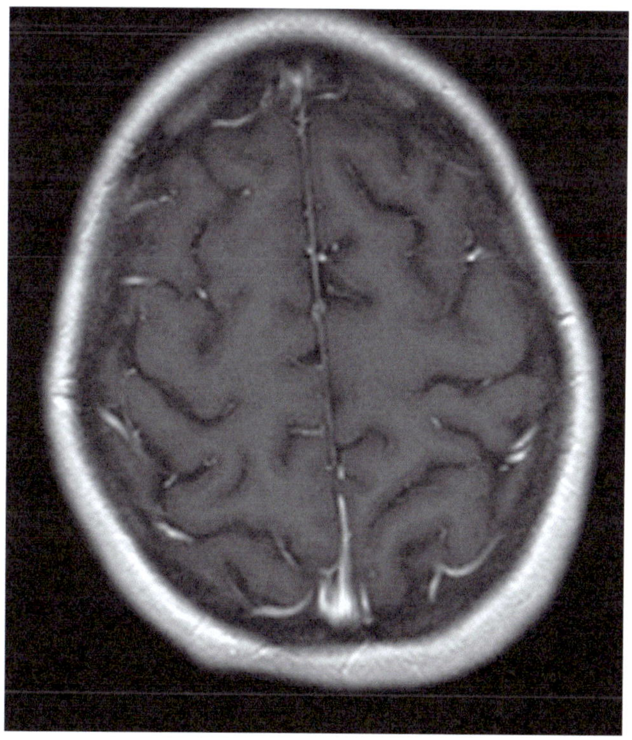

Fig. 70.8 MRI axial T1 sequence after contrast administration at the same high convexity level as Fig. 70.4 and obtained 3 weeks later. No abnormal contrast enhancement is present. The image is normal due to interval resolution of the global edema. The sulcal vessels are not as apparent

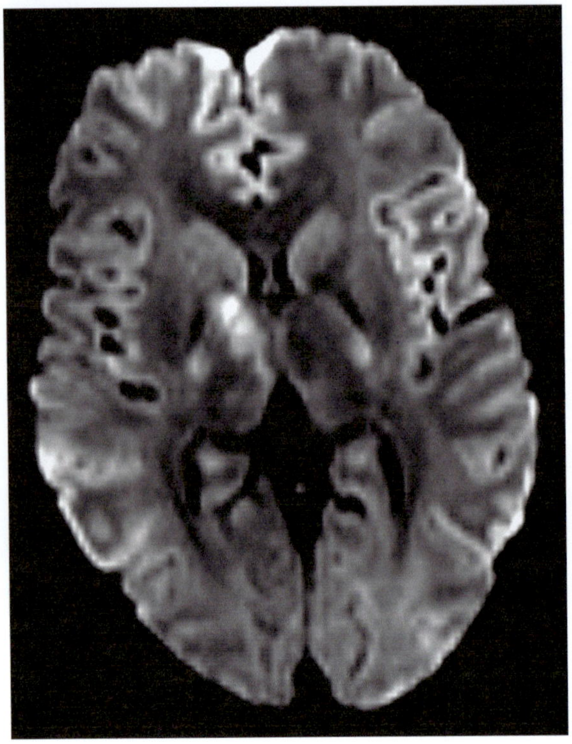

Fig. 70.9 MRI axial diffusion-weighted sequence at a thalamus level and obtained at the time of Figs. 70.1, 70.2, 70.3 and 70.4. Restricted diffusion is evident in the anterior, right thalamus and genu of the right internal capsule. The hyperintensity along cortical ribbon and bilaterally in the posterior limb of internal capsule is due to signal inhomogeneity. These structures are normal

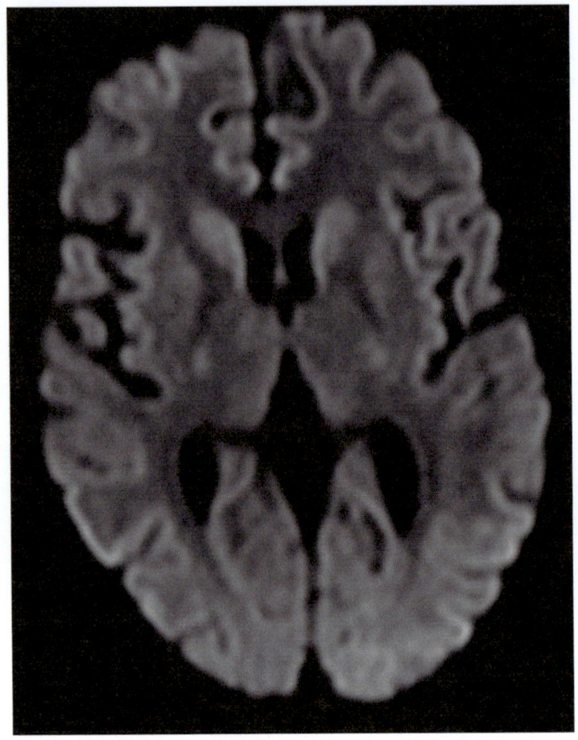

Fig. 70.11 MRI axial diffusion-weighted sequence at the same thalamus level as Fig. 70.9 and obtained 3 weeks later. The image is normal with complete resolution of the restricted diffusion

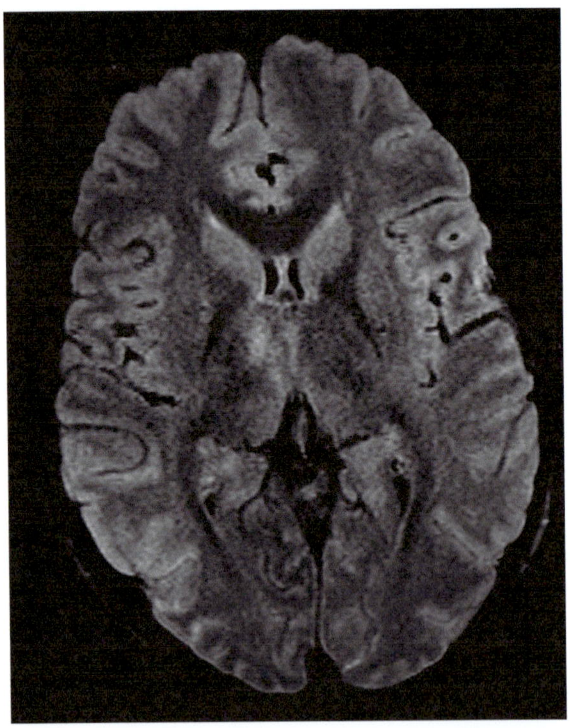

Fig. 70.10 MRI axial FLAIR sequence at the same thalamus level as Fig. 70.9 and also obtained at the time of Figs. 70.1, 70.2, 70.3, and 70.4. Abnormal hyperintensity is present in the right anterior thalamus with extension into the genu of the right internal capsule. The remaining brain is normal. The varying signal in the cortical ribbon is artifact

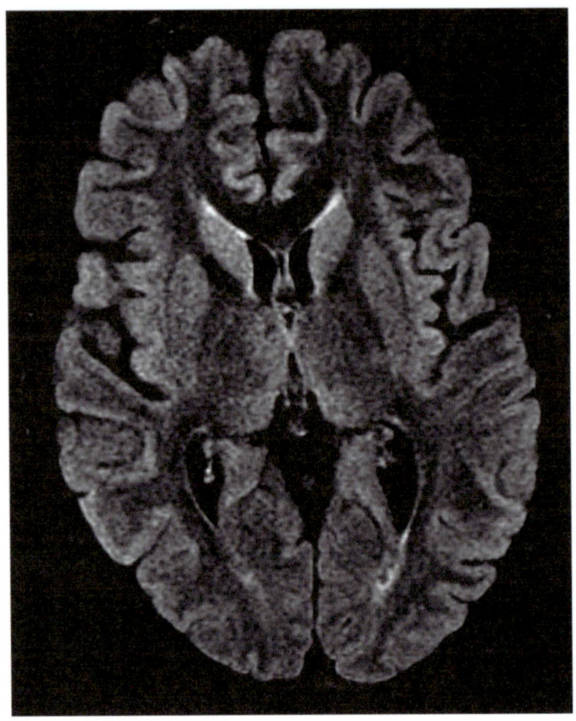

Fig. 70.12 MRI axial FLAIR sequence at a thalamus level similar to Fig. 70.10 and obtained three weeks later. Subtle signal asymmetry is evident in the anterior portion of thalamus with greater signal on the right, but the right anterior thalamus signal has clearly decreased over the interval. The signal abnormality in the genu of the right internal capsule has completely resolved

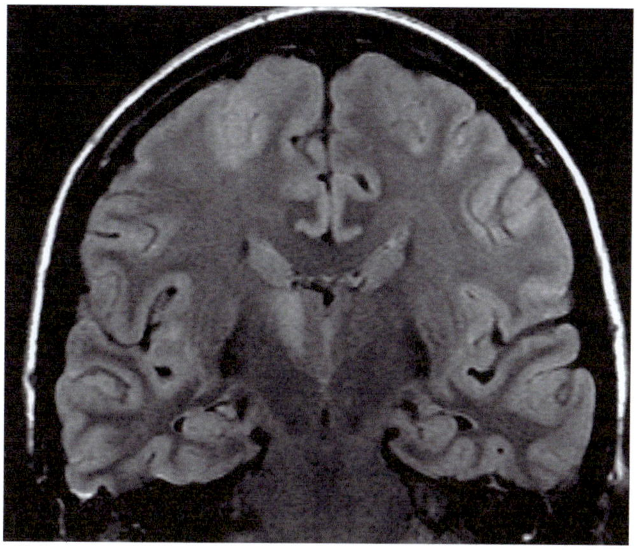

Fig. 70.13 MRI coronal FLAIR sequence at a hippocampal head level and obtained at the time of Figs. 70.1, 70.2, 70.3, and 70.4). Abnormal hyperintensity and edema are evident in the right superior and middle frontal gyri. An additional focal abnormality is evident as an oval-shaped hyperintensity in the right anterior superior portion of thalamus. Diffuse edema is present across the high convexity, as evident in the bilateral effacement of the cortical sulci. The temporal lobes are normal

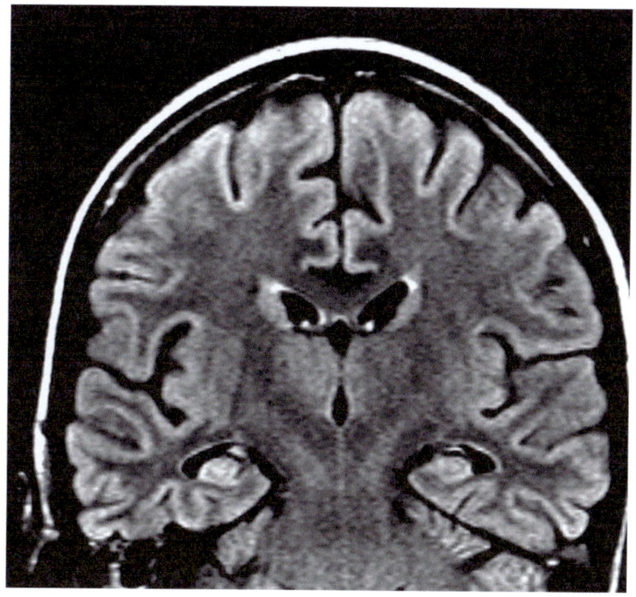

Fig. 70.14 MRI coronal FLAIR sequence at the same hippocampal head level as Fig. 70.13 and obtained 3 weeks later. The signal abnormality of the right superior and middle frontal gyri has resolved along with the diffuse high convexity edema. The cortical sulci and the lateral ventricles are larger and now normal. The thalamus has subtle asymmetry with right-sided hyperintensity, but the signal and asymmetry have decreased

Status Epilepticus Due to Inflammation

71

Clinical History

The first recognized seizure occurred at age 7 years as a tonic-clonic seizure that lasted 8 minutes and was followed by 4 hours of impaired awareness and intermittent right arm shaking. Emergent care was obtained, and admission to an intensive care unit soon followed.

At presentation, focal seizures were diagnosed retrospectively based on a history of episodic impaired awareness with staring and oral-facial automatisms over the preceding few months. After hospital admission, similar focal seizures recurred with accompanying tachycardia and durations of up to 1 minute. The frequency was one to five times each hour with persistence of the impaired mentation between the seizures. Treatment for status epilepticus was provided and advanced to include anesthesia. When anesthesia was reduced over the subsequent weeks, focal seizures returned with durations of up to 8 minutes.

An epilepsy risk factor was not present. Neurologic development was normal.

Neurological examination when not sedated identified somnolence with orientation to self and birthdate but not to the hospitalization. Cooperation with simple commands was not present. The neurological examination was otherwise normal. Medical history was normal. Routine laboratory tests, cerebrospinal fluid (CSF), and autoimmune antibody assays were normal.

Video-EEG monitoring recorded focal seizures manifested as repeated episodes of staring with oral automatisms. Ictal EEG's seizure onset was across the right temporal region.

MRI upon presentation and after 1 week of treatment identified edema of the right mesial temporal lobe. PET identified hypermetabolism of the right mesial temporal lobe with surrounding hypometabolism.

The history and evaluation indicate focal status epilepticus with EEG and imaging evidence of a right mesial temporal epileptogenic zone. The evaluation did not indicate an etiology.

A resection was performed approximately 1 month after the onset of status epilepticus because of continued medication resistance. Histopathological examination identified lymphoid inflammation consistent with either viral or autoimmune etiology no seizures or auras have occurred for the 2 years since surgery. Anti-seizure medication treatment has continued at a lower dose.

J. M. Stern, N. Salamon, *Imaging of Epilepsy*, https://doi.org/10.1007/978-3-030-86672-3_71

Imaging

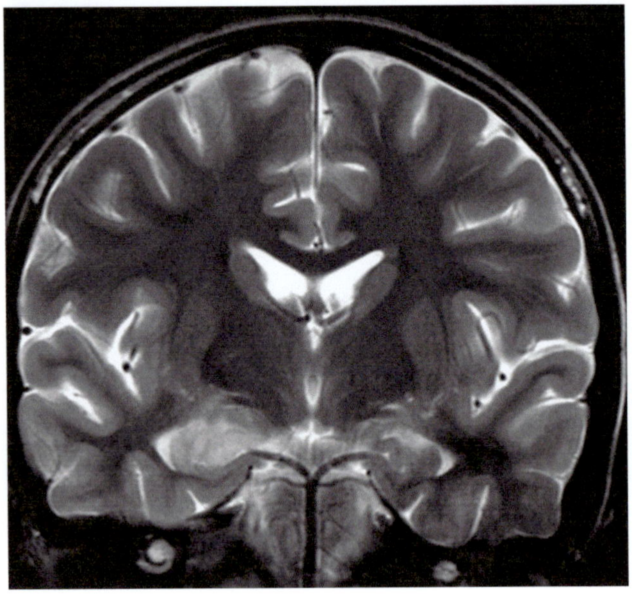

Fig. 71.1 MRI coronal T2 sequence at a hippocampal head level. The right hippocampal head is enlarged and has hyperintense signal abnormality, but its internal structure is maintained without abnormality of the architecture. The left hippocampal head has normal signal intensity and size. No other abnormalities are evident, including the remaining right temporal lobe

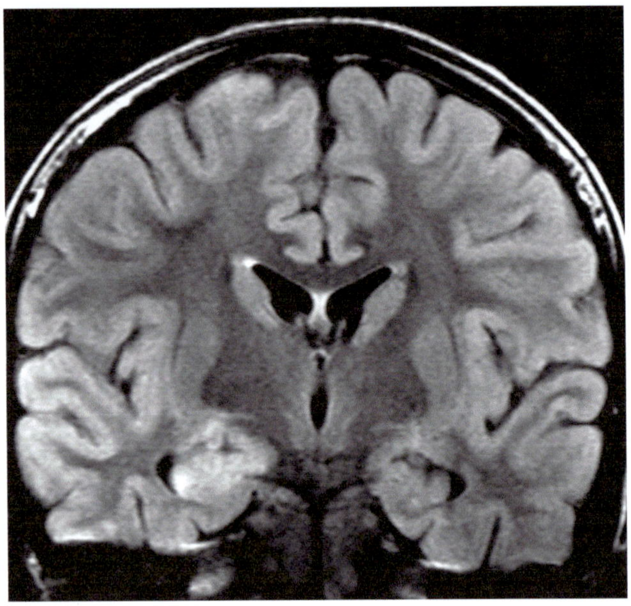

Fig. 71.2 MRI coronal FLAIR sequence at the same hippocampal head level as Fig. 71.1. The right hippocampal head is enlarged and has hyperintense signal abnormality, especially when compared to the left hippocampal head, which has normal size and signal. The right temporal lobe gray matter has hyperintense signal with gray-white junction differentiation when compared to the left temporal lobe, which suggests right temporal lobe cortical edema. The symmetry of the white matter signal in the right and left temporal lobes indicates that the gray matter signal asymmetry is not due to field inhomogeneity. No other abnormality is evident

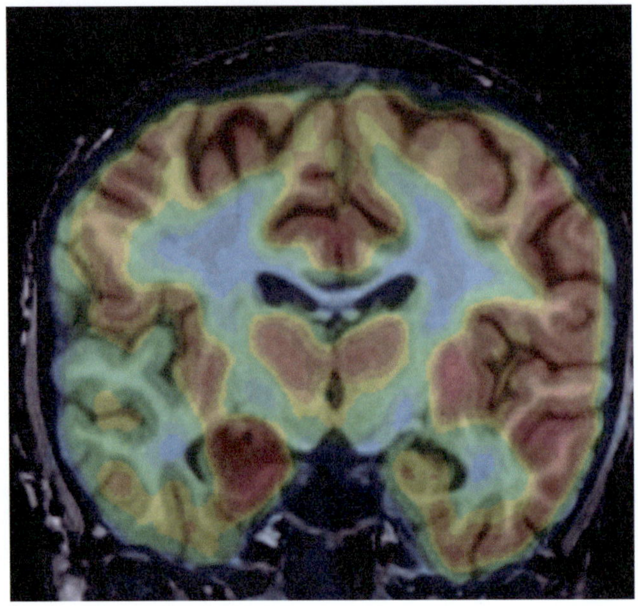

Fig. 71.3 PET-MRI co-registration with color-scale FDG tracer in a coronal plane at the same hippocampal head level as Figs. 71.1 and 71.2. Marked hypermetabolism is evident of the right hippocampal head and parahippocampal gyrus, which supports the PET as an ictal image. The right superior temporal gyrus and frontal operculum are hypometabolic, which is consistent with the ictal PET's seizure localization. The thalami and left temporal lobe are normal

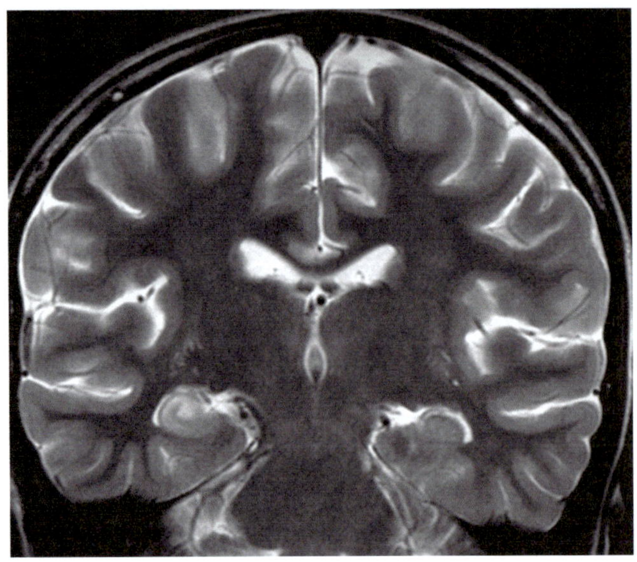

Fig. 71.4 MRI coronal T2 sequence at a hippocampal body level. The right hippocampus is enlarged and abnormally hyperintense with normal internal architecture, but internal structure is accentuated by the swelling. The right parahippocampal gyrus is normal along with remaining right temporal lobe. The left hippocampus has normal size and signal

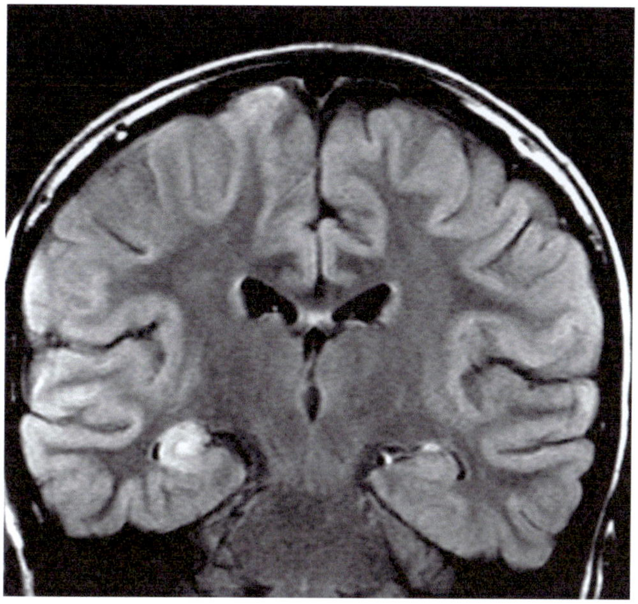

Fig. 71.5 MRI coronal FLAIR sequence at the same hippocampal body level as Fig. 71.4. Similar to Fig. 71.4, the right hippocampus is abnormally hyperintense and enlarged but has normal internal architecture. The left hippocampus' internal architecture is clearer in this figure than Fig. 71.4, which is unusual because the architecture is typically clearer with T2 than FLAIR. The right temporal lobe's cortical ribbon has a minor hyperintense signal abnormality compared to the left

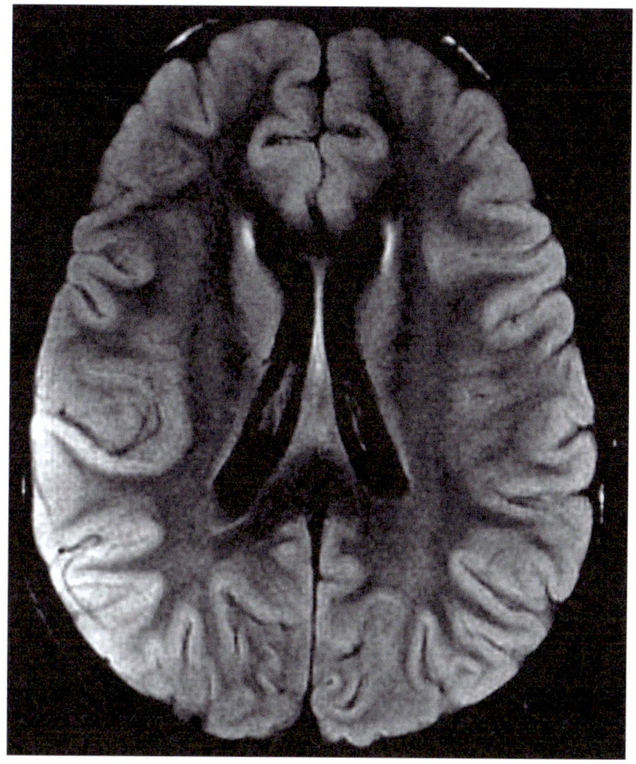

Fig. 71.7 MRI axial FLAIR sequence at a lateral ventricle level. Abnormal hyperintensity is evident along the cortical ribbon of the right supramarginal and angular gyri. No other abnormality is present

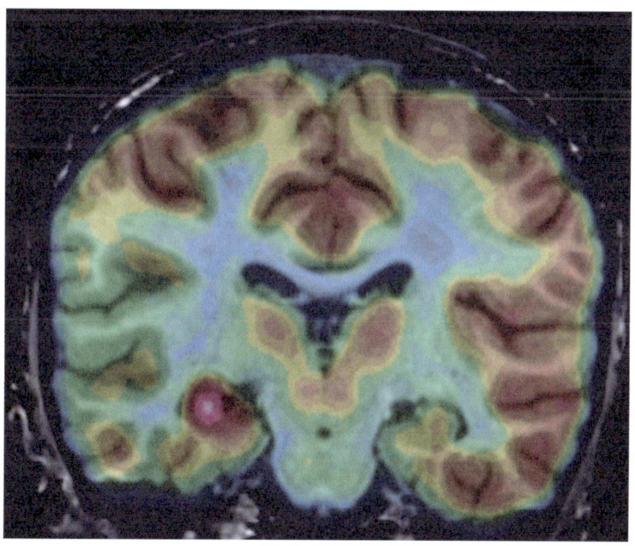

Fig. 71.6 PET-MRI co-registration with color-scale FDG tracer in a coronal plane at a hippocampal body level similar to Figs. 71.4 and 71.5. Abnormal hypermetabolism is evident within the right hippocampal body and subiculum. The right parahippocampal gyrus is less abnormal than in Fig. 71.3. Hypometabolism extends across the right temporal lobe and operculum. The thalami are normal and symmetric

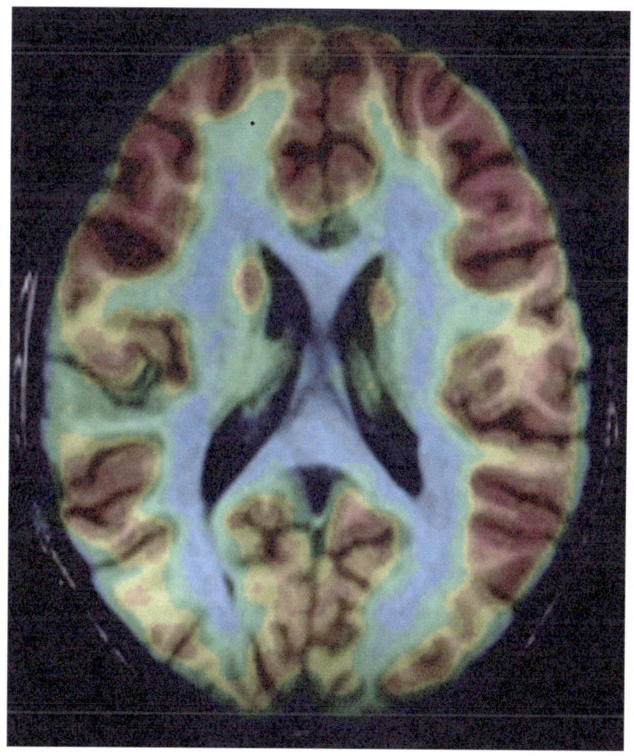

Fig. 71.8 PET-MRI co-registration with color-scale FDG tracer in an axial plane at a lateral ventricle level similar to Fig. 71.7. Abnormal hypometabolism extends across the right supramarginal gyrus and, to a lesser extent, across the right parietal lobe. The frontal lobes are symmetric. No regions of hypermetabolism are present

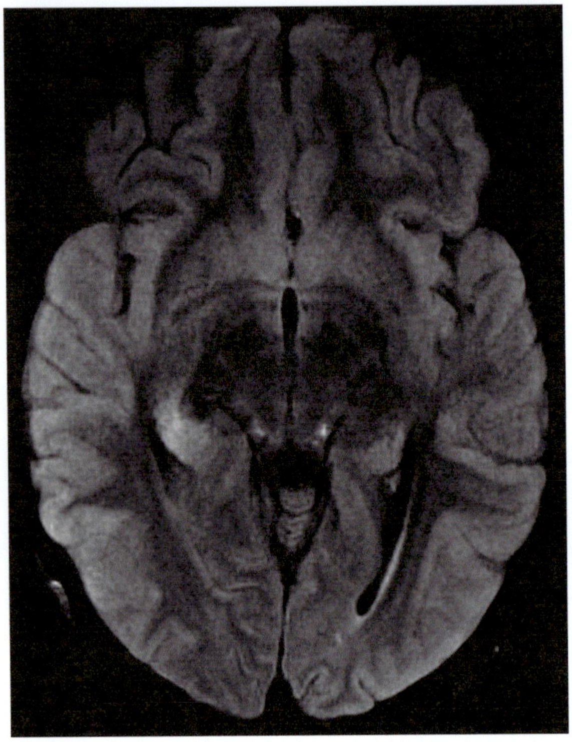

Fig. 71.9 MRI axial FLAIR sequence at a hippocampus level. Abnormal enlargement and hyperintense signal are evident in the right hippocampus from the body to the tail. The right temporal lobe's cortical ribbon also is abnormally hyperintense. The left hippocampus and bilateral frontal lobes are normal

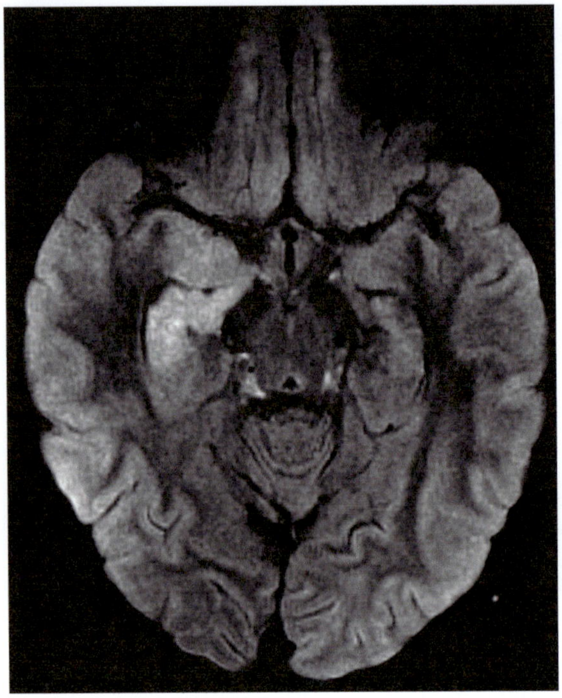

Fig. 71.11 MRI axial FLAIR sequence at an amygdala and hippocampal head level. The right hippocampal head, anterior hippocampal body, and the amygdala are abnormally enlarged and hyperintense. The right temporal lobe's cortical ribbon also is abnormally hyperintense but to a lesser degree overall. However, the ribbon varies in its hyperintense abnormality with greater cortical ribbon hyperintensity along the posterior aspect

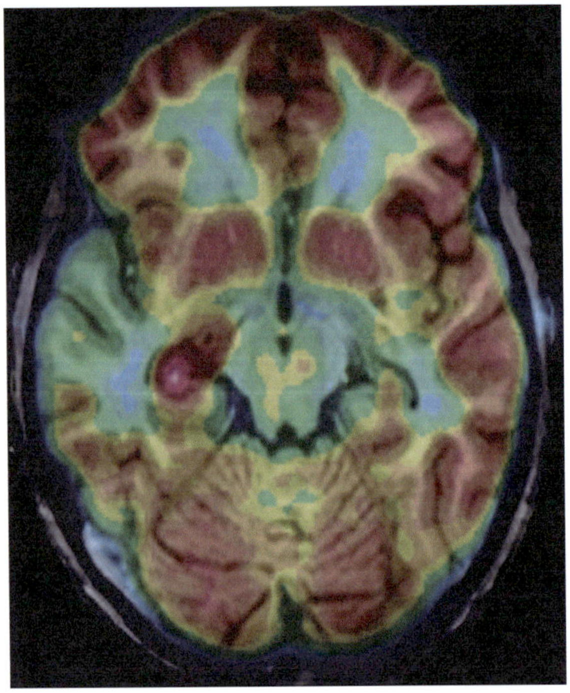

Fig. 71.10 PET-MRI co-registration with color-scale FDG tracer in an axial plane at a hippocampus level slightly differing in its angle from Fig. 71.9. Abnormal hypermetabolism is evident within the right hippocampal head. The remaining right temporal lobe is abnormally hypometabolic. No other metabolic abnormality or asymmetry is present

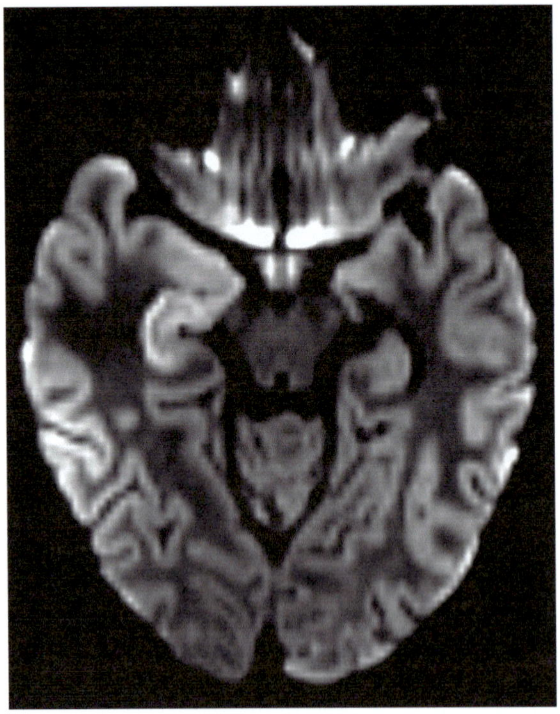

Fig. 71.12 MRI axial diffusion-weighted imaging sequence at the same amygdala and hippocampal head level as Fig. 71.11. Restricted diffusion that is particularly evident along the lateral aspect of the right hippocampal head and anterior hippocampal body corresponds to cornu ammonis. Restricted diffusion also is present within the right amygdala and right temporal lobe's cortical ribbon. The left hippocampus is incompletely visible because of the angle of the level

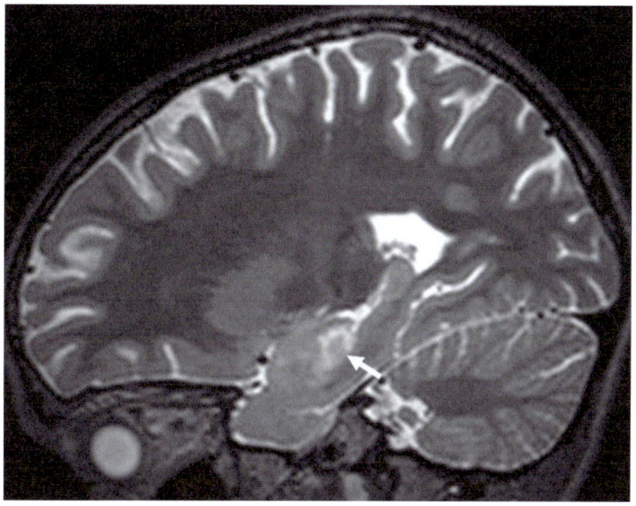

Fig. 71.13 MRI sagittal T2 sequence at a right hippocampus level. Abnormal hyperintense signal (arrow) is evident at the hippocampal head with the signal abnormality indicating the contour of the hippocampal head. The blurring of the temporal pole's gray-white junction is an additional abnormality. The hippocampal body is not in this image's level

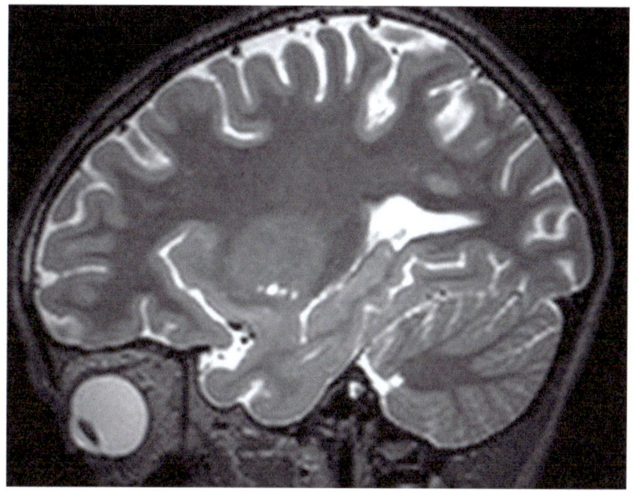

Fig. 71.15 MRI sagittal T2 sequence at a left hippocampus level. The hippocampal size and signal are normal. A sharp delineation of the temporal pole's gray-white junction is evident and clearly differs from Fig. 71.13

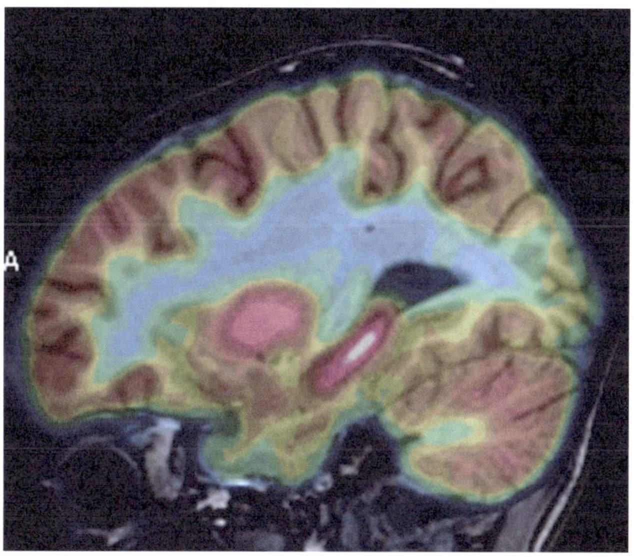

Fig. 71.14 PET-MRI co-registration with color-scale FDG tracer in a sagittal plane at a right hippocampus level similar to Fig. 71.13. Abnormal hypermetabolism of the right hippocampal body is evident along with hypometabolism of the temporal pole. No other abnormal metabolism is evident

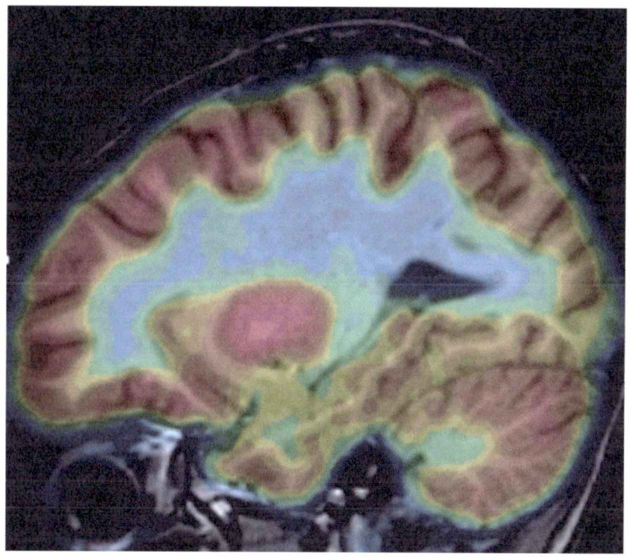

Fig. 71.16 PET-MRI co-registration with color-scale FDG tracer in a sagittal plane at a left hippocampus level similar to Fig. 71.15. The metabolic signal of the hippocampus and temporal pole are normal and clearly differ from Fig. 71.14

Status Epilepticus Due to Stroke

72

Clinical History

Presentation was decreased responsiveness accompanied by left gaze preference and involuntary eyelid and jaw movements. The neurological exam upon presentation also demonstrated the preexisting quadriplegia due to a pontine stroke, so seizure-related limb movements or a new deficit would not be manifested. Status epilepticus was diagnosed clinically, and an intravenous benzodiazepine produced temporary resolution to the gaze preference without improvement in responsiveness. Because of a history of multiple strokes, the evaluation included a head CT and CT angiogram, and a new infarct, hemorrhage, or vascular occlusion was not evident. Treatment was escalated to intravenous anesthesia and intubation with continuous EEG monitoring. During treatment, hypotension, metabolic acidosis, and sepsis of pulmonary origin developed. Ultimately, care was changed to palliation with transfer to a hospice.

The seizure risk factor was cerebral vascular disease.

Neurological examination at the time of presentation identified nonresponsiveness to voice and tactile stimuli, persistent left gaze deviation, leftward head deviation, diffuse hyperreflexia, no spontaneous movements, and no limb movements with tactile stimuli. Medical history did not include prior seizures or epilepsy, and it included hypertension, hyperlipidemia, diabetes, atrial fibrillation without anticoagulation, left hemiparesis due to two right middle cerebral artery strokes with one affecting the temporal-parietal cortex and the other the frontal-parietal cortex, and a later pontine stroke that produced dysphagia, dysarthric, and right hemiparesis that progressed to quadriplegia.

Ictal EEG during anesthesia depicted 1-Hz generalized periodic discharges occurring in bursts lasting several seconds and separated by suppressions. After 4 days, the anesthesia was reduced, and the EEG depicted diffuse delta slowing without epileptiform abnormality. Over the following few days, anesthesia was discontinued, and the EEG became a burst-suppression pattern without epileptiform features.

MRI was obtained 3 months prior to status epilepticus, when presenting with an acute basilar artery infarction. The cerebral levels from this earlier MRI provide comparisons to the MRI during status epilepticus. The earlier MRI identified regions of chronic ischemic injury within the territory of the right middle cerebral artery. MRI upon presenting with status epilepticus identified prominent restricted diffusion within the cortical ribbon of the left frontal lobe, anterior cingulate, insula, supramarginal gyrus, and thalamus. Head CT angiography and perfusion imaging identified increased blood flow within the left cerebral hemisphere.

The history and evaluation indicate focal status epilepticus with MRI and CT indicating maximal abnormality within the left frontal lobe with extension to include much of the left middle cerebral artery's territory. The seizure localization depended on the imaging because quadriplegia precluded motor signs in the limbs, and the EEG was obtained only after anesthesia was begun. The left gaze preference at presentation does not have lateralizing specificity, as gaze deviation is contralateral when seizures affect oculomotor function and is ipsilateral when seizures produce a sensory neglect.

J. M. Stern, N. Salamon, *Imaging of Epilepsy*, https://doi.org/10.1007/978-3-030-86672-3_72

Imaging

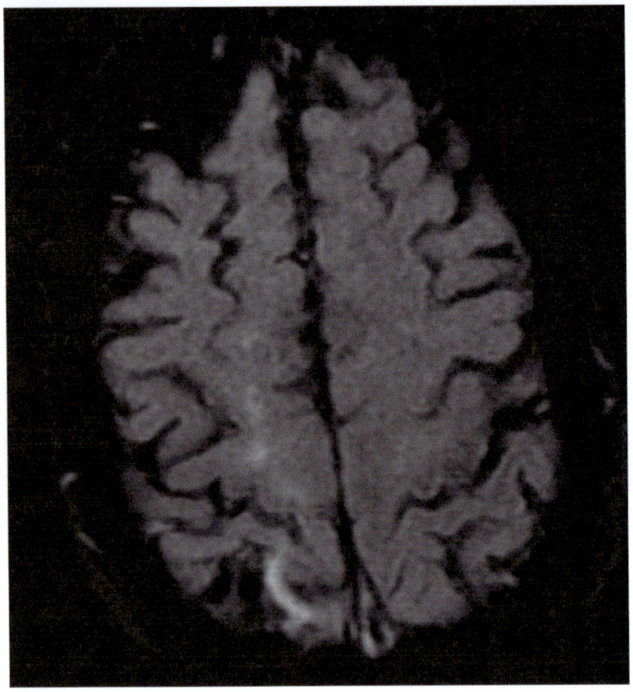

Fig. 72.1 MRI axial FLAIR sequence at a high convexity level. This figure and Figs. 72.2, 72.3, 72.4, and 72.5 were obtained 3 months prior to presentation. Encephalomalacia and abnormal subcortical hyperintensity are evident within the right parietal lobe. Additional abnormal hyperintensities have a linear appearance in the white matter from the right superior frontal gyrus to the paracentral lobule

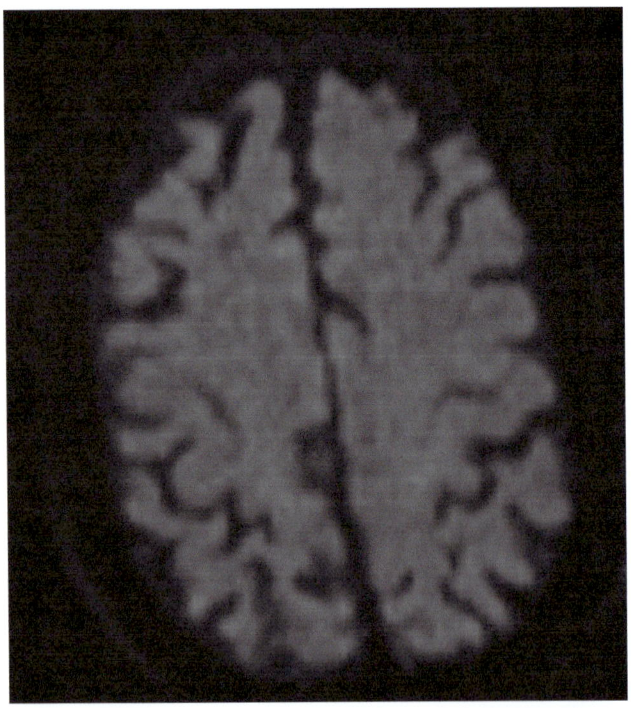

Fig. 72.2 MRI axial diffusion-weighted sequence at the same high convexity level as Fig. 72.1. No region of restricted diffusion is present, which is supportive of no acute abnormality. The MRI was obtained to evaluate for a cerebral infarction

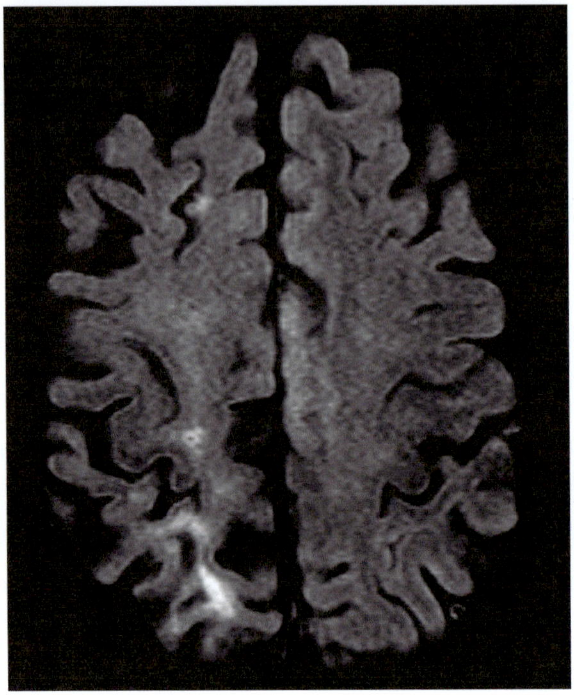

Fig. 72.3 MRI axial FLAIR sequence at a high convexity level that is slightly inferior to Fig. 72.1. Consistent with Fig. 72.1, abnormal hyperintensities are evident in the right parietal lobe and right frontal white matter. In addition, abnormal hyperintensity is evident along the medial aspect of left hemisphere along the gray matter surface of the left superior frontal and cingulate gyri

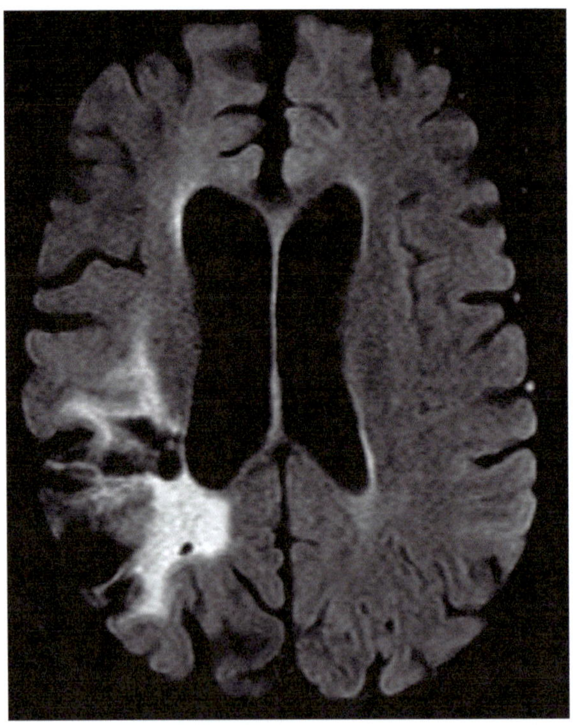

Fig. 72.4 MRI axial FLAIR sequence at a lateral ventricle level. The chronic infarction of right parietal lobe corresponds to a middle cerebral artery territory. The cortical sulci are effaced and abnormally hyperintense along the left anterior cingulate gyrus, left superior frontal gyrus, and left parietal lobe

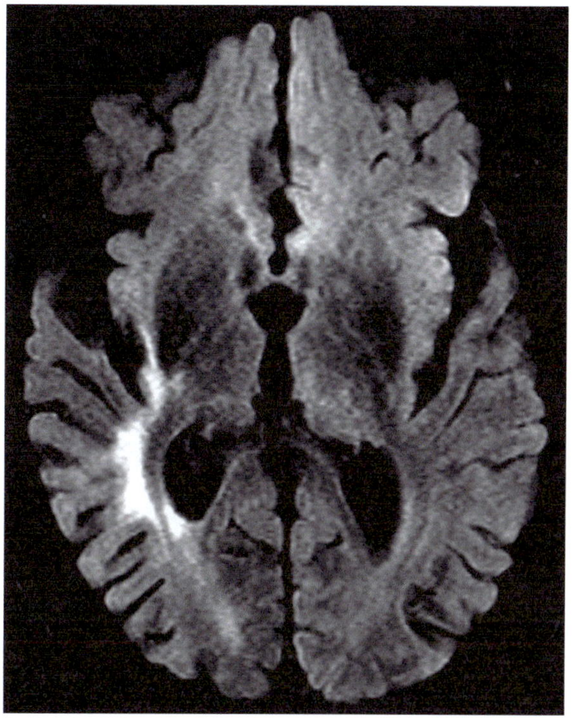

Fig. 72.5 MRI axial FLAIR sequence at a thalamus level. Chronic infarction is evident in the right temporal lobe and right posterior insula with volume loss of the right insula. Abnormal cortical hyperintensity spans the left hemisphere's gyrus rectus, orbitofrontal region, and anterior insula. In particular, the thalamus is asymmetric with a brighter signal on the left

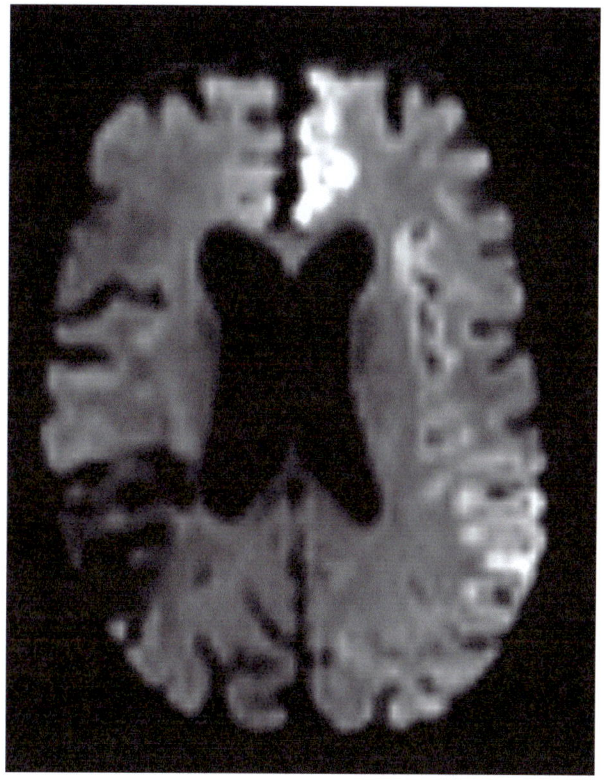

Fig. 72.7 MRI axial diffusion-weighted sequence at the same lateral ventricle level as Fig. 72.4. Restricted diffusion is evident on the left in the anterior cingulate, super frontal, and supramarginal gyri and in the left anterior insula. The right-sided hypointensity is due to the chronic right parietal lobe infarction

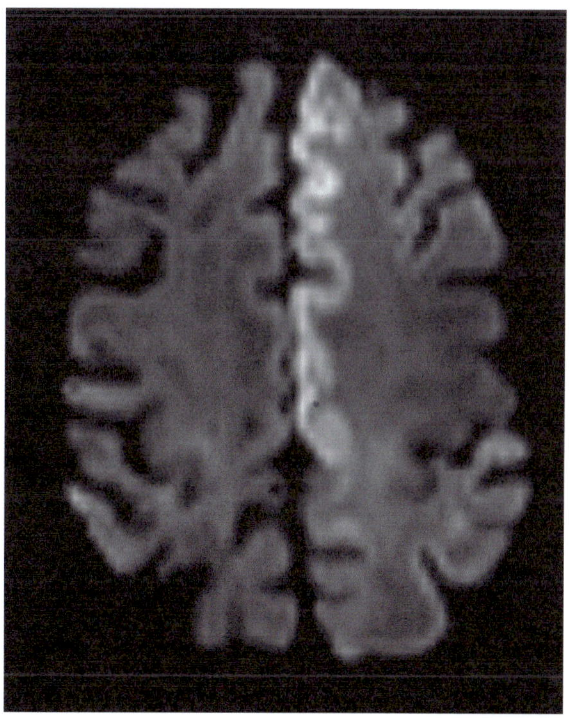

Fig. 72.6 MRI axial diffusion-weighted sequence at a high convexity level similar to Fig. 72.3 and obtained 3 months after Fig. 72.3 along with Figs. 72.7, 72.8, 72.9, 72.10, 72.11, and 72.12. Restricted diffusion is evident in the left hemispheric gray matter involving the left superior frontal and cingulate gyri and the lateral left parietal lobe

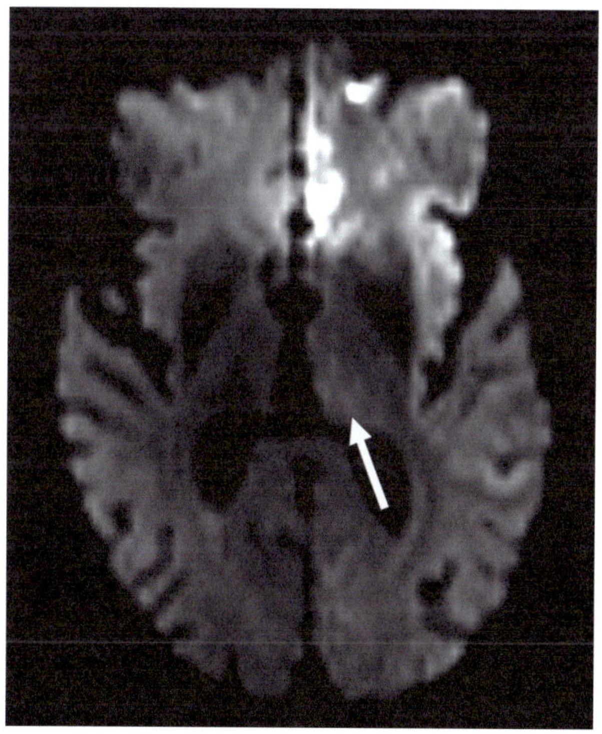

Fig. 72.8 MRI axial diffusion-weighted sequence at a thalamus level. Restricted diffusion is prominent in the left gyrus rectus and orbitofrontal region and present with lesser and varying signal intensity in the left anterior insula and left thalamus (arrow)

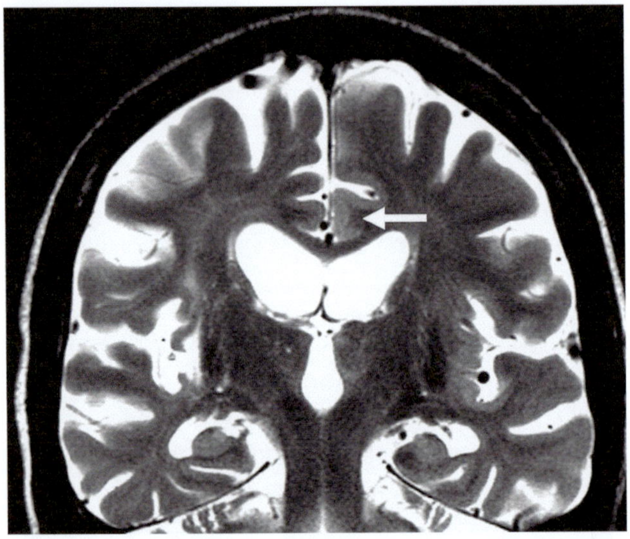

Fig. 72.9 MRI coronal T2 sequence at a hippocampal body level. Edema and abnormal hyperintensity are evident in the gray matter of the left middle cingulate (arrow) and left superior frontal gyri. A chronic infarction is present in the right insula, and the cerebrum is globally atrophic. The hippocampi are normal bilaterally

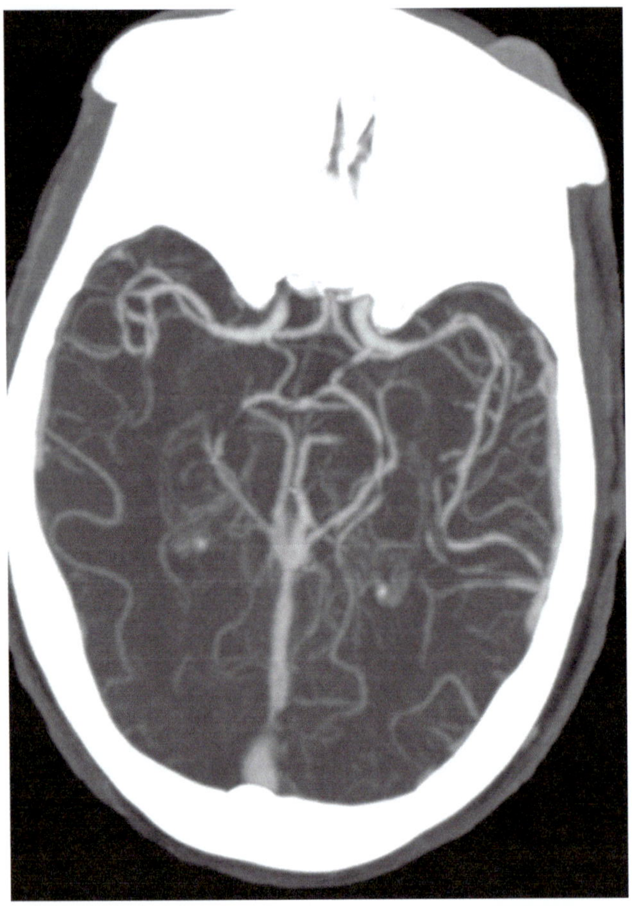

Fig. 72.10 CT angiogram in an axial plane at a circle of Willis level. Increased vascularity is evident across the left hemisphere. Intracranial vessels are patent bilaterally

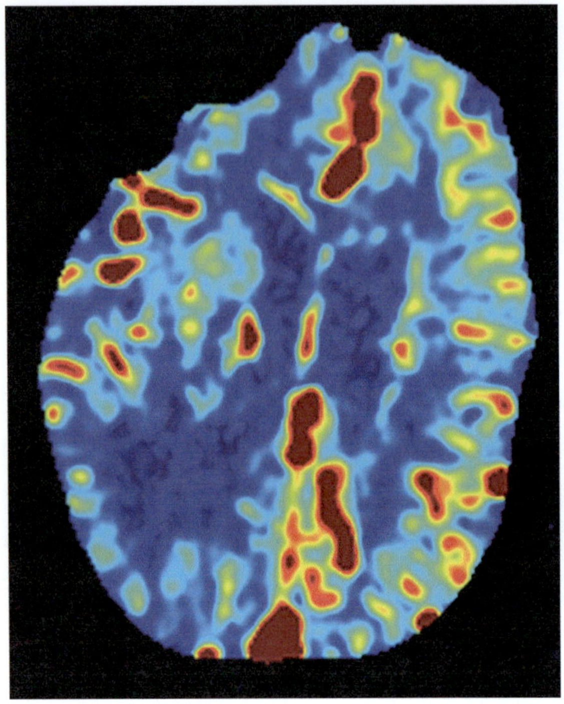

Fig. 72.11 Post-processed perfusion CT imaging of cerebral blood flow at a lateral ventricle level. Increased cerebral blood flow is evident across the left hemisphere compared to the right, but the parietal lobe asymmetry is partly due to diminished cerebral blood flow in the region of the right parietal lobe infarction

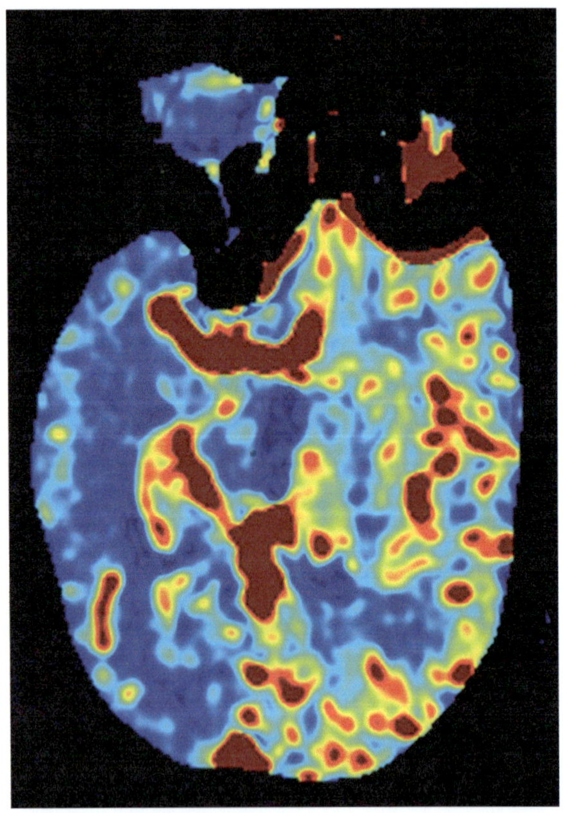

Fig. 72.12 Post-processed perfusion CT imaging of cerebral blood flow at a thalamus level. Increased perfusion is evident across the entire left hemisphere. The confluent red signal on the right is produced by normal vasculature

Part IX

Treatment Related Findings

Brain surgery
Epilepsy surgery
Anterior-mesial temporal lobe resection
Anterior temporal lobe resection
Focal cortical resection
Hemispherotomy
Hemispherectomy
Corpus callosotomy
Stereotactic thermoablation
Laser interstitial thermal therapy
Stereotactic radiosurgery
Neuromodulation devices
Vagus nerve stimulator/stimulation (VNS)
Responsive neurostimulator/stimulation (RNS)
NeuroPace
Deep brain stimulator/stimulation (DBS)
Resective surgery

A standard surgical treatment for mesial temporal lobe epilepsy includes resection of the temporal pole,a mygdala, anterior hippocampus, anterior superior temporal gyrus, and inferior temporal lobe. The extent of inclusion for each of these structures varies across surgeons and epilepsy surgery centers with the essential consideration of minimizing resection extent to minimize the risk of a neurologic deficit while maximizing the resection extent to maximize the likelihood of seizure freedom. As such, the anterior-mesial temporal lobe resection varies within a general anatomic framework.

Surgical treatment for focal epilepsies beyond the mesial temporal lobe may be considered as focal cortical resections. When focal cortical resections include a structural lesion, the resection often extends beyond the lesion and includes immediately adjacent tissue because this tissue often is part of the epileptogenic zone. If the resection is limited to a structural lesion, it is considered a lesionectomy. Non-lesional epilepsy surgery is typically defined by the absence of imaging evidence of a structural abnormality, but focal cortical resections may be provided if other diagnostic evidence indicates a likely localization for the epileptogenic zone. The resection margins for both lesional and non-lesional focal cortical resections are sometimes determined using intra-operative electrocorticography and functional mapping.

Hemispheric surgery

The anatomical hemispherectomy is the removal of an entire cerebral hemisphere and differs from the functional hemispherotomy, which is the removal of the hemisphere's central portion and disconnection of its remaining tissue. The functional hemispherotomy's intention is isolate a hemisphere and thereby eliminate its capacity to produce a clinical seizure while reducing the surgical risk of an anatomic hemispherectomy. Most patients who undergo either surgery are children and already have neurologic deficits related to a dysfunctional cerebral hemisphere.

Corpus callosotomy

When medication resistant epilepsy is bihemispheric, corpus callosotomy may provide a palliative treatment by impeding seizure propagation. The disconnection has greater effect on seizure severity than seizure frequency, and it may alter seizure manifestation with a reduction in sudden bilateral motor seizures that cause falls, which are collectively termed drop attacks. Conventionally, the anterior two thirds of the corpus callosum is sectioned, so sufficient interhemispheric connections are maintained to reduce the risk of language and motor dysfunction. When necessary for seizure control and the risk of neurologic deterioration is low, a complete corpus callosotomy may be indicated.

Stereotactic ablation

Laser interstitial thermal therapy allows surgical treatment to regions that are not accessible with conventional resection techniques without unacceptable risk. The treatment is based on thermal ablation through a stereotactically placed catheter that contains optical fibers. The fibers deliver the tissue-heating light directly into the target, heating it to temperatures that are sufficient to cause tissue necrosis. During the laser exposure, magnetic resonance thermography provides monitoring of the tissue heating. The volume of the ablated tissue is more limited than resection, so candidates are patients whose potentially epileptogenic zone is both deep and not extensive.

Stereotactic radiosurgery can target lesions throughout the brain and is similar to laser ablation by being a less invasive approach than conventional resection. It differs from laser ablation by delivering the therapy's energy as focused radiation, which allows treatment without a breach of the skull. The radiation-induced necrosis develops over months, so the resultant seizure control often requires more than a year before plateauing.

Implanted stimulation devices

Implanted stimulation devices are considered palliative approaches because of the lower rates of seizure freedom when compared to resective or ablative surgery. The three devices now available are sometimes considered neuromodulatory because of the gradual change to epileptogenicity over extended periods of treatment. Regardless of the similarities, the devices have substantial differences that are important when considering patient candidacy.

Vagus nerve stimulation is provided by a stimulator that is placed subcutaneously in the left chest and connected by a subcutaneous lead to a cuff electrode that encircles the left vagus nerve in the neck. The stimulation is provided as a cycle that commonly is 30 seconds of stimulation every 5 minutes, but other duty cycles are also used. The stimulation also can be initiated by a magnet placed near the generator and, for the more recent models, a change to the heart rhythm that often occurs with seizure onset. Vagus nerve stimulation is provided for both focal and generalized epilepsies. The stimulation's efficacy depends brainstem nuclei connections and ultimately the release of norepinephrine from the locus coeruleus and effects on the thalamus.

Responsive neurostimulation, which is often called by the manufacturer's name NeuroPace, is provided by a stimulator that is placed on a ferrule within a craniotomy and connected to leads that traverse the subdural space to the seizure-onset zone. Because of the craniotomy, the outer surface of the stimulator is aligned with the surface of the skull and is covered by the scalp. The stimulator is connected to two leads, and the leads are available with either subdural or intra-parenchymal electrode contacts. The electrodes allow continuous monitoring of the electrocorticogram for specific epileptiform abnormalities by the stimulator's microprocessor. When the microprocessor identifies the physician-specified epileptiform features, stimulation is provided to the location generating the abnormality. In this way, the neurostimulation is responsive to abnormality and provides efficacy through interruption of the generation of epileptic abnormality. Based on this design, the responsive neurostimulator is intended for well-localized focal seizures.

Deep brain stimulation for epilepsy employs the same devices used for treatment of other neurologic disorders, but the anatomic targets differ. The stimulator is placed subcutaneously in the chest and connects by two leads that extend through subcutaneous tissue in the neck to surgical openings in the skull, through which stereotactically targeted electrodes reach the brain. Most commonly, the anterior nucleus of the thalamus is the stimulation target with an electrode placed in each hemisphere's thalamus. This target is intended to interrupt the propagation of focal seizures regardless of the seizure-onset localization. With this approach, the efficacy was established for focal seizures and does not depend upon identifying a localization. However, other brain regions are being investigated for stimulation and are being clinically targeted, and these regions may provide benefit for seizures that are generalized at their onset.

References

Barbaro NM, Quigg M, Ward MM, et al. Radiosurgery versus open surgery for mesial temporal lobe epilepsy: the randomized, controlled ROSE trial. Epilepsia. 2018;59:1198–207.

Englot D. A modern epilepsy surgery treatment algorithm: Incorporating traditional and emerging technologies. Epilepsy Behav. 2018;80:68–74.

Graham D, TIsdall MM, Gill D. Corpus callosotomy outcomes in pediatric patients: a systematic review. Epilepsia. 2016;57:1053–68.

Gooneratne IK, Green AL, Dugan P, et al. Comparing neurostimulation technologies in refractory focal-onset epilepsy. J Neurol Neurosurg Psychiatry. 2016;87:1174–82.

Marras CE, Granata T, Franzini A, et al. Hemispherotomy and functional hemispherectomy: Indications and outcome. Epilepsy Res. 2010;87:104–12.

Youngerman BE, Save AV, McKhann GM. Magnetic resonance imaging-guided laser interstitial thermal therapy for epilepsy: Systematic review of technique, indications, and outcomes. Neurosurgery. 2020;86:E366–82.

73 Anterior Temporal Lobe Resection

Clinical History

The first recognized seizure occurred at age 14 years as an episode of aphasia and amnesia. Epilepsy was diagnosed at that time, but the details of the evaluation were not recalled.

The habitual seizures were identical to the first seizure and manifested as disrupted speech due to repetitions of sounds or words for about 30 seconds with awareness of the difficulty and retained memory. The language disruption episodes occurred in isolation with about half of the episodes progressed to impaired awareness. The impaired awareness was accompanied by behavioral arrest with staring, oral automatisms, and posturing of one or both arms for 1 to 2 minutes. Postictal recovery lasted about 10 minutes and included paraphasic errors. Treatment prior to epilepsy surgery included multiple anti-seizure medications with a seizure frequency of one weekly and a range of up to six seizures in a month and no seizures for two months.

The epilepsy risk factor was hippocampal sclerosis and anterior temporal lobe cortical dysplasia.

Neurological examination was normal. Neuropsychological testing identified deficits in naming and verbal memory.

Interictal EEG depicted bilateral, independent epileptiform discharges over the anterior temporal lobes with most discharges on the left. Video-EEG monitoring recorded focal seizures manifested as impaired awareness, rhythmic oral movements, manual automatisms, and then bilateral arm posturing. Ictal EEG's seizure onset was an alpha frequency range rhythm across the left anterior temporal lobe.

MRI identified signal abnormality of the left anterior temporal lobe and the left hippocampus. PET identified bilateral anterior temporal lobe hypometabolism with asymmetrically lower metabolism on the left. An intracarotid amobarbital test identified left hemispheric dominance for language and dependence on the right mesial temporal lobe for episodic memory. The left mesial temporal lobe structures provided no encoding.

The history and evaluation indicate left mesial temporal lobe epilepsy. The habitual occurrence of aphasia without impaired awareness is unusual for mesial temporal lobe epilepsy and more often suggests neocortical temporal lobe epilepsy, but the mesial temporal MRI, PET, and neuropsychological abnormalities along with the anterior temporal EEG abnormalities provided justification for an anterior temporal lobe resection.

A left anterior-medial temporal lobe resection and hippocampectomy was performed. Histopathological examination identified focal cortical dysplasia of the temporal pole evident in dyslamination with neuronal heterotopia. Neuronal dysmorphism was not present. No seizures or auras have occurred for the 1.5 years since surgery.

J. M. Stern, N. Salamon, *Imaging of Epilepsy*, https://doi.org/10.1007/978-3-030-86672-3_73

Imaging

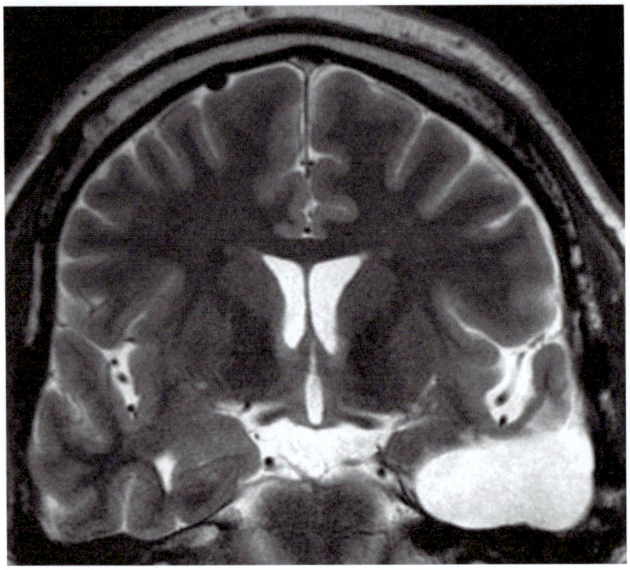

Fig. 73.1 MRI coronal T2 sequence at an amygdala level. A resection cavity includes the lateral and inferior portions of the left temporal lobe. The left superior temporal gyrus and amygdala remain. No other abnormality is present

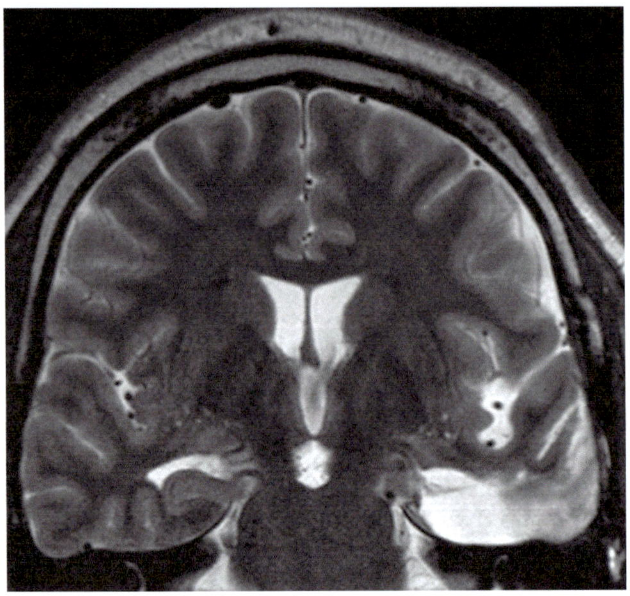

Fig. 73.2 MRI coronal T2 sequence at a hippocampal head level. A resection cavity includes the left hippocampus, inferior temporal gyrus, fusiform gyrus, and parahippocampal gyrus. The left superior temporal gyrus and a remnant of the left middle temporal gyrus remain

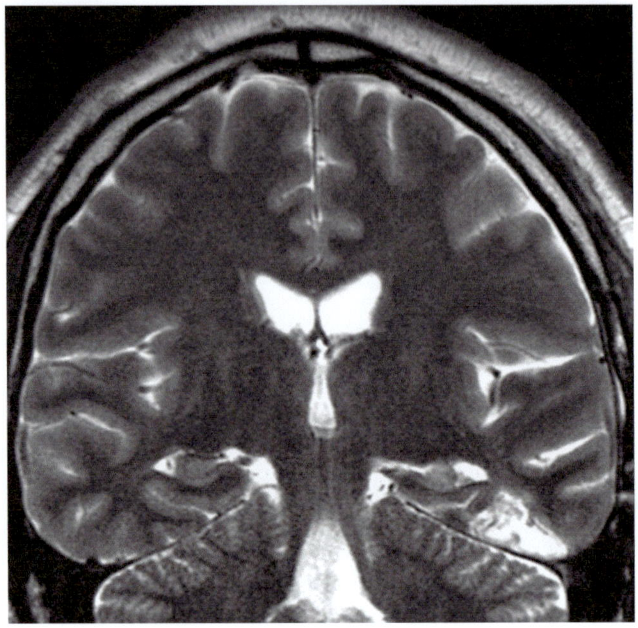

Fig. 73.3 MRI coronal T2 sequence at a hippocampal body level. A resection cavity includes the left fusiform gyrus. The left hippocampal abnormality is evident in atrophy and hyperintense signal. The left parahippocampal gyrus also is atrophic

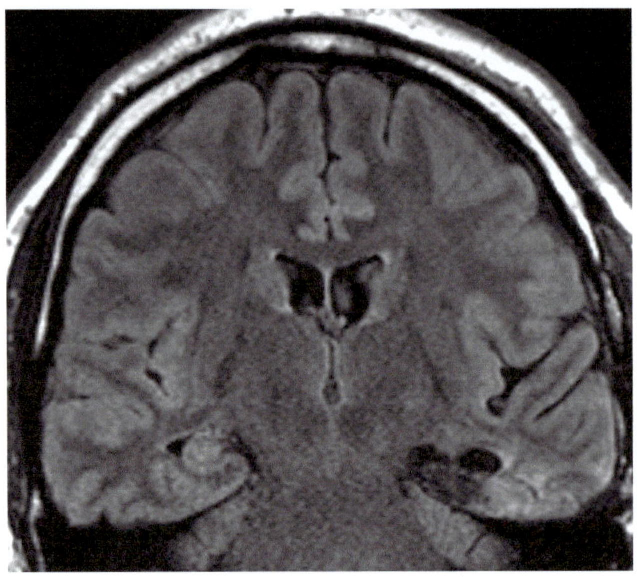

Fig. 73.4 MRI coronal FLAIR sequence at a hippocampal body level between the levels in Figs. 73.2 and 73.3. The left hippocampus has been resected. Postsurgical changes are evident in the hyperintense inferior temporal gyrus and fusiform gyrus. The hypointensity within the parahippocampal gyrus is likely related to volume averaging at the resection's margin

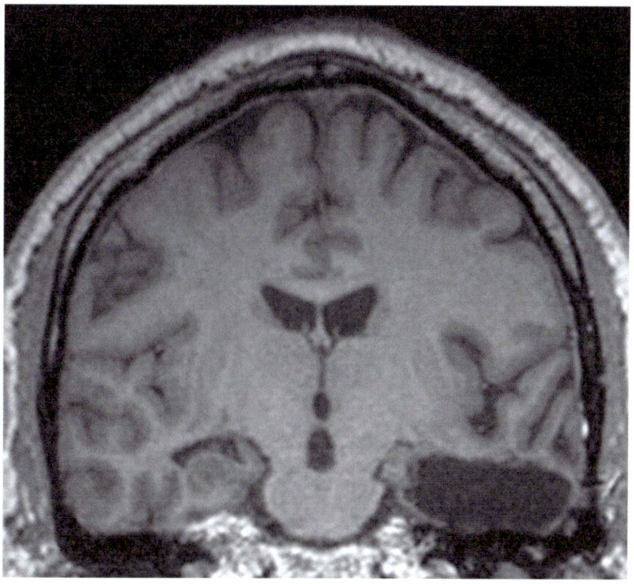

Fig. 73.5 MRI coronal T1 sequence at the same hippocampal head level as Fig. 73.2. A resection includes the left hippocampus, inferior temporal gyrus, and fusiform gyrus. A remnant of the left middle temporal gyrus is evident. The left superior temporal gyrus is normal

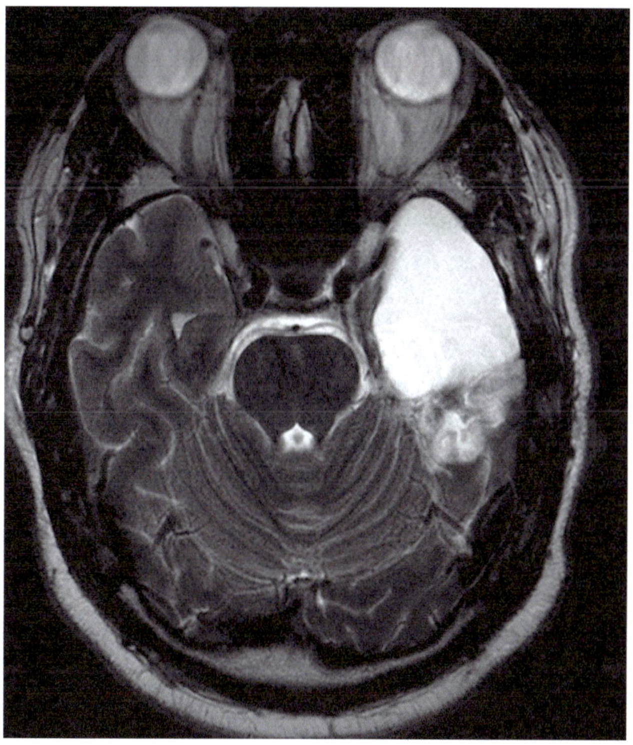

Fig. 73.6 MRI axial T2 sequence at a hippocampal head level. A resection cavity in the left middle cranial fossa includes the left anterior temporal lobe. Hyperintensity of the left posterior fusiform and inferior temporal gyri is due to postsurgical changes

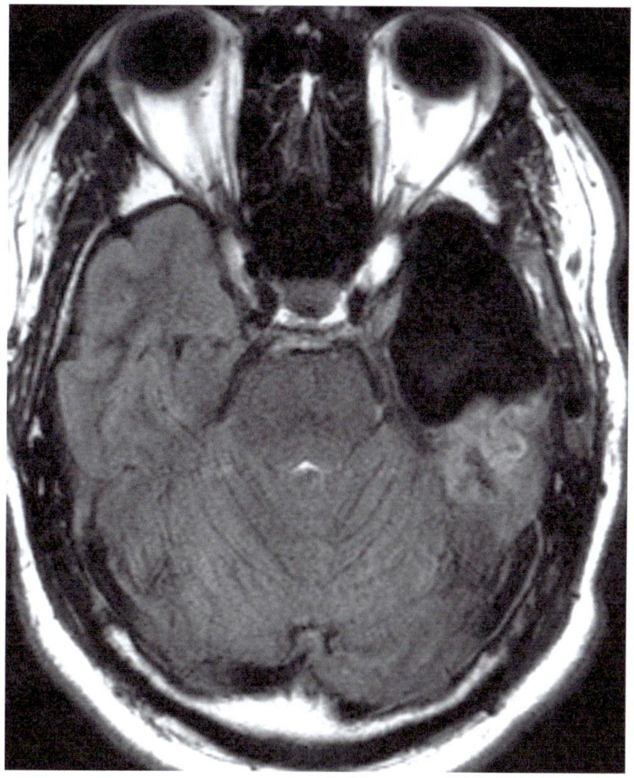

Fig. 73.7 MRI axial FLAIR sequence at the same hippocampal head level as Fig. 73.6. A resection cavity in the left middle cranial fossa and including the left anterior temporal lobe is indicated by signal with cerebrospinal fluid (CSF) intensity. The hyperintensity within the posterior inferior temporal gyrus is due to postsurgical changes

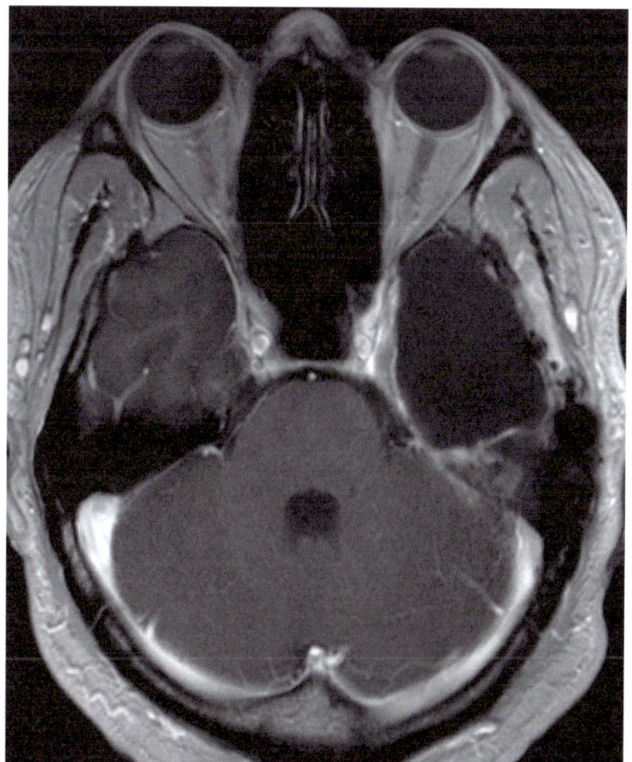

Fig. 73.8 MRI axial T1 sequence after contrast administration at the same hippocampal head level as Figs. 73.6 and 73.7. No abnormal enhancement is present

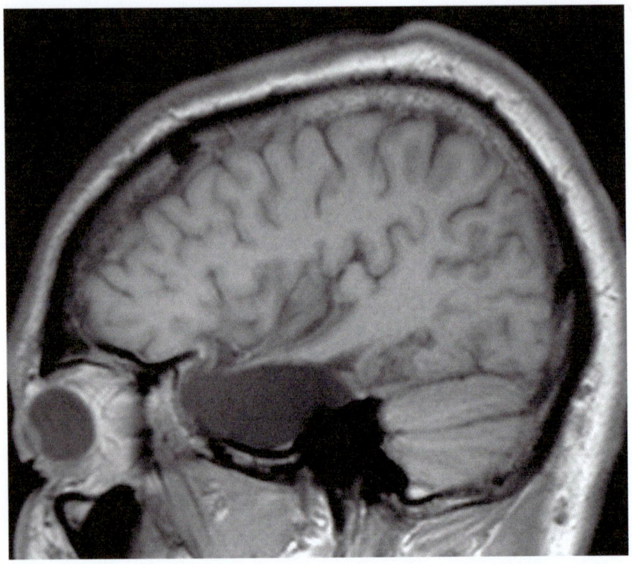

Fig. 73.9 MRI sagittal T1 sequence at a left hippocampus level. The resection cavity produced by a left anterior temporal lobe resection is evident in the CSF signal. The medial superior temporal gyrus tapers anteriorly and is normal posteriorly with Heschl's gyrus visible

Focal Cortical Resection

74

Clinical History

The first recognized seizure occurred at age 13 years as an episode of impaired awareness, repetitive chewing, and bilateral hand movements described as a combination of fidgeting and picking. The evaluation at that time was not recalled.

The habitual seizures manifested as an indescribable sensation for about 1 minute that was followed by impaired awareness with grimacing, bilateral manual automatisms, and repeated lateral head movements. The impairment's duration was about 1 minute, and recovery was quick and with minimal postictal fatigue or confusion. None of the seizures progressed to asymmetric posturing, and the only tonic-clonic seizure occurred after discontinuing all anti-seizure medication. Prior to epilepsy surgery, auras never occurred in isolation. Treatment included multiple anti-seizure medications and a vagus nerve stimulator with a seizure frequency of five seizures weekly prior to epilepsy surgery. Seizures often clustered with several in 1 day.

An epilepsy risk factor was not present.

Neurological examination was normal. Neuropsychological testing identified deficits in visuospatial memory, organizational inefficiencies, and naming. Phonologic sequencing and reading were normal.

Interictal EEG depicted left frontal-temporal epileptiform discharges. Video-EEG monitoring recorded focal seizures manifested as arising from the bed, lateral head turning, repeated tongue movements, and alternately lateralized manual automatisms. Ictal EEG's seizure onset was broadly across the left temporal region.

MRI identified a focal signal abnormality in the left posterior superior temporal gyrus. PET was normal.

The history and evaluation indicated focal seizures with auras and automatisms that progressed only once to tonic-clonic. The behavioral features suggest limbic involvement, but the quick recovery suggests a neocortical localization. The EEG indication of a left temporal lobe epilepsy does not differentiate between limbic and neocortical and neuropsychological testing did not indicate a single localization, but the MRI supported a posterior superior temporal localization. To localize with more certainty and identify language cortex boundaries, a subdural grid electrode video-EEG monitoring was performed with electrodes across the left anterior temporal lobe and left temporal-parietal region. The ictal subdural grid EEG's seizure onsets were localized to the superior temporal gyrus lesion. Extra-operative language mapping with electrical stimulation through the subdural grid identified languages areas adjacent to and separate from the seizure onset zone.

A left temporal lobe resection with intraoperative electrocorticographic mapping was performed. Histopathological examination identified a low-grade mixed glioma and focal cortical dysplasia, type 2. Several habitual seizures occurred during the first few months after surgery, and auras in isolation occurred over the subsequent 2 years; however, no seizures with impaired awareness have occurred in the past 3 years and no auras in the past 2 years.

J. M. Stern, N. Salamon, *Imaging of Epilepsy*, https://doi.org/10.1007/978-3-030-86672-3_74

Imaging

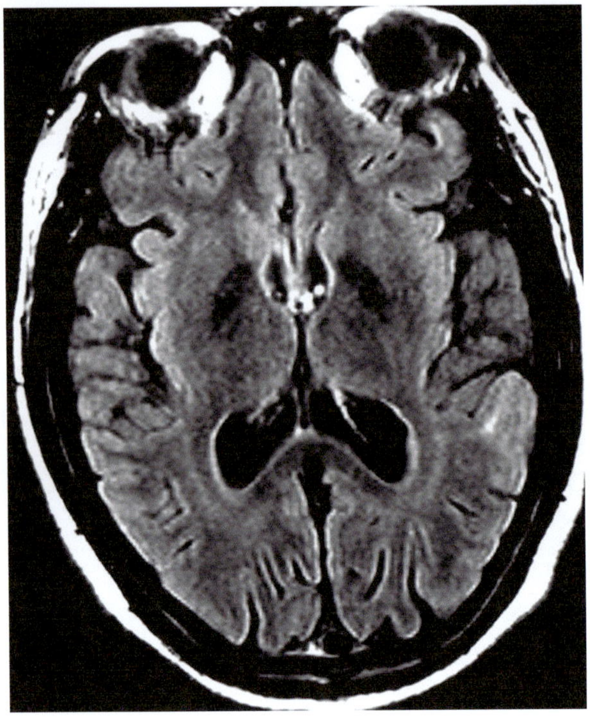

Fig. 74.1 MRI axial FLAIR sequence at a thalamus level. A focus of abnormal hyperintense signal is evident in the left posterior superior temporal gyrus and is consistent with a focal cortical dysplasia

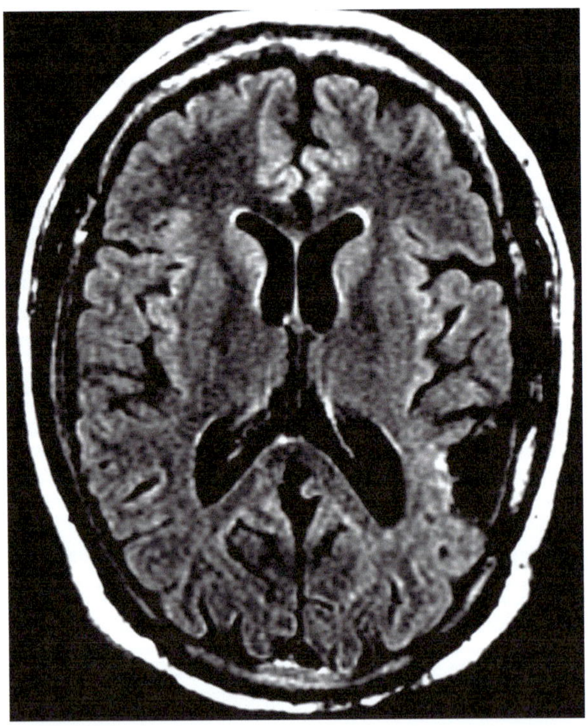

Fig. 74.2 MRI axial FLAIR sequence at a thalamus level slightly superior to Fig. 74.1 A resection cavity is evident in the left posterior superior temporal gyrus. The hyperintensity along the medial edges of the cavity are postsurgical changes

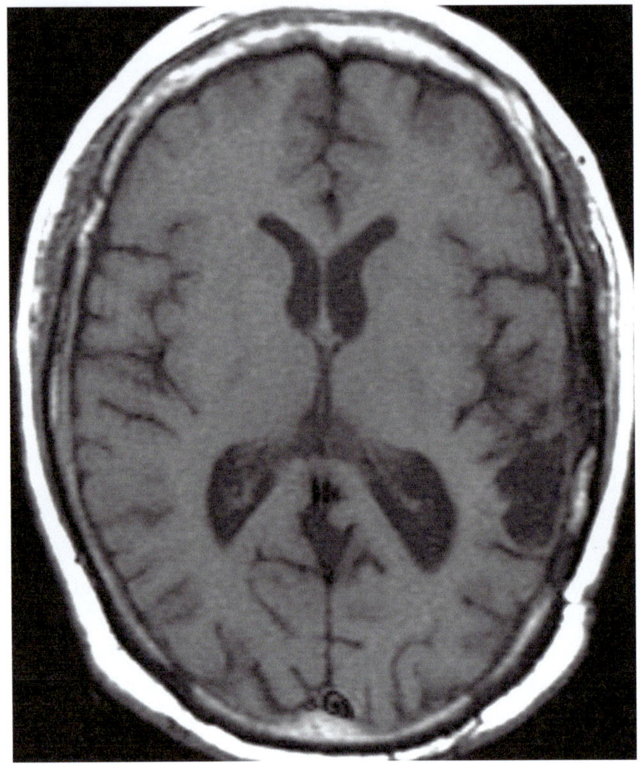

Fig. 74.3 MRI axial T1 sequence administration at the same thalamus level as Fig. 74.2. A resection cavity is evident in the left posterior superior gyrus. Because the image is based on a T1 sequence and not the FLAIR sequence in Fig. 74.2, the hyperintense signal along the medial edge is not evident. No abnormal enhancement is present

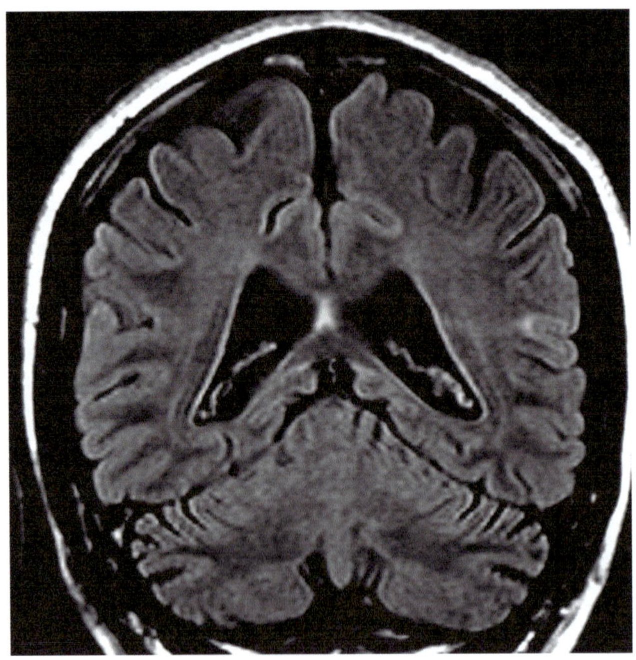

Fig. 74.4 MRI coronal FLAIR sequence at an atrium of the lateral ventricles level. A focus of abnormal hyperintense signal is evident in the subcortical white matter of the left posterior superior temporal gyrus and is consistent with a focal cortical dysplasia

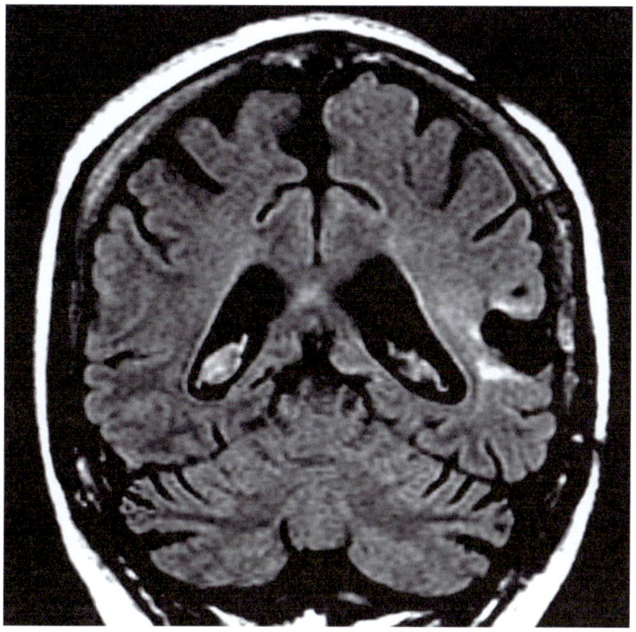

Fig. 74.5 MRI coronal FLAIR sequence at an atrium of the lateral ventricles level similar to Fig. 74.4. A resection cavity is evident in the left posterior superior temporal gyrus and is bounded by hyperintense signal indicating postsurgical gliosis

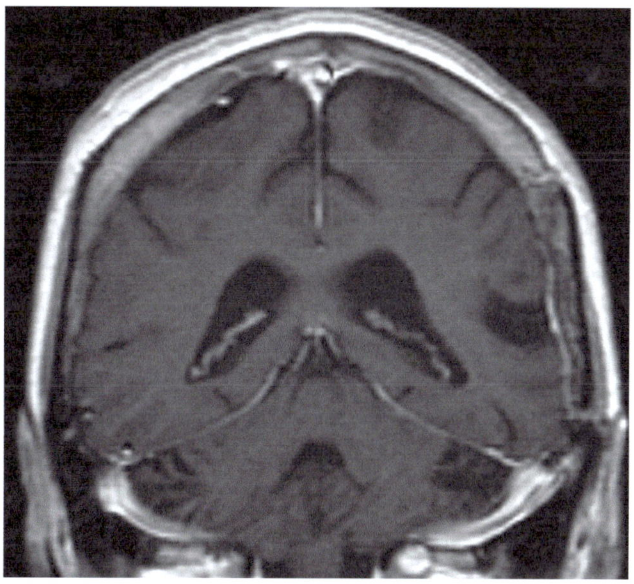

Fig. 74.6 MRI coronal T1sequence after contrast administration at an atrium of the lateral ventricles level similar to Figs. 74.4 and 74.5. A resection cavity is evident in the left posterior superior temporal gyrus, as is evident in Fig. 74.5. No abnormal enhancement is present

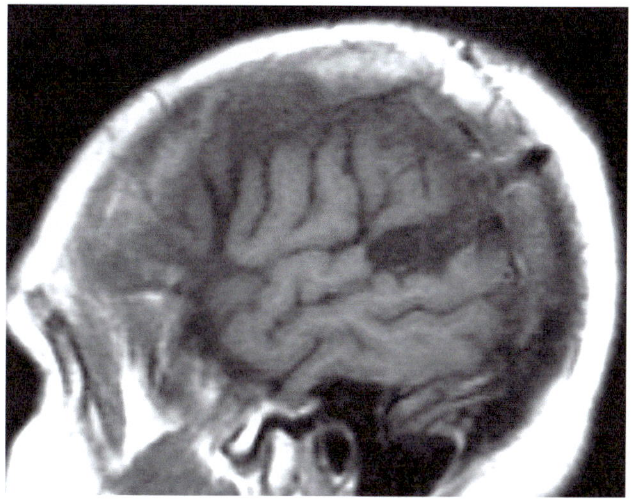

Fig. 74.7 MRI sagittal T1 sequence at a left Sylvian fissure level. A resection cavity is evident in the posterior portion of the superior temporal gyrus with a clear margin in the middle portion of the gyrus

Focal Cortical Resection and Extension

75

Clinical History

The first recognized seizure occurred at age 3 years as right leg cramping. Additional episodes occurred over the subsequent year with durations of about 15 second, and some produced a fall. At age 4 years, the frequency increased to several daily, and epilepsy was diagnosed when one episode was witnessed during routine pediatric care.

The habitual seizures manifested as right leg cramping followed by right arm contraction and eyelid fluttering with amnesia for a total seizure duration of 15 to 45 seconds. Postictal speech difficulty and right arm and leg weakness were present for 20 to 30 seconds. Treatment included multiple anti-seizure medications with a seizure frequency of 12 to 15 times daily prior to epilepsy surgery.

An epilepsy risk factor was not present.

Neurological examination was normal. Neurologic development was normal, and school performance was good.

Interictal EEG depicted generalized epileptiform discharges. Video-EEG monitoring recorded focal seizures manifested as tonic extension of the right arm and leg. Ictal EEG's seizure onset was over the left parasagittal region.

MRI identified focal cortical dysplasia within the left superior parietal lobule and medial precentral gyrus. PET identified hypometabolism in the superior aspect of the left parietal lobe.

The history and evaluation indicate focal seizures with ictal and postictal behavioral features suggesting the left central region. The ictal EEG and PET are concordant with lesion evident on MRI, but the proximity of the lesion to motor-sensory cortex constrained the size of a resection because of the risk of a deficit. The interictal EEG's generalized epileptiform discharges relate to rapid propagation of neocortical discharges close to the midline.

A focal resection within the left superior parietal lobule was performed at age 8 years with somatosensory evoked potentials and electrocorticographic guidance. Histopathological examination identified focal cortical dysplasia, type 1a. Postoperative motor-sensory function was unchanged, and seizure control was excellent with only two seizures during the first month after surgery and then seizure freedom for almost 2 years. With recurrence, the seizure frequency was initially about 1 monthly and then gradually increased to two to five daily with seizure manifestations that were described as identical to the habitual seizures before surgery.

Video-EEG monitoring after the recurrence of seizures recorded focal seizures with the same behavioral and electrographic features, so it supported the prior localization. MRI and PET depicted the resection with remaining focal cortical dysplasia at the margins that had been spared because of proximity to motor-sensory cortex. Upon reconsideration of the seizures and the risks of a motor or sensory deficit, an extension of the resection was performed. Histopathological examination identified focal cortical dysplasia, type 2b, with dysmorphic neurons, cytomegaly, and abundant balloon cells. No seizures have occurred for the 1.5 years since the extension of the resection, and treatment is now being reduced to two anti-seizure medications. Motor and sensory function was not affected by the second resection.

J. M. Stern, N. Salamon, *Imaging of Epilepsy*, https://doi.org/10.1007/978-3-030-86672-3_75

Imaging

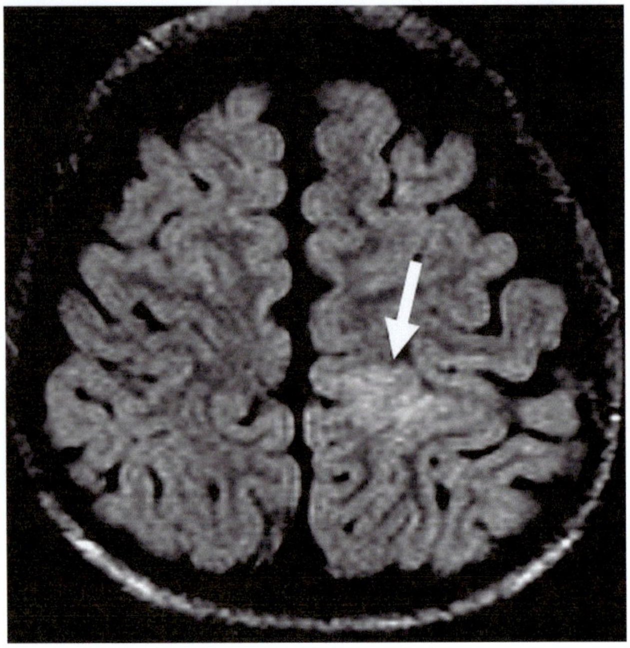

Fig. 75.1 MRI axial FLAIR sequence at a high convexity level. Hyperintense signal is evident in the left paracentral lobule (arrow) in the region of the leg sensorimotor cortex. The abnormality is consistent with focal cortical dysplasia

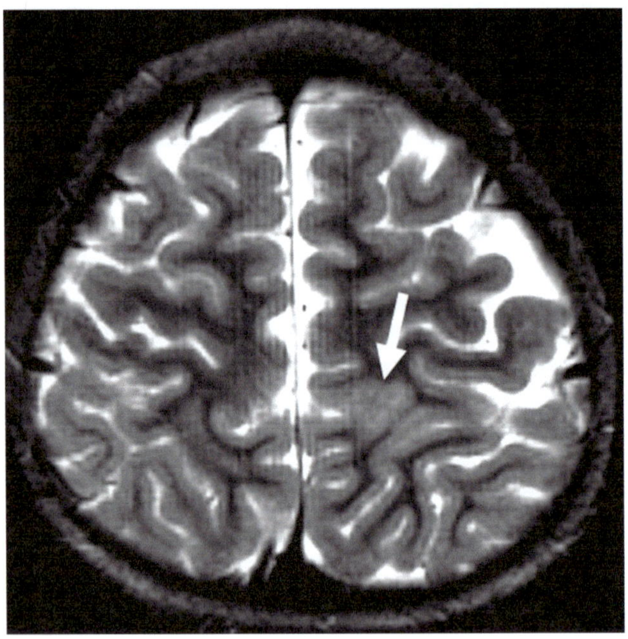

Fig. 75.2 MRI axial T2 sequence at the same high convexity level as Fig. 75.1. Abnormal, hyperintense signal (arrow) is evident in the left paracentral lobule but less apparent than in Fig. 75.1

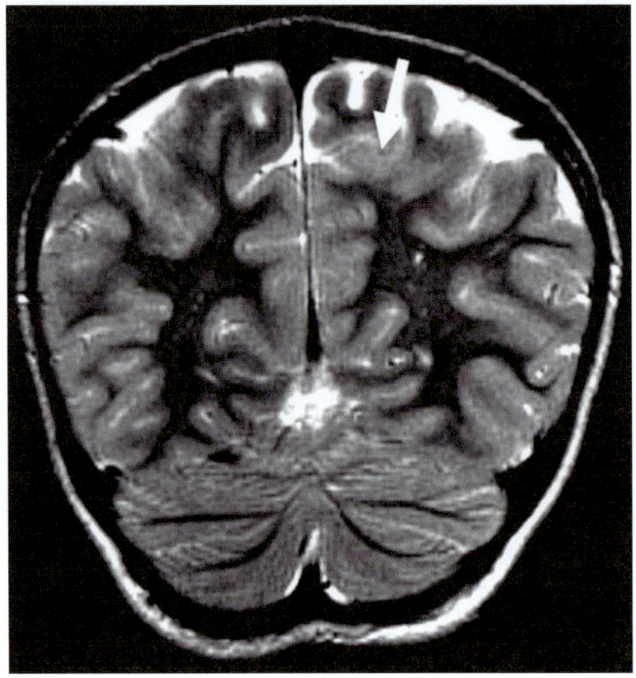

Fig. 75.3 MRI coronal T2 sequence at a level immediately posterior to the occipital horns of the lateral ventricles. Abnormal, hyperintense signal is evident in the left paracentral lobule and superior parietal lobule. The oblique angle of the level produces the appearance of a thickened cortical ribbon, but the signal abnormality is the indicator of the focal cortical dysplasia

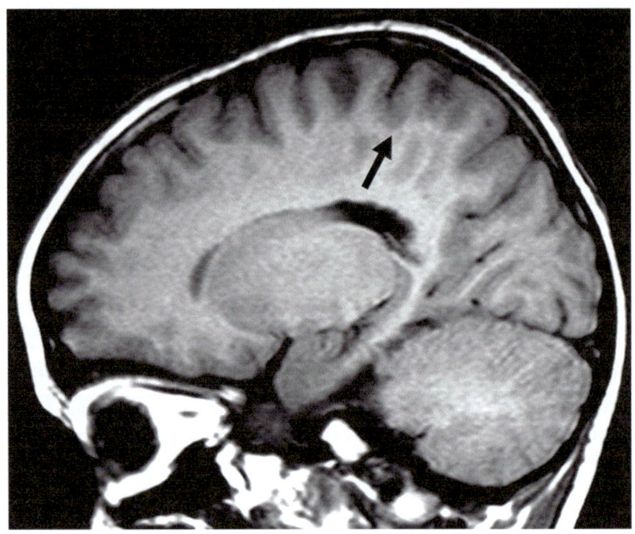

Fig. 75.4 MRI sagittal T1 sequence at a left hippocampal head level. The focal cortical dysplasia is evident at the depth of the parietal lobe sulcus (arrow) as abnormally thickened cortex with normal signal intensity

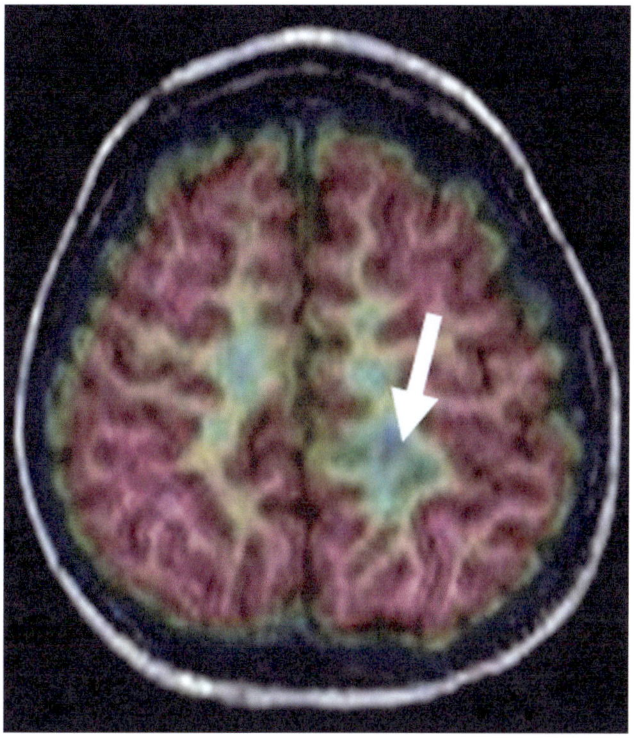

Fig. 75.5 PET-MRI co-registration with color-scale FDG tracer in an axial plane at the same high convexity level as Figs. 75.1 and 75.2. Abnormal hypometabolism is evident in the left paracentral lobule and corresponds to the T2 and FLAIR sequence signal abnormality in Figs. 75.1 and 75.2. The cortical ribbon metabolism is otherwise normal

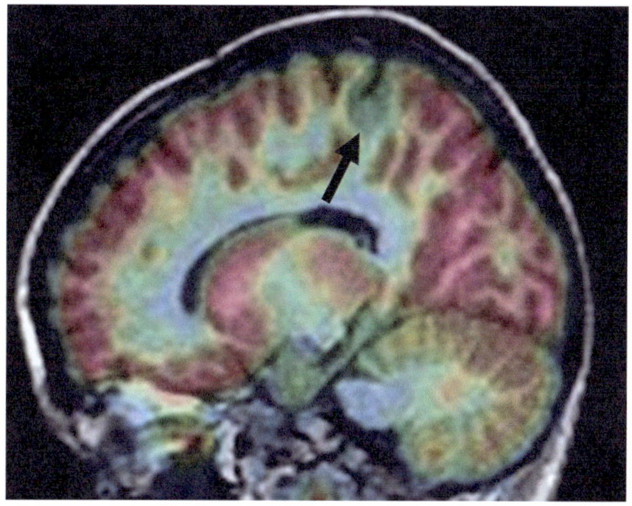

Fig. 75.7 PET-MRI co-registration with color-scale FDG tracer in a sagittal plane at the same left hippocampal head level as Fig. 75.4. The depth of the parietal lobe sulcus (arrow) is abnormally hypometabolic and thickened. The metabolism of the amygdala and parahippocampal cortex is normal. The regions of greater metabolism within the white matter are due to volume averaging with gray matter. The white matter is normal

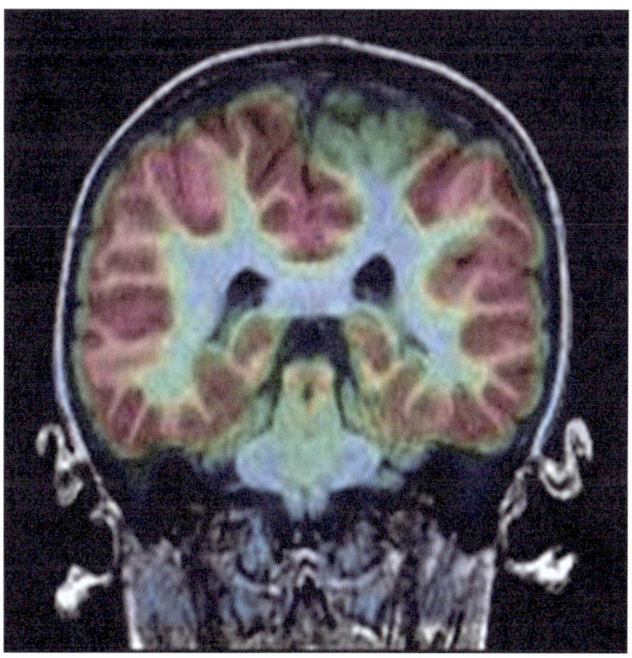

Fig. 75.6 PET-MRI co-registration with color-scale FDG tracer in a coronal plane at a splenium of the corpus callosum level anterior to Fig. 75.3. The left paracentral and superior parietal lobules are abnormally hypometabolic. The gray matter is normal in the remaining cortical ribbon

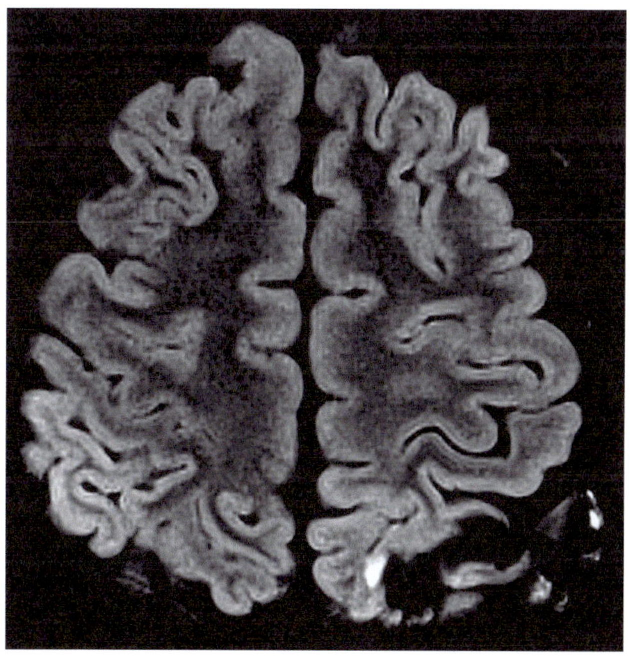

Fig. 75.8 MRI axial FLAIR sequence at a high convexity level slightly inferior to Fig. 75.1. A resection cavity is evident in the left superior parietal lobule. Hyperintensity within the left paracentral lobule is focal cortical dysplasia that was spared to preserve leg sensory function. The nodule of hyperintensity along the cavity's medial margin is postsurgical gliosis

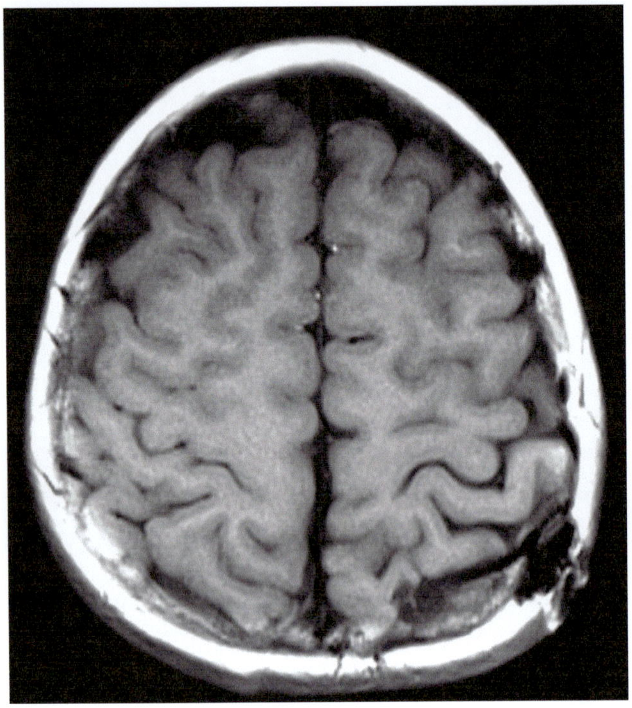

Fig. 75.9 MRI axial T1 sequence at the same high convexity level as Fig. 75.8. A resection cavity is evident in the left superior parietal lobule along the craniotomy changes in the neighboring left skull. Postsurgical gliosis is evident as hyperintense signal medial to the cavity at the posterior edge of the cerebrum at this level

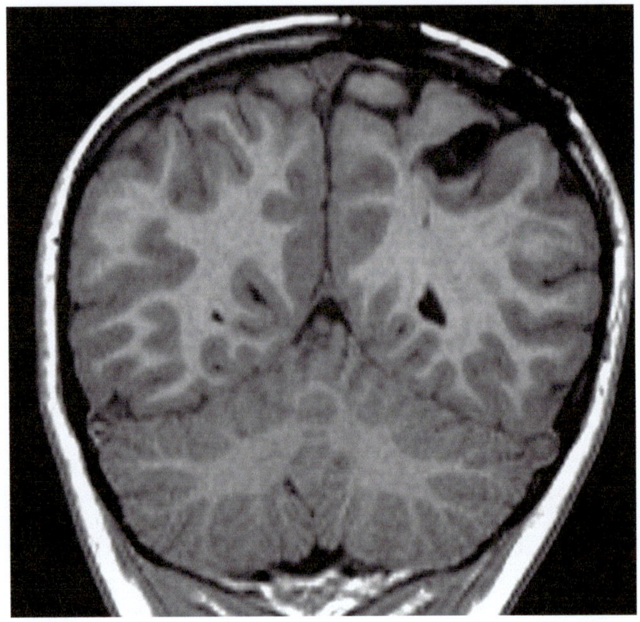

Fig. 75.11 MRI coronal T1 sequence at the same posterior to the occipital horns level as Fig. 75.3. The craniotomy changes in left parietal bone are evident along the resection cavity in the left superior parietal lobule

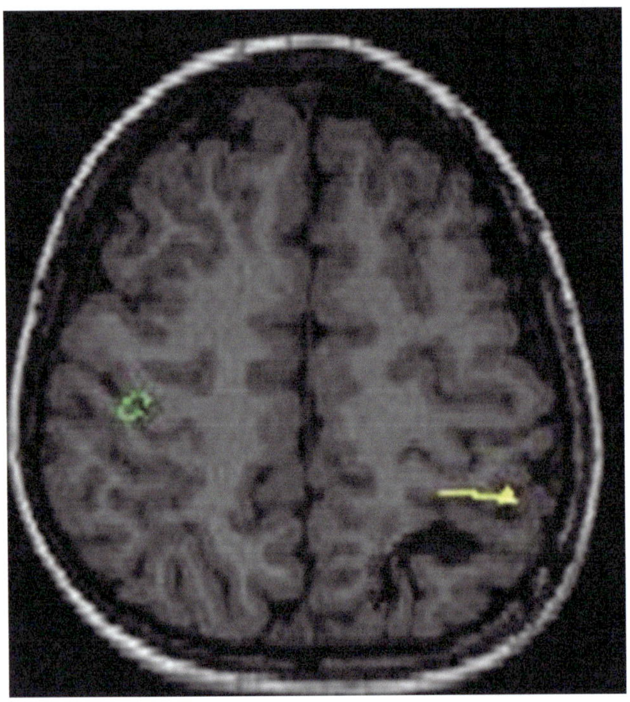

Fig. 75.10 MEG co-registered to axial T1 sequence MRI at the same high convexity level as Figs. 75.8 and 75.9. An epileptiform dipole is indicated in yellow along the left postcentral gyrus, anterior to the resection cavity. Right sensorimotor cortex is indicated by an evoked dipole in green

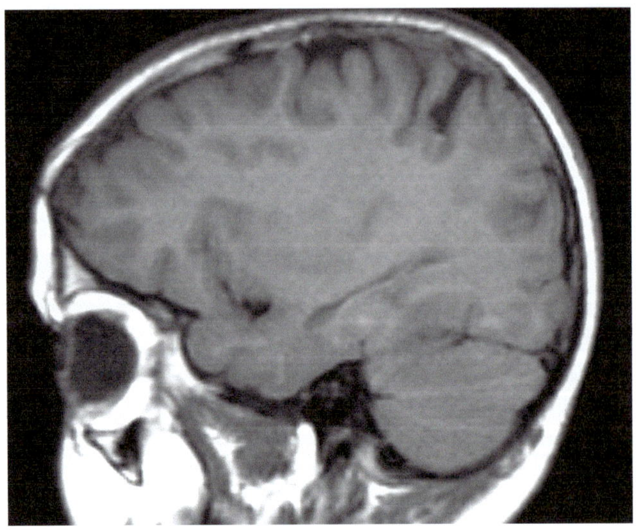

Fig. 75.12 MRI sagittal T1 sequence at a hippocampus level lateral to Fig. 75.4. In this sagittal orientation, the resection cavity in the left superior parietal lobule has a linear appearance

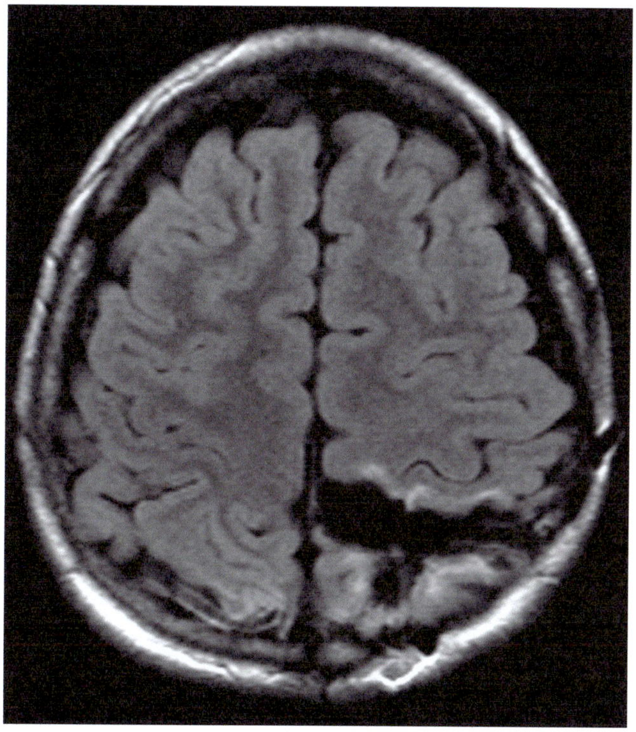

Fig. 75.13 MRI axial FLAIR sequence at the same high convexity level as Figs. 75.8 and 75.9. After the second operation, the resection cavity is extended medially and now includes the focal cortical dysplasia within the left paracentral lobule. The hyperintensity along the margins of the cavity is postsurgical gliosis

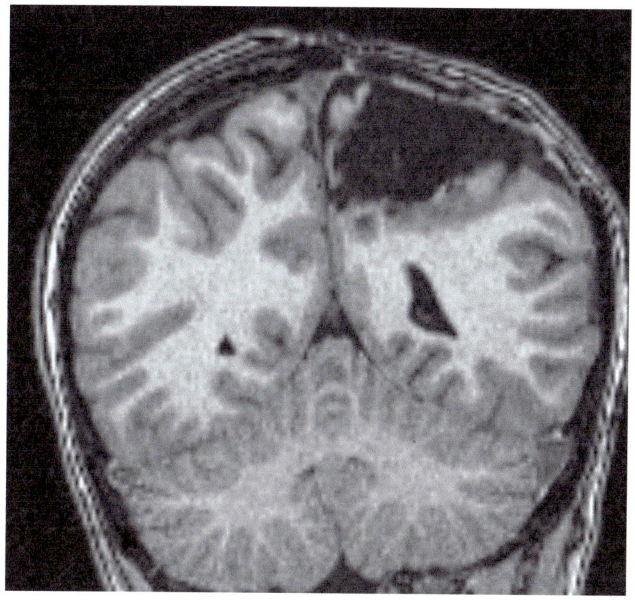

Fig. 75.15 MRI coronal T1 sequence at a similar level as Figs. 75.3 and 75.11. The left parietal resection cavity has been extended medially to the paracentral lobule. The residual tissue at the midline is a remnant of the paracentral lobule

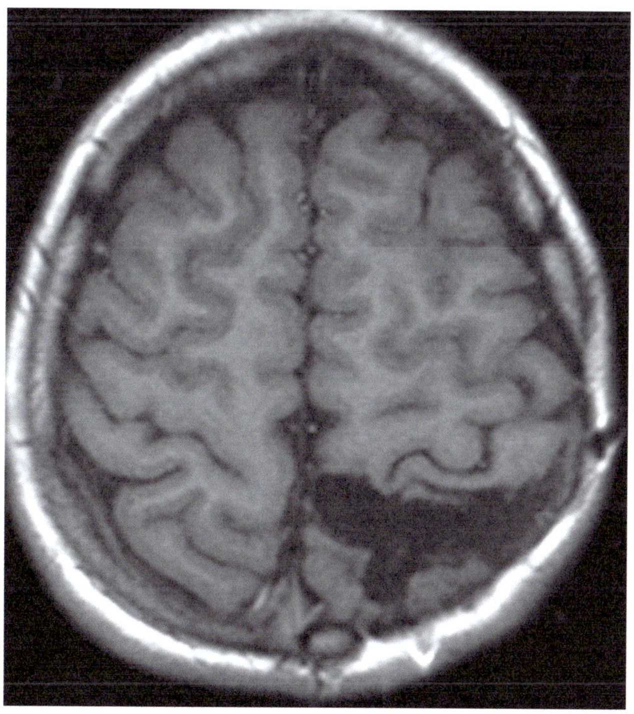

Fig. 75.14 MRI axial T1 sequence at the same high convexity level as Figs. 75.8, 75.9, and 75.13. The resection cavity has been extended into the left paracentral lobule. No other abnormality is present

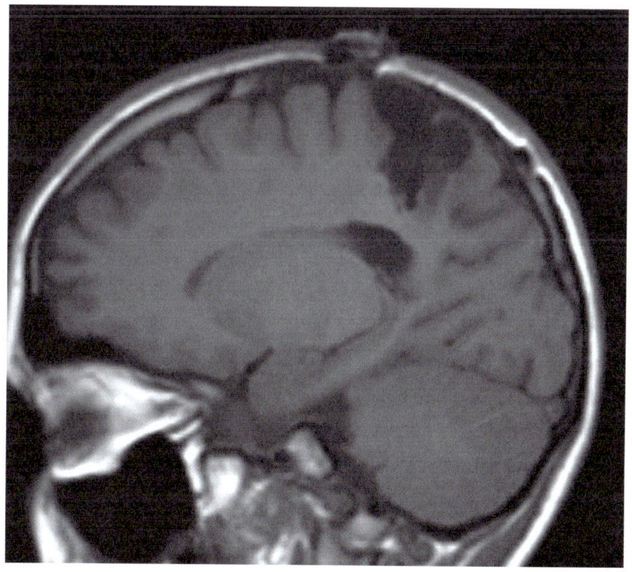

Fig. 75.16 MRI sagittal T1 sequence at the same hippocampal head level as Fig. 75.4 and slightly medial to Fig. 75.12. The resection cavity has been extended anteriorly, and the focal cortical dysplasia has been completely resected. The adjacent craniotomy changes are visible

Hemispherotomy

76

Clinical History

The first recognized seizure occurred at age 3 days as spasms with right eye deviation, drooling, and tonic extension of all limbs. An evaluation at that time identified right hemimegalencephaly.

The habitual seizures first manifested at age 20 days and were left hemibody clonus that sometimes progressed to left hemibody tonic spasms. Anti-seizure medications had benefit with up to 2 months of seizure freedom. At around age 3 years, the seizures changed to also include right gaze deviation and drooling, and the duration increased to 3–4 minutes with postictal fatigue lasting 2–3 hours.

Treatment included multiple anti-seizure medications with a seizure frequency of one seizure every few weeks to months. In addition to these seizures, a different seizure later presented with a manifestation of twitching of the left hand for seconds and recurrences multiple times daily.

The epilepsy risk factor was right hemimegalencephaly.

Neurological examination identified developmental delay and mild left hemiparesis. At age 3 years, spoken vocabulary was a few words, and walking was not possible without assistance. Medical history included Proteus syndrome with right hemibody hypertrophy.

Interictal EEG depicted diffuse abnormal slowing, frequent generalized attenuations, occasional left occipital epileptiform discharges, and very frequent epileptiform discharges and paroxysmal fast activity within the right frontal, temporal, central, and occipital regions. Video-EEG monitoring recorded both seizure manifestations with focal seizures occurring as nearly continuous twitching of the left eyelid, hand, and foot and as left-sided tonic seizures with 1-minute durations.

MRI identified right hemimegalencephaly with thickening of the cerebral cortex, band heterotopia, and dysplasia and hypertrophy of the cingulate gyrus. The left hemisphere was normal. PET identified hemimegalencephaly with a region of hypometabolism within the right parietal lobe.

The history and evaluation indicate infantile spasms that changed during infancy and early childhood to be left hemibody seizures with epilepsia partialis continua. The EEG and MRI identified a diffuse functional and structural abnormality of the right hemisphere, which indicated surgical treatment candidacy for seizure control and potentially to benefit neurologic development.

A right hemispherotomy was performed at age 3 years. The resection included the lateral hemisphere, temporal lobe, and orbitofrontal lobe and also included a corpus callosotomy. Histopathological examination of the central operculum, temporal lobe, and orbitofrontal cortex identified focal cortical dysplasia, type 1b, nodular and linear heterotopia in subcortical white matter, and foci of dystrophic calcification. No seizures have occurred for the 6 years since surgery, and anti-seizure medications were tapered to discontinuation after 2 years of seizure freedom. Neurological exam improved after surgery with increased vocabulary and spoken fluency and symmetric walking without assistance. Surgery produced left arm weakness with the left hand maintaining capacity for gripping tasks.

J. M. Stern, N. Salamon, *Imaging of Epilepsy*, https://doi.org/10.1007/978-3-030-86672-3_76

Imaging

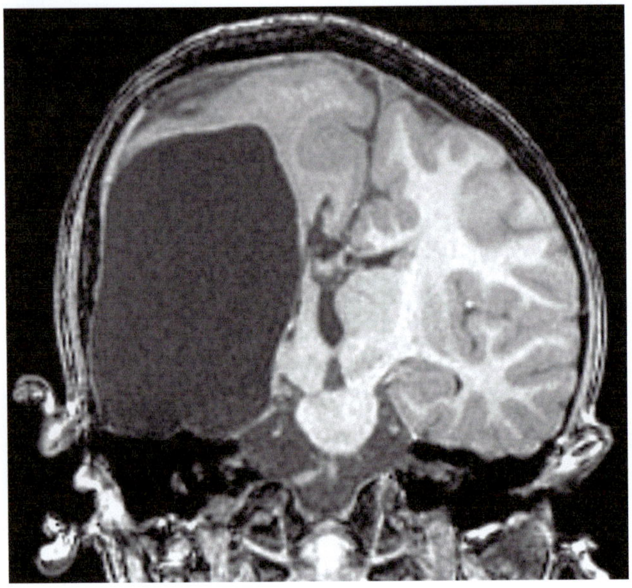

Fig. 76.1 MRI coronal T1 sequence at a thalamus level. A large resection cavity encompasses much of the right cerebral hemisphere including the right basal ganglia and the majority of the right thalamus. The residual right hemisphere has abnormally decreased gray-white differentiation. The interhemispheric fissure is shifted leftward, and the lateral ventricles are compressed. The third ventricle is midline and the left hemisphere is normal

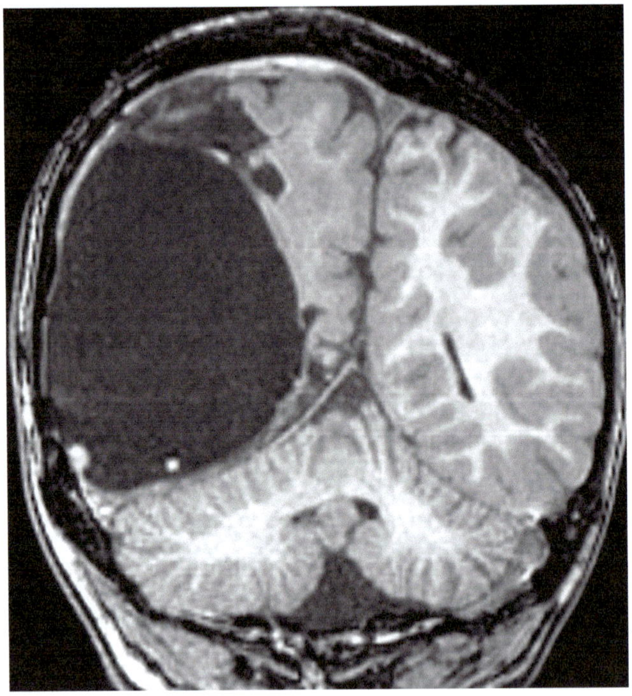

Fig. 76.2 MRI coronal T1 sequence at an occipital horn level. A large resection cavity includes most of the right parietal and occipital lobes. The residual right parietal lobe has decreased gray-white differentiation with abnormally decreased white matter signal. The cerebellum is asymmetric with left hemispheric atrophy due to diaschisis. The left cerebral hemisphere is normal

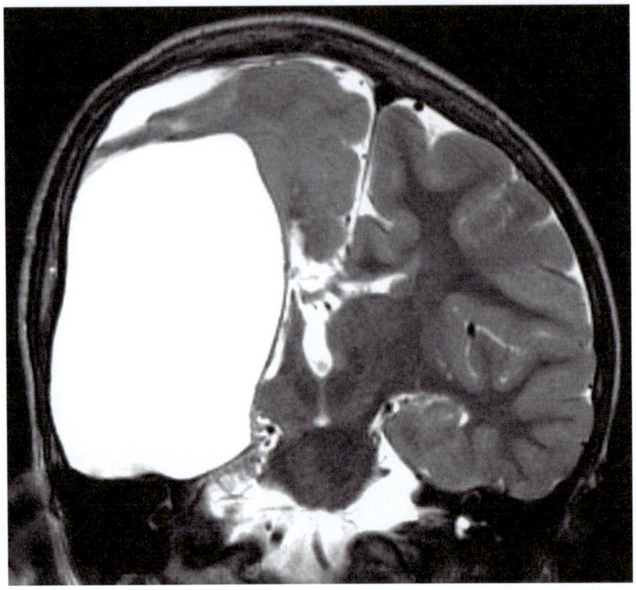

Fig. 76.3 MRI coronal T2 sequence at the same thalamus level as Fig. 76.1. A large resection cavity comprises much of the right cerebral hemisphere. The residual right frontal lobe's white matter has abnormally increased signal. The right lateral ventricle is distorted, and the left lateral ventricle is normal. The left hemisphere is normal

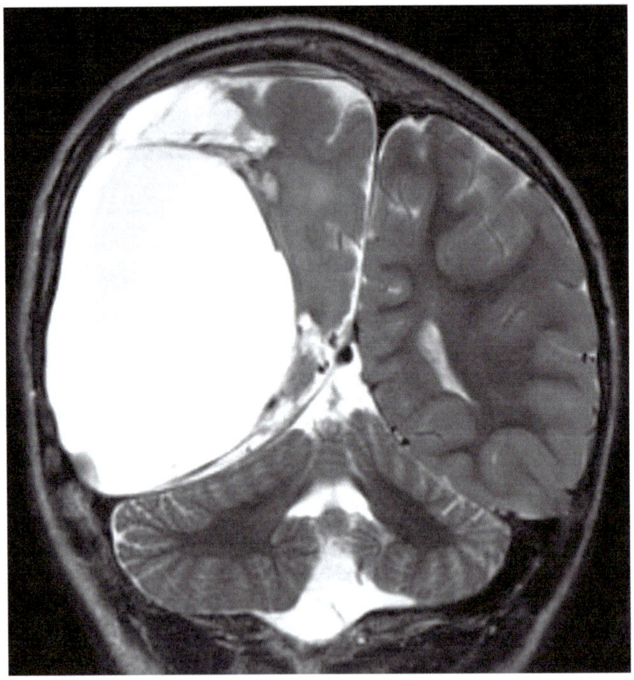

Fig. 76.4 MRI coronal T2 sequence at the same occipital horn level as Fig. 76.2. A large resection cavity includes the right parietal and occipital lobes with a septation evident in the superior aspect. The residual parietal lobe white matter has abnormally increased signal and abnormally decreased gray-white differentiation

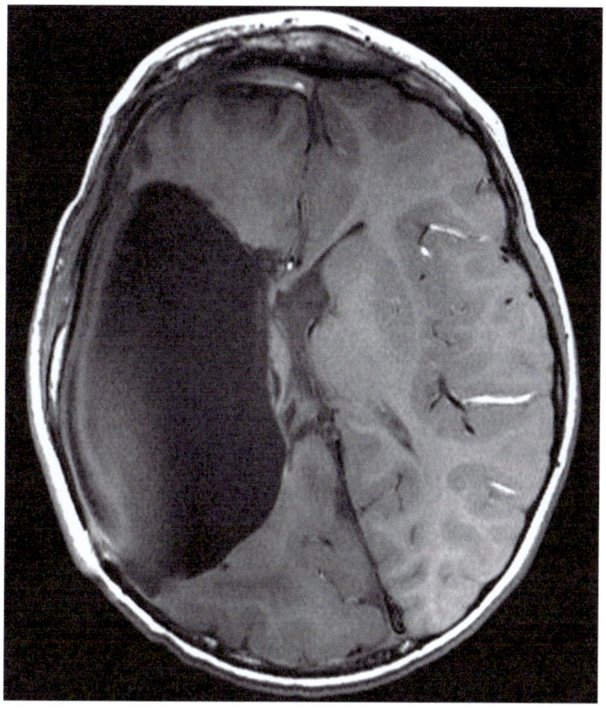

Fig. 76.5 MRI axial T1 sequence at a basal ganglia level. A resection cavity is evident within the central portion of right cerebral hemisphere, including the thalamus and basal ganglia. The right hemisphere is larger than the left, indicating hemimegalencephaly. The left hemisphere is normal, and no hydrocephalus is present. The linear hyperintensity within the left Sylvian fissure is flow artifact in this non-enhanced scan

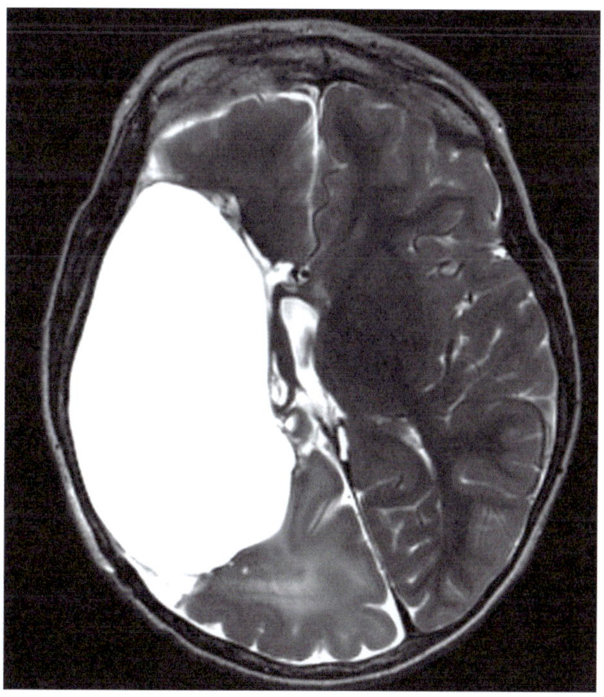

Fig. 76.6 MRI axial T2 sequence at the same basal ganglia level as Fig. 76.5. A resection cavity comprises the central portion of the right cerebral hemisphere and is prominent because of the high signal of the cerebrospinal fluid (CSF) filling the volume. The residual right hemisphere is dysmorphic and consistent with hemimegalencephaly, including the right frontal and occipital lobes' abnormally increased white matter signal and the poor gray-white differentiation. The ventricles and left hemisphere are normal

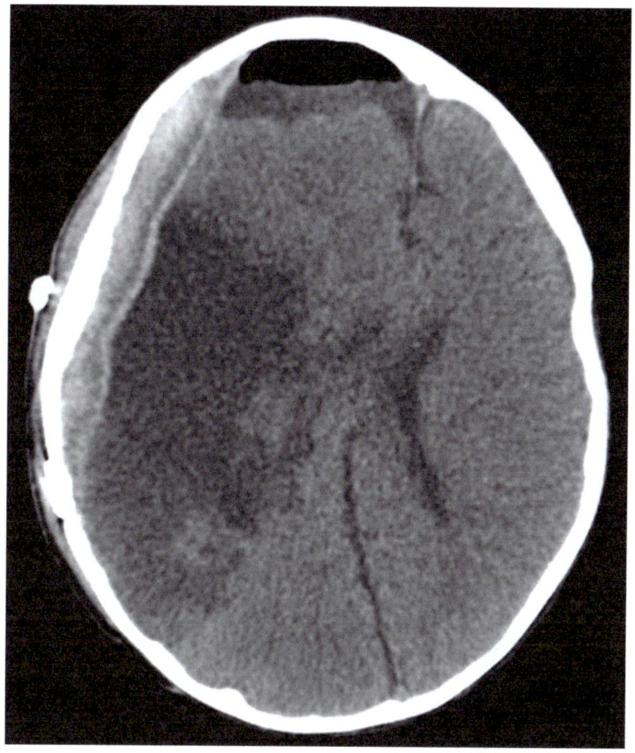

Fig. 76.7 CT in an axial plane at a lateral ventricle level. The CT was obtained postoperatively and depicts an extra-axial hematoma along the right convexity and pneumocephalus superficial to the right frontal lobe

77 Hemispherectomy

Clinical History

The first recognized seizures occurred at age 2 days as infantile spasms. An evaluation at that time identified hemimegalencephaly.

The habitual seizures manifested as sudden and brief right-hand grasping movements followed by hip flexion. The spasms repeated for about 5 minutes and were followed by 15 minutes of sleepiness or irritability. Treatment included multiple anti-seizure medications with 10 clusters of spasms daily for the first few months of life and then increasing to comprise about 6 hours daily. Around the time of the increasing seizures, seizures manifested solely as eyelid fluttering first developed and occurred several times weekly.

The epilepsy risk factor was left hemimegalencephaly.

Neurological examination in childhood identified diminished head control and preferential gaze to the left and inability to visually track.

Interictal EEG at age 2 months during both wakefulness and sleep depicted a modified hypsarrhythmia with excessive discontinuity, abnormally high amplitude across the left hemisphere, frequent epileptiform discharges across the left frontal and central regions, and paroxysmal fast activity across the left posterior quadrant. Video-EEG monitoring recorded seizures manifested as spasms with myoclonic jerks of right arm, bilateral legs, and occasionally the left arm after the right arm. Ictal EEG's seizure onset was left frontal central discharges followed by a generalized electrodecrement.

MRI identified a markedly enlarged left cerebral hemisphere with thickened gray matter and polymicrogyria of the perisylvian region. The left cerebellar hemisphere also is asymmetrically larger and included abnormal signal. The brainstem and right cerebral and cerebellar hemispheres were normal.

The history and evaluation indicate infantile spasms with asymmetric motor features and EEG abnormalities that are consistent with the cerebral hemisphere malformation. A left hemispherotomy with corpus callosotomy was performed at age 4 months. Histopathological examination identified focal cortical dysplasia, type IIa, and widespread polymicrogyria.

No seizures occurred for 1 year after surgery and neurologic development improved with the gaining of the previously delayed milestones. Seizures returned at age 18 months as slow, rhythmic left eyelid blinking. Over weeks, the seizure manifestation changed to a rapid eyelid flutter with an appearance of diminished awareness. Ictal EEG at that time was inconclusive. At about age 2 years, the seizure manifestation changed to include flushing of the upper body and left hemibody clonus. During an episode of status epilepticus with seizures lasting 30 minutes and recurring every 1–2 hours, EEG's seizure onset was focal at the left frontal pole.

Seizures changed at age 3 years to include brief staring behavior with an EEG seizure onset that was broadly across the left hemisphere, and an extension of the hemispherotomy was performed to include the remaining left cerebral cortex. This included the remaining frontal, parietal, and occipital lobes to provide an anatomic hemispherectomy. Histopathological examination identified polymicrogyria, widespread band and nodular heterotopia in subcortical gray matter, and cortex with neuronal dysmorphism and cytomegaly. Seizure freedom has been present for the 6 years since the hemispherectomy, and neurologic development has improved to include greater interaction and activity in the context of the global developmental abnormality.

J. M. Stern, N. Salamon, *Imaging of Epilepsy*, https://doi.org/10.1007/978-3-030-86672-3_77

Imaging

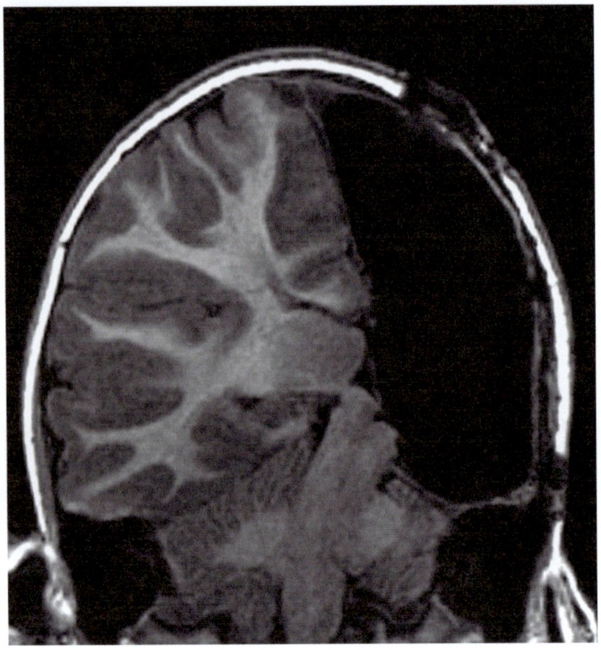

Fig. 77.1 MRI coronal T1 sequence at a posterior thalamus level. A large cavity has been produced by resection of the entire left cerebral hemisphere. Because of the resection, the brainstem and interhemispheric fissure are deviating leftward. The homogeneous signal within the cavity indicates only cerebrospinal fluid (CSF). The right cerebral hemisphere and the cerebellum are normal

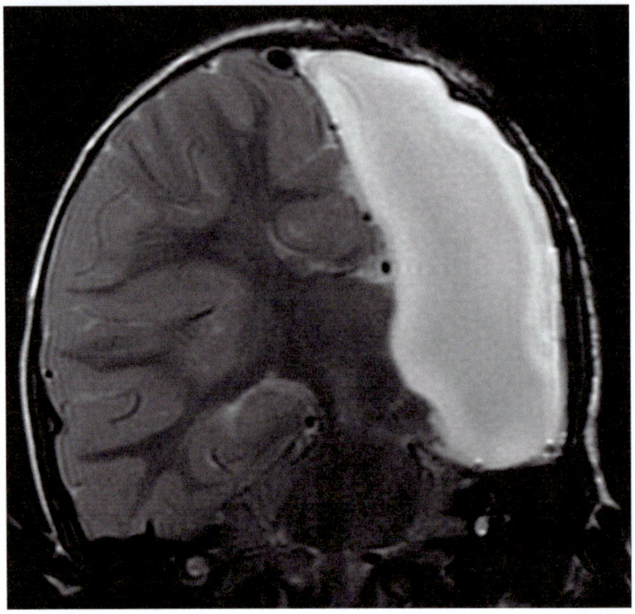

Fig. 77.3 MRI coronal T2 sequence at a thalamus level slightly anterior to Fig. 77.1. The left-sided resection cavity comprises the entire left cerebral hemisphere including the left thalamus and basal ganglia. The right cerebral hemisphere is normal, but its central structures protrude leftward and into the cavity

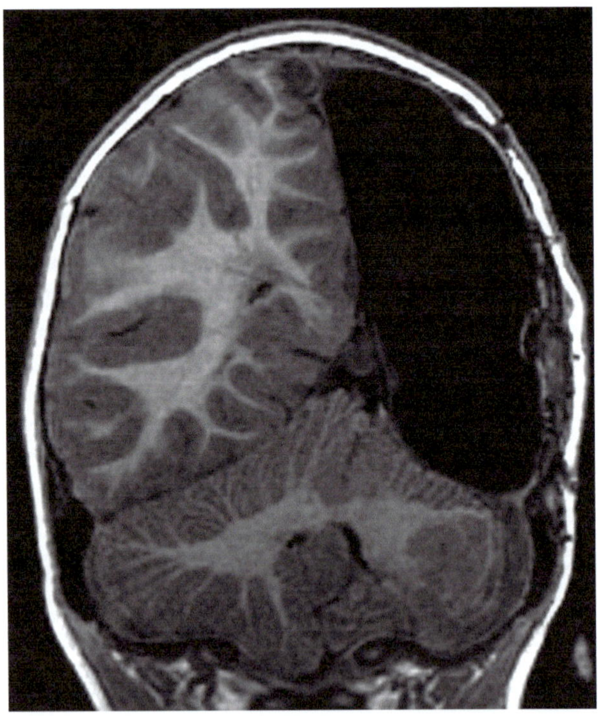

Fig. 77.2 MRI coronal T1 sequence at an occipital horn level. A large cavity has been produced by resection of the entire left cerebral hemisphere. The cerebellum is intact, but the left cerebellar hemisphere's gray matter is abnormal and is evident within the white matter, indicating cerebellar dysplasia. The right cerebral and cerebellar hemispheres are normal

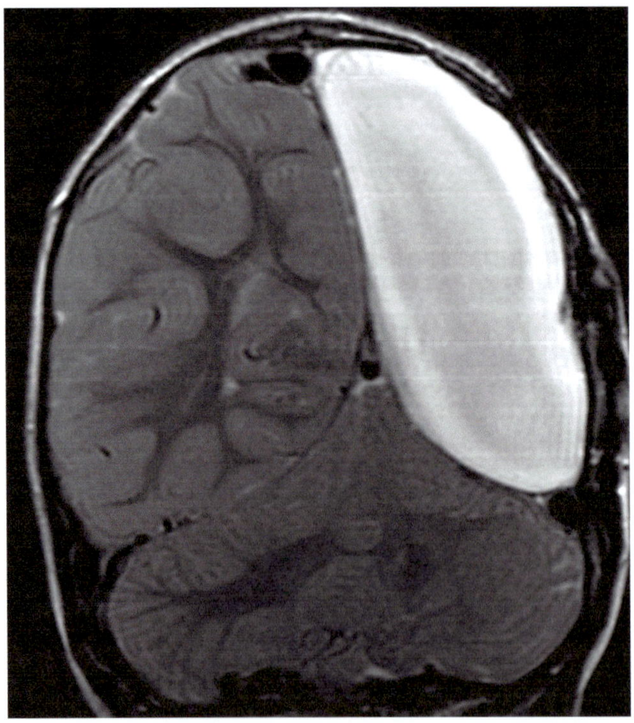

Fig. 77.4 MRI coronal T2 sequence at the same occipital horn level as Fig. 77.2. The left-sided resection cavity is evident as homogeneous signal indicating CSF. The left cerebellar hemisphere contains dysplastic tissue in the white matter. The right cerebral and right cerebellar hemispheres are normal

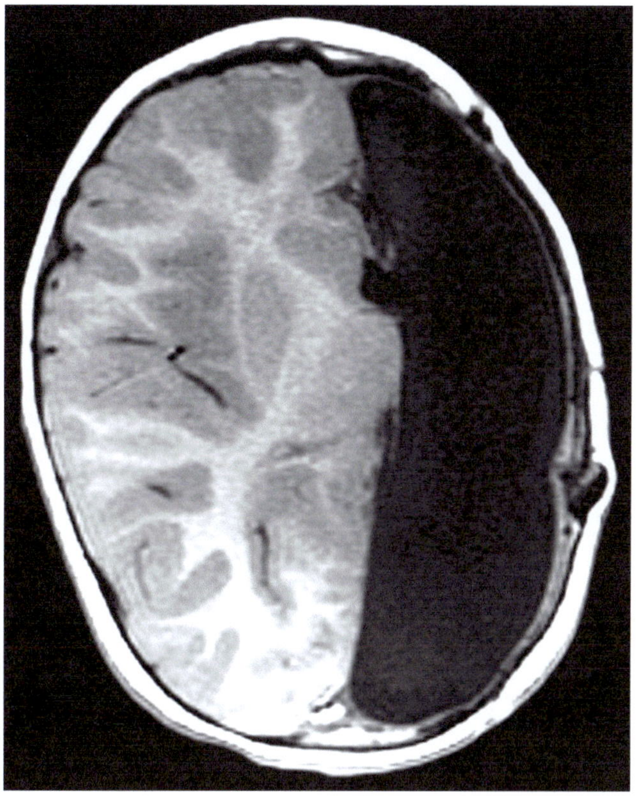

Fig. 77.5 MRI axial T1 sequence at a thalamus level. The entire left cerebral hemisphere has been resected, and the cavity's homogeneous signal indicates CSF. The right hemisphere's central structures have mild leftward shift with compensatory hypertrophy of right hemisphere. The right hemisphere is normal, and hydrocephalus is not evident

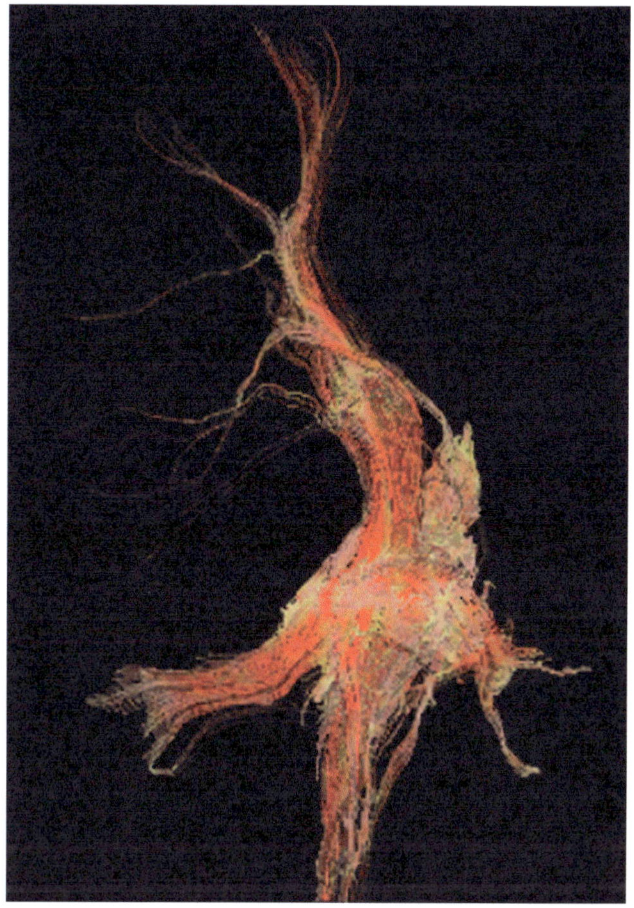

Fig. 77.6 MRI diffusion tensor imaging tractography with a coronal view. The left cerebrum's white matter tracts are absent, and the left cerebellum's white matter tracts are reduced. The white matter tracts in the right cerebrum are normal

Complete Corpus Callosotomy

78

Clinical History

The first recognized seizures occurred at age 2 months as infantile spasms. An evaluation at that time included video-EEG monitoring that identified a left hemispheric seizure onset. At that time, treatment included multiple anti-seizure medications and a ketogenic diet with a seizure frequency of one monthly.

The habitual seizures developed at age 9 years and occurred as two manifestations. Some seizures manifested as staring with unresponsiveness followed by a laugh, gaze deviation upward and leftward, and then followed by rightward gaze with tachypnea and tachycardia. The seizures had durations of several minutes. Other seizures manifested as bilateral tonic posturing with sudden falling and then hypotonia. Treatment included additional anti-seizure medications and a vagus nerve stimulator with a seizure frequency of eight daily.

The epilepsy risk factor was tuberous sclerosis.

Neurological examination identified marked developmental delay. Verbal communication and walking were not present until approximately age 7 years. At age 11 years, verbal expression was limited to several words and walking required assistance. Medical history included a cardiac rhabdomyoma identified at age 6 months and treated surgically.

Interictal EEG depicted abnormal, generalized slowing that was asymmetrically greater on the left, multifocal, independent epileptiform discharges with greater prominence on the left, and generalized paroxysmal fast activity during sleep with left-sided predominance. Video-EEG monitoring recorded seizures manifested as staring episodes and independently occurring episodes of epileptic myoclonus. Ictal EEG's seizure onset did not identify a focal epileptiform abnormality.

MRI identified multiple subcortical tubers and subependymal nodules. PET identified multiple regions of hypometabolism within the left prefrontal cortex and the right parietal-occipital cortex.

The history and evaluation indicate generalized epilepsy with atypical absence seizures and tonic seizures. Because of the generalized abnormality and failure of multiple treatments, an anterior corpus callosotomy was performed. Seizure control improved postoperatively for several months but then returned to the preoperative frequency and severity. Because of the initial improvement after the anterior callosotomy and the low risk of a clinically significant disconnection syndrome in the context of marked developmental delay, the callosotomy was then extended to be a complete transection. Unfortunately, seizure control did not improve. Video-EEG monitoring after the complete corpus callosotomy identified seizure onsets within the left frontal-temporal region.

J. M. Stern, N. Salamon, *Imaging of Epilepsy*, https://doi.org/10.1007/978-3-030-86672-3_78

Imaging

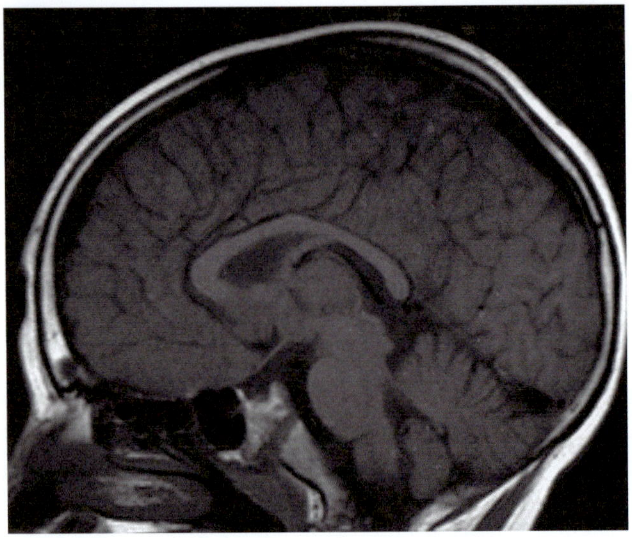

Fig. 78.1 MRI sagittal T1 sequence at a midline level. The image was obtained before a corpus callosotomy, and a normal corpus callosum is present. The cerebrum, cerebellum, and brainstem also are normal

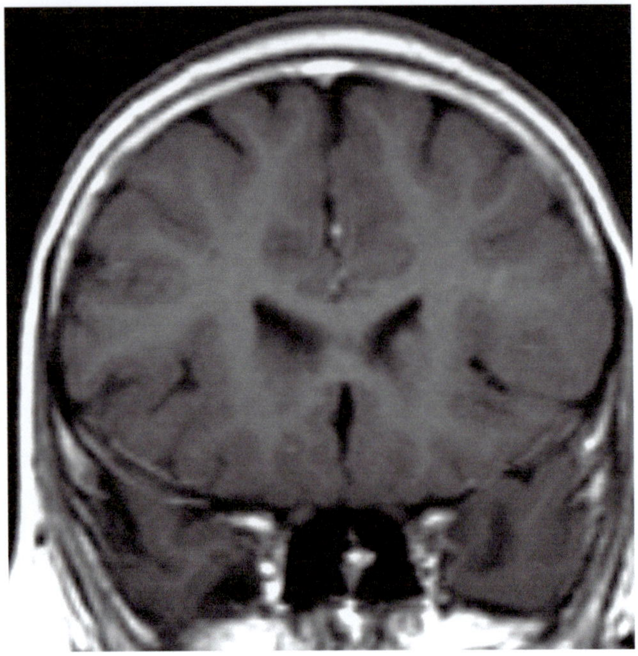

Fig. 78.3 MRI coronal T1 sequence at a genu of the corpus callosum level. The image was obtained before the anterior corpus callosotomy, and a normal corpus callosum is present. The lateral ventricles are normal. The curvilinear hypointensity in left temporal lobe is a tuber. No other abnormality is present

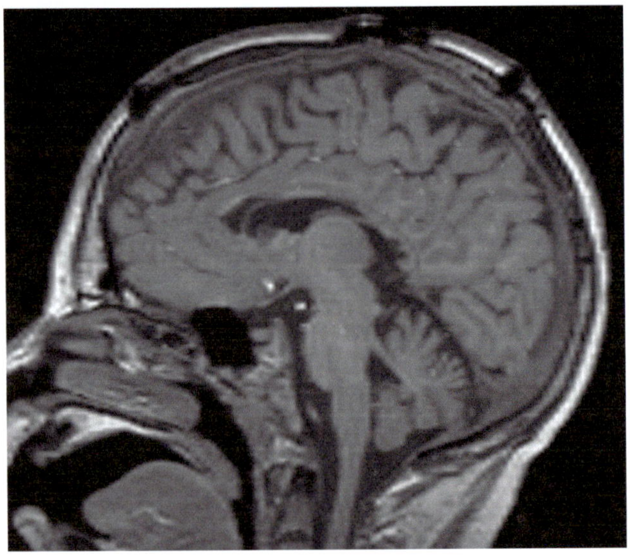

Fig. 78.2 MRI sagittal T1 sequence at the same midline level as Fig. 78.1. The image was obtained after a completion of the corpus callosotomy. Postsurgical hypointensity is evident within the corpus callosum from the genu to the splenium, indicating disconnection across this region. The two craniotomy locations are evident with skull changes. The remainder of the brain is normal.

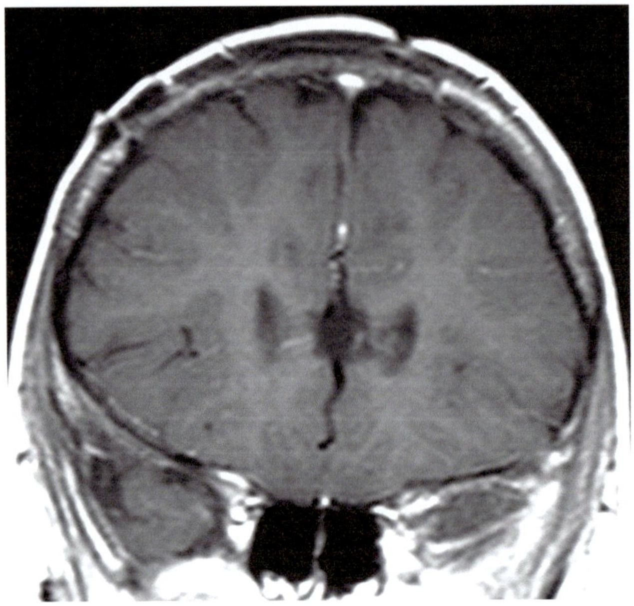

Fig. 78.4 MRI coronal T1 sequence at a genu of the corpus callosum sum level that is slightly anterior to Fig. 78.3. The image was obtained after the completion of the corpus callosotomy. A resection cavity is evident in the genu of the corpus callosum. Bifrontal craniotomy changes are present

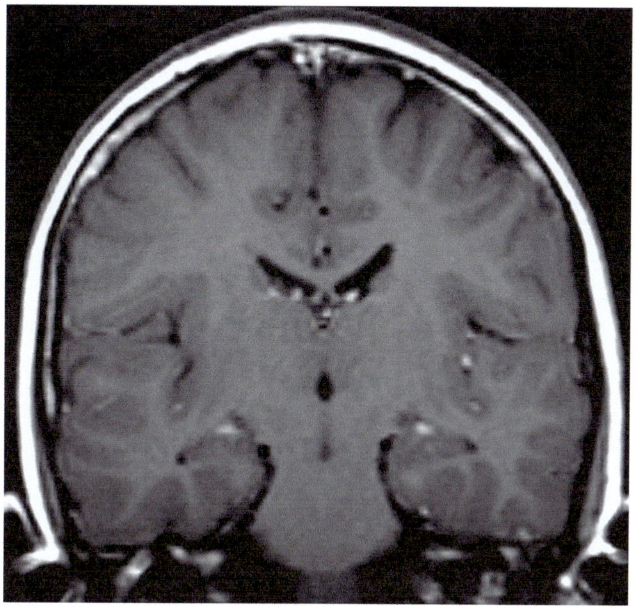

Fig. 78.5 MRI coronal T1 sequence at a body of the hippocampus level. The image was obtained before a corpus callosotomy. The body of the corpus callosum is normal. Three hyperintense subependymal nodules are projecting into the lateral ventricles with two on the right and one on the left. The ventricles are otherwise normal, and no other brain abnormality is evident.

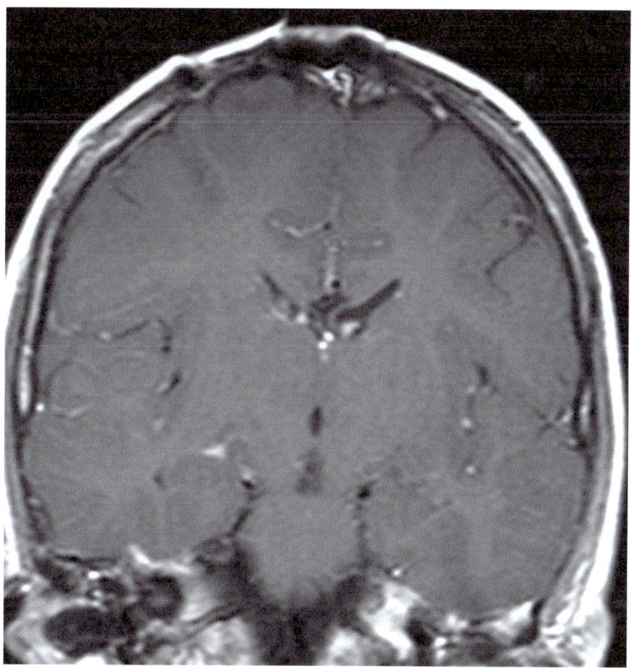

Fig. 78.6 MRI coronal T1 sequence at the same body of the hippocampus level as Fig. 78.5. The image was obtained after the completion of the corpus callosotomy, and a resection cavity is evident in the central portion of the body of the corpus callosum. The periventricular subependymal nodules are visible. The ventricles are otherwise normal

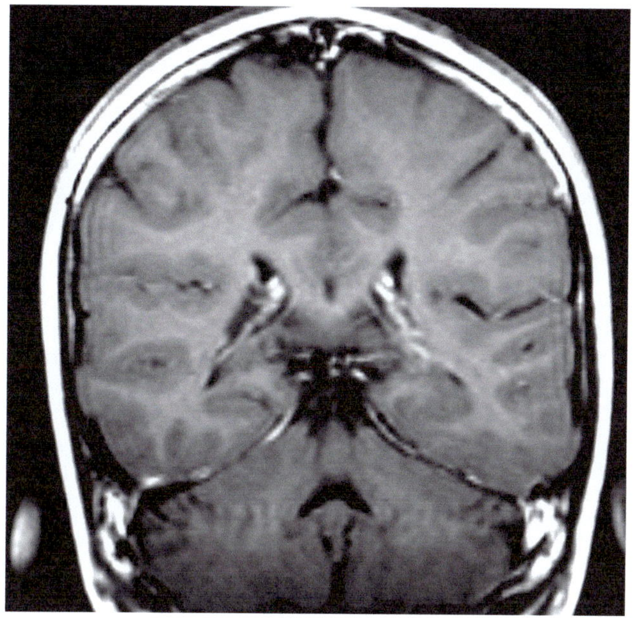

Fig. 78.7 MRI coronal T1 sequence at a splenium of the corpus callosum level. The splenium of the corpus callosum is normal. Two subependymal nodules are visible along the lateral margin of the right lateral ventricle. No other abnormality is present

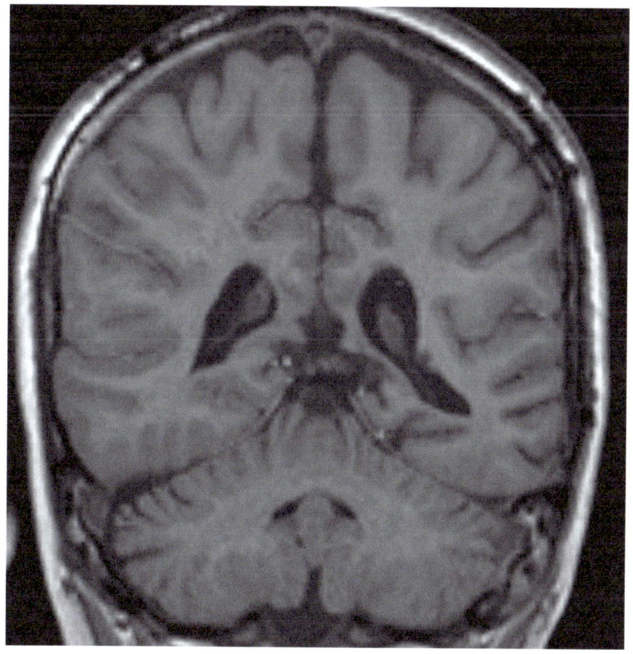

Fig. 78.8 MRI coronal T1 sequence at a splenium of the corpus callosum level similar to Fig. 78.7. A resection cavity is evident in the central portion of the splenium of the corpus callosum. The enlargement of the ventricles is related to overall brain atrophy compared to Fig. 78.7

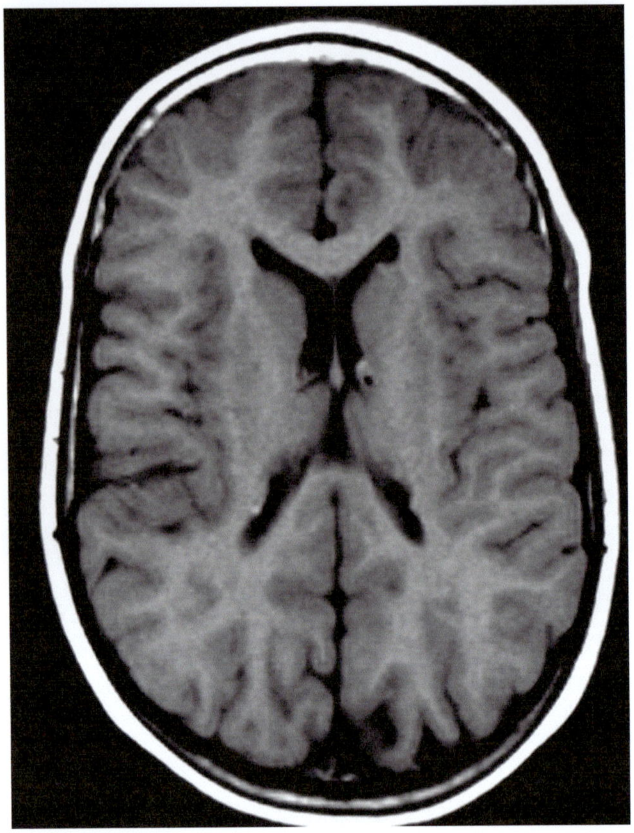

Fig. 78.9 MRI axial T1 sequence at a basal ganglia level. The image was obtained before a corpus callosotomy. The genu and splenium of the corpus callosum are normal. Subependymal nodules are evident along the posterior aspects of bilateral lateral ventricles. No other abnormality is present

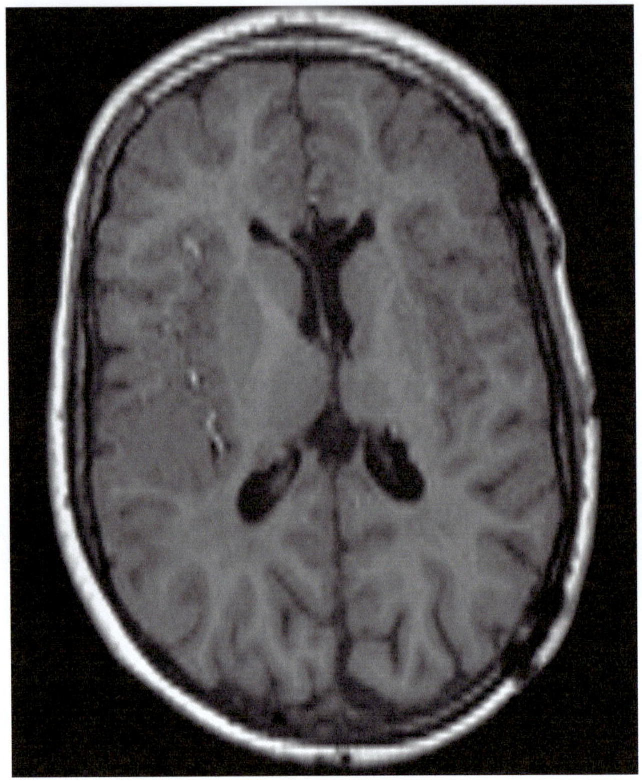

Fig. 78.10 MRI axial T1 sequence at a similar basal ganglia level as Fig. 78.9. Hypointensity indicating a resection cavity is evident in the genu and the splenium of the corpus callosum. The lateral ventricles are normal, and no other cerebral abnormality is evident

Anterior Corpus Callosotomy

79

Clinical History

The first recognized seizure occurred at age 8 years. The initial seizures were movements of the left arm that were diagnosed as tics until an episode progressed to left arm stiffening with leftward head turning. The episodes lasted 1 minute and did not include impaired awareness. An evaluation at that time included a brain MRI that identified bilateral cerebral encephalomalacia.

With diagnosis, treatment with anti-seizure medication began. Multiple anti-seizure medications and the vagus nerve stimulator were subsequently tried without success. Many seizures occurred daily.

The epilepsy risk factor was an intrauterine infarction of bilateral middle cerebral artery territories.

At age 9 years, video-EEG monitoring with scalp electrodes identified right frontal lobe seizure onsets. A subsequent video-EEG monitoring with subdural grid electrodes across the right frontal lobe provided additional mapping and led to a right frontal lobe resection. This reduced the seizure frequency to four weekly.

At age 12 years, the habitual seizures changed to become eyelid fluttering with gaze deviation upward, bilateral flexing of the arms, turning to the right, and tonic posturing of the legs. A fall resulted when a seizure occurred while standing. For most seizures, interaction was maintained, and postictal recall of the ictal period was intact. The seizures had durations ranging from 30 to 90 seconds and typically recurred in clusters with interictal periods of several minutes. Prolonged seizures and clusters produced confusion for approximately 15 seconds. Treatment at this time included multiple anti-seizure medications and a vagus nerve stimulator with a seizure frequency of an unknown number of seizures nightly during sleep and about 15 daily during wakefulness.

Neurological examination identified bilateral pronator drifts and a mild right hemiparesis with weakness and abnormally slowed fine movements of the right hand and circumduction of the right leg while walking. Medical history included normal development during infancy and toddler years. Learning difficulties were identified in preschool, and reading level was 3 years behind grade level.

Interictal EEG depicted symmetric, abnormal slowing and interictal epileptiform discharges broadly across the left temporal and right frontal regions. Video-EEG monitoring recorded seizures manifested as head dropping and generalized tonus for 10 seconds. Ictal EEG's seizure onset was across the parasagittal frontal lobes.

MRI identified volume loss of the right angular gyrus and left frontal-parietal operculum along with the postoperative changes related to the right frontal lobe resection. PET identified hypometabolism in the region of the right frontal lobe resection.

The history and evaluation indicate rapidly propagating motor seizures without lateralization and occurring in the context of congenital, bilateral frontal lobe structural abnormalities. The unilateral resection provided temporary benefit that was ultimately insufficient. Because of the evidence of a bihemispheric abnormality, an anterior corpus callosotomy was performed for additional palliative benefit with the goal of reducing the severity of the seizures and the injuries.

The anterior corpus callosotomy was performed at age 13 years. For the 2 years after the surgery, the frequency of the generalized motor seizures associated with falling decreased to about one daily. The improvement relates to the diminished propagation, and the more commonly occurring seizure is now focal motor without impaired awareness or change to tone with durations of 15 seconds and a frequency of about 30 occurrences daily.

J. M. Stern, N. Salamon, *Imaging of Epilepsy*, https://doi.org/10.1007/978-3-030-86672-3_79

Imaging

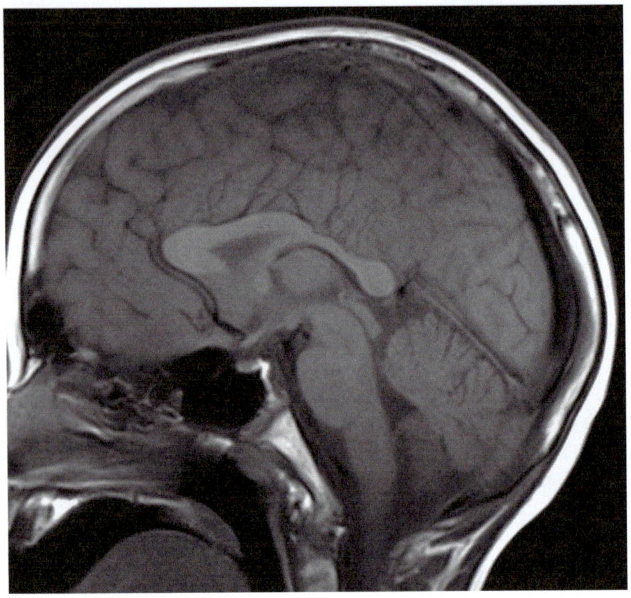

Fig. 79.1 MRI sagittal T1 sequence at a midline level obtained preoperatively. The corpus callosum is normal including the finding of thinning of its posterior body. The remainder of the brain also is normal

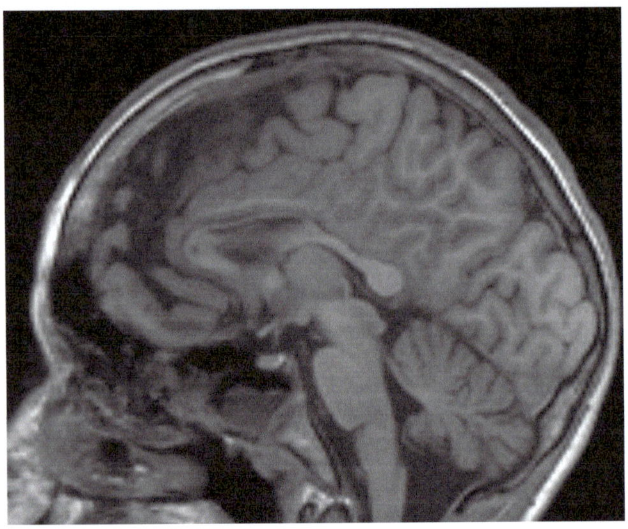

Fig. 79.2 MRI sagittal T1 sequence at a midline level obtained postoperatively. A linear resection cavity is evident in the corpus callosum's genu and anterior body. The frontal lobe changes, compared to Fig. 79.1, are due to widening of interhemispheric fissure and volume averaging

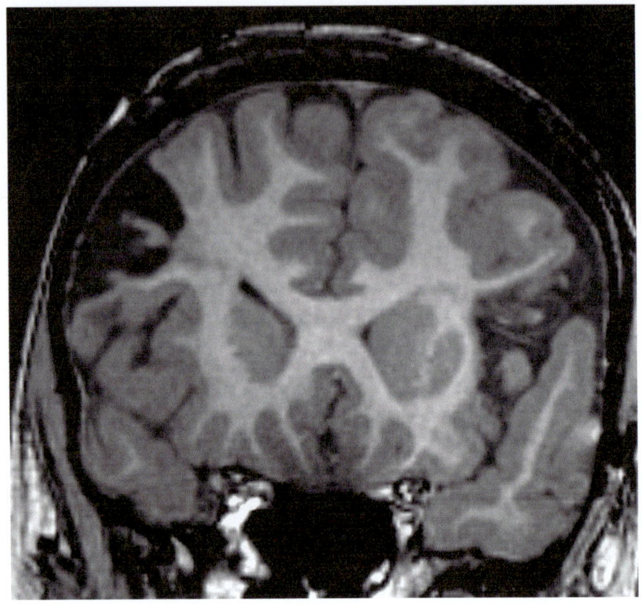

Fig. 79.3 MRI coronal T1 sequence at a genu of the corpus callosum level obtained preoperatively. The genu of the corpus callosum and the adjoining lateral ventricles are normal. Encephalomalacia of bilateral inferior frontal gyri is evident. The temporal lobes are normal

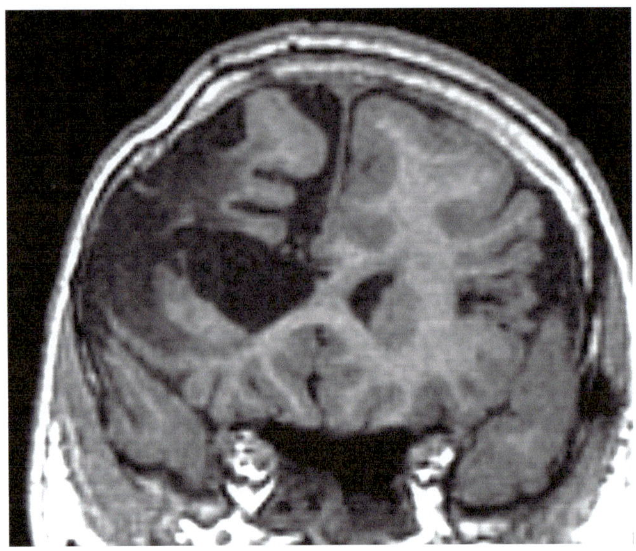

Fig. 79.4 MRI coronal T1 sequence at a genu of the corpus callosum level obtained postoperatively. A resection cavity is evident in the genu of the corpus callosum. The right lateral ventricle and the sulci of the right frontal lobe are markedly enlarged with associated, extensive encephalomalacia and gliosis of the right frontal lobe. The encephalomalacia of the left frontal lobe is unchanged

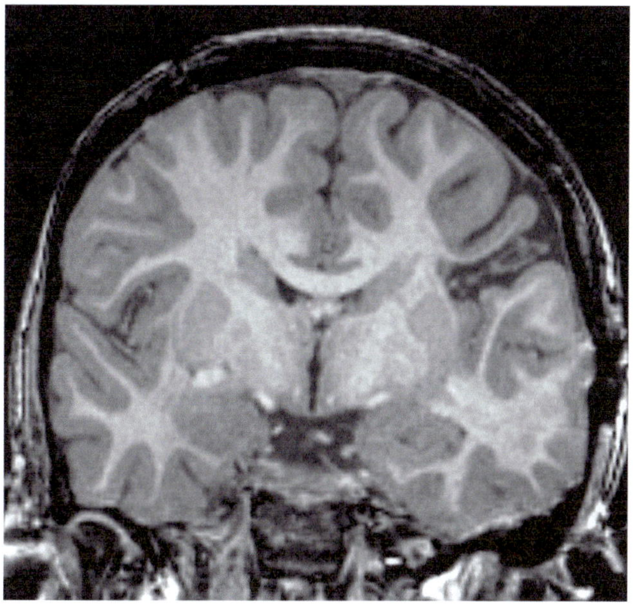

Fig. 79.5 MRI coronal T1 sequence at an anterior third ventricle level obtained preoperatively. The body of the corpus callosum is normal. Encephalomalacia of the left inferior frontal gyrus and the left insula is evident. The right hemisphere is normal

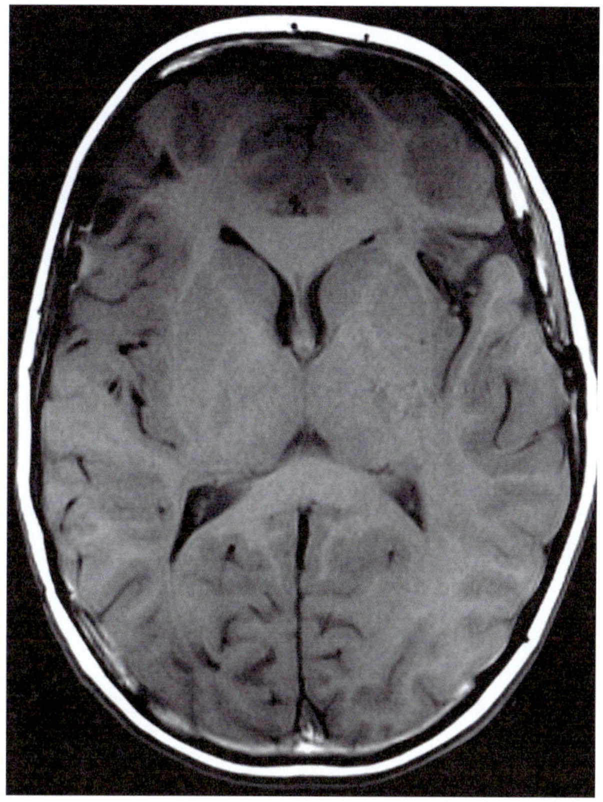

Fig. 79.7 MRI axial T1 sequence at a basal ganglia and thalamus level obtained preoperatively. The corpus callosum and lateral ventricles are normal. Encephalomalacia of bilateral inferior frontal gyri is evident

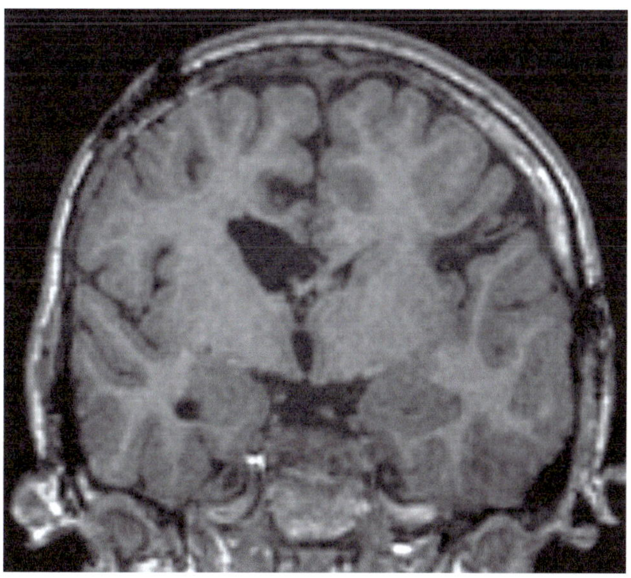

Fig. 79.6 MRI coronal T1 sequence at an anterior third ventricle level obtained postoperatively. A resection cavity is evident in the body of the corpus callosum with an associated enlarged right lateral ventricle. The remainder of the right hemisphere is normal. The left inferior frontal gyrus encephalomalacia is unchanged

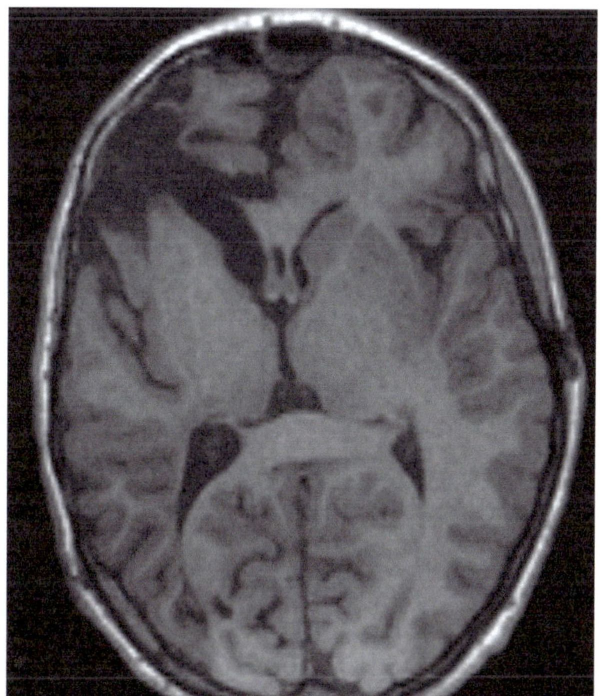

Fig. 79.8 MRI axial T1 sequence at a basal ganglia and thalamus level obtained postoperatively. The right lateral ventricle is enlarged with associated encephalomalacia or the right cingulate gyrus and lateral frontal lobe. The right side of the genu has been resected, but the central portion is not transected at this inferior level. The splenium of the corpus callosum is normal

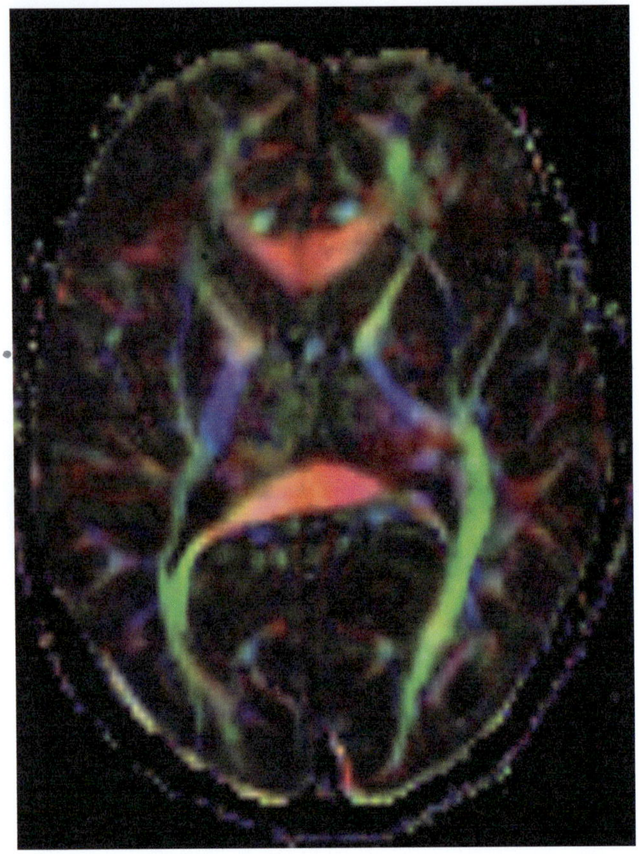

Fig. 79.9 MRI with axial diffusion tensor imaging obtained preoperatively at the same basal ganglia and thalamus level as Figs. 79.7 and 79.8. The white matter of the corpus callosum is normal. A subtle, abnormal decrease of the white matter in the right frontal lobe is evident as an asymmetry compared to the left frontal lobe

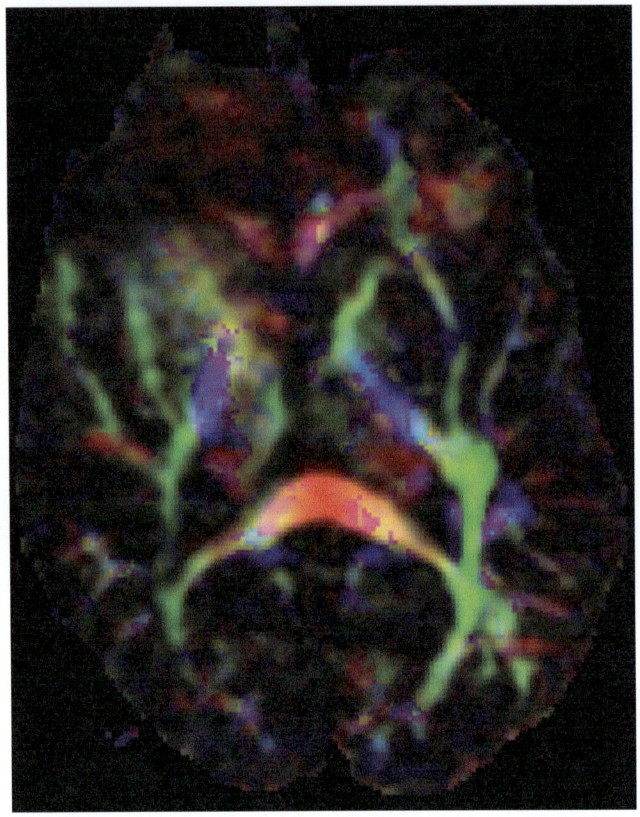

Fig. 79.10 MRI with axial diffusion tensor imaging obtained postoperatively at the same basal ganglia and thalamus level as Figs. 79.7 to 79.9. The white matter within the splenium of the corpus callosum is normal. The signal intensity within the genu of the corpus callosum is decreased compared to the preoperative image. The frontal lobe white matter is asymmetric with an abnormal decrease within the right frontal lobe

Stereotactic Thermal Ablation - Hypothalamic Hamartoma

80

Clinical History

The first recognized seizure occurred at age 3 months as unusual laughter. The evaluation at that time included a brain MRI that identified a hypothalamic hamartoma. MRI over the subsequent years demonstrated no change.

The habitual seizures during childhood manifested without an aura as laughter for about 5 seconds and occurred twice daily for many years before decreasing at age 9 years to once weekly. The frequency increased during adolescence and was once daily by age 14 years and twice daily by age 16 years. At 16 years, the seizure manifestation changed to include impaired awareness and several seconds of postictal confusion. This led to beginning anti-seizure medication and treatment produced a decrease in frequency to once weekly, but the seizures continued to impair awareness. At the time of the evaluation, the seizures manifested as laughter for 10–20 seconds either in isolation or followed by impaired awareness, slumping, or falling. Treatment included multiple anti-seizure medications with a frequency of seizures of laughter in isolation five times daily, seizures with impaired awareness three times weekly, and seizures with falls several times monthly.

The epilepsy risk factor was a hypothalamic hamartoma.

Neurological examination was normal.

Interictal EEG depicted normal activity. Video-EEG monitoring recorded focal seizures manifested as smiling and gesturing to indicate that a seizure is occurring. Some seizures progressed to non-responsiveness with right hand and oral automatisms for 1 minute. Ictal EEG's seizure onset was diffuse rhythmic slowing.

MRI identified a hypothalamic hamartoma with an 11-mm diameter and extension into the suprasellar cistern and third ventricle with displacement of the mammillary bodies.

The history and evaluation indicate gelastic epilepsy with an evident hypothalamic hamartoma. The increasing epilepsy burden with seizures that produced impairment and falls led to the evaluation that confirmed the diagnosis. In the context of the hypothalamic hamartoma, the confirmation of the seizure manifestation can be sufficient, as the EEG is often less informative.

A laser ablation of the hamartoma was performed. Seizure control was complete for 2 months after the ablation when a single seizure occurred, and this seizure is the only seizure after the ablation. Anti-seizure medications were continued for 2 years after the ablation and then were individually tapered. Seizure freedom has continued and has been present for the 6 months since anti-seizure medications were discontinued.

J. M. Stern, N. Salamon, *Imaging of Epilepsy*, https://doi.org/10.1007/978-3-030-86672-3_80

Imaging

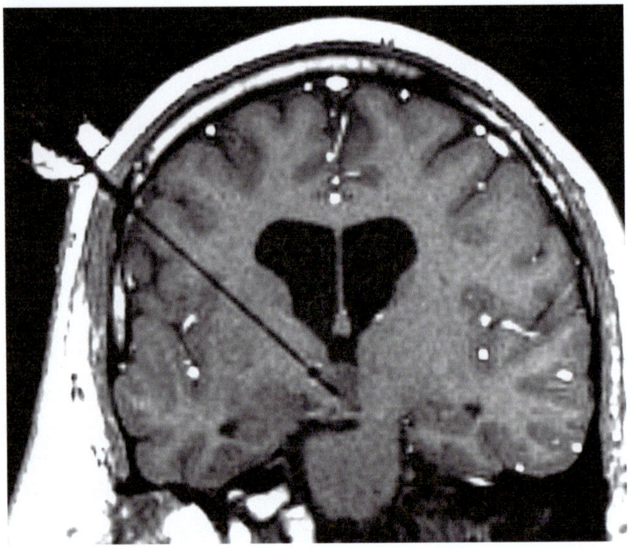

Fig. 80.1 MRI coronal T1 sequence at a hippocampus body level. The laser probe was placed stereotactically through the right frontal operculum with the tip at the center of the hypothalamic hamartoma. The hypointensity around the probe immediately lateral to the hamartoma is air artifact. The hamartoma is projecting into the third ventricle

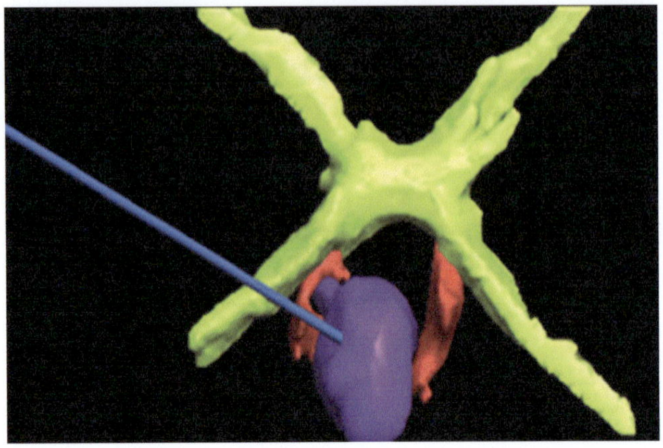

Fig. 80.3 MRI tractography from diffusion tensor imaging with processing to visualize structures. The optic chiasm is green, the hypothalamic hamartoma is purple, and the fornices are red. The tip of the probe, in blue, is within the hamartoma

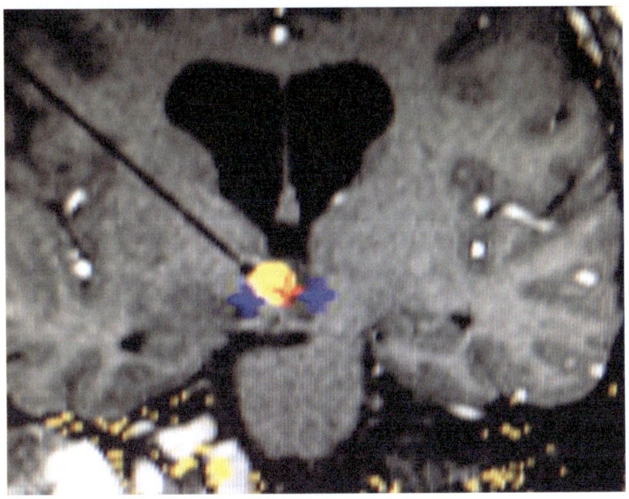

Fig. 80.2 MRI coronal phase contrast sequence at the same hippocampus body level as Fig. 80.1. Imaging is continuous during the procedure, so blood flow produces hyperintense signal within the vessels. The red cross indicates the laser at the probe's tip, and the yellow is MR thermography indicating the region of heating. The two blue crosses indicate safety points that are monitored for maximum acceptable heating for protection of the two fornices. The right fornix has been displaced by the hamartoma

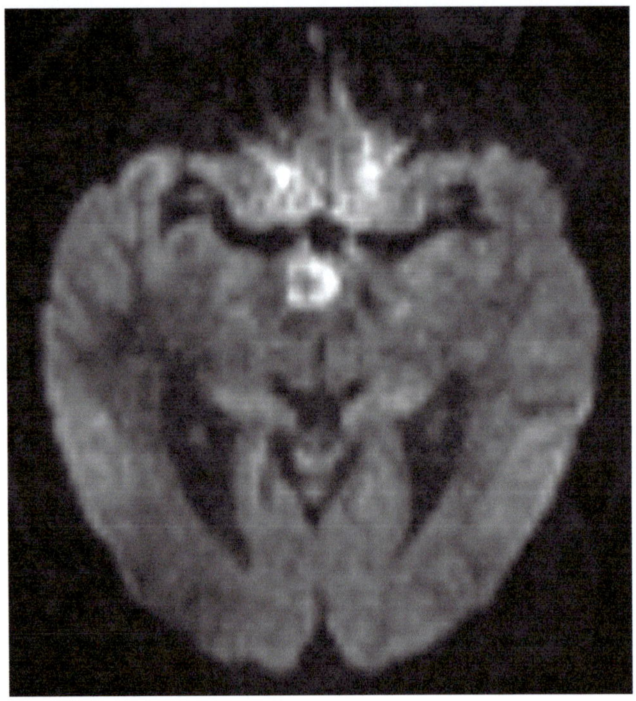

Fig. 80.4 MRI axial diffusion-weighted imaging sequence at the same midbrain level and obtained immediately after the ablation. Hyperintensity at the margins of the ablation indicates restricted diffusion. The hyperintensity in the anterior region is artifact from the paranasal sinus

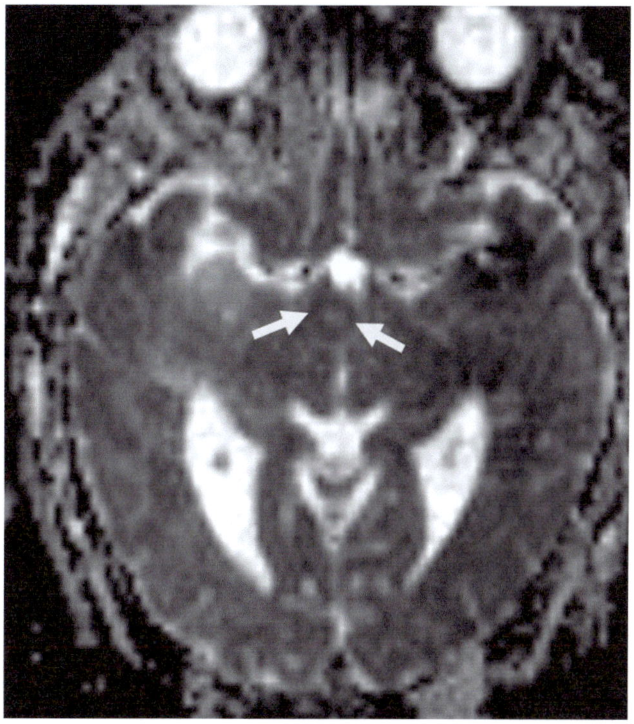

Fig. 80.5 MRI axial apparent diffusion coefficient map at a midbrain level slightly superior to Fig. 80.4 and obtained immediately after the ablation. A faint hypointense ring surrounds the ablation zone (arrows). Round hyperintensity anterior to the ablations in the third ventricle. Hypointensity of anterior medial left temporal poles is susceptibility artifact

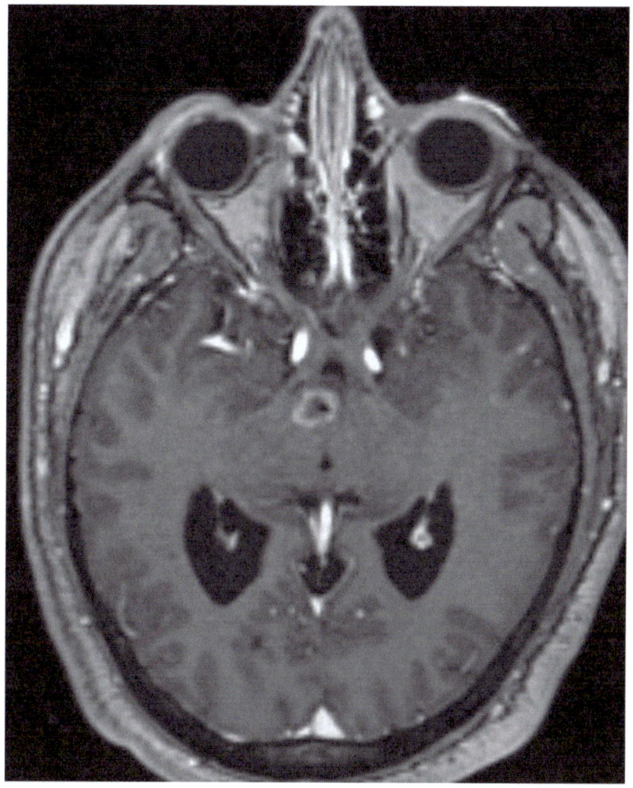

Fig. 80.7 MRI axial T1 sequence after contrast administration at a midbrain level inferior to Figs. 80.4 to 80.6 and obtained after the ablation. An enhancing ring indicates the ablation zone. The hypointensity within a portion of the ablation zone is susceptibility artifact from the probe's tip that was in place at the time of imaging

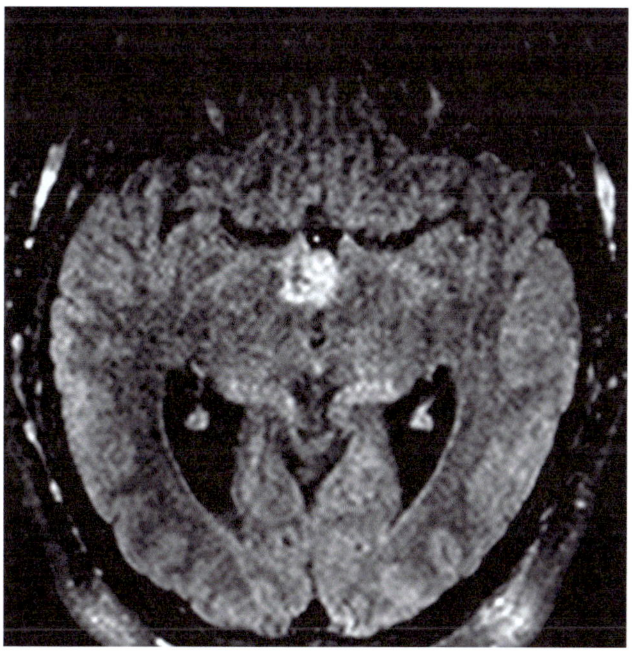

Fig. 80.6 MRI axial FLAIR sequence at the same midbrain level as Fig. 80.5 and obtained immediately after the ablation. Hyperintensity within hypothalamic hamartoma corresponds to the ablation. No edema is adjacent to the ablation

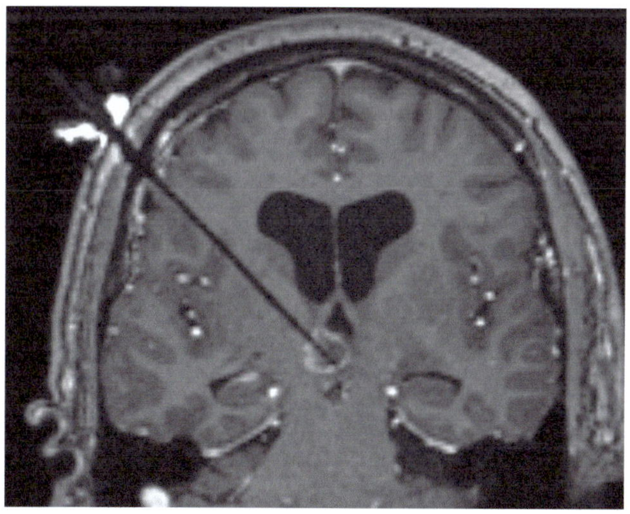

Fig. 80.8 MRI coronal T1 sequence after contrast administration at the same hippocampus body level as Figs. 80.1 and 80.2 and obtained after the ablation. The laser probe remains in place after the ablation. An enhancing rim at the probe's tip corresponds to the margins of the ablation zone

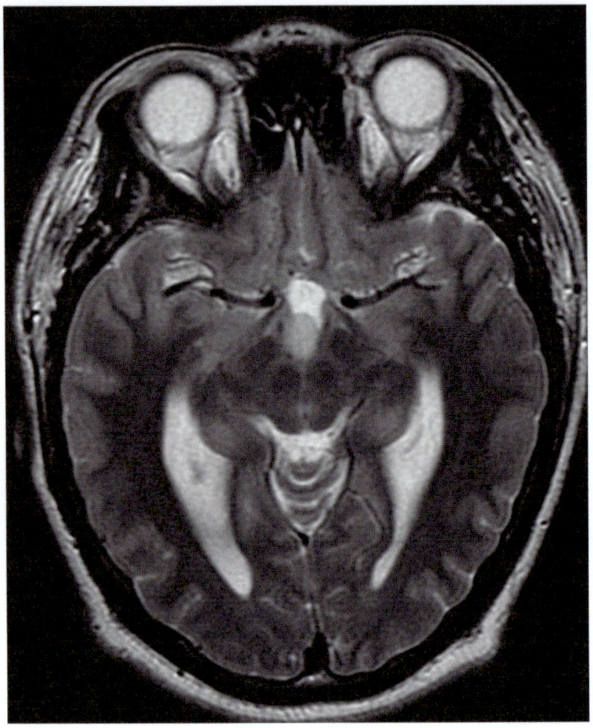

Fig. 80.9 MRI axial T2 sequence at a similar midbrain level as Fig. 80.5 and obtained before the ablation. A round hyperintense lesion is evident in the interpeduncular cistern and within the tuber cinereum. The lesion produces a minor displacement of the right cerebral peduncle. The cerebrospinal fluid (CSF) space anterior to the lesion is normal, and no signal abnormality is present posterior to the lesion in the midbrain

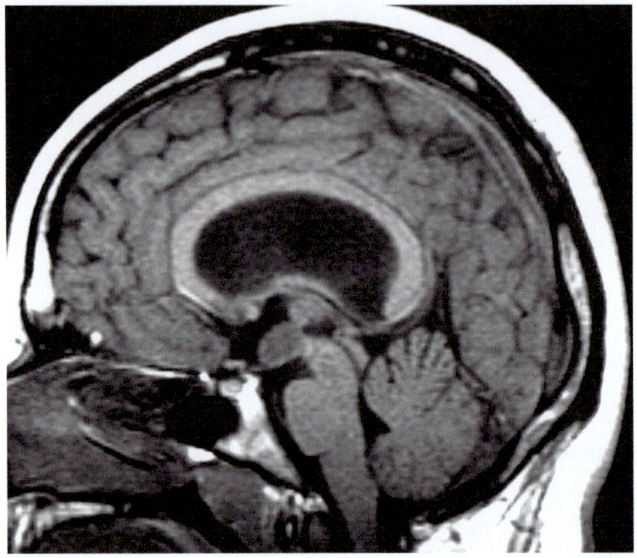

Fig. 80.11 MRI sagittal T1 sequence at a midline level and obtained before the ablation. A hypointense mass is evident in the tuber cinereum and protruding into the third ventricle. The lateral ventricle is enlarged and compressing the corpus callosum, which is an atypical finding with hypothalamic hamartomas

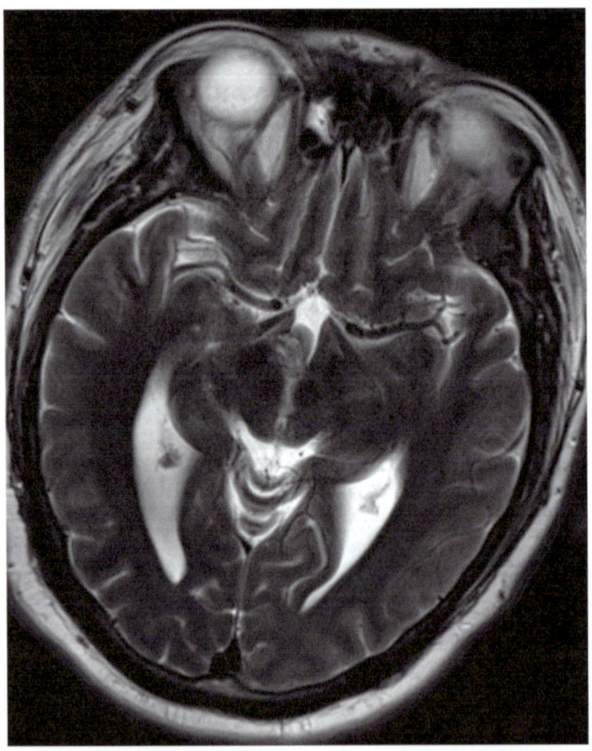

Fig. 80.10 MRI axial T2 sequence at a similar midbrain level as Fig. 80.9 and obtained 3 months after ablation. The ablation effect is evident as a reduction in the hamartoma's volume and a change to its signal characteristics. The signal within the hamartoma is decreased and more heterogeneous. The midbrain is otherwise normal

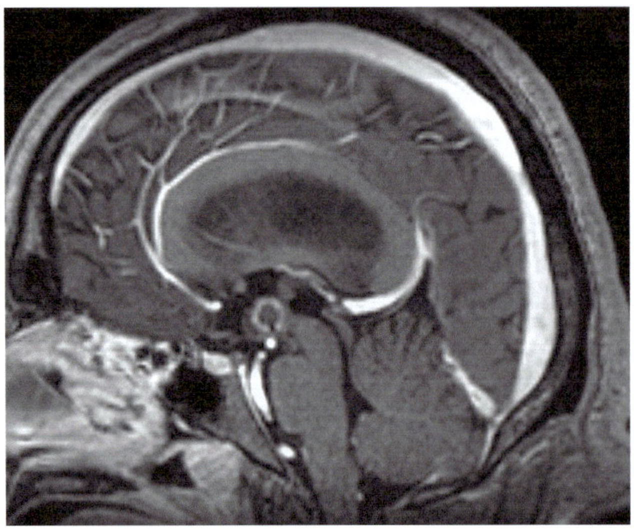

Fig. 80.12 MRI sagittal T1 sequence at a midline level after contrast administration and obtained after the ablation. An enhancing ring is evident at the location of the hypothalamic hematoma. No other abnormal enhancing is present

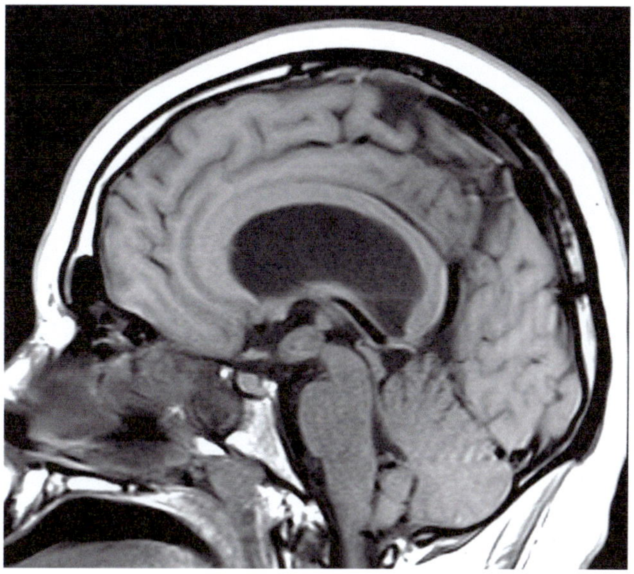

Fig. 80.13 MRI sagittal T1 sequence at a midline level and obtained 3 months after the ablation. The hypothalamic hamartoma's volume has decreased over the interval. The lateral ventricle is unchanged. No other abnormality is present

Stereotactic Thermal Ablation – Heterotopia

81

Clinical History

The first recognized seizure occurred at age 7 years as a sudden blackening of vision that recurred over months with each occurrence lasting several minutes and some including forced gaze to the right.

The subsequent habitual seizures manifested as either (1) a flash of light in the right visual field followed by a loss of vision for several seconds; (2) a dimming of central vision that expands outward and is associated with anxiety, amnesia, and repetitive questioning for 30–60 seconds; or (3) a bilateral tonic-clonic seizure. Treatment included multiple anti-seizure medications with focal visual seizures occurring about seven times daily and seizures with impaired awareness and memory occurring about five times monthly. Bilateral tonic-clonic seizures did not occur over the most recent 5 years.

An epilepsy risk factor was not present. Neurological examination was normal, including visual fields as assessed with automated testing.

Interictal EEG depicted intermittent and independent slowing over the temporal regions and the left posterior quadrant, multifocal epileptiform sharp waves across bilateral central and temporal regions and the left occipital region, and epileptiform discharges over the left occipital region during photic stimulation. Video-EEG monitoring recorded focal seizures manifested as right-sided vision changes due to blurring or hallucinations of flashes. Some seizures progressed to unresponsiveness with manual automatisms. Ictal EEG's seizure onset was evolving, rhythmic slowing that was maximal over the left occipital region.

MRI identified small foci of heterotopic gray matter along the ependymal surface of the occipital horns with a greater presence on the left. PET identified small, corresponding regions of hypometabolism along the ependymal surface of the occipital horns. See Chap. 18 in the Cerebral Malformations section for the diagnostic imaging figures.

The seizure experience of right-sided primary visual hallucinations and forced gaze and the ictal EEG's onset both suggest a left occipital epileptogenic region with seizure propagation to the mesial temporal lobes. This is supported by the structural and metabolic abnormality along the left occipital horn, but additional abnormality is present along the right occipital horn and the interictal EEG identifies more diffuse epileptiform abnormality. Based on this evidence, additional diagnostic testing was performed to further assess the localization and the deficit risk of a surgical treatment.

Interictal EEG source analysis localized 90% of the epileptiform discharges to either the left occipital lobe, left posterior parietal lobe, or left inferior-lateral temporal lobe. MEG identified epileptiform dipoles across the left temporal lobe and the left temporal-parietal-occipital junction.

Functional MRI of vision was normal and functional MRI of language identified left hemispheric dominance with the basal temporal naming area close to the heterotopia. Neuropsychological testing identified impairments in verbal and visual episodic memory and in visuospatial perception and reasoning.

The functional assessment provided further support for a left occipital epileptogenic region with likely involvement of the left occipital horn heterotopia. To avoid significant visual field deficits, the surgical treatment was stereotactic laser thermo-ablation. Following this treatment, the focal visual seizures and the seizures with impaired awareness were been reduced to about half of their preoperative frequency. At 1 year after surgery, automated visual field testing demonstrated no change, and neuropsychological testing identified improved visuospatial perception and reasoning.

J. M. Stern, N. Salamon, *Imaging of Epilepsy*, https://doi.org/10.1007/978-3-030-86672-3_81

Imaging

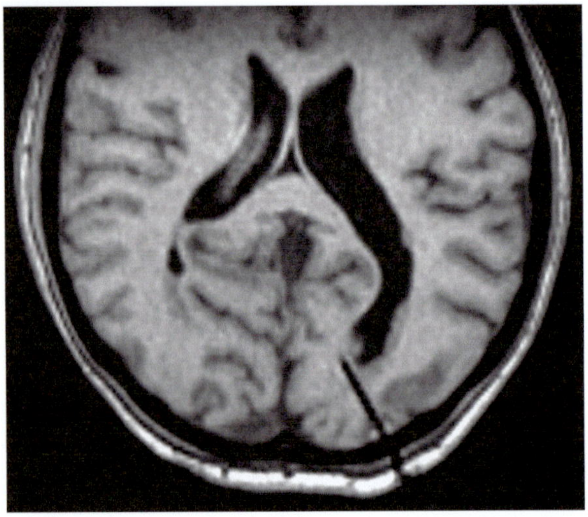

Fig. 81.1 MRI axial T1 sequence at a splenium of the corpus callosum level. The laser probe has been placed in the periventricular heterotopia along the occipital horn of the left lateral ventricle. Multiple additional periventricular heterotopia are evident along the wall of the left lateral ventricle

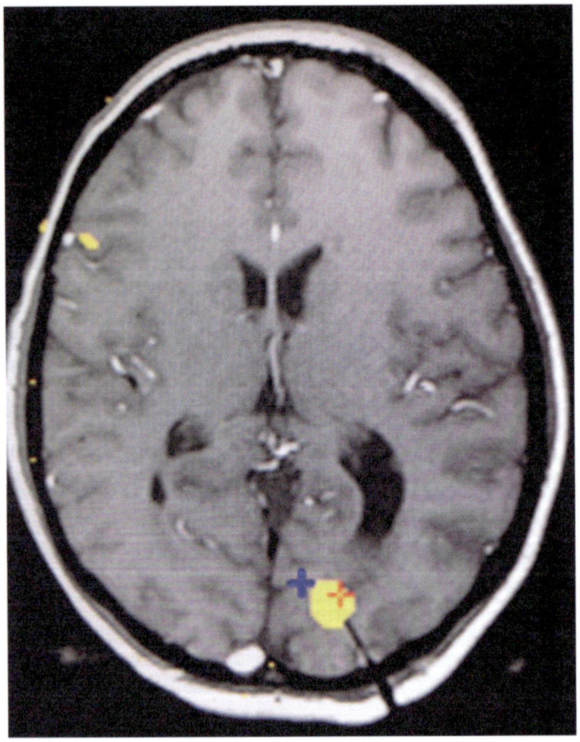

Fig. 81.2 MRI axial T1 sequence with a temperature map at an atrium of the lateral ventricle level that is slightly inferior to the level in Fig. 81.1. The yellow zone at the tip of the laser probe indicates an estimate of the ablation zone based on modeling of the heat transfer from the laser. The red cross within the yellow zone is close to the laser's tip and is the location where the temperature of the targeted tissue will be monitored during the heating. The blue cross at the edge of the yellow zone is a safety margin that was chosen because of proximity to the calcarine cortex, and excessive heating at blue cross will prompt discontinuation of the heating. The yellow signal in the right frontal lobe cortex is artifact, and the scattered hyperintense signal within the vasculature is due to the phase contrast sequence's depiction of blood flow

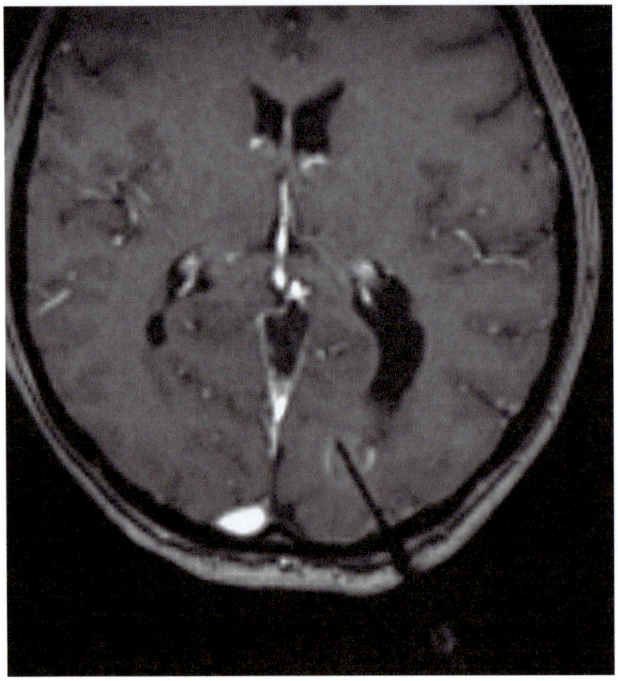

Fig. 81.3 MRI axial T1 sequence after contrast administration at the same atrium of the lateral ventricle level as Fig. 81.2. The image was obtained after thermal ablation. The laser tip's position has not changed, and the enhancing rim around the tip corresponds to the ablation's margins, which were predicted by the modeling and depicted by the yellow zone. No other abnormal enhancement is present

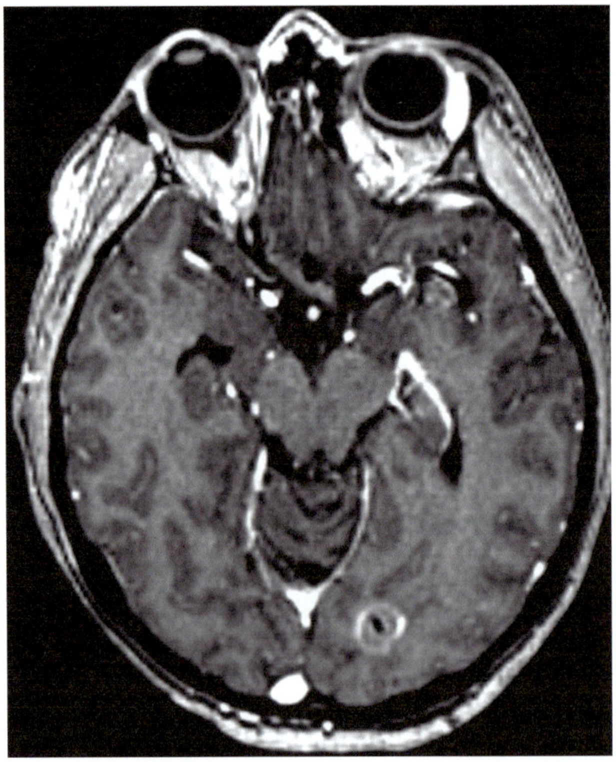

Fig. 81.4 MRI axial T1 sequence after contrast administration at a midbrain level. The image was obtained after thermal ablation. Only the tip of the laser probe is visible in this level, and the enhancing rim around the tip corresponds to the ablation's margins. No other abnormal enhancement is present

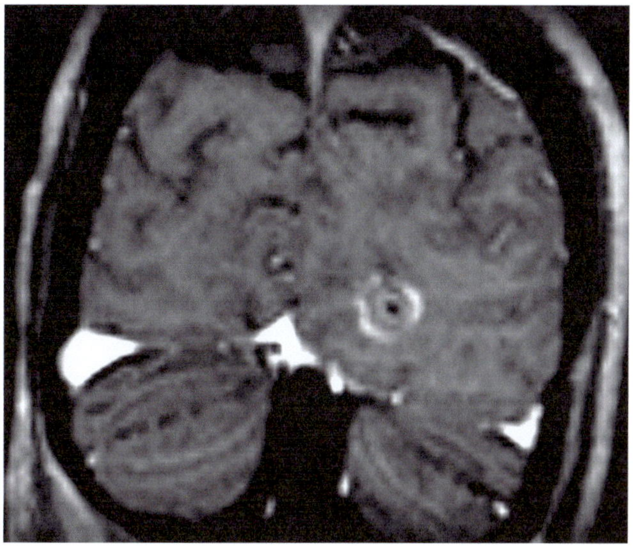

Fig. 81.5 MRI coronal T1 sequence after contrast administration at a level that is posterior to the occipital horn of the lateral ventricle. The laser probe's tip is evident as a hypointense circle, and the enhancing ring around it indicates the margins of the ablation. The circular margins in both the axial and coronal planes indicate the spherical shape of the ablation zone. No other abnormal enhancement is present

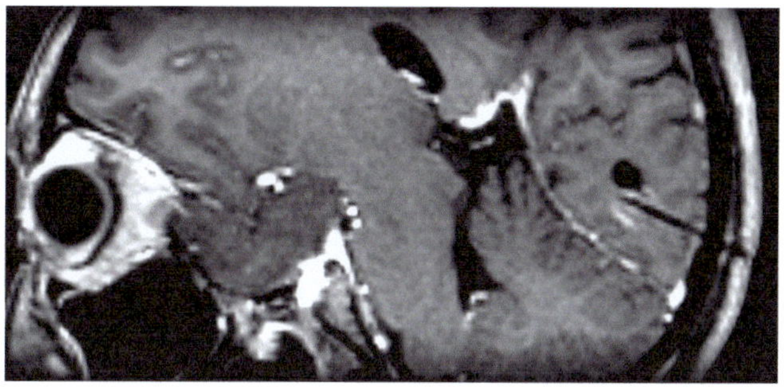

Fig. 81.6 MRI oblique sagittal T1 sequence after contrast administration at a left occipital lobe level. The laser probe's tip has been placed within periventricular heterotopia, and the lateral ventricle's occipital horn is visible immediately superior to the laser probe. The enhancing rim around the probe's tip indicates the ablation's margins. No other abnormal enhancement is present

82 Stereotactic Radiosurgery

Clinical History

The first recognized seizure occurred at age 22 years as a tonic-clonic convulsion. An evaluation at that time identified a left frontal lobe arteriovenous malformation (AVM).

The habitual seizures manifested as bilateral tonic-clonic convulsions that sometimes followed a stereotyped aura described as a heightened awareness of an imminent danger. The aura also occurred in isolation. Focal seizures with impaired awareness were rare and had a pattern of none occurring for years and several occurring within a day. When progressing to bilateral tonic-clonic, the seizures included asymmetric posturing of the arms, but the details of the asymmetry are not known. Treatment included multiple antiseizure medications with a seizure frequency of one bilateral tonic-clonic seizure every 1–3 months and one or a cluster of focal seizures once in several years.

The only epilepsy risk factor was the vascular malformation.

Neurological examination identified word finding and language fluency deficits. The deficit severity fluctuates and was most evident after a seizure. Neuropsychological testing identified borderline performance across multiple domains that suggested a decline from premorbid levels.

Interictal EEG depicted broad left-sided abnormal slowing that was maximal in the central-temporal region and epileptiform discharges over the left frontal and temporal regions. Video-EEG monitoring identified focal seizures manifested as left manual automatisms with clonic movements of the right arm and clonic turning of the head to the right. The ictal EEG's seizure onset was broadly across the left hemisphere with prominence in the left anterior frontal region before extending posteriorly.

MRI and CT identified a large, AVM with the superior frontal gyrus demonstrating the most prominent encephalomalacia. The temporal lobes were not affected. PET identified a large, left frontal, ametabolic region with a margin of hypometabolism. See Chap. 47 in the Vascular Abnormalities section for the diagnostic imaging figures.

The history and evaluation indicate focal seizures with ictal motor behavior that lateralizes the seizures to the left hemisphere and imaging that identifies a large, left, superior frontal lesion. Propagation into the limbic system is a possible explanation for the aura and focal seizures with impairment that do not progress to bilateral tonic-clonic, but an aura of sensing imminent danger is not necessarily limbic. Furthermore, the observed quick progression to asymmetric clonic movements is more suggestive of a neocortical onset and is referrable to the AVM location. Because of the AVM's features, two or more discrete epileptogenic regions may be present, which may explain the focal seizures and further complicates the epileptogenic zone localization.

The size of the AVM precluded complete resection, and the evaluation did not produce a reliable localization of a resectable epileptogenic zone within it. Stereotactic radiosurgery was provided without resultant neurologic deficits. Prior to the radiosurgery, seizures were exclusively bilateral tonic-clonic and occurred once every 3 weeks. One year after the radiosurgery, the seizures no longer progressed to bilateral tonic-clonic, and the frequency decreased to once every 3 months. Seizures at that time followed the same stereotyped aura and manifested as impaired awareness with posturing of the right arm for 30–60 seconds. Several years later, seizure control decreased and was bilateral tonic-clonic seizures with a frequency of one every 1–3 months. Although the residual AVM did not have evident imaging changes, the epilepsy change may still be related to minor hemorrhages.

J. M. Stern, N. Salamon, *Imaging of Epilepsy*, https://doi.org/10.1007/978-3-030-86672-3_82

Imaging

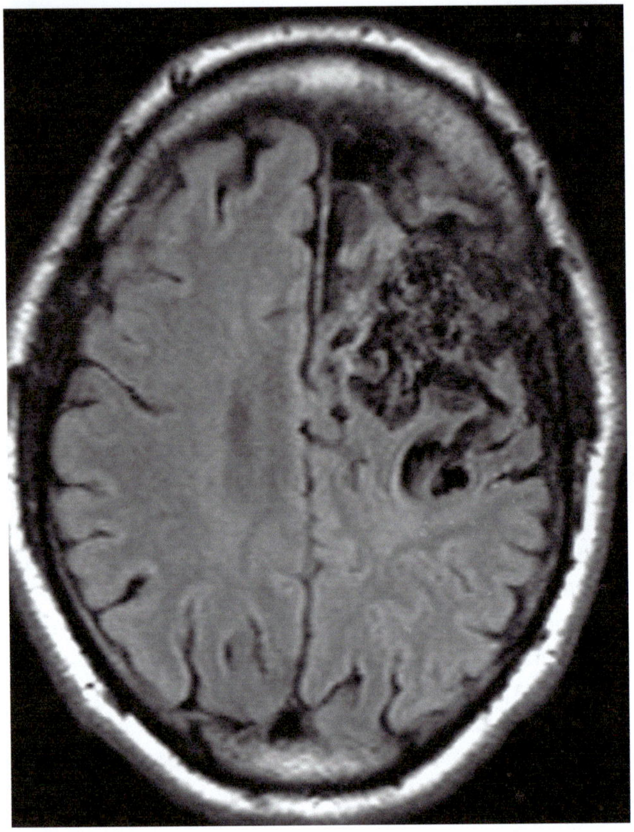

Fig. 82.1 MRI axial FLAIR sequence at a centrum semi-ovale level. Serpentine hypointensities are evident across much of the visible left frontal lobe and include the left precentral gyrus and indicate the nidus of an AVM. The left superior frontal gyrus is atrophic with abnormal hyperintensity suggesting gliosis

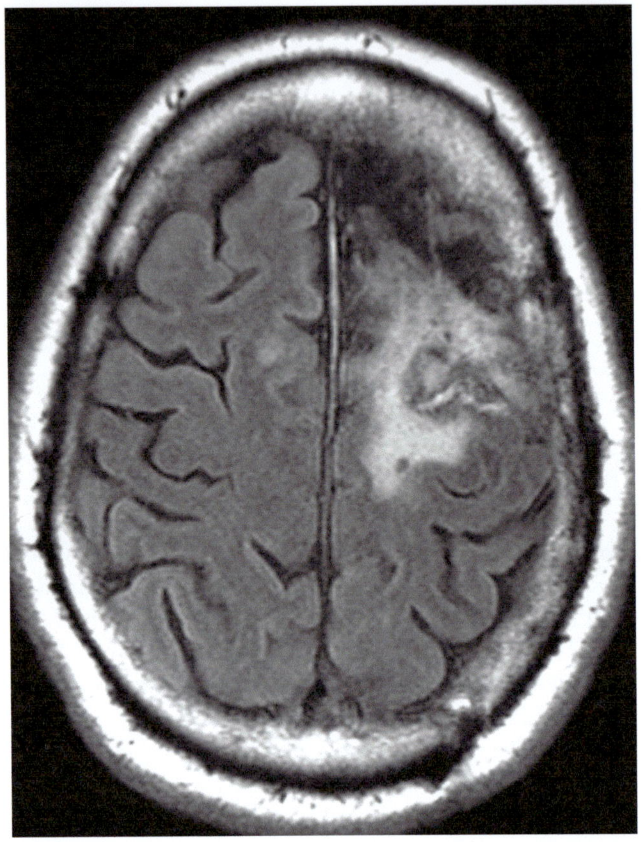

Fig. 82.2 MRI axial FLAIR sequence at a high convexity, centrum semi-ovale level that is slightly superior to the level in Fig. 82.1. The image was obtained 3 years after Fig. 82.1. The previously visible serpentine nidus of the AVM is no longer evident, and hyperintensity indicating gliosis has expanded across the left frontal lobe. The anterior margins of the frontal lobes are asymmetric due to encephalomalacia on the left. Within the subarachnoid space anterior to the left frontal lobe, a vessel is evident as a thin, hyperintense line. The vessel's hyperintensity is due to the slow flow within it. The round hyperintensity within the right superior frontal gyrus is gliosis that is unrelated to the AVM and possibly related to the radiosurgery

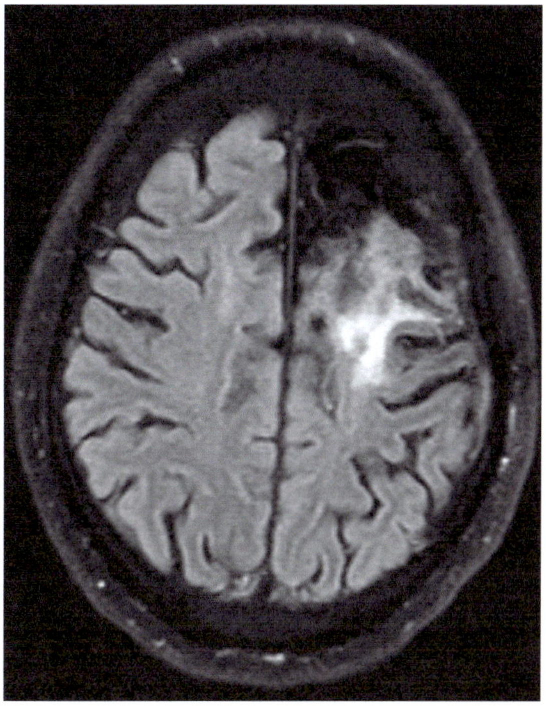

Fig. 82.3 MRI axial FLAIR sequence at the same high convexity, centrum semi-ovale level as Fig. 82.2. The image was obtained 8 years after Fig. 82.2. Left frontal lobe encephalomalacia and gliosis are evident with local volume loss and also generalized atrophy with more prominent cortical sulci bilaterally. The round hypointensity in the posterior portion of the left medial frontal lobe is volume averaging in the context of the atrophy. The subtle hyperintensity in right frontal white matter is mild gliosis related to the treatment

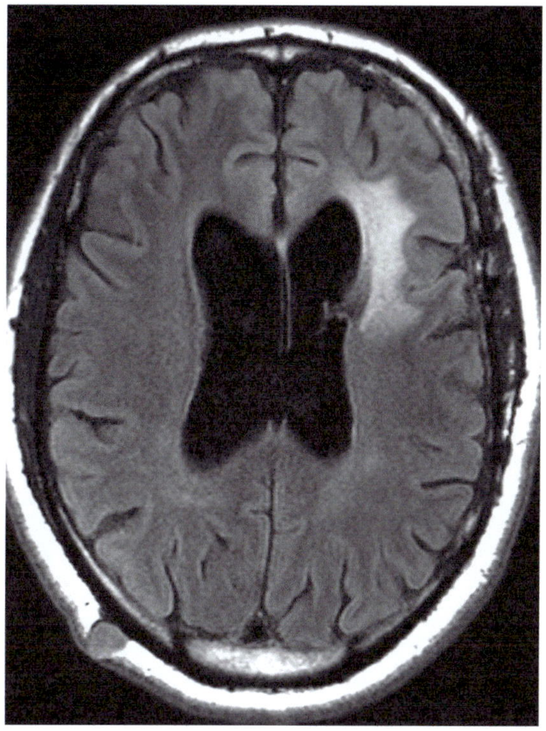

Fig. 82.5 MRI axial FLAIR sequence at the same lateral ventricle level as Fig. 82.4. The image was obtained 3 years later and at the same time as Fig. 82.2. The nidus in the left periventricular region is not present, but the gliosis in the surrounding region is similar. The lateral ventricles are slightly more enlarged. The protruding structure into the left lateral ventricle is choroid plexus

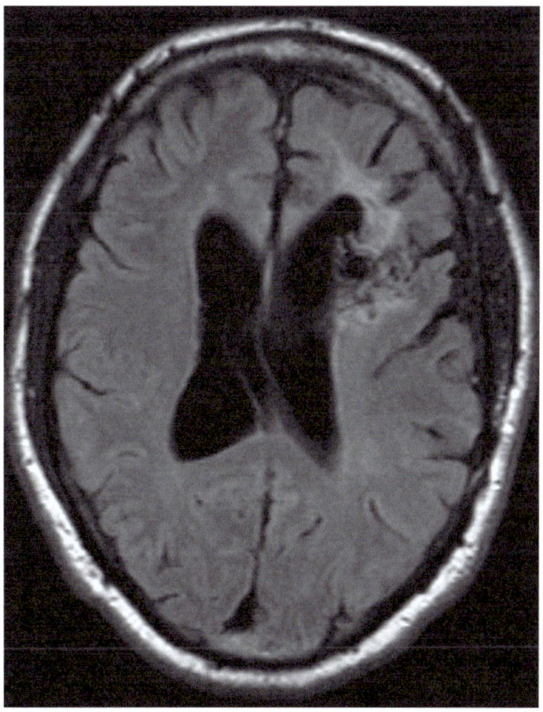

Fig. 82.4 MRI axial FLAIR sequence at a lateral ventricle level and obtained at the time of Fig. 82.1. The multiple, small, round hypointensities in the left periventricular region are the AVM's nidus. Gliosis is evident as hyperintensity within the same region and extending anterior to the nidus. The lateral ventricles are enlarged bilaterally

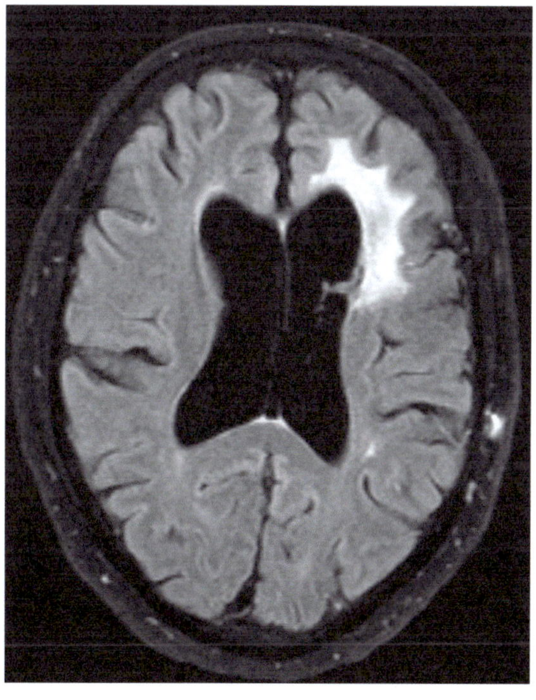

Fig. 82.6 MRI axial FLAIR sequence at the same lateral ventricle level as Figs. 82.4 and 82.5. The image was obtained 8 years later and at the same time as Fig. 82.3. The increased signal in the left periventricular white matter has expanded, indicating increased gliosis. The enlarged lateral ventricles are unchanged along with the choroid plexus along the left ventricular wall

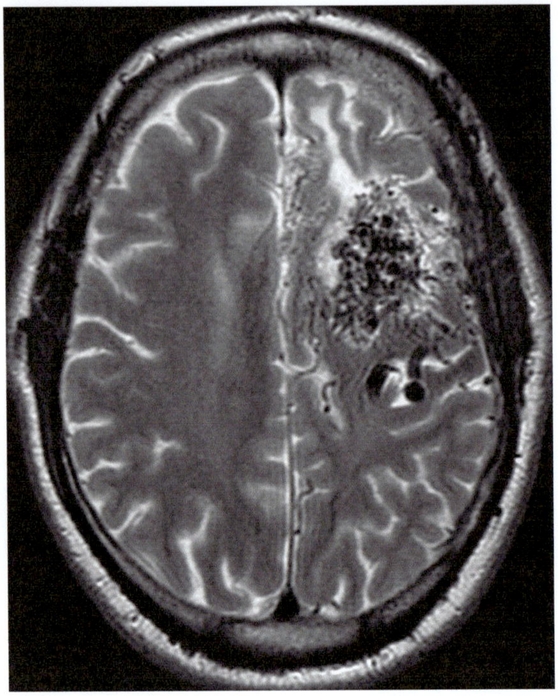

Fig. 82.7 MRI axial T2 sequence at a centrum semi-ovale level similar to Fig. 82.1 and obtained at the same time as Fig. 82.1. A tangle of vessels with hypointense signal are evident in the left frontal lobe white matter and are consistent with nidus of the AVM. Smaller but also enlarged vessels are evident medial and lateral to the nidus and are consistent with the AVM's feeding arteries. A dilated draining vein is within the left central sulcus region. The hyperintensity within the left superior frontal gyrus is due to gliosis

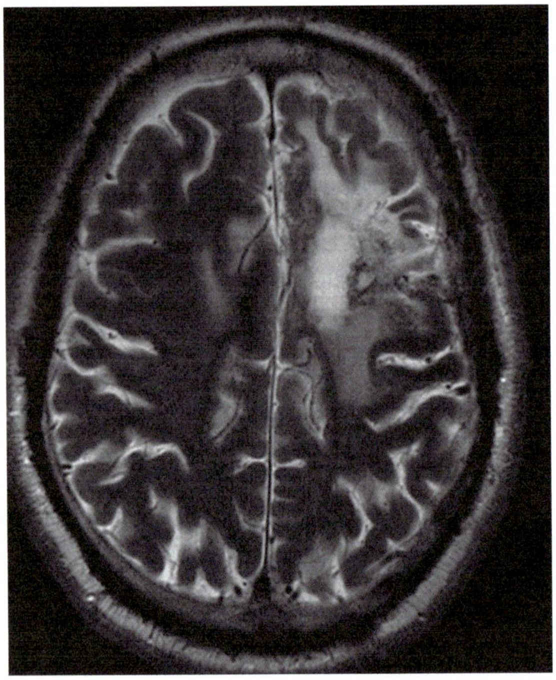

Fig. 82.8 MRI axial T2 sequence at the same centrum semi-ovale level as Fig. 82.7 and obtained 3 years later. The previously visible tangle of vessels within the left frontal lobe and the dilated draining vein in the left central sulcus region are no longer evident. The left frontal lobe hyperintensity indicating gliosis has increased

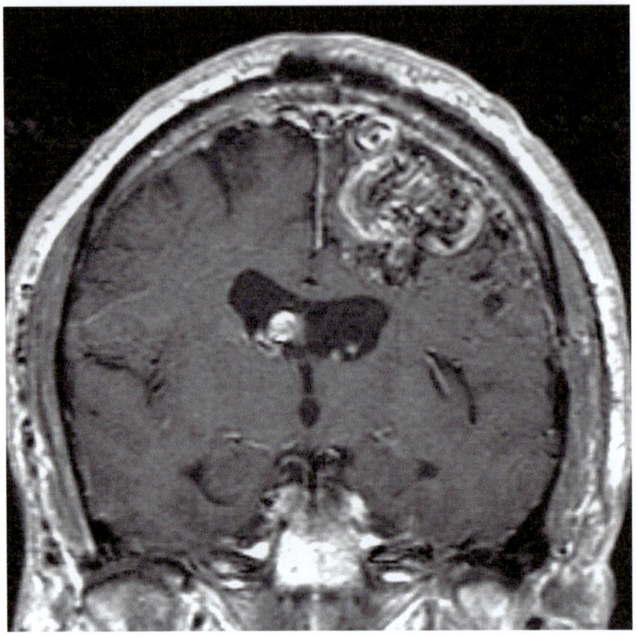

Fig. 82.9 MRI coronal T1 sequence after contrast administration at a third ventricle level. The image was obtained at the same time as Figs. 82.1, 82.4, and 82.7. A tangle of vessels is evident in the left frontal lobe with an enlarged draining vein in the periphery of the tangle. An enhancing deep draining vein is present in the frontal horn of the right lateral ventricle

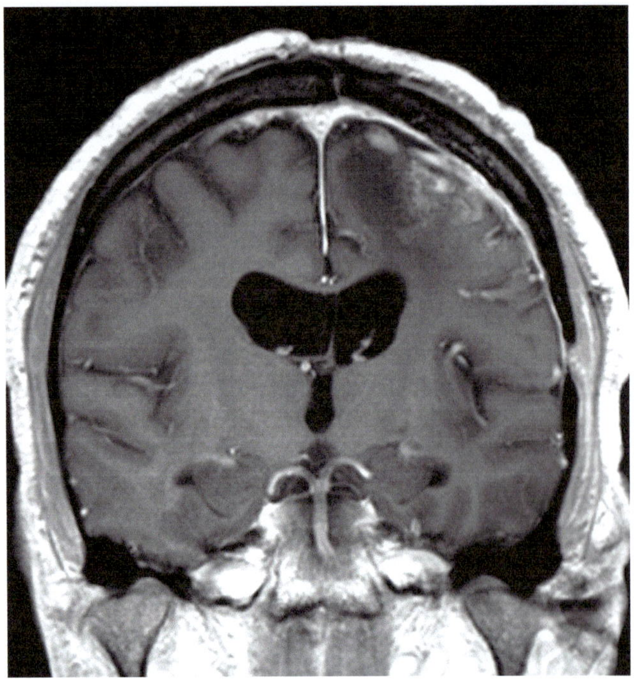

Fig. 82.10 MRI coronal T1 sequence after contrast administration at the same third ventricle level as Fig. 82.9. The image was obtained 3 years later and at the same time as Figs. 82.2, 82.5, and 82.8. The tangle of vessels in the left frontal lobe indicating the AVM's nidus is no longer visible. Minor enhancement is present in the left middle frontal gyrus due to the residual nidus, but the enhancement previously due to the draining veins is much reduced

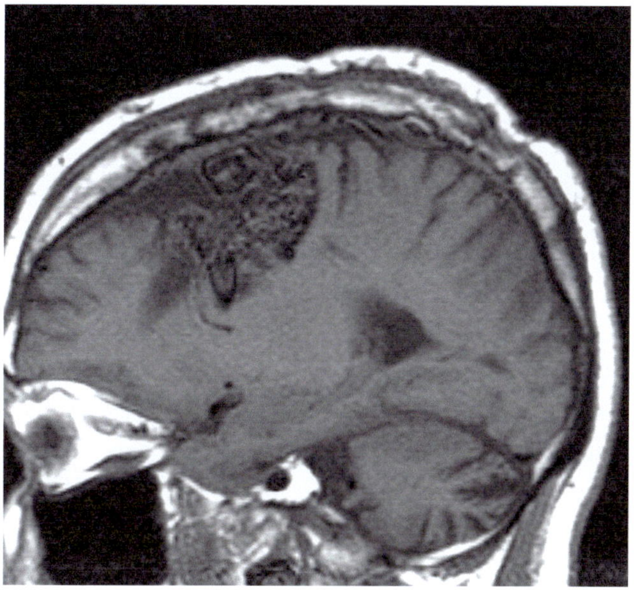

Fig. 82.11 MRI sagittal T1 sequence at a left hippocampus level and obtained at the same time as Figs. 82.1, 82.4, 82.7, and 82.9. A large tangle of vessels is evident in the frontal lobe with a dilated draining vein anterior superior to the nidus. Encephalomalacia is evident along the anterior aspect of the nidus and is due to previous surgery, which also is evident in the skull's postsurgical changes. Unrelated to the AVM findings, the inferior-posterior cerebellum is atrophic

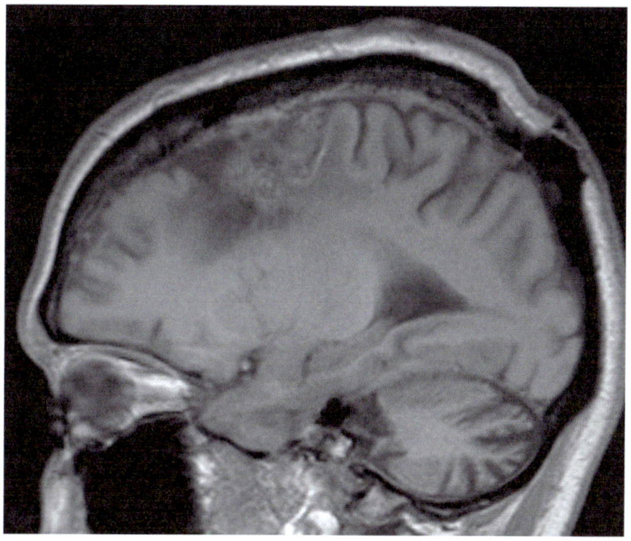

Fig. 82.12 MRI sagittal T1 sequence at the same left hippocampus level as Fig. 82.11. The image was obtained 3 years later and at the same time as Figs. 82.2, 82.5, 82.8, and 82.10. The previously seen nidus and draining veins are not evident. Signal within the region of the prior nidus is abnormal with gray matter hyperintensity and white matter hypointensity. The cerebellar atrophy is unchanged

83 Vagus Nerve Stimulator

Clinical History

The first recognized seizure occurred during infancy, and the details of the epilepsy history during childhood were not known.

In adulthood, the habitual seizures were most often tonic-clonic during sleep. The rare tonic-clonic seizures during wakefulness did not follow an aura and sometimes initially manifested with unilateral tonic posturing, but the unilateral posturing did not have a consistent lateralization. Every seizure in wakefulness progressed to bilateral tonic-clonic activity for several minutes and was followed by postictal confusion. Treatment included multiple anti-seizure medications with a seizure frequency of one seizure monthly.

An epilepsy risk factor was not present.

Neurological examination was normal. Medical history was unrelated to epilepsy.

Interictal EEG depicted bilaterally synchronous frontal-temporal epileptiform sharp waves that were more prominent on the left. Video-EEG monitoring recorded seizures manifested as gaze deviation rightward, extension of back and neck, tonic posturing of bilateral arms with an ictal cry, and then bilateral clonic activity. The ictal EEG's seizure onset was obscured by artifact, and the first visible ictal abnormality was bilateral rhythmic slow activity with frontal predominance and evolution with decreasing frequency.

MRI identified mild cerebellar atrophy and no other abnormality. PET was normal. Ictal SPECT identified possible hyperperfusion within the left insula. Interictal MEG depicted widespread epileptiform dipoles.

The history and evaluation indicate possibly left hemispheric onset with rapid progression to tonic-clonic, as was supported by the forced rightward gaze during the video-EEG monitoring and the ictal SPECT's suggestion of left-sided hyperperfusion. The lack of an aura and the ictal EEG's bilateral rhythmic slowing can be supportive of a focal neocortical onset but do not contribute to the identification of a putative epileptogenic zone, and the interictal EEG and MEG suggest the possibility of diffuse abnormality. Without an adequate hypothesis for evaluation with intracranial EEG, further evaluation for epilepsy surgery was not recommended.

Treatment was expanded to include a vagus nerve stimulator. The seizure frequency at the time of implantation was five monthly, and this initially decreased to two monthly. With adjustments to the stimulation settings, the frequency later decreased to one monthly. After 4 years, the generator's battery was depleted, and the seizure frequency increased to six monthly and then returned to one monthly after the generator was replaced.

J. M. Stern, N. Salamon, *Imaging of Epilepsy*, https://doi.org/10.1007/978-3-030-86672-3_83

Imaging

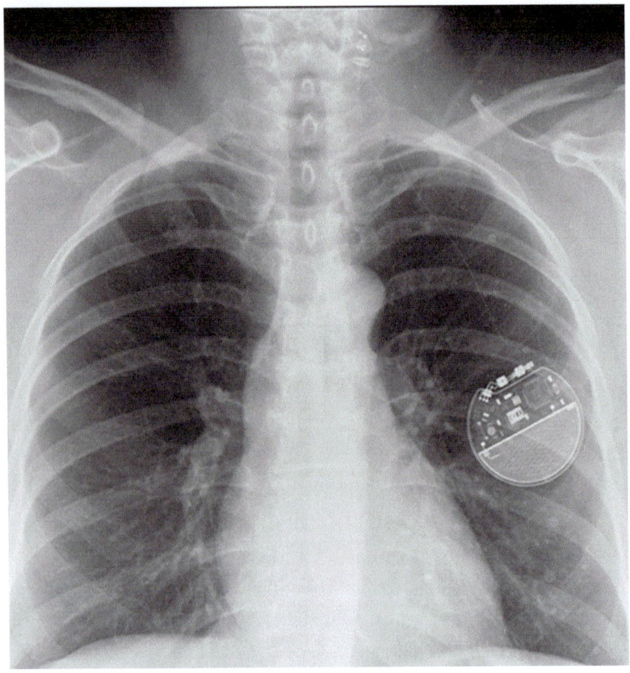

Fig. 83.1 Chest x-ray with an anterior-posterior view. The vagus nerve stimulator's generator, including internal circuitry and battery, is visible in the left anterior-lateral chest wall. The stimulator's electrode lead extends superiorly and medially from the lateral aspect of the generator's superior edge to the left lower neck

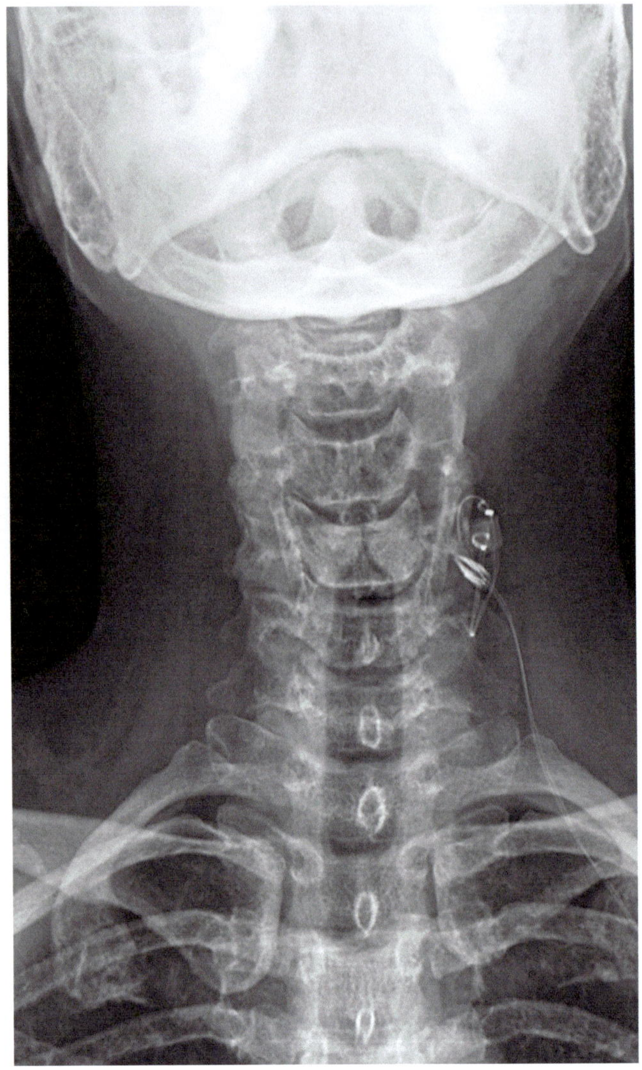

Fig. 83.2 Neck x-ray with an anterior-posterior view. The vagus nerve stimulator's electrode lead extends superiorly along the left lateral neck to the C5 level where it loops and then attaches at the vagus nerve's expected location. The electrode contacts are circular

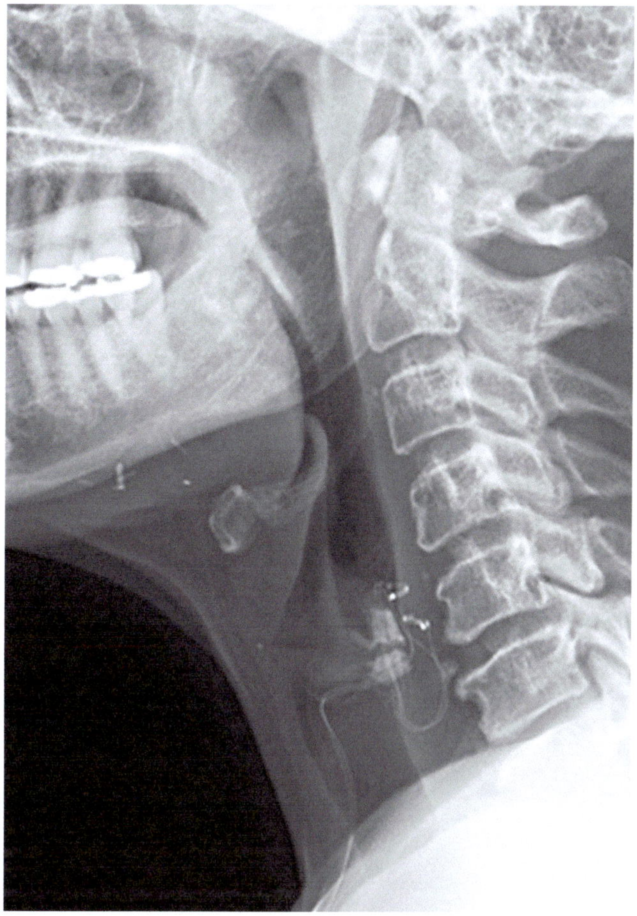

Fig. 83.3 Neck x-ray with a lateral view. The vagus nerve stimulator's electrode lead extends superiorly and is visible in the superficial soft tissue of the neck at the C5 level. It makes a loop before reaching two electrode cuffs that are hyperdense compared to the wire

84 Responsive Neurostimulator

Clinical History

The first recognized seizure occurred at age 17 years and retrospectively identified upon recalling an episode of regaining consciousness on the floor without memory of the circumstances. At age 18 years, two occurrences of oral injury during sleep were also retrospectively identified as seizures. At age 22 years, epilepsy was diagnosed after the development of stereotyped episodes of 1- to 2-second hallucinations of a metallic taste and a sense of spinning followed by impaired understanding of surroundings. After treatment was begun at this time, the stereotyped hallucinations ceased to occur, and witnessed tonic-clonic seizures occurred rarely for a few years before ceasing to occur.

The habitual seizures developed later and were initially manifested as the experience of hearing gibberish when listening to speech or music. During this time, speech was not possible, and attempts to write produced the repetition of a single letter. The seizure duration was usually 1–2 minutes and had a frequency of four to six daily. Another seizure manifestation was similar and replaced it as the habitual seizure by the time of the evaluation. Its manifestation was speech arrest without impairment of comprehension or memory for about 3 seconds that was followed by global aphasia for minutes. No other visible abnormality was present. Initially, the occurrence pattern was several seizures daily and then no additional seizures for about a week. Treatment included multiple anti-seizure medications with a seizure frequency that increased over several years to be about 100 seizures daily with postictal aphasia through much of each day.

The epilepsy risk factor was a family history of epilepsy. Several relatives had epilepsy, but no pattern of a specific epilepsy diagnosis was known.

Neurological examination was normal. Neuropsychological testing at a time without postictal aphasia identified normal memory and verbal function with verbal abilities superior to visuospatial function.

Interictal EEG depicted epileptiform discharges broadly across the left temporal and occipital lobes. Video-EEG monitoring recorded 21 focal seizures manifested as speech arrest. Of these, 18 occurred without impaired awareness and did not have an accompanying EEG abnormality, and three occurred with impaired awareness and the ictal EEG depicting an epileptiform rhythm across the posterior left temporal lobe that extended broadly to include the left middle temporal, occipital, and parietal lobes.

MRI and PET were both normal. Interictal MEG identified epileptiform dipoles across the middle and posterior left temporal lobe neocortex. Functional MRI identified left hemispheric dominance for language.

The history and evaluation indicate focal seizures with prominent ictal and postictal features of language cortex dysfunction. The initial seizures included a limbic feature with the gustatory hallucination and a posterior-lateral temporal cortex feature with vertigo. Because of the aphasia and vertigo, the epileptogenic region may be within the left posterior temporal lobe and the gustatory hallucination may be due to propagation into the mesial temporal lobe. The video-EEG recordings and MEG supported this left posterior temporal lobe localization, but the imaging did not depict an abnormality, and it indicated likely proximity to critical language areas. Therefore, determining epilepsy surgery candidacy required intracranial EEG.

To more accurately map the epileptic abnormality, video-EEG monitoring was performed with depth electrodes placed across the left temporal lobe and adjacent areas of the parietal and occipital lobes. To verify the seizure onset zone and map the seizure propagation, right item portal lobe depth electrodes also were placed. Nine focal seizures of speech arrest without impaired awareness were recorded, and the seizure onset was consistently at the left temporal-occipital junction electrode with rapid propagation to the left temporal-parietal electrode and then the left anterior hippocampus electrode. This confirmed the left posterior temporal seizure onset zone and proximity to language areas but did not identify margins for a resection or the anatomic relationship to language cortex.

J. M. Stern, N. Salamon, *Imaging of Epilepsy*, https://doi.org/10.1007/978-3-030-86672-3_84

To increase the anatomic detail, mapping of the region was performed with subdural grid electrodes that were placed across the left temporal lobe and the immediately adjacent portions of the parietal and occipital lobes with inclusion of the basal temporal-occipital junction. Focal seizures with speech arrest were recorded, and the seizure onset was localized to the inferior posterior temporal lobe with rapid propagation to the lateral posterior temporal lobe. Extra-operative language mapping with electrical stimulation identified co-localization of speech arrest, naming, and the seizure onset zone. As a resection would produce a language deficit, multiple subpial transections were performed across the seizure onset zone, and these produced a 90% reduction to interictal epileptiform discharges on the intraoperative electrocorticogram.

Over the 2 years after the multiple subpial transections, the seizure frequency decreased from the preoperative 100 seizures daily to about 10 seizures daily. When the responsive neurostimulator (RNS) became available, it was placed with strip electrode contacts. Three strips were placed across the basal temporal lobe covering the seizure onset zone and one across the temporal-parietal region covering the region demonstrating the early seizure propagation. The RNS allows for two strips to be connected, and the middle and posterior basal temporal strips were used. Programming adjustments during postoperative care found that stimulation with current flow between these two strips was the most effective.

Seizure frequency for the 5 years after RNS programming decreased from 10 daily to typically one weekly with periods of seizure freedom lasting up to 3 weeks. The impact of the individual seizures also improved. Although the seizures still lasted 3 seconds and manifested as speech arrest without impaired comprehension or memory, postictal aphasia did not occur, and the amount of time experiencing language dysfunction was been reduced. No abnormality was visible during or after the seizures.

Imaging

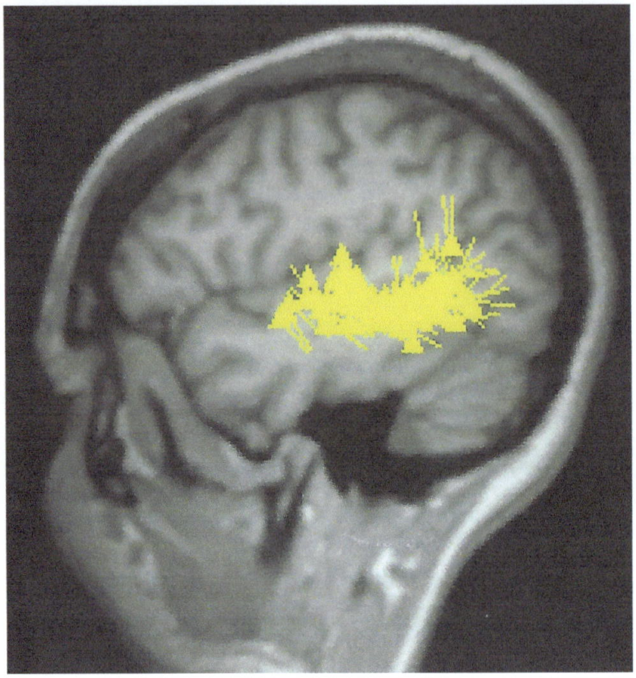

Fig. 84.1 MEG co-registered to MRI sagittal T1 sequence at a left Sylvian fissure level. A dense cluster of epileptiform dipoles are evident across the superior temporal gyrus, middle temporal gyrus, and extending to the supramarginal gyrus

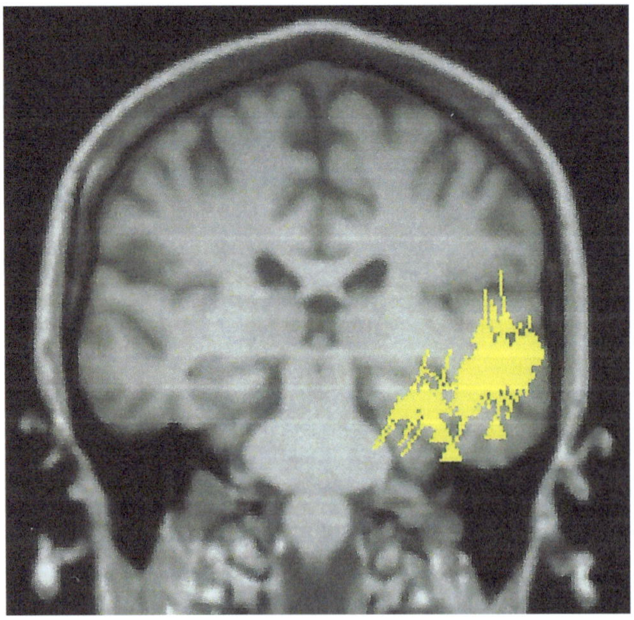

Fig. 84.2 MEG co-registered to MRI coronal T1 sequence at a pulvinar level. A dense cluster of epileptiform dipoles are evident across the superior temporal, middle temporal, inferior temporal, fusiform, and parahippocampal gyri

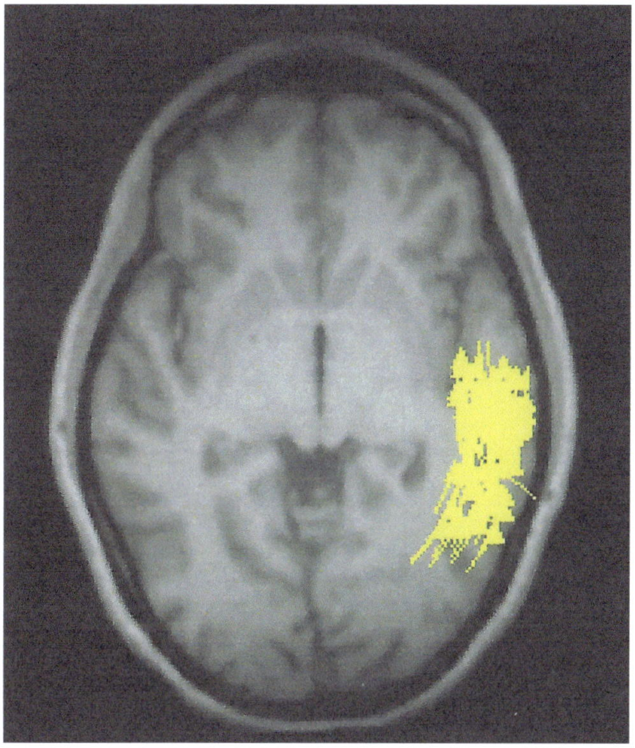

Fig. 84.3 MEG co-registered to MRI axial T1 sequence at a thalamus level. A dense cluster of epileptiform dipoles are evident across superior temporal gyrus and Heschl's gyrus

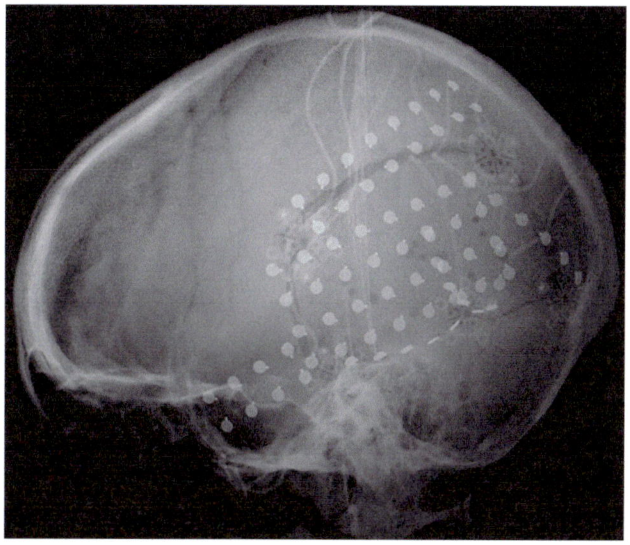

Fig. 84.5 X-ray with a lateral view of the skull obtained after the placement of a subdural grid electrodes across the left temporal-parietal region with additional subdural electrode strips extending superiorly, posteriorly, and anteriorly. The leads from the grid and strips are visible superiorly. The changes related to the craniotomy for placement of the electrodes also are visible. The electrodes were placed for extra-operative, inpatient mapping of seizure onsets and cortical function

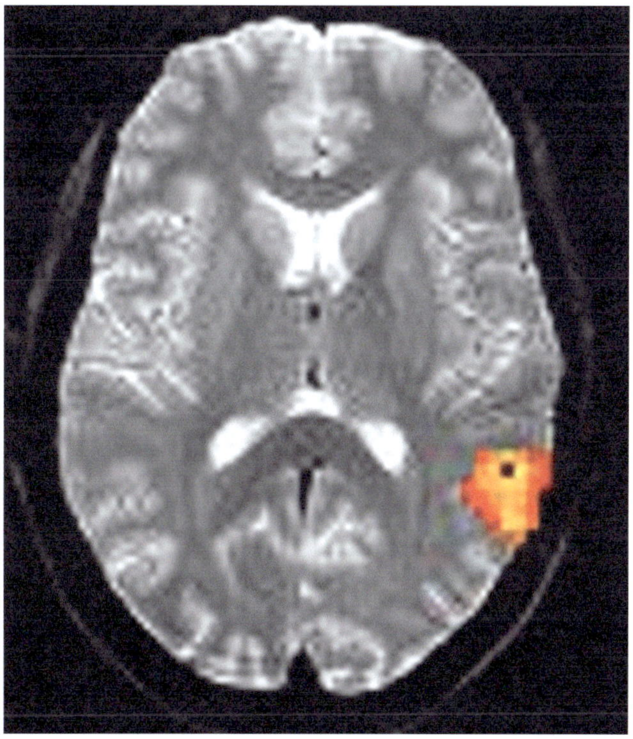

Fig. 84.4 Functional MRI with an axial view at a thalamus level. Language task correlation identifies Wernicke's area in the posterior portion of the left superior temporal gyrus

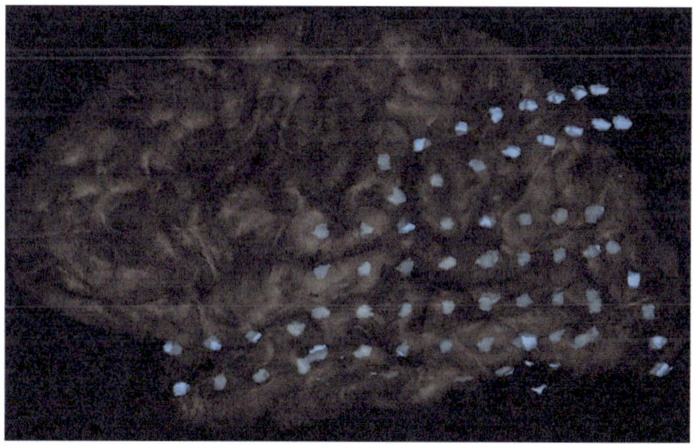

Fig. 84.6 MRI T1 sequence surface rendering of left hemisphere co-registered to head CT. The cortical surface electrode placement locations identified by CT are visible on the gyral anatomy identified by MRI. The electrode coverage includes the middle temporal gyrus, inferior temporal gyrus, temporal-parietal-occipital junction, supramarginal gyrus, angular gyrus, temporal-occipital junction, and basal temporal lobe

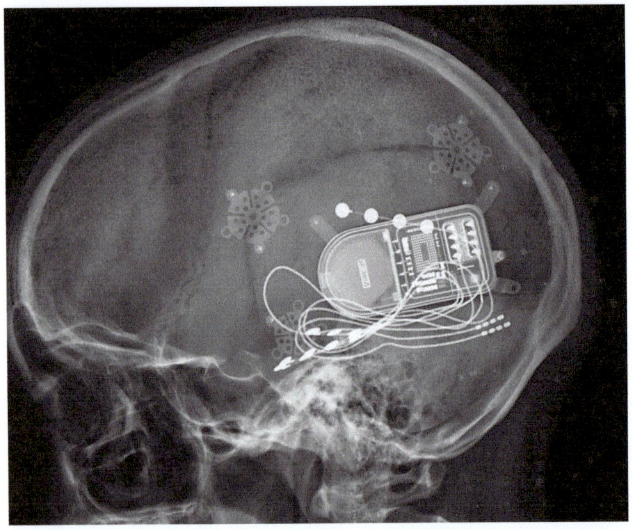

Fig. 84.7 X-ray with a lateral view of the skull obtained immediately after RNS implantation. The neurostimulator, with its internal components visible, has been placed on the ferrule within the craniectomy. Tabs at each of the ferrule's four corners affix the ferrule to the skull. A craniotomy extended beyond the craniectomy for placement of the electrode leads, and burr hole covers are visible at three of the craniotomy's corners. Four electrode strips were placed, and each has four electrode contacts. One strip was placed across the parietal lobe's lateral surface, and the other three strips are across the temporal lobe's inferior surface. Two electrode strip leads approach the neurostimulator at the posterior portion of its inferior edge and connect to it within its posterior portion. The other two leads are not connected to the neurostimulator, and the free ends are visible inferiorly

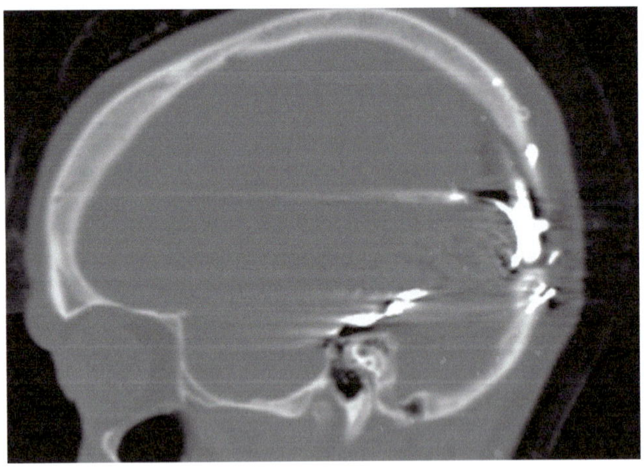

Fig. 84.8 CT of the head with bone windowing in a sagittal view at a left middle cranial fossa level. Streak artifact from the electrodes is visible. One electrode is prominent in the posterior inferior parietal region. Additional electrodes overlap in the middle cranial fossa beneath the temporal lobe. The high density at the surface of the parietal bone corresponds to the neurostimulator. Left temporal parietal craniotomy changes are also visible

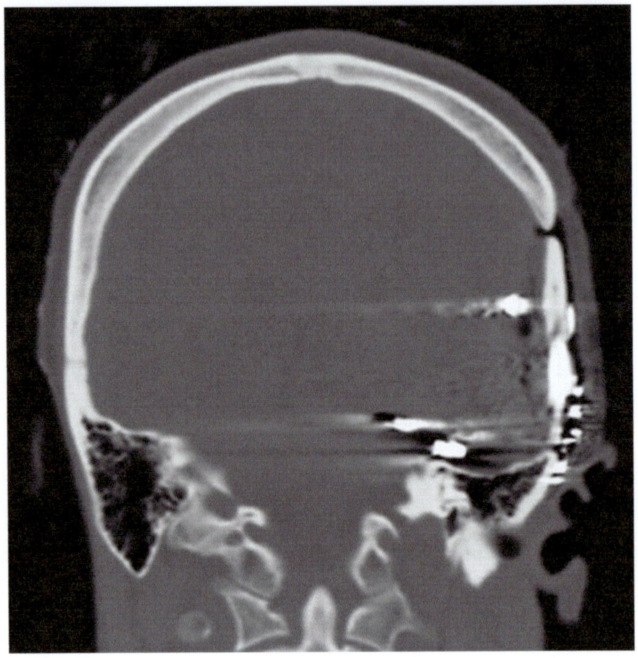

Fig. 84.9 CT of the head with bone windowing in a coronal view at a mastoid level. Streak artifact from the electrode contacts is evident along the left inferior parietal cortex and the left inferior temporal tentorium. Left temporal-parietal craniotomy changes are visible

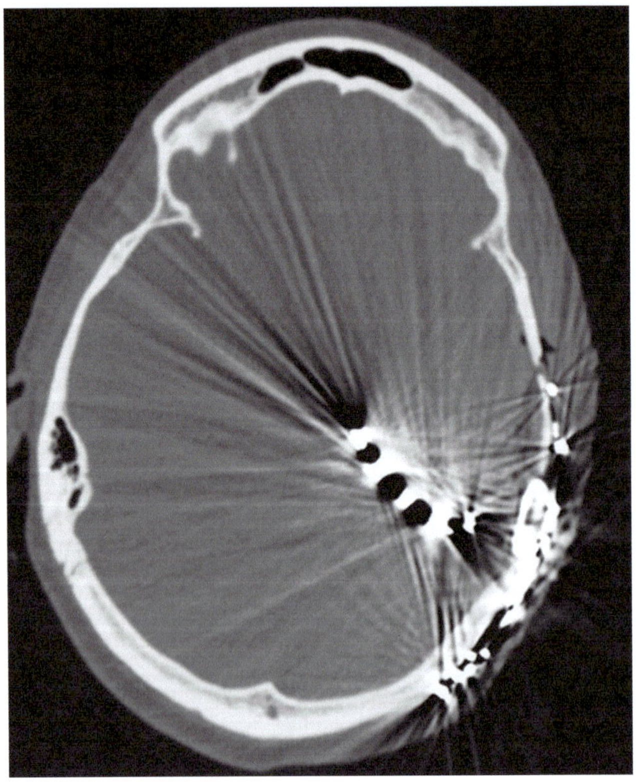

Fig. 84.10 CT of the head with bone windowing in an axial view at a middle cranial fossa level. Streak artifact is evident from the obliquely placed inferior temporal electrode contacts. Left temporal craniotomy changes are present with metal fastener artifact

Deep Brain Stimulator

85

Clinical History

The first recognized seizure occurred at age 12 years as a bilateral convulsion that lasted 2 minutes and resolved without postictal confusion.

The habitual seizures first occurred at age 27 years and manifested as an aura of right arm and leg sensory loss followed by falling and kicking of the right leg for several minutes. The seizures did not cause an impairment of awareness and were not followed by postictal confusion. Rarely, the seizures were similar to the first seizure and progressed to a bilateral convulsion without postictal confusion. Treatment included multiple anti-seizure medications with a seizure frequency of typically five daily.

The epilepsy risk factor was left-sided schizencephaly.

Neurological examination identified a mild right hemiparesis as evident in decreased right-sided fine finger movements and grip strength. The motor asymmetry was first noticed during early childhood as pathological left-handedness. Cognitive development was normal.

Interictal EEG depicted epileptiform discharges across the left hemisphere with prominence in the central, temporal, and posterior frontal regions. Interictal runs of rhythmic epileptiform discharges occurred across the left temporal region.

Video-EEG monitoring recorded focal seizures manifested as a sudden falling toward the left, extension of bilateral arms, and right arm or bilateral arm clonus. Awareness and interaction were normal upon immediate testing after the seizure onset. The ictal EEG's seizure onset was bilateral rhythmic slow waves.

MRI identified left hemispheric schizencephaly with polymicrogyria along the margins of the cleft from the posterior frontal lobe to the inferior parietal lobe and including the operculum. PET identified normal metabolism within the abnormal gray matter anatomy of the left-sided schizencephaly.

The history and evaluation indicate left-sided, central neocortical focal seizure onset based on the unilateral, sensorimotor focal features and either maintaining of awareness during the seizures or having immediate regaining of awareness after seizures that caused impaired awareness. The MRI and interictal EEG provide further evidence for this localization. Surgical treatment with resection was not offered because of the extensive region of structural abnormality and the significant risk of a postoperative motor deficit. As an alternative, deep brain stimulation of the anterior nucleus of the thalamus was provided. After 1 year of stimulation, the seizure frequency was five weekly, which was the lowest experienced in years.

J. M. Stern, N. Salamon, *Imaging of Epilepsy*, https://doi.org/10.1007/978-3-030-86672-3_85

Imaging

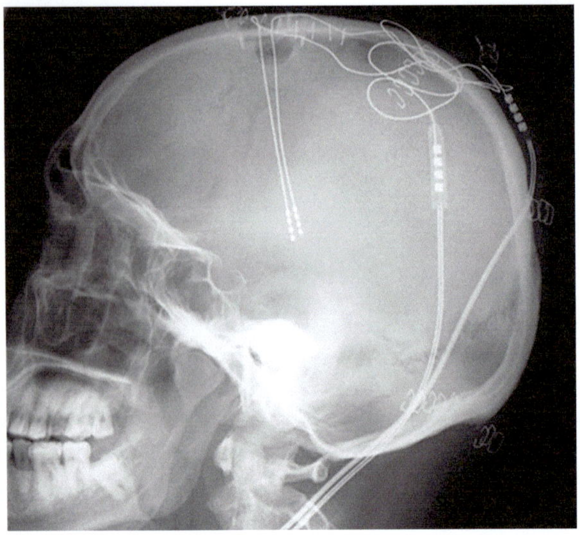

Fig. 85.1 Skull x-ray with a lateral view. Two electrode leads are evident from frontal bone burr holes to the brain's central structures, where four contacts are visible on each electrode. Superficial electrode wires extend along the scalp and are joined to the extension wires that continue to the neck. Because the x-ray was obtained immediately post-operatively, the extensions are external and staples within the scalp are present

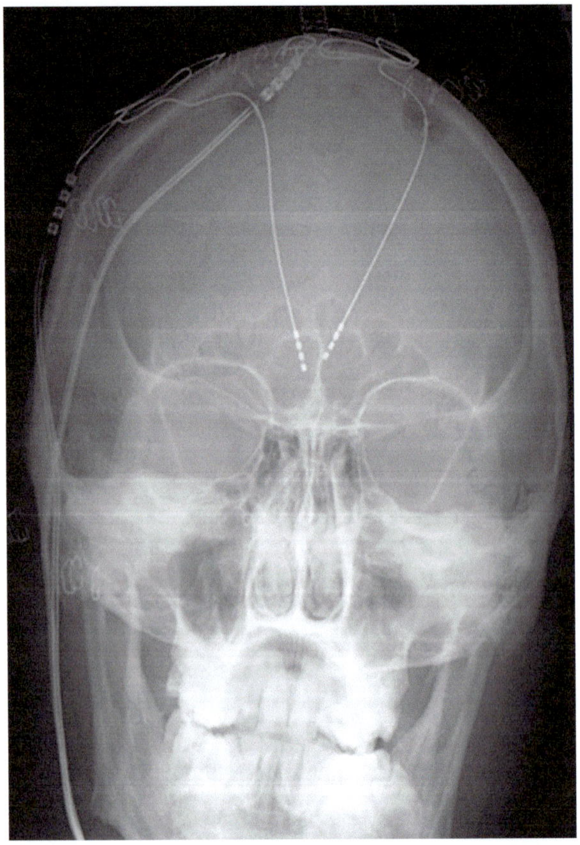

Fig. 85.2 Skull x-ray with an anterior-posterior view. Two frontal bone burr holes are evident with electrode leads extending through the skull toward the brain's central structures with four electrode contacts at the end of each lead. Electrode lead loops are evident across the skull, and the leads continue to the right lateral aspect of the head where they are connected to extensions that continue inferiorly

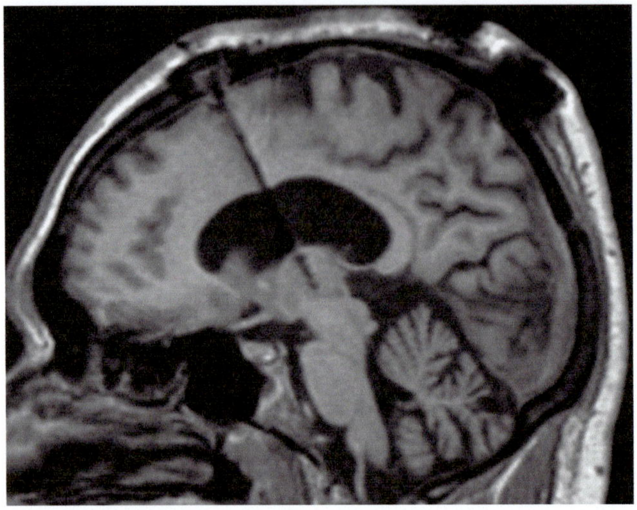

Fig. 85.3 MRI sagittal T1 sequence at a midline level. An electrode lead extends from a frontal bone burr hole through the frontal lobe and the lateral ventricle to reach the thalamus. Four round electrode contacts are evident at the electrode's tip with the superior contacts within the anterior nucleus of the thalamus

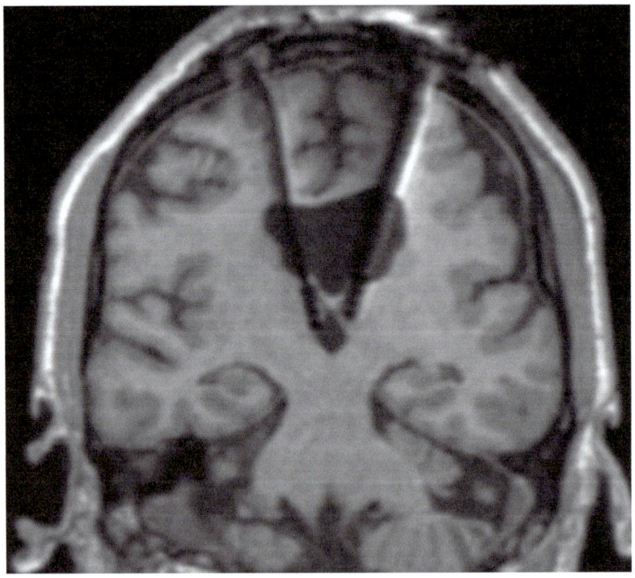

Fig. 85.4 MRI coronal T1 sequence at a hippocampal body level. Two electrode leads extend from two frontal bone burr holes through the frontal lobes and lateral ventricles to reach the thalamus. Of the four contacts at the end of each electrode, the most superior contact on the right and the second most superior on the left are within the anterior nucleus of the thalamus. Polymicrogyria is evident across the left superior temporal gyrus and perisylvian region

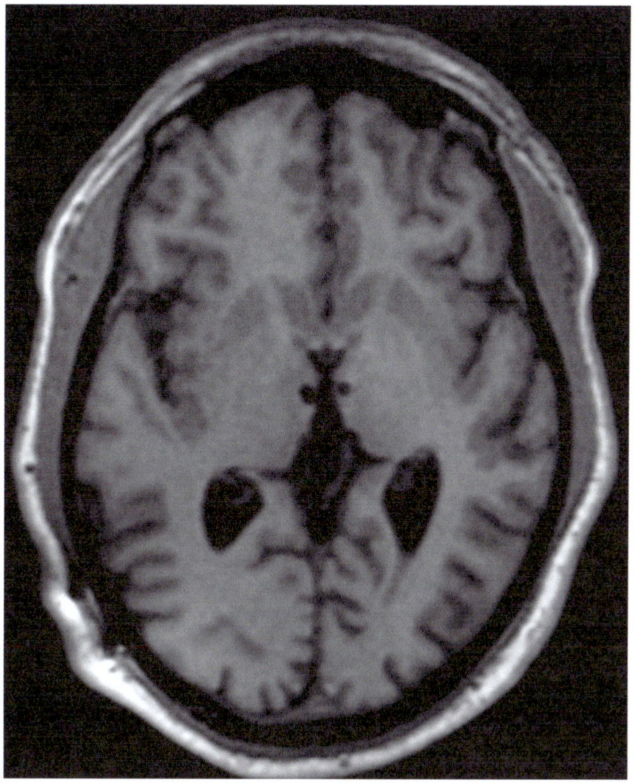

Fig. 85.5 MRI axial T1 sequence at a thalamus level. Each of the two electrodes is evident as a round hypointensity in an anterior nucleus of the thalamus. Polymicrogyria is evident along the left superior temporal gyrus

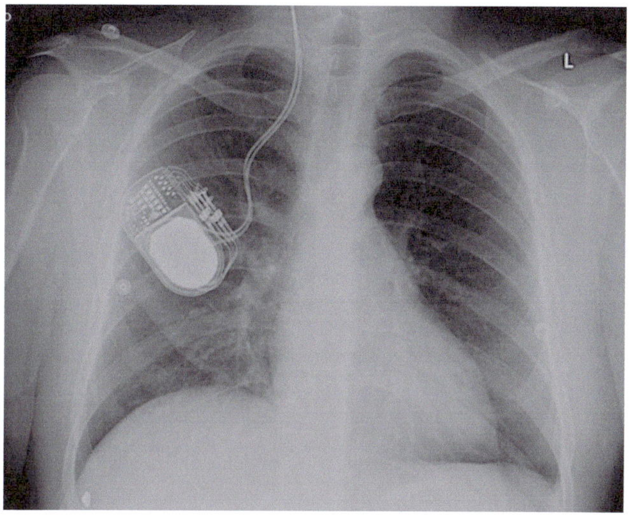

Fig. 85.6 Chest x-ray with an anterior-posterior view. The generator for the deep brain stimulation is along the right chest wall with two electrode extensions extending superiorly toward the right neck

Index

J. M. Stern, N. Salamon, *Imaging of Epilepsy*, https://doi.org/10.1007/978-3-030-86672-3

D

E

F

G

MIX
Papier aus verantwortungsvollen Quellen
Paper from responsible sources
FSC® C105338

If you have any concerns about our products,
you can contact us on
ProductSafety@springernature.com

In case Publisher is established outside the EU,
the EU authorized representative is:
Springer Nature Customer Service Center GmbH
Europaplatz 3, 69115 Heidelberg, Germany

Printed by Libri Plureos GmbH
in Hamburg, Germany